Application of Artificial Intelligence In Cardiovascular Medicine

notionpress.com

INDIA · SINGAPORE · MALAYSIA

ISBN
Paperback 979-8-89322-837-3
Hardcase 979-8-89363-362-7

Application of Artificial Intelligence In Cardiovascular Medicine

Prof.(Dr) K.C.VERMA

MBBS, DCH, MD, DM (CARDIOLOGY) FICP (USA),
FRSTM & H (Lond), FCSI (India)
Senior Consulting Heart Specialist and Formerly
Prof. in Cardiovascular and Thoracic Unit
Govt. Medical College, Jammu (J&K)

notionpress.com

INDIA · SINGAPORE · MALAYSIA

ACKNOWLEDGEMENT

I am indebted to the various scientific workers and research scholars whose names have been mentioned in respective chapter of bibliography and whose basic work became the foundation of each chapter of this book.

I am also very grateful to my wife Dr (Mrs) Urmil Kanta Verma, formerly Prof. in the department of blood transfusion medicine and pathology for providing me a perfect congenial atmosphere and all material and moral support needed for writing such a voluminous book : '**Application of Artificial Intelligence In Cardiovascular Medicine':**

To my grand children, Advita, Sidhant Leena, Meera and Deven.(USA)

(Author)

FOREWORD

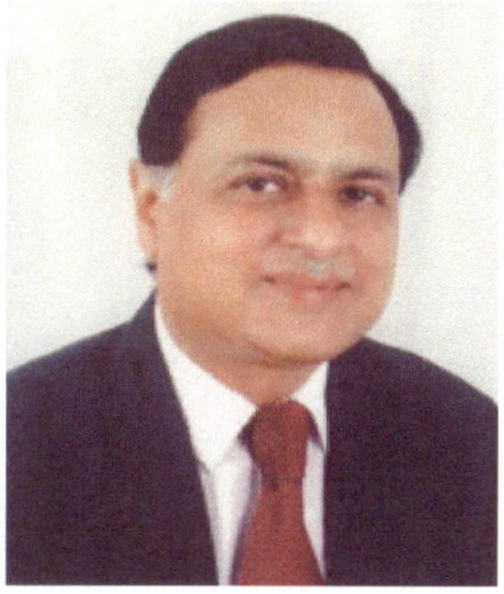

Dr KC Verma an eminent cardiologist practising in Jammu (J&K) has done a commendable job in writing a book ***"Application of Artificial Intelligence In Cardiovascular Medicine':*** "The book is an exhaustive work covering all aspects of Artificial intelligence in diagnosis , prediction of prognosis and guidance in a particular disease. It gives details of entire subject on the various innovations which have taken place over the past a few years ,especially on impotant topic of **"Ocular images-based on Artificial intelligence in diagnosis of Systemic diseases "**

I know Dr Verma for more than 3 decades and always found him a very inquisitive person very well read and always practising ethical medicine. He has been an excellent teacher for his younger colleagues.The book should be of a great help to the practising cardiologists/Reserch scholars /cardiac fellows /cardiology residents and DM cardiology scholars in revising and refreshing their already acquired knowledge . it would ,therefore,have a greater repurcussion in managing their patient with current techniques with mjnjmal cost and least morbidity and mortality. I recommend this very well written book for all the busy physicians and cardiologists who want evidence based guidance for treating their patients.

Prof. (Dr) Sanjay Tyagi,

MD,, DM, FAMS, FESC, FSCAI, FACC (USA)
Formerly Director Professor & Head of Cardiology Department G.B. Pant Institute of Postgraduate Medical Education & Research & Maulana Azad Medical College University of Delhi New Delhi, India
At present Director and chairman of cardiac sciences ,Appolo Hospital and Research center ,New Delhi

Dedication

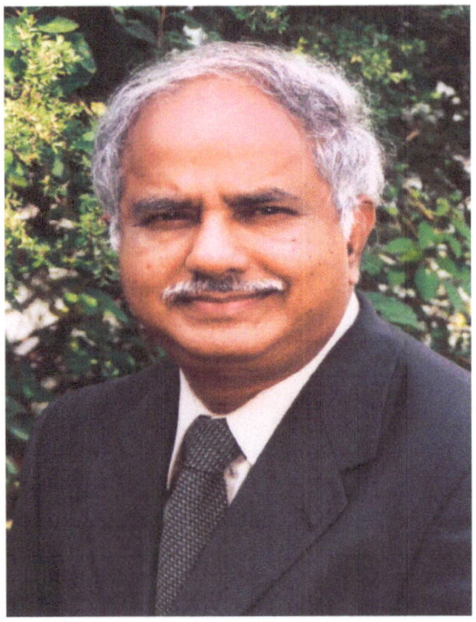

Dr.Dabbala Rajagopal "Raj" Reddy

Dabbala Rajagopal "Raj" Reddy (born 13 June 1937) is an Indian-born American computer scientist and a winner of the Turing Award. He is one of the early pioneers of artificial intelligence and has served on the faculty of Stanford and Carnegie Mellon for over 50 years. He was the founding director of the Robotics Institute at Carnegie Mellon University. He was instrumental in helping to create Rajiv Gandhi University of Knowledge Technologies in India, to cater to the educational needs of the low-income, gifted, rural youth. He is the chairman of International Institute of Information Technology, Hyderabad. He is the first person of Asian origin to receive the Turing Award, in 1994, known as the Nobel Prize of Computer Science, for his work in the field of artificial intelligence.

Reddy is the University Professor of Computer Science and Robotics and Moza Bint Nasser Chair at the School of Computer Science at Carnegie Mellon University. From 1960, he worked for IBM in Australia.He was an Assistant Professor of Computer Science at Stanford University from 1966 to 1969. He joined the Carnegie Mellon faculty as an associate professor of Computer Science in 1969. He became a full professor in 1973 and a university professor, in 1984.

Artificial Intelligence Research

Reddy's early research was conducted at the AI labs at Stanford, first as a graduate student and later as an assistant professor, and at CMU since 1969.His AI research concentrated on perceptual and motor aspect of intelligence such as speech, language, vision and robotics. Over a span of five decades, Reddy and his colleagues created several historic demonstrations of spoken language systems, e.g., voice control of a robot,large vocabulary connected speech recognition, speaker independent speech recognition, and unrestricted vocabulary dictation.Reddy and his colleagues have made seminal contributions to Task Oriented Computer Architectures, Analysis of Natural Scenes,Universal Access to Information, and Autonomous Robotic Systems.Hearsay I was one of the first systems capable of continuous speech recognition. Subsequent systems like Hearsay II, Dragon, Harpy, and Sphinx I/II developed many of the ideas underlying modern commercial speech recognition technology as summarized in his recent historical review of speech recognition with Xuedong Huang and James K. Baker. Some of these ideas—most notably the "blackboard model" for coordinating multiple knowledge sources—have been adopted across the spectrum of applied artificial intelligence

Awards and honors

He is a fellow of the AAAI, ACM, Acoustical Society of America, IEEE[and Computer History Museum.. Reddy is a member of the United States National Academy of Engineering, American Academy of Arts and Sciences, Chinese Academy of Engineering, Indian National Science Academy, and Indian National Academy of Engineering. He has been awarded honorary doctorates (Doctor Honoris Causa) from SV University, Universite Henri-Poincare, University of New South Wales, Jawaharlal Nehru Technological University, University of Massachusetts, University of Warwick, Anna University, IIIT (Allahabad), Andhra University, IIT Kharagpur, Hong Kong University of Science and Technology, Rajiv Gandhi University of Knowledge Technologies, and Carnegie Mellon University.\ In 1994 he and Edward Feigenbaum received the Turing Award, "for pioneering the design and construction of large scale artificial intelligence systems, demonstrating the practical importance and potential commercial impact of artificial intelligence technology."In 1984, Reddy was awarded the French Legion of Honour by French President François Mitterrand. Reddy also received Padma Bhushan, from the President of India in 2001,the Okawa Prize in 2004, the Honda Prize in 2005, and the Vannevar Bush Award in 2006

(Dr K C VERMA MD DM)

Preface

Artificial intelligence (AI) is a growing phenomenon, and will soon facilitate wide-scale changes in many professions, including medical education. In order for medical educators to be properly prepared for AI, they will need to have at least a fundamental knowledge of AI in relation to learning and teaching, and the extent to which it will impact on medical education. This Guide book begins by introducing the broad concepts of AI by using fairly well-known examples to illustrate AI's implications within the context of education. It then considers the impact of AI on medicine and the implications of this impact for educators trying to educate future doctors. Drawing on these strands, it then identifies AI's direct impact on the methodology and content of medical education, in an attempt to prepare medical educators for the changing demands and opportunities that are about to face them because of AI. The names of various chapters which have been discussed in this book "Application of Artificial Intelligence In Cardiovascular Medicine" are as follows:-

What is Artificial Intelligence? , Artificial intelligence-enhanced Electrocardiography in cardiovascular disease management , Artificial intelligence in advances in the World of Cardiovascular Imaging , Artificial intelligence in hypertension management ,Artificial intelligence in Atherosclerotic CardioVascular Disease,. AI in cardiovascular imaging for risk stratification in CAD, Current and future applications of Artificial intelligence in Coronary artery disease , Machine Learning and Artificial intelligence to improve Peripheral artery disease management, Artificial intelligence and automation in Valvular heart diseases, Artificial intelligence in diagnosis and Management of Cardiac arrhythmias , Ocular images-based Artificial intelligence in diagnosis of Systemic diseases including cardiovascular ailments,Artificial intelligence in Pediatric Cardiology, The future of Cardiothoracic surgery in Artificial intelligence, Artificial intelligence in the diagnosis and detection of heart failure, Artificial intelligence in guidance of advanced heart failure therapies: Artificial Intelligence and cardiac Magnetic Resonance imaging in myocardial Infarction(CAD), Artificial Intelligence / Machine learning for predicting cardiac events What does the future hold? Artificial intelligence-based Smart Comrade Robot for elders healthcare ,.Emerging role of Artificial intelligence in cardiac electrophysiology , Applications of ChatGPT in medical practice, education and research, Educating future physicians in Artificial intelligence.,Will AI eventually replace Doctors?, Artificial intelligence advancements in the cardiovascular imaging of Coronary atherosclerosis,Artificial intelligence-(AI) empowered Echocardiography interpretation , AI empowered diagnosis of Epicardial ,Pericardial Fat and Pericardial effusion., Implantable cardiac Pacemakers embedded with Artificial intelligence.Artificial Intelligence,wearables & remote monitoring for heart failure. The role of Artificial intelligence(AI) in clinical practice, Artificial intelligence in the differential diagnosis of Cardiomyopathy phenotypes and Artificial intelligence in cardiovascular medicine: current insights and future prospects. Since it was not possible to accommodate the detailed descriptions of the other newer innovations in the field of Cardiology,hence brief notes have been added in the last chapter of this book.

This book in its present format and educative contents of various selective chapters ,is certainly would be very informative particularily better understanding of recently introduced Artificial intelligence technology, to research scholars, practicing cardiologists, post-gradutes including DM cardiology ,senior residents of cardiology and medicine

KCVERMA

Contents

CHAPTER

1

What Is Artificial Intelligence? Definition, Uses, and Types.

Over- view

Artificial intelligence (AI) refers to computer systems capable of performing complex tasks that historically only a human could do, such as reasoning, making decisions, or solving problems

Today, the term "AI" describes a wide range of technologies that power many of the services and goods we use every day – from apps that recommend TV shows to chatbots that provide customer support in real time. But do all of these really constitute artificial intelligence as most of us envision it? And if not, then why do we use the term so often?

In this Chapter, you'll learn more about artificial intelligence, what it actually does, and different types of it. In the end, you'll also learn about some of its benefits and dangers and explore flexible courses that can help you expand your knowledge of AI even further

What is artificial intelligence?

Artificial intelligence (AI) is the theory and development of computer systems capable of performing tasks that historically required human intelligence, such as recognizing speech, making decisions, and identifying patterns. AI is an umbrella term that encompasses a wide variety of technologies, including machine learning, deep learning, and natural language processing (NLP).

Although the term is commonly used to describe a range of different technologies in use today, many disagree on whether these actually constitute artificial intelligence. Instead, some argue that much of the technology used in the real world today actually constitutes highly advanced machine learning that is simply a first step towards true artificial intelligence, or "general artificial intelligence" (GAI).

Yet, despite the many philosophical disagreements over whether "true" intelligent machines actually exist, when most people use the term AI today, they're referring to a suite of machine learning-powered technologies, such as Chat GPT or computer vision, that enable machines to perform tasks that previously only humans can do like generating written content, steering a car, or analyzing data.

Artificial intelligence examples

Though the humanoid robots often associated with AI (think Star Trek: The Next Generation's Data or Terminator's T-800) don't exist yet, you've likely interacted with machine learning-powered services or devices many times before.

At the simplest level, machine learning uses algorithms trained on data sets to create machine learning models that allow computer systems to perform tasks like making song recommendations, identifying the fastest way to travel to a destination, or translating text from one language to another. Some of the most common examples of AI in use today include:

- ChatGPT: Uses large language models (LLMs) to generate text in response to questions or comments posed to it.
- Google Translate: Uses deep learning algorithms to translate text from one language to another.
- Netflix: Uses machine learning algorithms to create personalized recommendation engines for users based on their previous viewing history.
- Tesla: Uses computer vision to power self-driving features on their cars.

AI in the workforce

Artificial intelligence is prevalent across many industries. Automating tasks that don't require human intervention saves money and time, and can reduce the risk of human error. Here are a couple of ways AI could be employed in different industries:

- Finance industry. Fraud detection is a notable use case for AI in the finance industry. AI's capability to analyze large amounts of data enables it to detect anomalies or patterns that signal fraudulent behavior.
- Health care industry. AI-powered robotics could support surgeries close to highly delicate organs or tissue to mitigate blood loss or risk of infection.

What is artificial general intelligence (AGI)?

Artificial general intelligence (AGI) refers to a theoretical state in which computer systems will be able to achieve or exceed human intelligence. In other words, AGI is "true" artificial intelligence as depicted in countless science fiction novels, television shows, movies, and comics.

As for the precise meaning of "AI" itself, researchers don't quite agree on how we would recognize "true" artificial general intelligence when it appears. However, the most famous approach to identifying whether a machine is intelligent or not is known as the Turing Test or Imitation Game, an experiment that was first outlined by influential mathematician, computer scientist, and cryptanalyst Alan Turing in a 1950 paper on computer intelligence. There, Turing described a three-player game in which a human "interrogator" is asked to communicate via text with another human and a machine and judge who composed each response. If the interrogator cannot reliably identify the human, then Turing says the machine can be said to be intelligent . To complicate matters, researchers and philosophers also can't quite agree whether we're beginning to achieve AGI, if it's still far off, or just totally impossible. For example, while a recent paper from Microsoft Research and OpenAI argues that Chat GPT-4 is an early form of AGI, many other researchers are skeptical of these claims and argue that they were just made for publicity . Regardless of how far we are from achieving AGI, you can assume that when someone uses the term artificial general intelligence, they're referring to the kind of sentient computer programs and machines that are commonly found in popular science fiction.

Strong AI vs. Weak AI

When researching artificial intelligence, you might have come across the terms "strong" and "weak" AI. Though these terms might seem confusing, you likely already have a sense of what they mean.

Strong AI is essentially AI that is capable of human-level, general intelligence. In other words, it's just another way to say "artificial general intelligence."

Weak AI, meanwhile, refers to the narrow use of widely available AI technology, like machine learning or deep learning, to perform very specific tasks, such as playing chess, recommending songs, or steering cars. Also known as Artificial Narrow Intelligence (ANI), weak AI is essentially the kind of AI we use daily.

The 4 Types of AI

As researchers attempt to build more advanced forms of artificial intelligence, they must also begin to formulate more nuanced understandings of what intelligence or even consciousness precisely mean. In their attempt to clarify these concepts, researchers have outlined four types of artificial intelligence.

Here's a summary of each AI type, according to Professor Arend Hintze of the University of Michigan:

1. Reactive machines

Reactive machines are the most basic type of artificial intelligence. Machines built in this way don't possess any knowledge of previous events but instead only "react" to what is before them in a given moment. As a result, they can only perform certain advanced tasks within a very narrow scope, such as playing chess, and are incapable of performing tasks outside of their limited context.

2. Limited memory machines

Machines with limited memory possess a limited understanding of past events. They can interact more with the world around them than reactive machines can. For example, self-driving cars use a form of limited memory to make turns, observe approaching vehicles, and adjust their speed. However, machines with only limited memory cannot form a complete understanding of the world because their recall of past events is limited and only used in a narrow band of time.

3. Theory of mind machines

Machines that possess a "theory of mind" represent an early form of artificial general intelligence. In addition to being able to create representations of the world, machines of this type would also have an understanding of other entities that exist within the world. As of this moment, this reality has still not materialized.

4. Self-aware machines

Machines with self-awareness are the theoretically most advanced type of AI and would possess an understanding of the world, others, and itself. This is what most people mean when they talk about achieving AGI. Currently, this is a far-off reality.

AI benefits and dangers

AI has a range of applications with the potential to transform how we work and our daily lives. While many of these transformations are exciting, like self-driving cars, virtual assistants, or wearable devices in the healthcare industry, they also pose many challenges. It's a complicated picture that often summons competing images: a utopia for some, a dystopia for others. The reality is likely to be much more complex. Here are a few of the possible benefits and dangers AI may pose: These are just some of the ways that AI provides benefits and dangers to society. When using new technologies like AI, it's best to keep a clear mind about what it is and isn't. With great power comes great responsibility, after all.

Over the last few years, artificial intelligence (AI) has worked its way into every area of our lives. If you're a programmer, chances are you've started working with GitHub's Copilot, an AI tool that turns natural language prompts into coding suggestions to expedite programming. If you're a writer, you might have come across OpenAI's GPT-3 or similar autoregressive language models that use deep learning to create human-like text. It was just a few years ago such AI programs were in their infancy. Now they are becoming ubiquitous tools in writing and coding.As the founder of a technology investment firm, I've seen firsthand just how much AI has advanced in such a short period of time. The underlying building blocks of the technology are getting astonishingly better at an exponential rate, far outpacing our expectations. Techniques like deep learning allow us to run complex AI models to solve the most difficult problems. But while those who work in technology-centric careers are aware of AI's explosive capabilities, the public at large is still largely unaware of the depth of AI's potential.

Table 1.1 A few of the possible benefits and dangers AI may pose:

Potential Benefits	Potential Dangers
Greater accuracy for certain repeatable tasks, such as assembling vehicles or computers.	Job loss due to increased automation.
Decreased operational costs due to greater efficiency of machines.	Potential for bias or discrimination as a result of the data set on which the AI is trained.
Increased personalization within digital services and products.	Possible cybersecurity concerns.
Improved decision-making in certain situations	Lack of transparency over how decisions are arrived at, resulting in less than optimal solutions.
Ability to quickly generate new content, such as text or images.	Potential to create misinformation, as well as inadvertently violate laws and regulations

Recent Advancements In Artificial Intelligence

- Improvements in natural language processing, speech recognition and generation, and chatbots
- Advances in computer vision and image classification, such as self-driving cars and road safety
- Applications of AI in medical diagnosis, such as big data for compiling possible diagnoses
- Innovations in augmented reality and virtual production, such as de-aging and deep fakes
- Development of AI robots, such as Boston Dynamics' machines

The Growth Of AI

Many of us have spent a few hours playing around with DALL-E 2, the AI text-to-image generator that can create detailed images out of the most bizarre requests (think Obi-Wan Kenobi eating a hot fudge sundae). But how many of us realize the level of technology that goes into the creation of one of those images? This app doesn't create images out of existing internet images but rather uses a complicated process called diffusion to refine a series of pixels until the visual rendering matches the text description. Not only is DALL-E 2 exponentially more powerful than its predecessor released the year before, but it has the potential to revolutionize the world of digital art. Think about it—if you are a digital artist, illustrator or graphic designer, how much would your career change if you could use an app to create a realistic-looking image within seconds? These technologies tie to real-world applications with serious implications.

The sheer velocity and magnitude of AI innovation have also led to impacts in fields such as commerce or digital healthcare. The development of AlphaFold, an AI system that descended from AlphaGo, was originally a deep learning model trained to beat human beings at the board game Go. When AlphaGo was released five years ago, few predicted that this deep learning model would one day lead to a revolutionary discovery in molecular biology. AlphaFold uses a deep neural network to predict the 3-D structures of proteins. The AI is a great advance in what scientists call the "protein-folding problem" and ended up predicting the structure of more than 200 million proteins, which is almost all that are currently known to exist. AlphaFold's capabilities have opened the floodgates for medical researchers to develop countless drugs and vaccines to help humankind.

S A Competitive Advantage

As AI continues to develop at an exponential rate, it is transforming the business world. Leveraging AI technologies can be a source of durable competitive advantage for businesses. Consider which repetitive tasks you might be able to automate using AI or how you can use AI to amplify your workers' capabilities. Enterprise functions such as marketing, sales, finance and HR are all areas that can utilize new AI-enabled applications; these applications include providing customers with 24/7 financial guidance, predicting and assessing loan risks and collecting and analyzing client data. In my view, we're reaching escape velocity when it comes to AI. Who knows what will be possible a few years from now? As AI innovations become relevant to nearly every economic sector and industry, I believe that companies that don't adopt AI are going to be severely disadvantaged.Newer companies hold a distinct advantage in this area. Whereas existing businesses have to replace old technology, up-and-coming entrepreneurs can more naturally invest in the latest technologies right from the start. I recommend executives keep up with evolving AI technological trends in order to avoid the risk of being leapfrogged by newer entrants

Final Thoughts

AI is the single biggest paradigm shift we've ever seen, and it's evolving much faster than prior shifts. Advancements such as the cloud, mobile and the internet all changed the game, but none of them have evolved quite as rapidly as AI. As artificial intelligence continues to grow, it will soon dwarf the impact of these prior technology enablers, even as it builds upon and expands the applicability and impact of those technologies. Our success depends on taking advantage of what AI has to offer. In spite of what some may believe, I see how AI is set to change our world. Rather than fretting about a dystopian future, we can see AI for what it really is—a potent amplifier of human potential. Our only task is to make the most of it.

25 Stunning advances in artificial intelligence

Artificial intelligence (AI) is defined as "a branch of computer science dealing with the simulation of intelligent behavior in computers; the capability of a machine to imitate intelligent human behavior," according to Webster's Dictionary. Recent advancements in the field, however, have proven that AI is so much more than a mere scientific curiosity. The technological advances attributed to AI have the potential to completely alter the world as we know it. Artificial intelligence used to be the stuff of science fiction; evidence of the concept being studied by real-life scientists dates back to the 1950s. The famous Alan Turing explored the theory in a research paper in the year 1950, but the fundamentals of computers weren't yet advanced enough to bring the idea of artificial intelligence to fruition. By 1955 The Logic Theorist program funded by the Research and Development (RAND) Corporation became what many believe to be the first example of AI. The program was designed to mimic the human mind's ability to problem solve, eventually setting the stage for a historic conference called the Dartmouth Summer Research Project on Artificial Intelligence in 1956. As computers began to get faster, more powerful, and less expensive, AI began to pick up steam through the '70s. Successful projects began emerging in scientific communities, some even securing funding from government agencies. Then, for close to a decade, AI research hit a wall as funding lapsed and scientific theories began to outpace computer ability once again. The biggest exception was a Japanese government-funded, $400 million project aimed at improving artificial intelligence from 1982 to 1990.The 1990s and 2000s saw some huge advancements in artificial intelligence as the fundamental limits of computer storage yielded to new hardware innovations. As the applications of AI become more and more prevalent in the daily lives of humans, it is essential to have the context of some of the most important advances in AI history.Stacker explored 25 advances in artificial intelligence from all different uses, applications, and innovations. Whether it's robots, supercomputers, health care, or search optimization, AI is coming up strong.

1.Boston Dynamics

Known for their AI robots and resulting viral videos, Boston Dynamics truly changed the public's understanding of what robots with AI technology are capable of. Videos of their first big robot "Big Dog" went viral in 2005, and since then millions of people have enjoyed watching the company grow from smaller four-legged robots to full-fledged humanoids with the ability to perform parkour and backflips.

2.ProFound AI

First launched in the U.S. in December 2018, ProFound AI is a cancer-detection software that assists radiologists in finding early digital breast tomosynthesis (DBT) in patients. While the technology has only reached select high-profile hospitals so far, the innovation is a great precursor to what's to come in the medical world of AI.

3.AI artwork

October 2018 marked the first piece of AI-generated artwork sold at a world auction, signaling the emergence of AI into the art world. The portrait was created by a Paris-based collective that is studying the interface between art and AI and sold at world-renowned Christie's auction house for $432,500 (almost 45 times its estimate).

4.AI-generated human faces

The Japanese startup DataGrid began creating AI-generated faces in 2018, but didn't go viral until April 2019. It was then that a press release revealed a series of photorealistic images of what appeared to be humans but were, in fact, created by AI. This advance utilizes a whole new level of deep learning algorithms that create realistic images so good that they can fool other humans.

5.TensorFlow

TensorFlow, the deep-learning library that Google uses in its products (search engines, translation, recommendations, etc), was first released to the public in 2015. TensorFlow is open source—meaning that anyone can download it and use it for free—and symbolizes the importance of making machine learning and AI available to anyone for any purpose.

6.AlphaGo

DeepMind Technologies' AlphaGo first made headlines when it defeated the European champion in the complex Chinese board game "Go" in 2015, before going on to beat the world champion in 2016. AlphaGo famously marked a new age in advanced AI programs combining traditional methods with deep neural networks

7.GAN

Generative adversarial networks (GANs) were first introduced in 2014 at the Neural Information Processing Systems Conference. The new GAN machine learning framework was innovative, consisting of two artificial neural networks able to compete and subsequently train one another, creating better results. An example of an updated version of GAN is the popular This Person Does Not Exist website, which uses AI to generate human faces.

8. Autonomous driving

In 2015 the first cross-country road trip performed by an autonomous car was completed in nine days. The Audi SQ5 was equipped with autonomous driving technology and software from Delphi Technologies to allow the car to make human-like decisions from merging onto highways to parking and everything in between. Though the safety driver (seated in the front seat per the law) reportedly had to interfere a few times, the trip marked a huge advancement in the future of driverless car technology.

9. IBM's Watson

When IBM's Watson computer running software defeated two "Jeopardy!" all-stars in February of 2011, it breached a gap between technology and popular culture in a big way. Watson could hold about one million books' worth of information in its software and storage, and when posed with a question, the AI ran several different algorithms to rank the best answer. This was different than traditional computer searching keyword-based software, as "Jeopardy!" questions are inherently human in nature, mixing colorful wordplay with puns and cultural references.

10. Siri

Siri may be present in most modern Apple products today, but when the automated voice assistant technology first came out commercially in 2010, it was cutting-edge. After being released as an app, Siri caught the eye of Steve Jobs, who bought the technology for $200 million and employed two of its inventors. The third inventor went on to co-found Viv Labs, acquired by Samsung for $215 million in 2016.

11. AI Glass

In July 2019, scientists from the University of Wisconsin-Madison created artificially intelligent glass with the ability to recognize images without a power source. One of the utilizations of this AI "smart glass" is creating face ID-locking security software on your phone without using the battery. Potentially, the glass could create a biometric lock that could stand the test of time without the need for an internet or battery source.

12. Deep Density Displacement Model

2019 saw a huge advancement for artificial intelligence in astrophysics with the development of the Deep Density Displacement Model. In June, astrophysicists were able to use AI to generate 3D simulations of the universe for the first time, shaving down the time it previously took to create complex simulations from minutes to milliseconds.

13."Ghost Population"discovery

In February of 2019, a report released by Nature Communications revealed that machine learning technology had found evidence in the human genome of unknown human ancestors, or a "ghost population." Somewhere down the line of human evolutionary history, a previously undiscovered group of hominins bred with homo sapiens leaving behind traces of DNA. The study is one of the first to directly illuminate how AI can actually help humans understand our own origins.

14.AI predicts death

In a chilling artificial intelligence development, health care data scientists and doctors found in March of 2019 that AI could accurately predict death in patients. The study tested a new system of machine learning algorithms designed to predict the risk of chronic illness and early death in middle-aged patients. These computer-based techniques have the potential to improve preventative health care and assist doctors in taking account of biometrics, lifestyle, and more.

15.AI in mobile phones

Chinese technology company Huawei claimed one of the first smartphones with artificial intelligence capabilities in September 2017, becoming the first company to base its key appeal for a cell phone around AI. The Huawei Mate 10's Kirin 970 chipset was specially designed for the fast processing required for taking photos on your phone, all while utilizing more bandwidth. Though Huawei has since come out with new models of phones with the tech, the original Mate 10 marked a leap towards the future of mobile AI

16.Facebook chatbots

In 2016, Facebook announced that the company would be placing chatbots on their messenger platform, giving businesses the opportunity to provide automatic customer support, interactive content, and more. The ability to replace real people with AI capable of performing tasks like making reservations, reviewing orders, and responding to human users with structured messages was a game-changer for businesses at the time. Facebook has continued to develop chatbot technology with its FAIR (Facebook Artificial Intelligence Research) program.

17.OpenAI language model

OpenAI, the artificial intelligence research company founded by Elon Musk, unveiled an AI system that can generate text in February 2019. The language model became available to the public in a limited form shortly thereafter and proved what was previously believed to be untrue—that AI had the capability to be creative

18.Deepfakes

The term "deepfake" is believed to have been coined in 2017 by a Reddit user, and describes the AI-based machine learning technology used to realistically superimpose mages or videos onto a source with incredible accuracy. While the tech is usually used playfully, deepfaking goes far beyond simply altering video footage and has the U.S. government concerned about its future misuse and weaponization.

19.Nautilus

Nautilus Labs entered the scene in 2016 when it began building AI technology platforms for the maritime shipping industry. By using machine learning programs to make predictions about shipping routes, the tech developed by Nautilus will maximize profit and minimize fuel consumption (a big win for the environment, too).

20.Cyc

With its initial development beginning in 1984, Cyc is the longest-running artificial intelligence program in history. The AI engine spent over 30 years gathering general knowledge to build a base before becoming commercialized in 2016 by Lucid AI. Cyc represents the longevity of AI systems, and only time will tell what the future holds for the program.

21.Amazon

The rise of Alexa and the Amazon Echo changed the world of smart home artificial intelligence when the product first launched in November 2014. One of its advantages over similar AI assistant services is the Echo's far-field microphone, which can pick up sound from larger distances when users use the wake word (usually "Alexa") to wake-up the virtual assistant.

22.Deep Blue

In 1997 IBM's Deep Blue computer became the first machine in history to beat a world champion at chess, famously proving to the world that AI could actually be developed to surpass humans in certain intellectual tasks. Deep Blue paved the way for IBM's future AI superstar computer, Watson, and changed the world of technology forever.

23.The DARPA Grand Challenge

TThe inaugural Defense Advanced Research Projects Agency (DARPA) driverless car competition in 2004 was the first of its kind. It was also generally considered a failure, due to the fact that none of the cars that qualified made it past the finish line. At the competition the following year, however, a few cars managed to finish the journey and create the momentum for three more important DARPA AI competitions: the Spectrum Challenge for radio, the Robotics Challenge, and the Cyber Grand Challenge tournament for automated network defense.

24.Waymo

Google's autonomous vehicle program, Waymo, made history in December 2018 when it announced a commercial self-driving taxi program in Arizona. Though the service will initially only be available to select customers and the cars will still have safety drivers in the front seats in case things go awry, the app-based program is completely original.

25. ELIZA

Before the days of Siri and Alexa, a language processing computing system called ELIZA started it all. The MIT Artificial Intelligence Laboratory developed ELIZA from 1964 to 1966 as a simulated Rogerian psychotherapist, where users could type out questions and receive a response back. The tech wasn't nearly as advanced as the artificial language processing systems of today, but ELIZA laid down AI-enhanced Safety of Prescription

Artificial intelligence in medicine

AI-enhanced Safety of Prescription

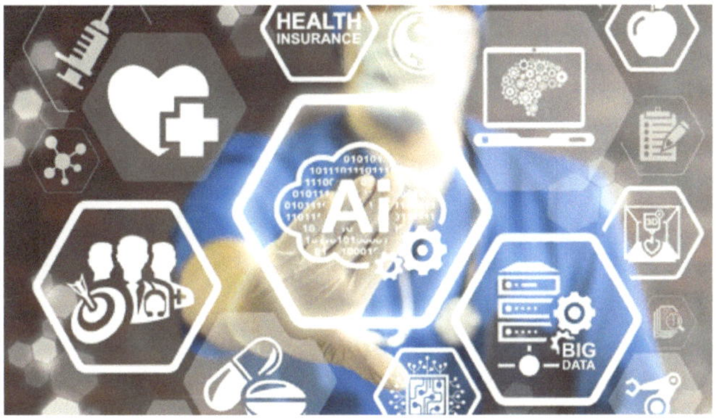

Fig.1.1 Research team leader : Prof. Yu-Chuan Li

Research briefing

Though the idea of an artificial thinking machine has been around since ancient Greek writings of mechanical men, it was the early computer age that made the concept seem obtainable When the term artificial intelligence – AI – was coined in 1955 Dr. Yu-Chuan Li was'nt yet born.. For Dr. Li, growing up with early portrayals of artificial thinking technology in movies was fascinating, and access to early computers made it possible to begin working with AI in high school.

Biomedical Signal AI Machine Learning

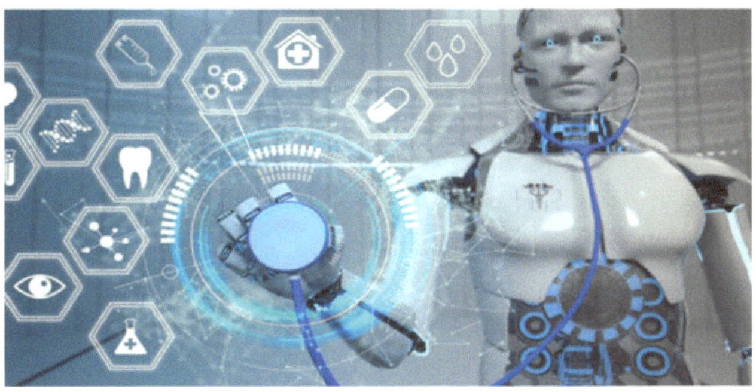

Fig.1.2 Research team leader : Prof. Yu-Chuan Li

Research briefing

Though the idea of an artificial thinking machine has been around since ancient Greek writings of mechanical men, it was the early computer age that made the concept seem obtainable When the term artificial intelligence – AI – was coined in 1955 Dr. Yu-Chuan Li was'nt yet born.. For Dr. Li, growing up with early portrayals of artificial thinking technology in movies was fascinating, and access to early computers made it possible to begin working with AI in high school.

Biomedical Signal AI Machine Learning

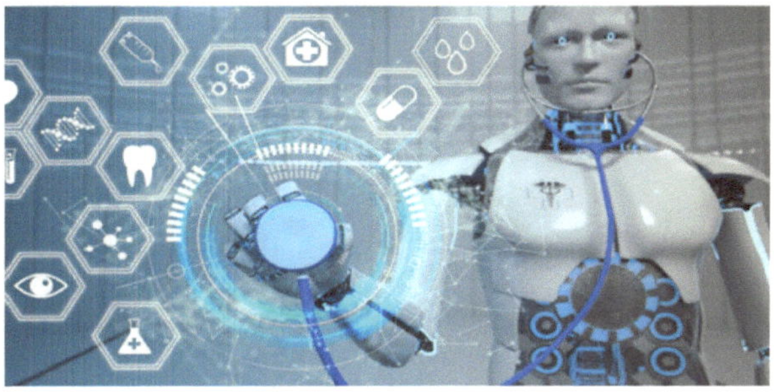

Fig 1.3 Research team leader : Dr. Jiunn-Horng Kang

Research briefing

Physiatrist Dr. Jiunn-Horng Kang has the calm demeanor of someone used to reassuring patients. At the same time, a somewhat mischievous smile and glasses make seem like he's be just as at home at a video game exhibition as at a patient's bedside. Between his time as a physiatrist, researcher, and associate professor, he has his assistants and students test out popular tech devices to find discrepancies between interpretations of physiological data and people's real world experiences. On his wrist is a new model smartwatch. "I wear a lot watches to see the signals I can get from different devices. Actually in our lab we have more than ten kinds of watches.

IBM Watson for Oncology

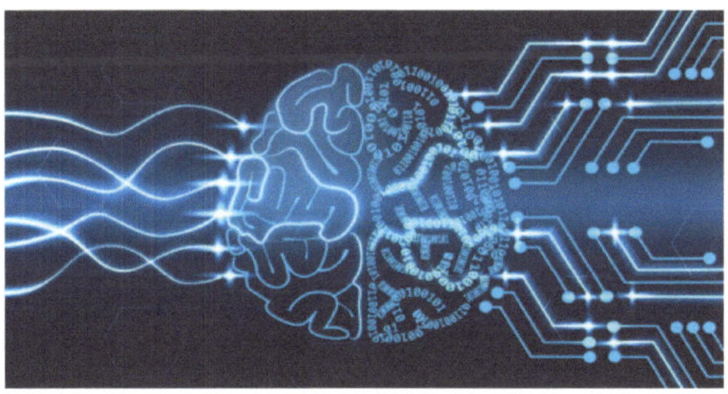

Fig. 1.4 Research team leader : Dr. Chun-You Chen

Research briefing

When facing a life threatening health crisis, it might sound good to have an intelligent supercomputer help inform your care, especially one that's been trained by some of the worlds' top oncologists. That's the goal for IBM's new AI based technology, which was brought to TMU hospitals last year. Spotlight spoke about the technology and its applications with Dr. Chun-You (Jim) Chen, radiation oncologist, self-taught programmer, and Chief Medical Information Officer at Wanfang Hospital. Dr. Chen created and continues to develop Wanfang Hospital's "One Page" patient information system, and is in charge of clinical adoption and EMR system integration of Watson for Oncology in the Taipei Cancer Center of Taipei Medical University.

AI in Imaging

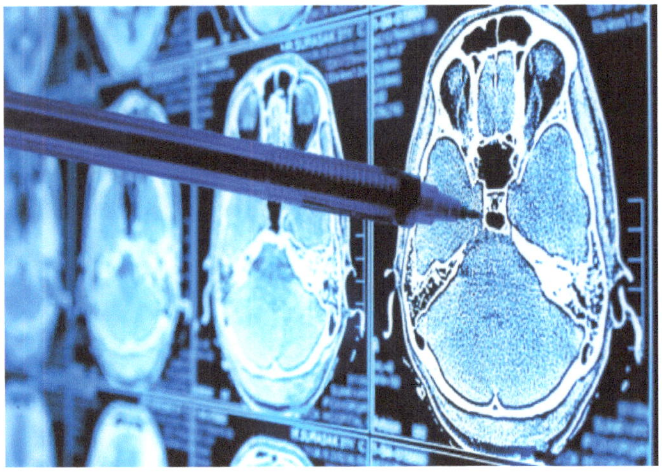

Fig.1.5 Research team leader : Dr. Wing-Pang Chan

Research briefing

At a time when artificial intelligence is being hyped as a solution to a multitude of health related problems is running high, some people are worried that tasks once done by humans may be better suited to machines – transferring health care responsibilities to computers and putting doctors out of work. In fact, this same question was being asked 27 years ago when Dr. Wing-Pang Chan, now Professor and Director of Radiology at Taipei Medical University and Chief of Radiology at Wanfang Hospital, was rained as research fellow in MSK Radiology, supervised by Professor Harry K. Genant, at the University of California, San Francisco. Dr. Genant and his team were working on a machine learning classification system for vertebral compression fractures. Machine learning was at that time in its early stages, and viewed by many medical practitioners as a promising technology for interpreting medical imaging data. But the hope for new technology brought with it reservations: would this technology eventually replace doctors' eyes and brains?

Box 1.1 There are different types of Artificial Intelligence (AI) Here are some of them:

- **Reactive Machines:** These are purely reactive machines that do not have memory and cannot use past experiences to inform future ones
- **Limited Memory:** These machines are reactive machines with combined capabilities of learning from historical data for decision making
- **Theory of Mind :** These machines can understand human emotions, beliefs, and thoughts.
- **Self Aware:** These machines have consciousness and can understand their own existence.

- **Artificial Narrow Intelligence (ANI):**These are AI tools designed to carry out very specific actions or commands.
- **Artificial General Intelligence (AGI):**These machines can perform any intellectual task that a human can.
- **Artificial Super Intelligence (ASI):** . These machines can surpass human intelligence and perform tasks that are beyond human capabilities

Artificial Intelligence to Enhance Clinical Value: Key Points

The following are key points to remember from this state-of-the art review on artificial intelligence (AI) to enhance clinical value across the spectrum of cardiovascular health care:

1. A step-wise framework for applying AI can improve the use of AI in clinical research. This should start by determining the appropriate methods and data sets to address the research hypotheses. It is recommended to develop a clear hypothesis when selecting the data to be included in the analysis. Data type and collection method can be considered unstructured, semi-structured, structured, and structured as information such as demographics or blood biomarkers. Semi-structured includes text-based or continuously measured data, while unstructured includes imaging data.

2.Adequate data pre-processing is essential for allowing AI methods to deliver accurate, meaningful results. The output of any AI model is only as good as the data inputted. Missingness is important to consider in this step. Considering standardizing or normalized data, imputation, and dimensionality reduction is also important.

3. Choosing the appropriate machine learning (ML) approach is based on the clinical question or hypothesis and the setting in which learning is performed. Supervised learning uses ML approaches with labeled data to train in prediction, while unsupervised learning's computational algorithms have no ground truth for comparison. Overfitting is a concern for prediction models during the training stage of any ML approach. A wide variety of ML algorithms are available, including decision trees, random forests, neural networks, deep neural networks, and autoencoders.

4. Validation is a critical next step to allow an understanding of how generalizable the findings are between data sets and real-world clinical practice. External validation is recommended for all AI studies. Currently, many studies do not validate their findings. It is recommended that investigators provide clear details on their methods, guided by the FAIR principles (Findability, Accessibility, Interoperability, and Reusability), and allow others to independently validate their findings.

5. Investigators must be mindful of relevant social constructs, data privacy, and health care equality.

AI in Health Care: Applications, Benefits, and Examples

Artificial intelligence (AI) has already changed much of the world as we know it – from automating systems to improving the decisions we make and the ways we go about making them. Yet, perhaps the most impactful and personal ways AI is changing our world are within the field of health care, where it's being used to diagnose, create personalized treatment plans, and even predict patient survival rates. In this article, you'll learn more about the types of AI used in health care, some of their applications and the benefits of AI within the field, as well as what the future might hold. You'll also explore relevant jobs and online courses that can help you get started using AI for health care purposes today.

How is AI used in health care?

Artificial Intelligence (AI) uses computers and machine processes to simulate human intelligence and perform complex automated tasks. While they seek to reflect the abilities of the human mind, AI-enabled machines are also capable of exceeding it in a number of ways, particularly by sifting through large volumes of big data efficiently in order to identify patterns, anomalies,and trends.

Unsurprisingly, AI presents a wealth of opportunities to health care, where it can be used to enhance a variety of common medical processes – from diagnosing diseases to identifying the best treatment plans for patients facing critical illnesses like cancer. Robotic surgical equipment outfitted with AI can help surgeons better perform surgeries by decreasing their physical fluctuations and providing updated information during the operation.

Types of AI in health care

AI is an umbrella term covering a variety of distinct, but interrelated processes. Some of the most common forms of AI used within health care include:

•**Machine learning (ML):** training algorithms using data sets, such as health records, to create models capable of performing such tasks as categorizing information or predicting outcomes.

Deep learning: A subset of machine learning that involves greater volumes of data, training times, and layers of ML algorithms to produce neural networks capable of more complextasks.

Neural language processing (NLP): the use of ML to understand human language, whether it be verbal or written. In health care, NLP is used to interpret documentation, notes, reports,andpublishedresearch.

Robotic process automation (RPA): the use of AI in computer programs to automate administrative and clinical workflows. Some health care organizations use RPA to improve the patient experience and the daily function of their facilities.

AI applications in health care

As artificial intelligence becomes more widely adopted, so too does the number of ways the technology is being used across industries. Researchers don't expect AI to replace health care professionals just yet. Instead, they see it as supporting and improving the work of health providers and professionals in the near future. Here are some of the most common applications of AI in the field today:

- **Health care analytics:** ML algorithms are trained using historical data to produce insights, improve decision-making, and optimize health outcomes.
- **Precision medicine:** AI is used to produce personalized treatment plans for patients that take into account such factors as their medical history, environmental factors, lifestyles, and genetic makeup.
- **Predict diseases and illness:** Using predictive models, health care professionals can determine the likelihood that someone might develop a particular condition or contract a disease.
- **Interpret tests and diagnose diseases:** ML models can be trained using common medical scans, like MRIs or X-rays, to interpret and diagnose such conditions as cancerous lesions.

Benefits of AI in health care

AI provides a number of benefits to the field of health care, the professionals working within it, and the patients that interact with it every day. While health care professionals can expect lower operational costs due to improved decision-making and more efficient automated services, providers can leverage the technology to design bespoke treatment plans

Table 1.2. Explanation of terms used in Artificial Intelligence

Term	Explanation
Artificial Intelligence (AI)	A branch of computer science in which the machines attempt to emulate what the human intelli-gence might do in the same situation.
Machine Learning (ML)	A branch of AI where, to emulate human predictions, machines are fed with data and learn by them.
Deep learning (DL)	A type of ML based on the use of artificial representation of human neural architecture, known as artificial neural networks.
Neural Network (NN)	An artificial representation of human neural architecture, characterized by the presence several layers, including an input and an output separated by several hidden layers.
Convolutional Neural Network (CNN)	A DL model characterized by the presence of several convolutional layers which are not fully connected each other but only with certain part of specific layers; they are mostly used to aggre-gate information for a global prediction.
Fully Convolutional Network (FCN)	A DL model characterized by a hierarchical communication among different layers; they are used to highlight information obtained from each pixel.
Recurrent Neural Network (RNN)	A DL model which, unlike CNN and FCN, can take into account inputs at different time points; they are used to learn task which might benefit from a dynamic contribution of information
Generative Adversarial Networks (GAN)	A DL model which use simultaneously two NN: the first generating data from input, the second checking the agreement between original and generated data; they are used to decrease the degree of mistakes.

and diagnose conditions more quickly and accurately than they could alone. Patients can expect potentially improved health outcomes and lower costs resulting from more efficienthealthservices.

AI jobs in health care

Both AI and health care are growing fields that are projected to have a big impact in the coming decade. It's little surprise, then, that AI-oriented positions are becoming increasingly common within the field of health care. If you're interested in pursuing one of these careers, here are some of the positions you should consider exploring:

1. Health informatics specialist
2. Machine learning engineer
3. Data scientist
4. AI engineer

The future of AI in health care

As with many other industries, AI is poised to change the health care landscape over the coming years. In addition to improving health facility operations, patient diagnoses, treatment plan development, and overall health outcomes, AI is also expected to help with the development and discovery of new medical cures.

The use of artificial intelligence in health care is expected to grow significantly over the next decade. According to Grand View Research, AI in health care is forecasted to be valued at $208.2 billion in 2030, which is many times higher than its 2022 market size value of $15.4 billion While some research indicates that AI could lead to significant job cuts as technology automates tasks like interpreting radiologic images, others believe that this is unlikely to be the case. One 2019 research paper, for instance, asserts that actual job loss is likely to be just five percent or less over the next ten to twenty years, indicating that most job seekers have little to worry about for the foreseeablefuture . Cardiovascular disease (CVD) represents a significant and increasing burden on healthcare systems. Artificial intelligence (AI) is a rapidly evolving transdisciplinary field employing machine learning (ML) techniques, which aim to simulate human intuition to offer cost-effective and scalable solutions to better manage CVD. ML algorithms are increasingly being developed and applied in various facets of cardiovascular medicine, including and not limited to heart failure, electrophysiology, valvular heart disease and coronary artery disease. Within heart failure, AI algorithms can augment diagnostic capabilities and clinical decision-making through automated cardiac measurements. Occult cardiac disease is increasingly being identified using ML from diagnostic data. Improved diagnostic and prognostic capabilities using ML algorithms are enhancing clinical care of patients with valvular heart disease and coronary artery disease. The growth of AI techniques is not without inherent challenges, most important of which is the need for greater external validation through multicenter, prospective clinical trials.

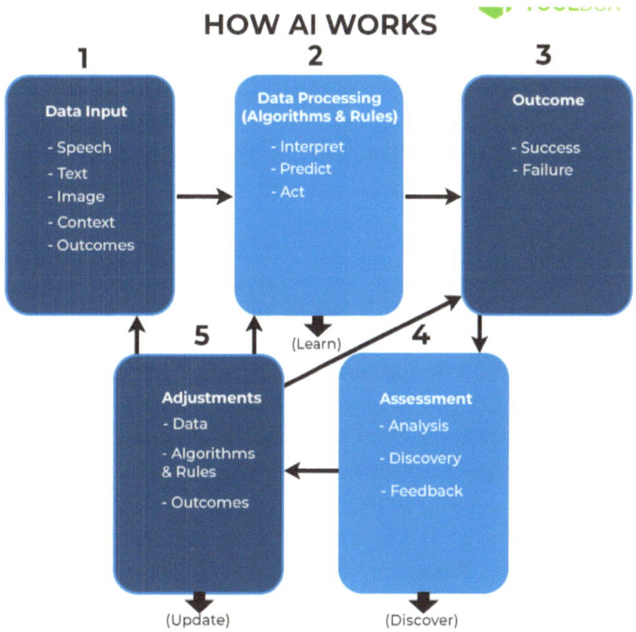

Fig.1.6 Illustration shows mechanism of AI Working

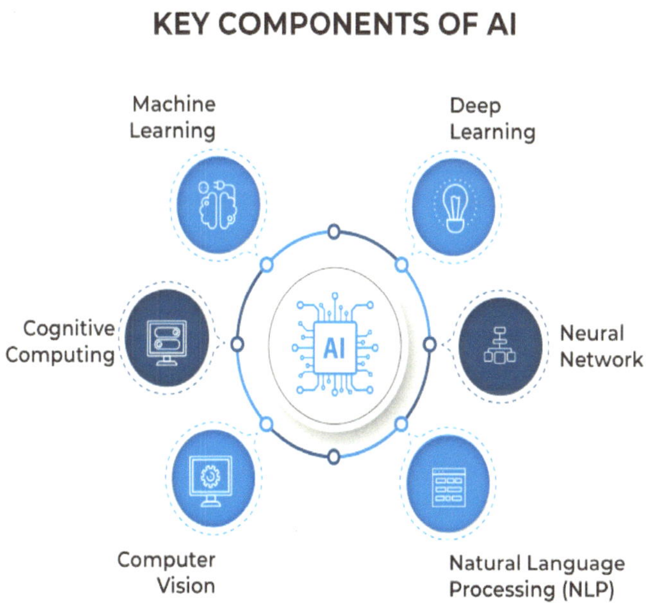

Fig.1.7 Illustration shows key components of AI

The types of AI based on capability.

1.Narrow AI

Narrow AI is a goal-oriented AI trained to perform a specific task. The machine intelligence that we witness all around us today is a form of narrow AI. Examples of narrow AI include Apple's Siri and IBM's Watson supercomputer.

Narrow AI is also referred to as weak AI as it operates within a limited and pre-defined set of parameters, constraints, and contexts. For example, use cases such as Netflix recommendations, purchase suggestions on ecommerce sites, autonomous cars, and speech & image recognition fall under the narrow AI category.

2. General AI

General AI is an AI version that performs any intellectual task with a human-like efficiency. The objective of general AI is to design a system capable of thinking for itself just like humans do. Currently, general AI is still under research, and efforts are being made to develop machines that have enhanced cognitive capabilities.

3. Super AI

Super AI is the AI version that surpasses human intelligence and can perform any task better than a human. Capabilities of a machine with super AI include thinking, reasoning, solving a puzzle, making judgments, learning, and communicating on its own. Today, super AI is a hypothetical concept but represents the future of AI.

4. Reactive machines

Reactive machines are basic AI types that do not store past experiences or memories for future actions. Such systems zero in on current scenarios and react to them based on the best possible action. Popular examples of reactive machines include IBM's Deep Blue system and Google's AlphaGo.

5. Limited memory machines

Limited memory machines can store and use past experiences or data for a short period of time. For example, a self-driving car can store the speeds of vehicles in its vicinity, their respective distances, speed limits, and other relevant information for it to navigate through the traffic.

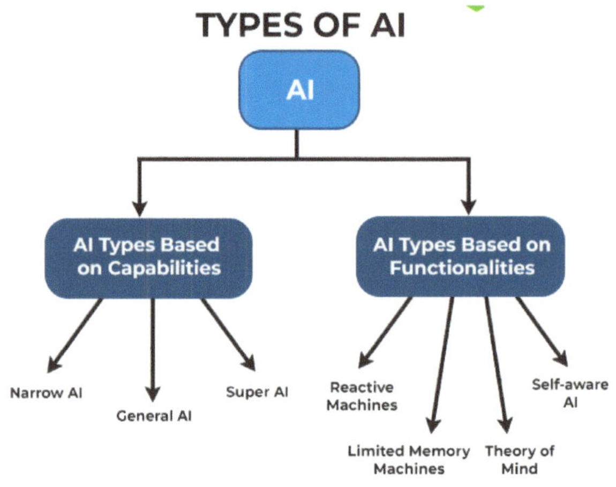

Fig. 1.8 Illustration shows various types of AI

6. Theory of mind

Theory of mind refers to the type of AI that can understand human emotions and beliefs and socially interact like humans. This AI type has not yet been developed but is in contention for the future.

7. Self-aware AI

Self-aware AI deals with super-intelligent machines with their consciousness, sentiments, emotions, and beliefs. Such systems are expected to be smarter than a human mind and may outperform us in assigned tasks. Self-aware AI is still a distant reality, but efforts are being made in this direction.

Goals of Artificial Intelligence

AI is primarily achieved by reverse-engineering human capabilities and traits and applying them to machines. At its core, AI reads human behavior to develop intelligent machines. Simply put, the foundational goal of AI is to design a technology that enables computer systems to work intelligently yet independently. The essential goals of AI are explained below.

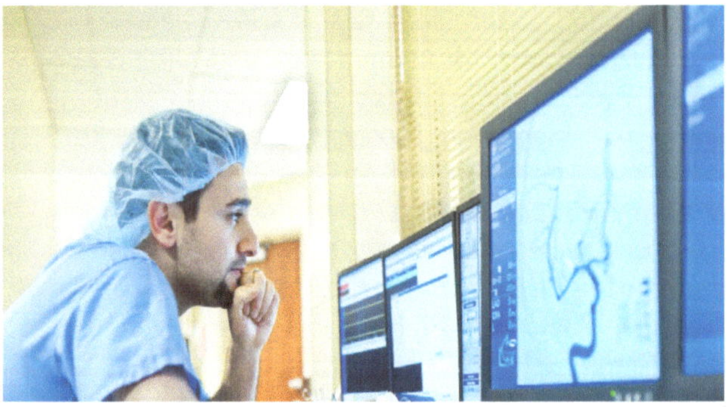

Fig 1.9 AI is changing how health care professionals provide care and how patients receive it.

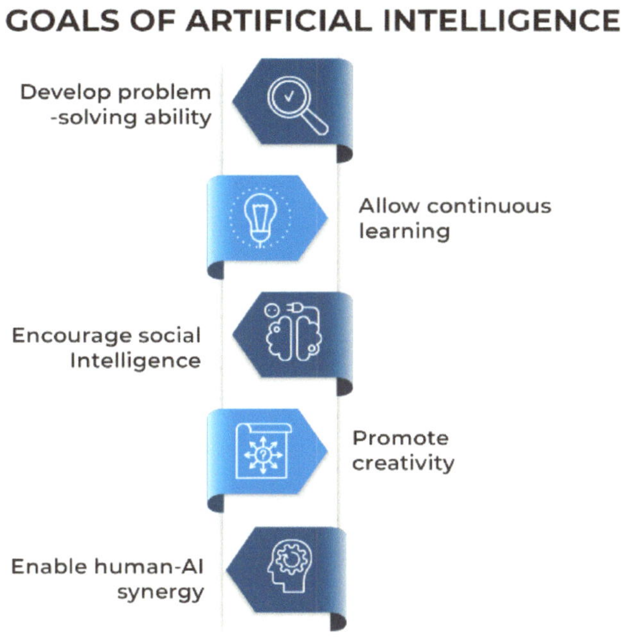

Fig. 1.10 Illustration shows various types of AI

Goals of Artificial Intelligence

1. Develop problem-solving ability

AI research is focused on developing efficient problem-solving algorithms that can make logical deductions and simulate human reasoning while solving complex puzzles. AI systems offer methods to deal with uncertain situations or handle the incomplete information conundrum by employing probability theory, such as a stock market prediction system. The problem-solving ability of AI makes our lives easier as complex tasks can be assigned to reliable AI systems that can aid in simplifying critical jobs.

2. Incorporate knowledge representation

AI research revolves around the idea of knowledge representation and knowledge engineering. It relates to the representation of 'what is known' to machines with the ontology for a set of objects, relations, and concepts.
The representation reveals real-world information that a computer uses to solve complex real-life problems, such as diagnosing a medical ailment or interacting with humans in natural language. Researchers can use the represented information to expand the AI knowledge base and fine-tune and optimize their AI models to meet the desired goals.

3. Facilitate planning

Intelligent agents provide a way to envision the future. AI-driven planning determines a procedural course of action for a system to achieve its goals and optimizes overall performance through predictive analytics, data analysis, forecasting, and optimization models. With the help of AI, we can make future predictions and ascertain the consequences of our actions. Planning is relevant across robotics, autonomous systems, cognitive assistants, and cybersecurity.

4.Allow continuous learning

Learning is fundamental to AI solutions. Conceptually, learning implies the ability of computer algorithms to improve the knowledge of an AI program through observations and past experiences. Technically, AI programs process a collection of input-output pairs for a defined function and use the results to predict outcomes for new inputs.
AI primarily uses two learning models–supervised and unsupervised–where the main distinction lies in using labeled datasets. As AI systems learn independently, they require minimal or no human intervention. For example, ML defines an automated learning process.

5.Encourage social Intelligence

Affective computing, also called 'emotion AI,' is the branch of AI that recognizes, interprets, and simulates human experiences, feelings, and emotions. With affective computing, computers can read facial expressions, body language, and voice tones to allow AI systems to interact and socialize at the human level. Thus, research efforts are inclined toward amplifying the social intelligence of machines.

6.Promote creativity

AI promotes creativity and artificial thinking that can help humans accomplish tasks better. AI can churn through vast volumes of data, consider options and alternatives, and develop creative paths or opportunities for us to progress. It also offers a platform to augment and strengthen creativity, as AI can develop many novel ideas and concepts that can inspire and boost the overall creative process.

7.Achieve general intelligence

AI researchers aim to develop machines with general AI capabilities that combine all the cognitive skills of humans and perform tasks with better proficiency than us. This can boost overall productivity as tasks would be performed with greater efficiency and free humans from risky tasks such as defusing bombs.

8.Promote synergy between humans and AI

One of the critical goals of AI is to develop a synergy between AI and humans to enable them to work together and enhance each other's capabilities rather than depend on just one system.

Key Challenges of AI

AI is poised at a juncture where its role in every industry has become almost inevitable, be it healthcare, manufacturing, robotics, autonomous systems, aviation, and plenty others. However, just because AI holds enormous potential, it does not mean that one can ignore the numerous challenges that come along with it. The critical challenges for AI that businesses can recognize and work toward resolving to propel its growth are:

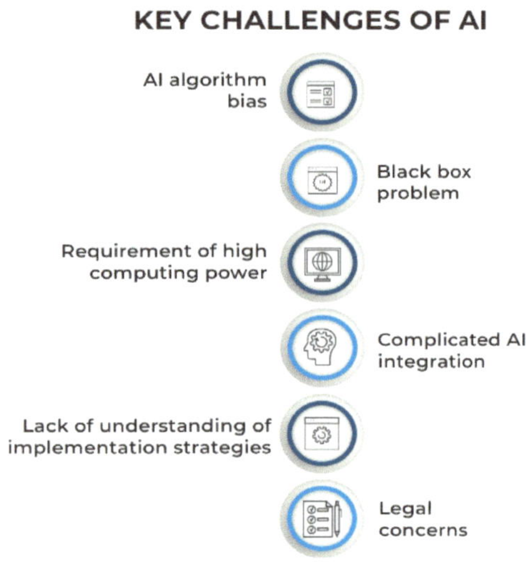

Fig.1.11 key Challenges of AI

1. AI algorithm bias

AI systems operate on trained data, implying the quality of an AI system is as good as its data. As we explore the depths of AI, the inevitable bias brought in by the data becomes evident. Bias refers to racial, gender, communal, or ethnic bias. For example, today's algorithms determine candidates suitable for a job interview or individuals eligible for a loan. If the algorithms making such vital decisions have developed biases over time, it could lead to dreadful, unfair, and unethical consequences.Hence, it is vital to train AI systems on unbiased data. Companies such as Microsoft and Facebook have already announced the introduction of anti-bias tools that can automatically identify bias in AI algorithms and check unfair AI perspectives.

2. Black box problem

AI algorithms are like black boxes. We have very little understanding of the inner workings of an AI algorithm. For example, we can understand what the prediction is for a predicting system, but we lack the knowledge of how the system arrived at that prediction. This makes AI systems slightly unreliable.

Techniques are being developed to resolve the black box problem, such as 'local interpretable model-agnostic explanations' (LIME) models. LIME provides additional information for every eventual prediction, making the algorithm trustworthy since it makes the forecast interpreta

3. Requirement of high computing power

AI takes up immense computing power to train its models. As deep learning algorithms become popular, arranging for an extra number of cores and GPUs is essential to ensure that such algorithms work efficiently. This is why AI systems have not been deployed in areas like astronomy, where AI could be used for asteroid tracking.

Moreover, complex algorithms require supercomputers to work at total capacity to manage challenging levels of computing. Today, only a few supercomputers are available globally but seem expensive at the outset. This limits the possibility of AI implementation at higher computing levels.

4. Complicated AI integration

Integrating AI with existing corporate infrastructure is more complicated than adding plugins to websites or amending excel sheets. It is critical to ensure that current programs are compatible with AI requirements and that AI integration does not impact current output negatively. Also, an AI interface must be put in place to ease out AI infrastructure management. That being said, seamless transitioning to AI is slightly challenging for the involved parties.

5. Lack of understanding of implementation strategies Even though AI is on the verge of transforming every industry, the lack of a clear understanding of its implementation strategies is one of the major AI challenges. Businesses need to identify areas that can benefit from AI, set realistic objectives, and incorporate feedback loops into AI systems to ensure continuous process improvement.

Additionally, corporate managers should be well-versed with current AI technologies, trends, offered possibilities, and potential limitations. This will help organizations target specific areas that can benefit from AI implementation.

6. Legal concerns

Organizations need to be wary of the legal concerns of AI. An AI system collecting sensitive data, irrespective of whether it is harmless or not, might very well be violating a state or federal law. Although the data collected by AI may be legal, organizations should consider how such data aggregation can have a negative impact.

In January 2020, the U.S. government set forth draft rules for AI regulation. Some critical legal issues raised relate to civil liability. For example, if a driverless car injures someone in an accident, who is the culprit in such a scenario? Who takes responsibility? Such use cases raise the question of criminal culpability.

Top 5 AI Trends

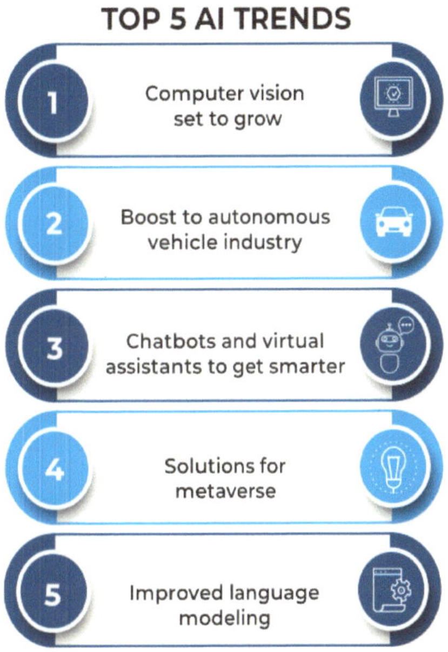

Fig.1.12 Illustration showing Top 5 AI Trends

1. Computer vision set to grow

In the race for AI supremacy, organizations and businesses are set to embrace computer vision technology at an unprecedented scale in 2022. According to a September 2021 survey by Gartner, organizations investing in AI are expected to make the highest planned investments in computer vision projects in 2022.

Computer vision refers to AI that uses ML algorithms to replicate human-like vision. The models are trained to identify a pattern in images and classify the objects based on recognition. For example, computer vision can scan inventory in warehouses in the retail sector. Similarly, the technology finds application in several other industries such as healthcare, agriculture & farming, manufacturing, autonomous vehicles, and more.

2. Boost to the autonomous vehicle industry

As more and more car manufacturers continue to invest in autonomous vehicles, the market penetration of driverless cars is expected to rise considerably. According to Statista's Dec 2021 projections, the global autonomous vehicle market is estimated to be valued at around $146.4 billion in 2022, a substantial rise from$105.7 billion in 2021. Self-driving cars enabled with computer vision are already being tested by companies like Tesla, Uber, Google, Ford, GM, Aurora, and Cruise. This trend is only expected to scale in the next 12 months. In August 2021, Tesla unveiled the 'Dojo' chip specifically designed to process large volumes of images collected by computer vision systems embedded in its self-driving cars. Around the same time, Waymo, Google's subsidiary, expanded its self-driving taxi services outside Arizona.

3. Chatbots and virtual assistants to get smarter

Another AI trend that is most talked about in 2022 is smarter chatbots and virtual assistants. This comes from the pandemic, as global industries are now comfortable giving their employees digital workplace experiences. Most chatbots and virtual assistants use deep learning and NLP technologies on the verge of automating routine tasks. Moreover, researchers and developers continue to add features and enhance these bots.For example, Amelia, a global leader in conversational AI, performs complex conversation tasks with supplemental training provided by developers. Amelia claims to achieve 90% accuracy in identifying customer intent and a customer satisfaction rate of 91%, which isat par with human assistants. Tech companies such as Nuance, IBM, and Amazon Lex are making significant efforts to improve their virtual assistance through smarter bots.

4. Solutions for metaverse

AI agents and virtual assistants will play a key role as the tech world plunges into the concept of the metaverse. Metaverse defines a virtual environment that allows users to interact with digital tools and gives them an immersive experience. In October 2021, Mark Zukerberg rebranded Facebook as 'Meta' and announced plans to build a metaverse. Virtual agents are expected to use AI to enable people to connect to the virtual environment. The famous humanoid AI robot Sophia is tokenized for metaverse appearance. Developers claim that tokenized Sophia, being AI, will interact with users from anywhere, at any time, and across devices and media platforms. Although metaverse may not reveal itself in a full-fledged version in 2022, the blend of virtual and augmented technologies and AI will continue to stay as a backbone of the metaverse. Metaverse is therefore expected to be one of the major AI research trends in the next 12 months.

5. Improved language modeling

Another AI trend that will continue to feature in 2022 is improved language modeling. Language modeling is a technology that allows computers to understand language semantics, complete sentences via word prediction, and convert text into computer codes.Generative Pre-trained Transformer 3 (GPT-3), by OpenAI, is a comprehensive language modeling tool available today. It uses 175 billion parameters to process and generate human-like language. Also, OpenAI, in August 2021, released a better version of its tool, Codex, which parses natural language and generates programming code in response. The company is also working on the next version of GPT-3 (i.e., GPT-4), and it is expected that GPT-4 will be 500 times the size of GPT-3 in terms of the parameters that it may use to parse a language.Apart from the trends listed above, other popular AI trends that could grab attention in 2022 include hyperautomation in modern businesses, the rise of artificial intelligence as a service (AIaaS), AI in cybersecurity, and increased sophistication in AIoT (merger of AI and the internet of things (IoT).

Table 1.3 Current applications of artificial intelligence in health care

Technology	Application scheme	Application area
Robotics	Provide high-quality treatment by improving the precision andaccuracy of the surgical procedures.	MMedical device, Health IT
Digital secretary	Find the golden hour of appropriate intervention by continuously monitoring the patient condition indicators and alerting the nurse when necessary.	Medical device, Health IT
Machine learning	Predict and analyze patterns based on the data affecting treatment results. Reduce the uncertainty in the medical treatment decision-making by processing large volumes of diagnostic medical images through self-learning	Diagnostic medical image, Health IT
Image processing	Quickly process large amounts of medical images and apply the findings in judging the disease type and negative and positive test results.	Diagnostic medical image, Health IT
Natural language processing	Convert long unstructured text data, such as medical charts, to be easily read and interpreted.	Medical device, Health IT
Voice recognition	Capture patient voice and language and store important information in electronic medical records.	Medical device, Health IT
Statistical analysis	Predict patient treatment results through rapidly analyzing large amounts of patient health record data.	Medicine, Health IT
Big data analysis	Provide personalized recommendations to the patients and therapeutics by processing large amounts of data maintained by healthcare institutions	Medicine, Health IT
Predictive modeling	Predict treatment outcomes, such as predicting risky diseases, by applying mathematical models.	Medicine, Health IT

WHO Report: AI in Health - 6 Guiding Principles for its Design and Use

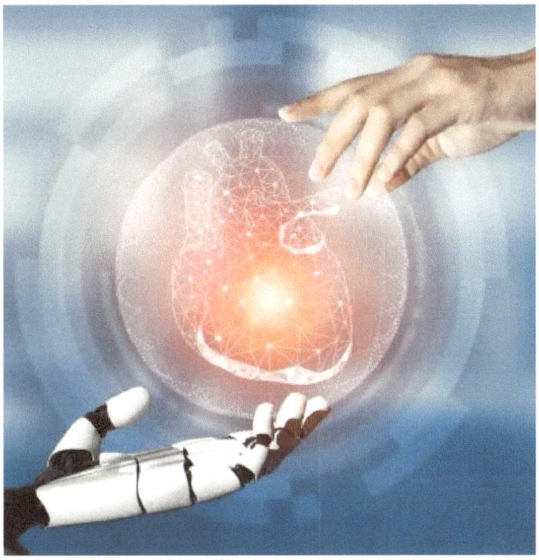

Fig. 1.13 Ethics and human rights must be a part of the design, deployment, and use of Artificial Intelligence (AI) in the delivery of healthcare, according to the World Health Organisation's first global report on AI in health. The WHO report, Ethics and governance of artificial intelligence for health, wasreleased June 28th, and is the result of two years of consultations by international experts.
"Like all new technology, artificial intelligence holds enormous potential for improving the health of millions of people around the world, but like all technology it can also be misused and cause harm," said Dr Tedros Adhanom Ghebreyesus, WHO Director-General. "This important new report provides a valuable guide for countries on how to maximise the benefits of AI, while minimising its risks and avoiding its pitfalls."

WHO provides the following six principles to ensure AI works for the public interest:

1. Protecting human autonomy: In the context of healthcare, this means that humans should remain in control of health-care systems and medical decisions; privacy and confidentiality should be protected, and patients must give valid informed consent through appropriate legal frameworks for data protection.
2. Promoting human well-being and safety and the public interest. The designers of AI technologies should satisfy regulatory requirements for safety, accuracy and efficacy for well-defined use cases or indications. Measures of quality control in practice and quality improvement in the use of AI must be available.
3. Ensuring transparency, explainability and intelligibility. Transparency requires that sufficient information be published or documented before the design or deployment of an AI technology. Such information must be easily accessible and facilitate meaningful public consultation and debate on how the technology is designed and how it should or should not be used.
4. Fostering responsibility and accountability. Although AI technologies perform specific tasks, it is the responsibility of stakeholders to ensure that they are used under appropriate conditions and by appropriately trained people. Effective mechanisms should be available for questioning and for redress for individuals and groups that are adversely affected by decisions based on algorithms.
5. Ensuring inclusiveness and equity. Inclusiveness requires that AI for health be designed to encourage the widest possible equitable use and access, irrespective of age, sex, gender, income, race, ethnicity, sexual orientation, ability or other characteristics protected under human rights codes.
6. Promoting AI that is responsive and sustainable. Designers, developers and users should continuously and transparently assess AI applications during actual use to determine whether AI responds adequately and appropriately to expectations and requirements. AI systems should also be designed to minimise their environmental consequences and increase energy efficiency. Governments and companies should address anticipated disruptions in the workplace, including training for healthcare workers to adapt to the use of AI systems, and potential job losses due to use of automated systems.

Bibliography and Acknowledgement

- Ahmed MR, Zhang Y, Feng Z, Lo B, Inan OT, Liao H. Neuroimaging and machine learning for dementia diagnosis: recent advancements and future prospects. IEEE Rev Biomed Eng. 2019;12:19–33. [PubMed] [Google Scholar]
- Aldeen YA, Salleh M, Razzaque MA. A comprehensive review on privacy preserving data mining. Springerplus. 2015;4(1):694. [PMC free article] [PubMed] [Google Scholar]
- Azencott CA. Machine learning and genomics: precision medicine versus patient privacy. Philos Trans A Math Phys Eng Sci. 2018;376(2128):20170350. [PubMed] [Google Scholar]
- Beccaria M, Mellors TR, Petion JS, Rees CA, Nasir M, Systrom HK, et al. Preliminary investigation of human exhaled breath for tuberculosis diagnosis by multidimensional gas chromatography - time of flight mass spectrometry and machine learning. J Chromatogr B Analyt Technol Biomed Life Sci. 2018;1074-1075:46–50. [PubMed] [Google Scholar]
- Cruz JA, Wishart DS. Applications of machine learning in cancer prediction and prognosis. Cancer Inform. 2007;2:59–77. [PMC free article] [PubMed] [Google Scholar]
- Currie G, Hawk KE, Rohren E, Vial A, Klein R. Machine learning and deep learning in medical imaging: intelligent imaging. J Med Imaging Radiat Sci. 2019;50(4):477–487. [PubMed] [Google Scholar]
- Dankwa-Mullan I, Rivo M, Sepulveda M, Park Y, Snowdon J, Rhee K. Transforming diabetes care through artificial intelligence: the future is here. Popul Health Manag. 2019;22(3):229–242. [PMC free article] [PubMed] [Google Scholar]
- Erickson BJ, Korfiatis P, Akkus Z, Kline TL. Machine learning for medical imaging. Radiographics. 2017;37(2):505–515. [PMC free article] [PubMed] [Google Scholar]
  EvidNet. [Updated 2020]. [Accessed August 20, 2020]. https://en.evidnet.com/
- Executive Office of the President (US) Artificial intelligence, automation, and the economy. [Updated 2016]. [Accessed August 20, 2020]. https://www.whitehouse.gov/sites/whitehouse.gov/files/images/EMBARGOED%20AI%20Economy%20Report.pdf.
- Executive Office of the President (US) The national artificial intelligence research and development strategic plan: 2019 update. [Updated 2019]. [Accessed August 20, 2020]. https://www.nitrd.gov/pubs/National-AI-RD-Strategy-2019.pdf.
- Fernández-Caramés TM, Froiz-Míguez I, Blanco-Novoa O, Fraga-Lamas P. Enabling the internet of mobile crowdsourcing health things: a mobile fog computing, blockchain and IoT based continuous glucose monitoring system for diabetes mellitus research and care. Sensors (Basel) 2019;19(15):E3319. [PMC free article] [PubMed] [Google Scholar]
- Fischer AM, Varga-Szemes A, Martin SS, Sperl JI, Sahbaee P, Neumann D, et al. Artificial intelligence-based fully automated per lobe segmentation and emphysema-quantification based on chest computed tomography compared with global initiative for chronic obstructive lung disease severity of smokers. J Thorac Imaging. 2020;35(Suppl 1):S28–34. [PubMed] [Google Scholar]
- Gulshan V, Peng L, Coram M, Stumpe MC, Wu D, Narayanaswamy A, et al. Development and validation of a deep learning algorithm for detection of diabetic retinopathy in retinal fundus photographs. JAMA. 2016;316(22):2402–2410.
- Hannun AY, Rajpurkar P, Haghpanahi M, Tison GH, Bourn C, Turakhia MP, et al. Cardiologist-level arrhythmia detection and classification in ambulatory electrocardiograms using a deep neural network. Nat Med. 2019;25(1):65–69. [PMC free article] [PubMed] [Google Scholar]
- He J, Baxter SL, Xu J, Xu J, Zhou X, Zhang K. The practical implementation of artificial intelligence technologies in medicine. Nat Med. 2019;25(1):30–36. [PMC free article] [PubMed] [Google Scholar]
  Healthcare IT News. Next up for EHRs: vendors adding artificial intelligence into the workflow. [Updated 2018]. [Accessed August 20, 2020].https://www.healthcareitnews.com/news/next-ehrs-vendors-adding-artificial-intelligence-workflow.
- Hripcsak G, Duke JD, Shah NH, Reich CG, Huser V, Schuemie MJ, et al. Observational health data sciences and informatics (OHDSI): opportunities for observational researchers. Stud Health Technol Inform. 2015;216:574–578. [PMC free article] [PubMed] [Google Scholar]
- Hu W, Cai B, Zhang A, Calhoun VD, Wang YP. Deep collaborative learning with application to the study of multimodal brain development. IEEE Trans Biomed Eng. 2019;66(12):3346–3359. [PMC free article] [PubMed] [Google Scholar]
- IBM. Clinical trial recruitment with AI. [Updated 2020]. [Accessed August 20, 2020]. https://www.ibm.com/watson-health/learn/clinical-trial-recruitment.
- Jiang F, Jiang Y, Zhi H, Dong Y, Li H, Ma S, et al. Artificial intelligence in healthcare: past, present and future. Stroke Vasc Neurol. 2017;2(4):230–243. [PMC free article] [PubMed] [Google Scholar]
  John B. Are you ready for general data protection regulation? BMJ. 2018;360:k941. [PubMed] [Google Scholar]
- Kayaalp M. Patient privacy in the era of big data. Balkan Med J. 2018;35(1):8–17. [PMC free article] [PubMed] [Google Scholar]
  Kelly CJ, Karthikesalingam A, Suleyman M, Corrado G, King D. Key challenges for delivering clinical impact with artificial intelligence. BMC Med. 2019;17(1):195. [PMC free article] [PubMed] [Google Scholar]
- Kim JK, Choi MJ, Lee JS, Hong JH, Kim CS, Seo SI, et al. A Deep Belief Network and Dempster-Shafer-Based Multiclassifier for the Pathology stage of prostate cancer. J Healthc Eng. 2018;2018:4651582. [PMC free article] [PubMed] [Google Scholar]
- Kim JP, Kim J, Park YH, Park SB, Lee JS, Yoo S, et al. Machine learning based hierarchical classification of frontotemporal dementia and Alzheimer's disease. Neuroimage Clin. 2019;23:101811. [PMC free article] [PubMed] [Google Scholar]
- Kim K, Kim S, Lee YH, Lee SH, Lee HS, Kim S. Performance of the deep convolutional neural network based magnetic resonance image scoring algorithm for differentiating between tuberculous and pyogenic spondylitis. Sci Rep. 2018;8(1):13124. [PMC free article] [PubMed] [Google Scholar]
- Komura D, Ishikawa S. Machine learning approaches for pathologic diagnosis. Virchows Arch. 2019;475(2):131–138.
- Lee J, An JY, Choi MG, Park SH, Kim ST, Lee JH, et al. Deep learning-based survival analysis identified associations between molecular subtype and optimal adjuvant treatment of patients with gastric cancer. JCO Clin Cancer Inform. 2018;2(2):1–14. [PMC free article] [PubMed] [Google Scholar]
- Lee J, Sun J, Wang F, Wang S, Jun CH, Jiang X. Privacy-preserving patient similarity learning in a federated environment: development and analysis. JMIR Med Inform. 2018;6(2):e20. [PMC free article]

- Long NP, Jung KH, Yoon SJ, Anh NH, Nghi TD, Kang YP, et al. Systematic assessment of cervical cancer initiation and progression uncovers genetic panels for deep learning-based early diagnosis and proposes novel diagnostic and prognostic biomarkers. Oncotarget. 2017;8(65):109436–109456. [PMC free article] [PubMed] [Google Scholar]
- Mobihealthnews. Medtronic, IBM Watson launch Sugar.IQ diabetes assistant. [Updated 2018]. [Accessed August 19, 2020]. https://www.mobihealthnews.com/content/medtronic-ibm-watson-launch-sugariq-diabetes-assistant.
- Mooney SJ, Pejaver V. Big data in public health: terminology, machine learning, and privacy. Annu Rev Public Health. 2018;39(1):95–112. [PMC free article] [PubMed] [Google Scholar]
- Mori Y, Kudo SE, Misawa M, Saito Y, Ikematsu H, Hotta K, et al. Real-time use of artificial intelligence in identification of diminutive polyps during colonoscopy: a prospective study. Ann Intern Med. 2018;169(6):357–366. [PubMed] [Google Scholar]
- Nikkei Asian. New rules to speed AI-based medicine in Japan. [Updated 2018]. [Accessed August 20, 2020]. https://asia.nikkei.com/Economy/New-rules-to-speed-AI-based-medicine-in-Japan.
- Obermeyer Z, Emanuel EJ. Predicting the future - big data, machine learning, and clinical medicine. N Engl J Med. 2016;375(13):1216–1219. [PMC free article] [PubMed] [Google Scholar]
- Park HJ, Kim SM, La Yun B, Jang M, Kim B, Jang JY, et al. A computer-aided diagnosis system using artificial intelligence for the diagnosis and characterization of breast masses on ultrasound: added value for the inexperienced breast radiologist. Medicine (Baltimore) 2019;98(3):e14146. [PMC free article] [PubMed] [Google Scholar]
- Patel V, Armstrong D, Ganguli M, Roopra S, Kantipudi N, Albashir S, et al. Deep learning in gastrointestinal endoscopy. Crit Rev Biomed Eng. 2016;44(6):493–504. [PubMed] [Google Scholar]
- Pelayo S, Bras Da Costa S, Leroy N, Loiseau S, Beuscart-Zephir MC. Software as a medical device: regulatory critical issues. Stud Health Technol Inform. 2013;183:337–342. [PubMed] [Google Scholar]
- Pesapane F, Codari M, Sardanelli F. Artificial intelligence in medical imaging: threat or opportunity? Radiologists again at the forefront of innovation in medicine. Eur Radiol Exp. 2018;2(1):35. [PMC free article] [PubMed] [Google Scholar]
- Pipersburgh J. The push to increase the use of EHR technology by hospitals and physicians in the United States through the HITECH Act and the Medicare incentive program. J Health Care Finance. 2011;38(2):54–78. [PubMed] [Google Scholar]
- Price WN, 2nd, Gerke S, Cohen IG. Potential liability for physicians using artificial intelligence. JAMA. 2019;322(18):1765. [PubMed]
- Rajkomar A, Dean J, Kohane I. Machine learning in medicine. N Engl J Med. 2019;380(14):1347–1358. [PubMed] [Google Scholar]
- Reed C. How should we regulate artificial intelligence? Philos Trans A Math Phys Eng Sci. 2018;376(2128):20170360.
- Ryu SM, Seo SW, Lee SH. Novel prognostication of patients with spinal and pelvic chondrosarcoma using deep survival neural networks. BMC Med Inform Decis Mak. 2020;20(1):3. [PMC free article] [PubMed] [Google Scholar]
- Sajid A, Abbas H. Data privacy in cloud-assisted healthcare systems: state of the art and future challenges. J Med Syst. 2016;40(6):155.
- Shimizu H, Nakayama KI. Artificial intelligence in oncology. Cancer Sci. 2020;111(5):1452–1460. [PMC free article]
- Soffer S, Ben-Cohen A, Shimon O, Amitai MM, Greenspan H, Klang E. Convolutional neural networks for radiologic images: a radiologist's guide. Radiology. 2019;290(3):590–606. [PubMed] [Google Scholar]
- Tariq RA, Hackert PB. Patient Confidentiality. Treasure Island, FL: StatPearls Publishing LLC.; 2020. [Google Scholar]
- The Korea Industry Daily. [Updated 2017]. [Accessed August 20, 2020]. http://www.kidd.co.kr/news/198013.
- The Lancet. Artificial intelligence in health care: within touching distance. Lancet. 2018;390(10114):2739. [PubMed] [Google Scholar]
- Ting DS, Cheung CY, Lim G, Tan GS, Quang ND, Gan A, et al. Development and validation of a deep learning system for diabetic retinopathy and related eye diseases using retinal images from multiethnic populations with diabetes. JAMA. 2017;318(22):2211–2223. [PMC free article] [PubMed] [Google Scholar]
- Ting DS, Pasquale LR, Peng L, Campbell JP, Lee AY, Raman R, et al. Artificial intelligence and deep learning in ophthalmology. Br J Ophthalmol. 2019;103(2):167–175. [PMC free article] [PubMed] [Google Scholar]
- Topol EJ. High-performance medicine: the convergence of human and artificial intelligence. Nat Med. 2019;25(1):44–56. [PubMed] [Google Scholar]
- U.S. Food and Drug Administration. Software as a Medical Device (SaMD) [Updated 2018]. [Accessed August 20, 2020]. https://www.fda.gov/medical-devices/digital-health/software-medical-device-samd.
- Vahlsing T, Delbeck S, Leonhardt S, Heise HM. Noninvasive monitoring of blood glucose using color-coded photoplethysmographic images of the illuminated fingertip within the visible and near-infrared range: opportunities and questions. J Diabetes Sci Technol. 2018;12(6):1169–1177. [PMC free article] [PubMed] [Google Scholar]
- Veeranki SP, Kramer D, Hayn D, Jauk S, Eggerth A, Quehenberger F, et al. Is regular re-training of a predictive delirium model necessary after deployment in routine care? Stud Health Technol Inform. 2019;260:186–191. [PubMed] [Google Scholar]
- WELCOMEAI. Arterys - Cardio AI. [Updated 2020]. [Accessed August 19, 2020]. https://www.welcome.ai/tech/healthcare/arterys-cardio-ai.
- You SC, Lee S, Cho SY, Park H, Jung S, Cho J, et al. Conversion of National Health Insurance Service-national sample cohort (NHIS-NSC) database into observational medical outcomes partnership-common data model (OMOP-CDM) Stud Health Technol Inform. 2017;245:467–470. [PubMed] [Google Scholar]

CHAPTER

2

Artificial intelligence-enhanced Electrocardiography In Cardio-Vascular Disease Management

The electrocardiogram (ECG) is a ubiquitous tool in clinical medicine that has been used by cardiologists and non-cardiologists for decades. The ECG is a low-cost, rapid and simple test that is available even in the most resource-scarce settings. The test provides a window into the physiological and structural condition of the heart but can also give valuable diagnostic clues for systemic conditions (such as electrolyte derangements and drug toxic effects). Although the acquisition of the ECG recording is well standardized and reproducible, the reproducibility of human interpretation of the ECG varies greatly according to levels of experience and expertise. In this setting, computer-generated interpretations have been used for several years. However, these interpretations are based on predefined rules and manual pattern or feature recognition algorithms that do not always capture the complexity and nuances of an ECG. However, artificial intelligence (AI) in the form of deep-learning convolutional neural networks (CNNs), which have been used mostly in computer vision, image processing and speech recognition, has now been adapted to analyse the routine 12-lead ECG. This development has resulted in fully automated AI models mimicking human-like interpretation of the ECG, with potentially greater diagnostic fidelity and workflow efficiency than traditional rule-based computer interpretations.Indeed, the ECG is an ideal substrate for deep-learning AI applications. The ECG is widely available and yields reproducible raw data that are easy to store and transfer in a digital format. In addition to fully automated interpretation of the ECG, rigorous research programmes using large databanks of ECG and clinical datasets, coupled with powerful computational capabilities, have been able to demonstrate the utility of the AI-enhanced ECG (referred to as the AI–ECG in the remainder of this Review) as a tool for the detection of ECG signatures and patterns that are unrecognizable by the human eye. These patterns can signify cardiac disease, such as left ventricular (LV) systolic dysfunction, silent atrial fibrillation (AF) and hypertrophic cardiomyopathy (HCM),), but might also reflect systemic physiology, such as a person's age and sex or their serum potassium levels, as reviewed in detail herein. Among several potential clinical applications, a single 12-lead ECG might therefore allow the rapid phenotyping of an individual's cardiovascular health and help to guide targeted diagnostic testing in an efficient and potentially cost-effective manner.

This transformative progress has not occurred without potential limitations and challenges that require attention. Challenges with AI applications are not necessarily unique to the ECG and include the need for data quality control, external validity, data security and the demonstration of superior patient outcomes with the implementation of AI-enabled tools, such as the AI–ECG. In this Review, we focus on the promise, clinical capabilities, research opportunities, gaps and risk of the application of AI to the ECG for the diagnosis and management of cardiovascular disease. Finally, we discuss the numerous challenges to the development, validation and implementation of the AI–ECG in medicine.

Deep-learning methods applied to the ECG

Deep learning is a subfield of machine learning that uses neural networks with many layers (hence the term 'deep') to learn a function between a set of inputs and a set of outputs. The training is done by presenting to the network a set of input data with their corresponding output labels, and the model learns certain rules by applying and adjusting the network weights to minimize an error function until the model outputs are as close as possible to the actual data values. The strength of deep neural networks lies in using their ability to identify novel relationships in the data independent of features selected by a human. In the past, conventional statistical models, such as linear and logistic regression, and even neural networks with few layers (sometimes called 'shallow models') were developed on the basis of inputs using human-selected data features. For example, in ECG analysis, the inputs were morphological and temporal features, such as the QT, QRS and RR intervals or QRS and/ or T-wave morphology, and the outputs would be the ECG rhythm, the serum potassium level or the LV ejection fraction (LVEF). As the inputs are features that were selected by humans, the model is limited to those features alone. In addition, any random or systematic error in calculating features will propagate to the output and will limit the accuracy of the model.

Conversely, in deep-learning networks, the representation of the input is learned by the network itself. The most common model for this type of representation learning is a subtype of neural networks called 'CNNs'. CNNs were originally designed to solve computer vision tasks such as image recognition because they use a set of convolutional filters to select features used to represent the input into the model1. These filters start with random weights and, as the network self-trains, the architecture optimizes both the features used as a representation of the data and the rules applied to this representation and the outputs. Therefore, a neural network can be thought of as having two sequential components: the feature extraction layers (typically convolutional filters) and the mathematical model (such as pooling layers), which take feature output as their input to perform analysis and create the ultimate output. The number and the shape of the convolutional filters are selected by the model architect and will affect the learned representation. In the ECG, one dimension is the spatial axis (each row in the input represents a time series from one of the leads) and the second dimension is the temporal axis (each column represents the voltage sampled at a specific time point across all leads). Therefore, a convolution can be horizontal (combining information from more than one time point but only within one lead), vertical (combining information from many leads but at a single time point) or both horizontal and vertical (combining information on both axes

Using deep learning, the model can learn a representation of the input data that includes features that are relevant to the task that we are trying to accomplish without any human bias and without the need for human selection and engineering of features, which can be time-consuming, inaccurate and dependent on expertise and current physiological theories.The agnostic approach in a neural network is an optimal representation, but this approach is also non-linear, and the learned associations between input and output data are unexplainable at present, making the model a black box — humans cannot understand how the network makes its decisions — which is one of the concerns raised regarding the clinical application of deep-learning CNNs2. Therefore, less agnostic machine-learning models, such as the more traditional logistic regression, e. reinforcement learning and random forest models, still hold promise and can help to inform research and clinical practic For example, reinforcement learning is a field of AI providing the framework for training of a clinical decision model in which certain decisions (model input) under specific conditions are linked to long-term outcomes. The optimal reinforcement learning model is built through a continuous process of updating of inputs and outcomes (or rewards)3. In addition, CNNs are supervised models, which require data to have a label assigned during training. Conversely, unsupervised machine-learning methods, such as clustering models, do not require labelling of input data for their development, thereby minimizing the risk of random or systematic error introduced by a human.

In this Review, the natural language processing applications has also been discussed . The field of natural language processing integrates AI, computer science and linguistics methodology to structure unstructured data (such as free text in clinical notes in electronic health records), thereby making these data analysable. These methods include rule-based recognition of word patterns, text vectorization and topic modelling.

Fully automated interpretation of ECGs

One of the top priorities for the application of AI to the interpretation of ECGs is the creation of comprehensive, human-like interpretation capability. Since the advent of the digital ECG more than 60 years ago4, ongoing effort has been towards rapid, high-quality and comprehensive computer-generated interpretation of the ECG. The problem seems tractable; after all, ECG interpretation is a fairly circumscribed application of pattern recognition to a finite dataset. Early programs for the interpretation of digital ECGs could easily recognize fiducial points, make discrete measurements and define common quantifiable abnormalities.Modern technologies have moved beyond these rule-based approaches to recognize patterns in massive quantities of labelled ECG data. Several groups have worked to create AI-driven algorithms, and some of these algorithms are already in limited clinical use10. Some studies have developed CNNs from large datasets of single-lead ECGs and then applied them to the 12-lead ECG.For instance, using 2 million labelled single-lead ECG traces collected in the Clinical Outcomes in Digital Electrocardiology study, one group used a CNN to identify six types of abnormalities on the 12-lead ECG9. This study demonstrated the feasibility of this approach, but widespread implementation or external validation in other 12-lead ECG datasets is forthcoming. Another group conducted a similar study of the application of CNNs to

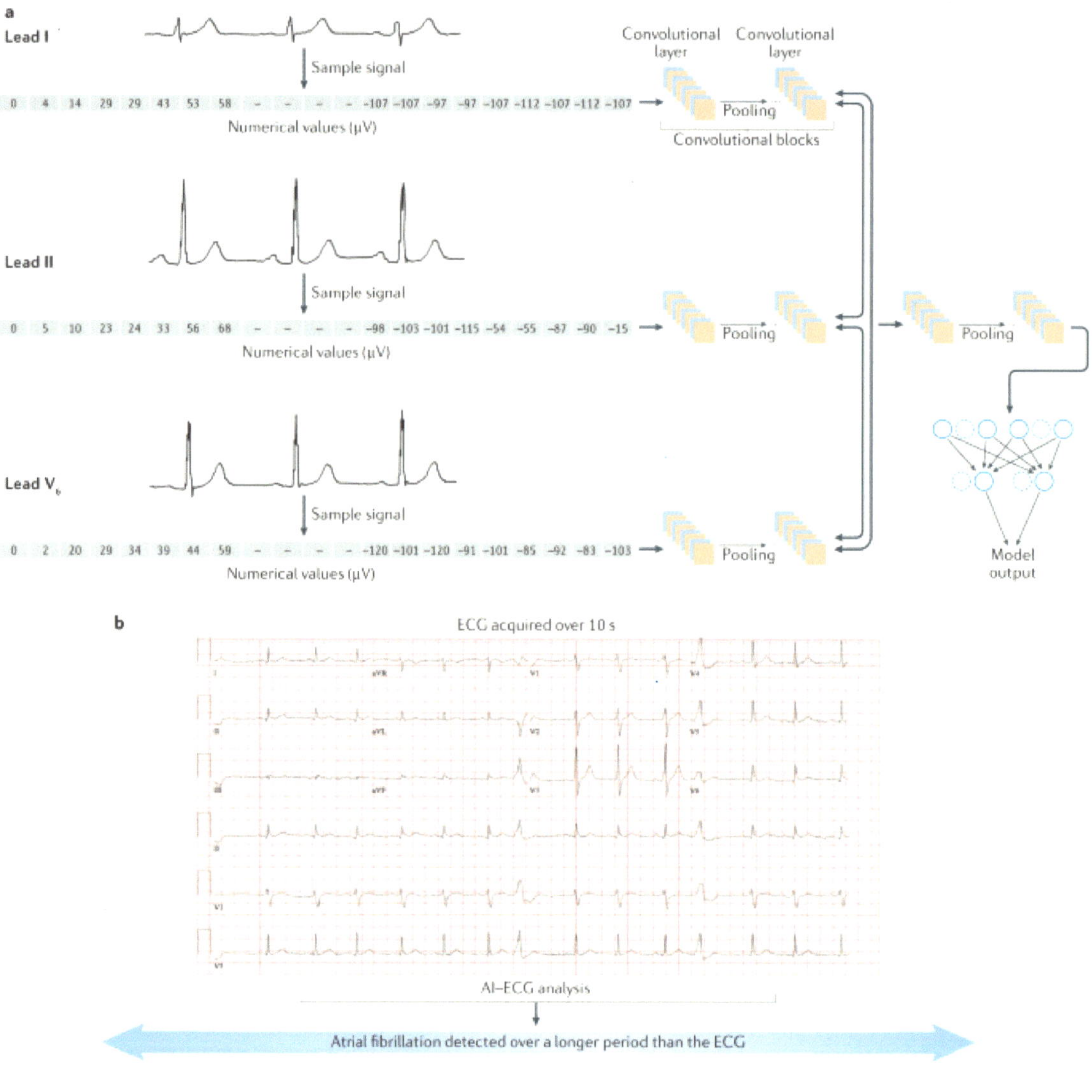

Fig. 2.1 Development of a convolutional neural network using the 12-lead ECG and application to detect silent atrial fibrillation.a | The analogue electrocardiogram (ECG) signal is converted to a digital recording, resulting in a list of numerical values corresponding to the amplitude of the signal. (The numerical values depicted are arbitrary and shown for illustrative purposes only.) These numerical values are then convolved with the network weights within each lead and across leads, feeding sequential layers of convolutions until the final model output is reached. b | With the use of a trained, deep-learning artificial intelligence-enhanced ECG (AI–EGG) model, a one-off, standard, 12-lead, sinus-rhythm ECG can become a surrogate for prolonged rhythm monitoring for the detection of silent atrial fibrillation. Part a adapted with permission from ref.70, Elsevier.

to single-lead ECGs and demonstrated that the CNN could outperform practising cardiologists for some diagnoses8. However, whether this approach will translate to clinically useful software for 12-lead ECG interpretation remains to be seen

In an evaluation published in 2020, a CNN was developed for the multilabel diagnosis of 21 distinct heart rhythms based on the 12-lead ECG using a training and validation dataset of >80,000 ECGs from >70,000 patients11. The reference standard consisted of consensus labels by a committee of cardiologists. In a test dataset of 828 ECGs, the optimal network exactly matched the gold standard In infrastructure. abels in 80% of the ECGs, significantly exceeding the performance of a single cardiologist interpreter. The model had a mean area under the curve (AUC) receiver operating characteristic score of 98%, sensitivity of 87% and specificity of 99%. Our group has worked with our internal dataset of >8 million ECGs performed for clinical indications (which have all been labelled by expert ECG readers and are linked to the respective electronic health record) to generate a comprehensive ECG-interpretation infrastructure. It was found that a CNN can identify 66 discrete codes or diagnosis labels, with favourable diagnostic performance. Lately, we have developed a novel method that uses a CNN to extract ECG features and a transformer network to translate ECG features into ECG codes and text strings.This process creates a model output that more closely resembles that of a human ECG reader — presenting information in a similar order, with similar language — and also makes sense of associated codes, thereby avoiding the presentation of contradictory or mutually exclusive interpretations that would not be presented by a human reader. This technology will be particularly important as we increasingly rely on ECG data obtained through novel, consumer-facing applications, which are massively scalable. For instance, AI–ECG algorithms have been applied to single-lead ECG traces obtained through mobile, smartwatch-enabled recordings for the detection of AF. This democratization of ECG technology will exponentially increase the volume of signals that demand interpretation, which might quickly outstrip the capacity of human ECG readers. We anticipate that these models will be essential in facilitating telehealth technologies (that is, automatic, patient-facing or consumer-facing technologies) and could allow the creation of core laboratory facilities capable of ingesting and processing massive quantities of data. However, we caution that the signal quality obtained with these devices can be inconsistent, and AI–ECG might be less able than human expert over-readers to classify the heart rhythm using poor-quality tracings, as noted in the aforementioned smartwatch study. Similarly, in another study, a deep neural network developed using ECG recordings from smartwatches demonstrated good performance for passive detection of AF compared with the reference standard of AF diagnosed from 12-lead ECGs, but its performance was much less robust in reference to a self-reported history of persistent AF. Nevertheless, although great progress has been made towards a comprehensive, human-like ECG-interpretation package, the realization remains on the horizon. Even in its most modern incarnation, the package lacks the accuracy needed for implementation without human oversight. Additionally, computer-derived ECG interpretation has the potential to influence human over-readers and, if inaccurate, can serve as a source of bias or systematic error. This concern is particularly relevant if the algorithms are derived in populations that are distinct from those in which the algorithms are applied. This limitation underscores the need for a diverse derivation sample (ideally including a diverse patient population and varied means of data collection that reflect real-world practices), rigorous external validation studies andphased implementation with ongoing assessment of model performance and effectiveness. Quality control systems based on regular over-reads by expert interpreters of ECGswho are blinded to the outputof the CNN will allow continuous calibration of the model.

The ECG as a deep phenotyping tool

Interpretation of an ECG by a trained cardiologist relies on established knowledge of what is normal or abnormal on the basis of more than a century of experience with assessing the ECG in patient care and based on our understanding of the electropathophysiology of various cardiac conditions. Despite the enormous potential to gain insights into cardiac health and disease from an expert interpretation of the ECG, the information gain is limited by the interpreter's finite ability to detect isolated characteristics or patterns fitting established rules. However, hidden in plain sight might be subtle signals and patterns that do not fit traditional knowledge and that are unrecognizable by the human eye. Harnessing the power of deep-learning AI techniques together with the availability of large ECG and clinical datasets, developing tools for systematic extraction of features of ECGs and their association with specific cardiac diagnoses has become feasible. Of course, some conditions are not reflected in the ECG, which even an AI–ECG cannot resolve — even if these technologies can see beyond an expert reader's capacity, they cannot see what is not there. In this section, we review the latest advances in the application of deep-learning AI techniques to the 12-lead ECG for the detection of asymptomatic cardiovascular disease that might not be readily apparent, even to expert eyes.

Detection of LV systolic dysfunction

The systolic function of the left ventricle, traditionally quantified as the LVEF by echocardiography, is a key measure of cardiac function. A reduced LVEF defines a large subgroup of patients with heart failure, but a decline in LVEF can be asymptomatic for a long time before any symptoms trigger evaluation. Indeed, up to 6% of people in the community might have asymptomatic LV dysfunction (LVEF <50%)16. A low LVEF has both prognostic and management implications17. Detection of a low LVEF should trigger a thorough evaluation for any reversible causes that should be addressed in a timely fashion to minimize the extent of permanent myocardial damage. The early initiation of optimal medical therapy can result in improvements in systolic LV function and quality of life, but can also reduce heart failure-related morbidity and mortality18. However, in the absence of symptoms, identifying these patients remains a challenge and, therefore, asymptomatic LV dysfunction might be under-recognized. Several approaches to screening patients for asymptomatic LV systolic dysfunction have been investigated, including risk factors, the standard 12-lead ECG, echocardiography and measuring the levels of circulating biomarkers. However, none of these approaches has sufficient diagnostic accuracy or cost-effectiveness to justify routine implementation clinically. The potential of the AI–ECG as a marker of asymptomatic LV dysfunction has been demonstrated. With the use of linked ECG and echocardiographic data from 44,959 patients at the Mayo Clinic (Rochester, MN, USA), a CNN was trained to identify patients with LV dysfunction, defined as LVEF of ≤35% by echocardiography, on the basis of the ECG alone. The model was then tested on a completely independent set of 52,870 patients, and its AUC was 0.93 for the detection of LV dysfunction, with corresponding sensitivity, specificity and accuracy of 93.0%, 86.3% and 85.7%, respectively. In individuals in whom the CNN seemingly incorrectly detected LV dysfunction (apparent false positive tests), those with a positive AI screen were fourfold more likely to develop LV dysfunction over a mean follow-up of 3.4 years than those with a negative AI screen, suggesting the ability of the model to detect LV dysfunction even before a decline in LVEF measured by echocardiography. Akin to the paradigm of the ischaemic cascade in myocardial infarction and ischaemic heart disease, the preclinical cascade of cellular-level alterations (such as changes to calcium homeostasis) and mechanical function alterations (such as abnormal lusitropy and strain rate) might be reflected in the ECG and detectable by a trained deep-learning CNN AI–ECG model. This observation raises the possibility that this model could be used to identify patients with early or subclinical LV dysfunction or even those with normal ventricular function who are at risk of heart failure. In a subsequent prospective validation from our group, the AI–ECG algorithm was applied in 3,874 patients who underwent transthoracic echocardiography and an ECG recording within 30 daysIn these patients, the algorithm was able to detect an LVEF of ≤35% with 86.8% specificity, 82.5% sensitivity and 86.5% accuracy (AUC 0.918). This algorithm has been validated externally in patients presenting with dyspnoea to the emergency department24. A validation effort in a multicentre, international cohort is also under way. Of note, the algorithm has also demonstrated high accuracy for detecting low LVEF when applied to a single-lead ECG, thereby allowing its application with the use of smartphone-based or even stethoscope-based electrodes. Although further rigorous clinical testing for patient outcomes is required, these data highlight the AI–ECG as a potential means to overcome the limitations of previously tested screening biomarkers for asymptomatic LV dysfunction. Other future applications of the AI–ECG algorithm for the detection of LV dysfunction might include the longitudinal monitoring of patients with established congestive heart failure who are receiving medical therapy, the prognostication of the risk of incident cardiomyopathy in patients receiving cardiotoxic chemotherapy in whom cardioprotective therapy might be instituted prophylactically or the longitudinal monitoring of patients with valvular heart disease in whom the development of LV dysfunction would signify an indication for surgical intervention. Additionally, the FDA issued an Emergency Use Authorization for the 12-lead AI–ECG algorithm to detect LV dysfunction in patients with coronavirus disease 2019 (COVID-19)25. Broad clinical application across other specialties might also be possible. Detection of silent AF from a sinus-rhythm ECG AF portends an increased risk of impaired quality of life, stroke and heart failure, and results in frequent visits to the emergency department and frequent inpatient admissions. Among patients with an embolic stroke of undetermined source (ESUS), previously called 'cryptogenic stroke', who undergo 30-day rhythm monitoring, about 15% are found to have previously undiagnosed paroxysmal AF26. In these patients, anticoagulation lowers the recurrence of stroke and might lower mortality, whereas in the absence of documented AF, anticoagulation offers no clinical benefit and increases the risk of bleeding. However, the diagnosis of AF can be elusive because up to 20% of patients are completely asymptomatic, and another approximately one-third of patients have atypical symptoms. Moreover, AF is only intermittent (or paroxysmal) in many patients. Despite extensive research on the topic, the value of screening individuals for AF remains a matter of debate, and the US Preventive Services Task Force states that the data are currently insufficient to recommend routine AF screening in general populations In the recent Apple Heart Study. the largest pragmatic evaluation of AF screening in a general population using a smartwatch-enabled photoplethysmography technology, 0.52% of participants received notifications of possible AF over an average of >3 months of monitoring. In approximately one-third of these individuals, AF was later confirmed by week-long patch ECG monitoring. This finding suggests that, although mass screening of unselected populations is feasible with current technologies, the yield of this approach is low and the clinical effect is uncertain. Simple and highly accurate approaches to the detection of asymptomatic paroxysmal AF would be important for the selection of patients for early institution of oral anticoagulation for the prevention of AF-related morbidity and death.To assess the likelihood of silent AF, a group of investigators from the Mayo Clinic developed a CNN to predict AF on the basis of a standard 12-lead ECG obtained during sinus rhythm.The algorithm was developed using nearly half a million digitally stored ECGs from 126,526 patients and was validated and tested in separate internal datasets. The model applied convolutions on a temporal axis and across multiple leads to extract morphological and temporal features during the training and validation processes (Fig. 1a). Patients with at least one ECG showing AF within 31 days after the sinus-rhythm ECG were classified as being positive for AF. In the testing dataset, the algorithm demonstrated an AUC of 0.87, sensitivity of 79.0%, specificity of 79.5% and an accuracy of 79.4% in detecting patients with documentation of AF using only information from the sinus-rhythm ECG32. Therefore, the algorithm can detect nearly concomitant, unrecognized AF, rather than predict the long-term risk of AF. Conceptually, this AI tool converts a routine 10-s, 12-lead ECG into the equivalent of a prolonged rhythm-monitoring tool (Fig. 1b), although the duration of 'monitoring' and its yield require validation. Additionally, this tool can be applied retroactively to digitally stored ECGs from patients with a previous ESUS. This algorithm might facilitate targeted AF surveillance (such as using an ambulatory rhythm-monitoring patch or implantable loop recorder) in subsets of high-risk patients. This work is preliminary, but we are currently assessing the performance of this algorithm in identifying patients who might benefit from prospective AF screening or monitoring (with Holter or extended monitoring) and, ultimately, various stroke-prevention strategies. We also note that other groups have derived similar AF risk-prognostication tools that examine other electrophysiological parameters, such as signal-averaged ECG-derived P-wave analysis ECGs are ubiquitously performed for a variety of screening, diagnostic and monitoring purposes, thereby providing ample opportunities for the application of this algorithm. The ultimate clinical utility of this approach will be determined by the observed positive and negative predictive values of the algorithm when applied to a given population and by the cost and downstream consequences, particularly for patient outcomes, related to follow-up diagnostic testing and therapies.

Unlike the traditional risk-prediction models that comprise predefined variables, the CNN described above is agnostic, because we do not know what ECG features the CNN is 'seeing' and which factors drive its performance.

The performance of the algorithm is likely to be based on a combination of ECG signatures that are known risk factors for AF (such as LV hypertrophy, P-wave amplitude, atrial ectopy and heart rate variability) as well as others that are currently unknown or are not obvious to the human eye, in combination, in a non-linear manner34. The ECG is also likely to contain information that correlates with known clinical risk factors.

AI-enabled ECG and rhythm tools in AF care

In addition to screening individuals for silent AF, CNNs can also be developed from ECGs or other rhythm-monitoring data (including those derived from permanently implanted cardiac devices) for the stratification of stroke risk and the refinement of decision-making about oral anticoagulant use. In an analysis using data from implanted cardiac devices in >3,000 patients with AF (including 71 patients with stroke), three different supervised machine-learning models of AF burden signatures were developed to predict the risk of stroke (random forest, CNN and L1 regularized logistic regression. In the testing cohort, the random forest model had an AUC of 0.66, the CNN model had an AUC of 0.60 and the L1 regularized logistic regression model had an AUC of 0.56. By contrast, the CHA2DS2–VASc score, the most widely used stroke-prediction scheme in current practice36, had an AUC of 0.52 for stroke prediction. However, the highest AUC (0.63) was achieved when the CHA2DS2–VASc score was combined with the random forest and CNN models, indicating the prognostic strength of approaches that combine AI-enriched models with traditional clinical tools. The performance of this model is still quite modest. The integration of additional information from the clinical history, imaging tests and circulating biomarkers might further improve risk stratification but this task is beyond current AI capabilities. For example, in an unsupervised cluster analysis of approximately 10,000 patients with AF in the ORBIT-AF registry, including patient-specific clinical data, medications, and laboratory, ECG and imaging data, four clinically relevant phenotypes of AF were identified, each with distinct associations with clinical outcomes (low comorbidity, behavioural comorbidity, device implantation and atherosclerotic comorbidity clusters. However, although this finding offers a proof of concept, the clinical utility of these clusters has not yet been demonstrated. The hope is that phenotype-specific treatment strategies will lead to superior patient outcomes, but testing is required

A fully automated, electronic health record-embedded platform powered with AI–ECG capabilities and other advanced machine-learning methods, including natural language processing, could be trained to collect data from the ECG, AF patterns and other diagnostic tests or even clinical notes in order to continuously assess the risk of stroke. When a high risk of stroke is detected, the clinician is alerted and the timely initiation of anticoagulation could prevent a potentially devastating adverse clinical event. Similarly, real-time modelling of the risk of stroke could be realized on the basis of information collected via wearable ECG technologies or consumer-facing, smartphone-based ECG technologies. Ultimately, developing an easy-to-implement tool that provides clinically actionable data that are fully vetted and validated will be required to allow interventions for stroke prevention.

Detection of HCM

CM is infrequent in the general population, with an estimated prevalence of 1 in 200 to 1 in 500 individuals38,39. However, HCM is one of the leading causes of sudden cardiac death among adolescents and young adults. HCM is also associated with substantial morbidity in all age groups40. Over the past 15 years, interest has focused on the screening of at-risk populations for HCM. This interest is often rekindled by highly publicized sudden deaths of athletes and other young adults, events that are devastating and potentially preventable if a diagnosis of HCM had been established. In most cases, a diagnosis of HCM can be established with echocardiography combined with the clinical history, but the widespread use of echocardiography for the detection of HCM in otherwise asymptomatic individuals is impractical. Therefore, alternative modalities, such as the ECG, have been considered as a means for screening. More than 90% of patients with HCM have electrocardiographic abnormalities41, but these abnormalities are non-specific and can be indistinguishable from LV hypertrophy. Generally, ECG screening has relied on manual or automated detection of particular features, such as LV hypertrophy, left axis deviation, prominent Q waves and T-wave inversions. However, these approaches have insufficient diagnostic performance to justify routine ECG screening42. Moreover, several sets of ECG criteria have been proposed to distinguish between HCM and athletic heart adaptation, but their diagnostic performance has been inconsistent when external validations have been attempted43,44. The nature of a deep-learning AI approach might offer the advantage of an agnostic and unbiased approach to the ECG-based detection of HCM that does not rely on traditional criteria for LV hypertrophy. With use of the ECGs of 2,500 patients with a validated diagnosis of HCM and >50,000 age-matched and sex-matched control individuals without HCM, an AI–ECG CNN was trained and validated to diagnose HCM on the basis of the ECG alone. In an independent testing cohort of 612 patients with HCM and 12,788 control individuals, the AUC of the CNN was 0.96 (95% CI 0.95–0.96) with sensitivity of 87% and specificity of 90%. The performance of the model was robust in subgroups of patients meeting the ECG criteria for LV hypertrophy and among those with normal ECGs. Importantly, performance was even better in younger patients (aged <40 years) but declined with increasing age. Furthermore, the performance of the model did not seem to be affected by the sarcomeric mutation status of the patient,

given that the model-derived probabilities for a diagnosis of HCM were a median of 97% and 96% in patients with HCM who either had or did not have confirmed variants in sarcomere-encoding genes, respectively45. The algorithm developed had equally favourable performance when implemented on the basis of a single lead (rather than all 12 leads of the ECG), meaning that this algorithm could be applied as a screening test on a large scale and across various resource settings. Figure 2 shows an example of a woman aged 21 years with massive septal hypertrophy who underwent surgical septal myectomy45. Despite only modest abnormalities on her ECG before myectomy, the AI–ECG algorithm indicated a probability of HCM of 72.6%, whereas after myectomy, the AI–ECG algorithm indicated a probability of HCM of only 2.5%, despite more obvious and striking ECG abnormalities.

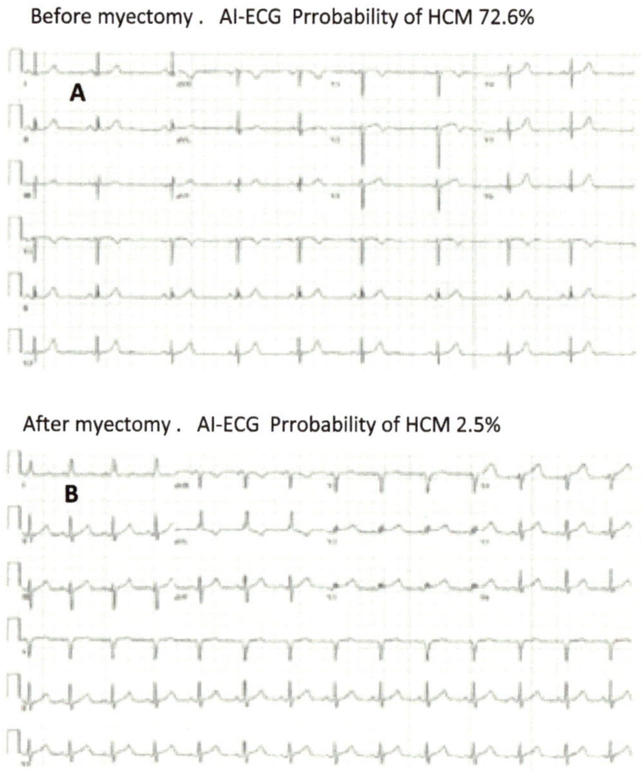

Fig.2.2: The AI–ECG to detect HCM.Use of an artificial intelligence-enhanced electrocardiogram (AI–ECG) model to detect obstructive hypertrophic cardiomyopathy (HCM) in a woman aged 21 years before (part a) and after (part b) septal myectomy. Adapted with permission from ref.45, Elsevier.T

Another group of investigators used a large, 12-lead ECG dataset to train machine-learning models for the detection of HCM together with other elements of cardiac structure (LV mass, left atrial volume and early diastolic mitral annulus velocity) and disease (pulmonary arterial hypertension, cardiac amyloidosis and mitral valve prolapse)

Although a different model architecture was applied from that in the aforementioned study, including a novel combination of CNNs and hidden Markov models, the performance of the model for the detection of HCM was also quite favourable, with an AUC of 0.91. Of note, the researchers also reported good performance for the detection of pulmonary arterial hypertension (AUC 0.94), cardiac amyloidosis (AUC 0.86) and mitral valve prolapse (AUC 0.77). The favourable diagnostic performance of these models suggests that HCM screening based on fully automated AI–ECG algorithms might be feasible in the future. External validations in other populations with greater racial diversity, as well as in athletes and in adolescents, will be crucial in the evaluation of the AI–ECG algorithm as a future screening tool for HCM in individuals at risk of adverse outcomes, particularly sudden cardiac death. Direct comparisons with other possible screening methods and cost-effectiveness and other practical implementation issues also need to be evaluated.

Detection of hyperkalaemia

Numerous studies have shown that either hyperkalaemia or hypokalaemia is associated with increased mortality, and evidence suggests that the mortality associated with hyperkalaemia might be linked to underdosing of evidence-based therapies47. Our group has evaluated the performance of an AI–ECG CNN for the detection of hyperkalaemia in patients with chronic kidney disease48,49. In the latest large-scale evaluation, the model was trained to detect serum potassium levels of ≥5.5 mmol/l using >1.5 million ECGs from nearly 450,000 patients who underwent contemporaneous assessment of serum potassium levels. This level of potassium was chosen because this threshold was thought to be clinically actionable. At this cut-off point, the model demonstrated 90% sensitivity and 89% sensitivity in a multicentre, external validation cohort49. This algorithm could be applied to detect clinically silent but clinically significant hyperkalaemia without a blood draw and could facilitate remote patient care, including diuretic dosing, timing of haemodialysis or adjustment of medications such as angiotensin-converting enzyme inhibitors or angiotensin-receptor blockers in the setting of heart failure or chronic kidneydisease.

Antiarrhythmic drug management

Dofetilide and sotalol are commonly used for the treatment of AF. Their antiarrhythmic effect is exerted on the myocardium by prolonging the duration of the repolarization phase, meaning that QT prolongation is an anticipated effect of these drugs.Owing to the ensuing risk of substantial QT prolongation and potentially fatal ventricular proarrhythmia, patients require close monitoring with a continuous ECG in the hospital setting when these drugs are used, particularly for dofetilide. In addition, with the long-term use of these medications, the QT interval should be intermittently assessed because dose adjustments might be necessary in cases of substantial QT prolongation, concomitant medications with QT-prolonging effects and fluctuations in renal function (both sotalol and dofetilide are primarily metabolized through the kidneys). Using serial 12-lead ECGs and linked information on plasma dofetilide concentrations in 42 patients who were treated with dofetilide or placebo in a crossover randomized clinical trial, a deep-learning algorithm predicted plasma dofetilide concentrations with good correlation (r = 0.85)50. By comparison, a linear model of the corrected QT interval correlated with dofetilide concentrations with a coefficient of 0.64 (ref.50). This finding suggests that the QT interval might not accurately reflect the plasma dofetilide concentration in some patients and so might underestimate or overestimate the proarrhythmic risk. Machine-learning approaches, including supervised, unsupervised and reinforcement learning, have also been used to determine the optimal dosing regimen during dofetilidetreatment.

In the future, patients treated with dofetilide, sotalol or other antiarrhythmic medications might avoid the need for hospitalization for drug loading or office visits for routine surveillance ECGs by monitoring their own ECG using smartphone-based tools powered with AI capabilities to determine the plasma concentrations of the drug or the risk of drug-related toxic effects. The development of these AI algorithms applied to a single-lead ECG is still in progress.

Wearable and mobile ECG technologies

AI algorithms can be applied to wearable technologies, enabling rapid, point-of-care diagnoses for patients and consumers. Although many algorithms have been derived using 12-lead ECG data, some studies have demonstrated favourable performance even when algorithms are deployed on single-lead ECGs8. The performance of AI–ECG algorithms for the detection of HCM or the determination of serum potassium levels when applied to single-lead ECGs has been shown not to be significantly different from the performance when applied to 12-lead ECGs45,52. Additionally, signals other than the ECG can also be analysed using AI approaches. For instance, a deep neural network has been developed to detect AF passively from photoplethysmography signals obtained from the Apple Watch14. Newer iterations of the Apple

Watch now allow users to confirm the presence of AF using electrophysiological signals obtained through a single bipolar vector

The COVID-19 pandemic has highlighted the need for rapid, point-of-care diagnostic testing. For instance, early interest in the use of hydroxychloroquine or azithromycin for the treatment of the infection resulted in a marked increase in the use of these medications. Given the potential for these medications to prolong myocardial repolarization and increase the risk of dangerous ventricular arrhythmias, the FDA issued an Emergency Use Authorization for the use of mobile devices to record and monitor the QT interval in patients taking these medications. The FDA also issued an Emergency Use Authorization for the detection of low LVEF as a potential complication of COVID-19 using the AI–ECG algorithm integrated in the digital Eko stethoscope (Eko Devices). Furthermore, an international consortium is currently evaluating the ECG as a potential means to diagnose COVID-19, cardiac involvement or the risk of cardiac deterioration, given the known ECG changes and cardiac involvement in patients with COVID-19 . Although results are not yet available, these types of investigation emphasize the potential power of digitally delivered AI technologies for timely deployment at the point of care and large-scale implementation.

including screening, diagnosis, prognostication, and personalized treatment selection and monitoring. The preliminary data on the performance of the AI–ECG algorithms are clearly promising, but these technologies will be meaningful only inasmuch as they improve our clinical practice and patient outcomes.To this end, several AI technologies are currently being tested in various clinical applications.

Current, versatile electrocardiogram (ECG)-recording technologies (wearable and implantable devices, smartwatches and e-stethoscopes) coupled with the ability to store, transfer, process and analyse large amounts of digital data are increasingly allowing the deployment of artificial intelligence (AI)-powered tools in the clinical arena, addressing the spectrum of patient needs. The science of AI-enhanced ECG (AI–ECG) implementation, including the interface between patients and the AI–ECG output, integration of AI–ECG tools with electronic health records, patient privacy, and cost and reimbursement implications, is in its infancy and continues to evolve The algorithm to identify LV dysfunction using the ECG is currently being evaluated in a large-scale, pragmatic, cluster randomized clinical trial56. The EAGLE trial57 randomly assigned >100 clinical teams (or clusters) either to have access to the new AI screening tool results or to usual care at nearly 50 primary care practices

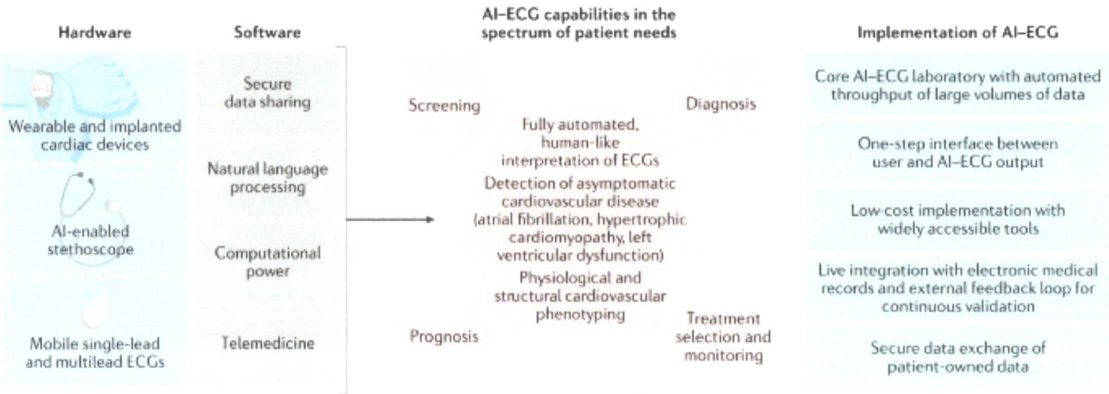

Fig. 2.3: Framework for AI–ECG applications in clinical practice

Implementation of AI–ECG

In contrast to data obtained through the clinical history, medical record review or imaging tests, the ease and consistency with which ECG data can be obtained and analysed for the development and implementation of AI models are likely to accelerate the uptake of the AI–ECG in clinical applications, with ensuing increases in workflow efficiency. The demonstrated capabilities of the AI–ECG described in the previous sections have the potential to influence the spectrum of patient care, (which will encompass >400 clinicians and >24,000 patients) in the Mayo Clinic Health System. Eligible patients include adults who undergo ECG for any reason and in whom low LVEF has not been previously diagnosed. The primary outcome is the detection of low LVEF (<50%), as determined by standard echocardiography. The objective of this study is twofold: to evaluate the real-world efficacy of the algorithm in identifying patients with asymptomatic or previously unrecognized LV dysfunction in primary care practices and to understand how information derived from AI algorithms is interpreted and acted on by clinicians — how do humans and machines interact? This study will validate (or refute) the utility of this approach and will help us to understand potential barriers and opportunities for the implementation of AI in clinical practice. Regardless of its results, the EAGLE trial57 will be an important study because it will be the prototype study for the implementation of AI-enabled tools.Similarly, we are developing a protocol to assess the algorithm to identify concomitant silent AF or the risk of near-term AF using a 12-lead ECG obtained during normal sinus rhythm. The BEAGLE trial58 will seek to evaluate the utility of this AI algorithm for targeted AF screening in patients who would have at least a moderate risk of stroke if they had AF. Subsequent follow-up studies will test the role of empirical anticoagulation in selected patients without known documented AF who have a high probability of AF according to the AI–ECG. In the first pilot phase, patients at various levels of risk of AF on the basis of their AI–ECG will be fitted with cardiac event monitors to provide surveillance for incident AF. We anticipate that the AI–ECG output will help us to identify patients who are at risk of AF and that the AI–ECG might increase the diagnostic yield of screening. Another application of this algorithm might be in guiding treatment decisions for patients with ESUS. We postulate that these patients might benefit from intensified screening or even empirical anticoagulation on the basis of a high probability of AF, as indicated by the AI–ECG algorithm. Several studies have shown no benefit of empirical anticoagulation in patients with ESUS but the AI–ECG might help to identify a subset of patients with ESUS in whom recurrent strokes can be prevented. At this point, this concept is speculative, but we intend to pursue this hypothesis by examining existing datasets and possibly in a prospective clinical trial.We have demonstrated the potential utility of the AI–ECG for the diagnosis of HCM45. Screening individuals for HCM has attracted considerable controversy, driven mostly by the poor diagnostic performance of the ECG and the downstream consequences of false positive or equivocal findings. External validation of this algorithm in completely independent cohorts of patients with HCM is currently in progress. Evaluations of this algorithm in various populations, including family members of patients with HCM, patients with undifferentiated syncope, athletes oreven unselected patients through retrospective medicalrecord review, are also being planned. These studies are likely to demonstrate the utility and limits of the AI–ECG for screening individuals for rare conditions and will help us to understand how to apply appropriate thresholds based on Bayesian concepts of pretest risk and downstream effects of a test, including costs. In addition to straightforward diagnostic tests, the AI–ECG might help to refine the clinical workflow. One such application might be the initiation and monitoring of antiarrhythmic medications that carry a risk of cardiotoxicity or proarrhythmia and require close monitoring for QT prolongation and new ventricular arrhythmias in order to guide initial and subsequent dosing50. Other potential future applications of the AI–ECG in various settings with direct effects on cardiac clinical care

At the Mayo Clinic, we have developed an internal website (AI–ECG Dashboard) where the medical record number of any patient of interest can be entered for all their ECGs to be retrospectively analysed, with probabilities reported for the presence of LV systolic dysfunction, silent AF and HCM, and their AI–ECG age and sex prediction also reported. ECG-derived probability of AF on an ECG that preceded the thromboembolic event by 12 years.At 5 years after the initial stroke, this patient had a recurrent stroke and was clinically documented to have AF shortly thereafter, which was 17 years after the first ECG had indicated an elevated risk of AF by AI analysis60. Figure 4b depicts an example of a different patient with a history of cardiomyopathy who underwent heart transplantation in 2005, at which time the probability of low LVEF dropped precipitously and remained low until 2020, when the patient experienced graft rejection with LV dysfunction. At that point, the AI–ECG reported a high probability of low LVEF, correlating accurately with the clinical syndrome. The AI–ECG Dashboard has now been integrated into the electronic medical record, and clinicians can rapidly access the results of the AI analysis on all of a patient's available ECGs. Other tools, such as those for AI–ECG detection of valvular heart disease, cardiac amyloidosis and pulmonary arterial hypertension, have been developed and are undergoing testing before their addition to the dashboard.

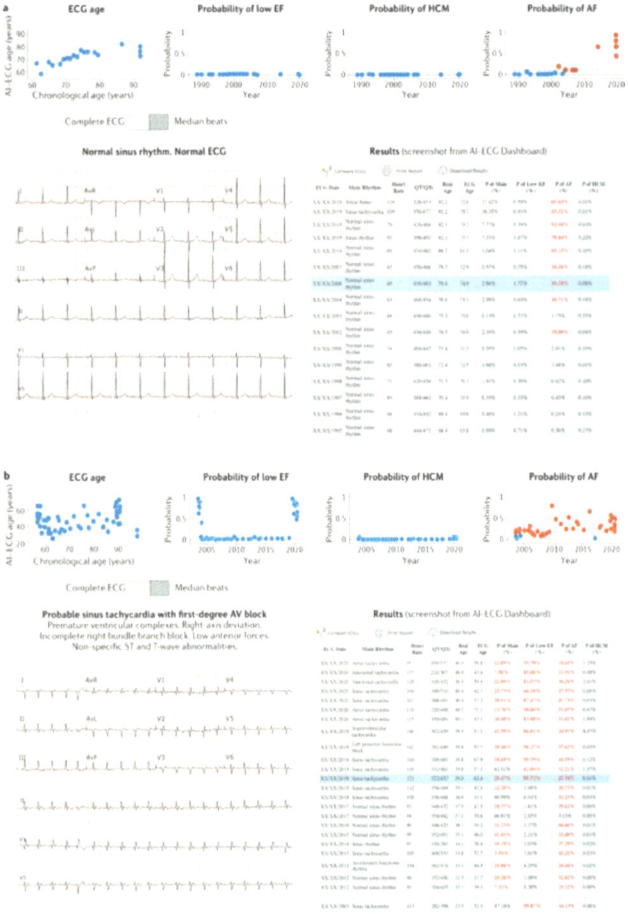

Fig.2.4: AI–ECG Dashboard linked from within the electronic health record for point-of-care application.

a | A patient with embolic stroke of undetermined source had an increased probability of silent atrial fibrillation (AF; red data points) that predated the clinical documentation of atrial flutter. b | A patient with a history of heart transplantation in 2005 who experienced graft rejection with left ventricular systolic dysfunction in 2020. At that point, the artificial intelligence-enhanced electrocardiogram (AI–ECG) reported a high probability of low ejection fraction (EF), correlating with the graft rejection. AV, atrioventricular; HCM, hypertrophic cardiomyopathy.

Box 2.1 Potential future applications of the AI–ECG

1. **Atrial Fibrillation**

- Beyond the CHA2DS2–VASc score —electrocardiogram (ECG) markers of stroke risk integrated with electronic health record-based clinical information, imaging and biomarkers
  Rhythm-pattern recognition (implantable and wearable
- Cardiovascular electronic devices) to predict atrial fibrillation events and artificial intelligence-enhanced ECG (AI–EGG)-guided 'pill-in-pocket' (oral anticoagulation or class Ic antiarrhythmic drugs) in patients with paroxysmal atrial fibrillation
- dofetilide or other medications that can affect repolarization is initiated or for patients longitudinally treated with sotalol, dofetilide or other medications that can affect repolarization

2. **Sudden cardiac death:**
identifying which patients should receive an implantable cardioverter–defibrillator and integration with clinical and imaging markers

- Beyond the left ventricular ejection fraction in patients with ischaemic or non-ischaemic cardiomyopathy
- Risk stratification in patients with hypertrophic cardiomyopathy or inherited arrhythmia syndromes

3. **Predicting the exacerbation of congestive heart failure**
on the basis of continuous ECG ambulatory data to prevent emergency department visits and hospitalizations

4. **Severity and staging of heart failure, valvular heart disease and pulmonary arterial hypertension to guide clinical decision-making, prognosis and monitoring**

5. **Angina and stress ECG analysis** — identifying high-risk patients who will benefit from invasive coronary evaluation and possible intervention

Potential challenges and solutions

The AI–ECG technologies offer great promise, but it is important to acknowledge several potential challenges. Given that models are often derived from high-quality databases with meticulously obtained ECGs and well-phenotyped patients, their application to ECGs obtained in routine clinical practice in real-world settings might be poor. Similarly, although the models might perform well in one population, they require rigorous evaluation for external validity in diverse populations. The aforementioned AI–ECG model for low LVEF has been validated in racially diverse cohorts, but validation data for the other AI–ECG model algorithms are pending. Although models might perform well in terms of their individual performance characteristics, this performance does not always translate into meaningful and actionable clinical information. For instance, screening tests for very rare conditions might be limited by low positive predictive value when applied to populations with low pretest probability of the disease. Although an algorithm might seem to predict a disease state well, if this information does not add to other readily available data (such as age, sex and comorbidities), the algorithm will add very little to clinical risk stratification. Many routinely used screening and diagnostic tests often do not produce consistent improvements in downstream patient outcomes, thereby offering little incremental value to clinical care61. Similar assessments of the effects of routinely integrating the AI–ECG into clinical practice and its implications for patient outcomes and costs will be important. Clearly, the delivery of AI-related applications in the clinical environment generates a new set of previously unrecognized challenges.

As with most other AI-enabled tools, the development of AI–ECG models requires large datasets for training, validation and testing. In some cases, multicentre collaborations might be necessary to assemble the sample sizes required for the development of high-fidelity models. Such collaboration is particularly pertinent when the condition of interest is rare or when an urgent clinical need dictates the rapid development of a model, such as the AI–ECG tools for the diagnosis and risk stratification of COVID-19 during the current pandemic. In this process and during external validation of any AI–ECG model, large amounts of patient data are exchanged between research teams worldwide, generating concerns for the security and protection of sensitive patient information that might be susceptible to cyberattacks or other threats. In the current environment, the use of traditional encryption methods might not be sufficient to alleviate these concerns. Among other possible novel data-protection solutions, block chain technology might allow the secure and traceable sharing of patient data between investigators and institutions for the development, validation and clinical implementation of AI tools by generating a decentralized marketplace of securely stored patient data specifically intended to be used in AI applications. Of note, even a miniscule artificial perturbation of the input data (such as a single pixel in an image or an ECG) that is unrecognizable by the human eye might lead an otherwise well-trained CNN to misclassify the data and generate false output. CNNs are clearly vulnerable to adversarial perturbations of input data, and shielding against these vulnerabilities will be important for their future widespread implementation.

We must also acknowledge that a risk of perpetuating bias exists with AI. Algorithms that are derived using current clinical practice patterns and outcomes will reflect the disparity present and pose a risk of reinforcing and perpetuating these inequities. To address this risk, investigators and consumers of these algorithms must consider how the data are collected (in what population and of what quality), how the models perform, how the model should best be applied and how the findings fit within existing knowledge.Clinical and technical challenges also exist to the application of the AI–ECG to patient care. AI analysis relies on standardized digital ECG acquisition that is not universal in current clinical environments, even in high-resource settings. Poor-quality data can prevent the effective development and application of AI–ECG technologies. Current AI tools cannot analyse ECGs stored as images (such TIFF or PDF file types), which limits generalizability in some clinical environments. Furthermore, the infrastructure to integrate AI–ECG results into electronic health records and make them available at the point of clinical care is not widely available.

An evidence base for the real-world effects of AI–ECG analysis on clinical care and ultimately on important patient outcomes remains to be established. Outcomes to be considered are the uptake by clinicians, effect on clinical decision-making (how does the result of AI analysis affect downstream testing and therapies?) and ultimately whether AI–ECG analysis improves the provider and patient experience and patient-specific clinical outcomes. Similarly, how does the AI–ECG algorithm complement existing clinical or laboratory markers of disease? For example, can we use the AI–ECG algorithm to detect LV systolic dysfunction in addition to using measurements of plasma levels of N-terminal prohormone of B-type natriuretic peptide and what does it add? Randomized clinical trials of the pragmatic implementation of the AI–ECG, such as the EAGLE56,57 and BEAGLE58 trials discussed previously, are now being conducted and will provide unique insights. Rigorous testing of AI–ECG tools in randomized trials is crucial for demonstrating their value, as with any other form of clinical intervention. Lastly, the regulatory aspects of incorporating AI–ECG-derived diagnoses for direct clinical care are now starting to be formulated. The barrier to approval by regulatory bodies might be quite different from that for devices or medications and might vary according to the ability of a clinician to 'over-read' the AI–ECG findings. For algorithms that streamline workflow but perform a task that is usually done by humans (for example, rhythm determination), the algorithm might be approved as a tool to aid clinician workflow. However, if the models perform an analysis that cannot be done by expert clinicians (for example, determination of 'ECG age' or the risk of future AF), additional approval complexities might exist. Similarly, if algorithms are meant to be applied for patients and consumers at the point of care (without clinician oversight), a higher bar for performance of the model might be required. A legal framework to support AI-based clinical decision-making has not yet been established.

Conclusion

The true potential of deep-learning AI applied to the ubiquitous 12-lead ECG is starting to be realized. The utility of the AI–ECG is being demonstrated as a tool for comprehensive human-like interpretation of the ECG, but also as a powerful tool for phenotyping of cardiac health and disease that can be applied at the point of care. The implementation of the AI–ECG is still in its infancy, but a continuously growing clinical investigation agenda will determine the added value of these AI tools, their optimal deployment in the clinical arena and their multifaceted and so-far largely unpredictable implications. As with any medical tool, the AI–ECG must be vetted, validated and verified, and clinicians must be trained to use it properly, but when integrated into medical practice, the AI–ECG holds the promise to transform clinical care.

Key points

1. *The feasibility and potential value of the application of advanced artificial intelligence methods, particularly deep-learning convolutional neural networks (CNNs), to the electrocardiogram (ECG) have been demonstrated.*
2. *CNNs developed with the use of large numbers of digital ECGs linked to rich clinical datasets might be able to perform accurate and nuanced, human-like interpretation of ECGs.*
3. *CNNs have also been developed to detect asymptomatic left ventricular dysfunction, silent atrial fibrillation, hypertrophic cardiomyopathy and an individual's age, sex and race on the basis of the ECG alone.*
4. *CNNs to detect other cardiac conditions, such as aortic valve stenosis and amyloid heart disease, are in active development.*
5. *These approaches might be applicable to the standard 12-lead ECG or to data obtained from single-lead or multilead mobile or wearable ECG technologies.*
6. *Evidence on patient outcomes, as well as the challenges and potential limitations from the real-world implementation of the artificial intelligence-enhanced ECG, continues to emerge.*

Bibliography and Acknowledgement

- Adedinsewo, D. et al. An artificial intelligence-enabled ECG algorithm to identify patients with left ventricular systolic dysfunction presenting to the emergency department with dyspnea. Circ. Arrhythm. Electrophysiol. 13, e008437 (2020).
- Attia, Z. I. et al. An artificial intelligence-enabled ECG algorithm for the identification of patients with atrial fibrillation during sinus rhythm: a retrospective analysis of outcome prediction. Lancet 394, 861–867 (2019).
- Attia, Z. I. et al. Noninvasive assessment of dofetilide plasma concentration using a deep learning (neural network) analysis of the surface electrocardiogram: a proof of concept study. PLoS ONE 13, e0201059 (2018).
- Attia, Z. I. et al. Novel bloodless potassium determination using a signal-processed single-Lead ECG. J. Am. Heart Assoc. 5, e002746 (2016).
- Attia, Z. I. et al. Prospective validation of a deep learning electrocardiogram algorithm for the detection of left ventricular systolic dysfunction. J. Cardiovasc. Electrophysiol. 30, 668–674 (2019).
- Attia, Z. I. et al. Screening for cardiac contractile dysfunction using an artificial intelligence-enabled electrocardiogram. Nat. Med. 25, 70–74 (2019).

Bangalore, S. et al. ST-segment elevation in patients with Covid-19 — a case series. N. Engl. J. Med. 382, 2478–2480 (2020).

- Bumgarner, J. M. et al. Smartwatch algorithm for automated detection of atrial fibrillation. J. Am. Coll. Cardiol. 71, 2381–2388 (2018).
- Caceres, C. A. & Rikli, A. E. The digital computer as an aid in the diagnosis of cardiovascular disease. Trans. NY Acad. Sci. 23, 240–245 (1961).

Caceres, C. A. et al. Computer extraction of electrocardiographic parameters. Circulation 25, 356–362 (1962).

- Chen, T. M., Huang, C. H., Shih, E. S. C., Hu, Y. F. & Hwang, M. J. Detection and classification of cardiac arrhythmias by a challenge-best deep learning neural network model. iScience 23, 100886 (2020).
- Corrado, D. et al. Recommendations for interpretation of 12-lead electrocardiogram in the athlete. Eur. Heart J. 31, 243–259 (2010).

Costello-Boerrigter, L. C. et al. Amino-terminal pro-B-type natriuretic peptide and B-type natriuretic peptide in the general community: determinants and detection of left ventricular dysfunction. J. Am. Coll. Cardiol. 47, 345–353 (2006).

- Dewland, T. A. et al. Atrial ectopy as a predictor of incident atrial fibrillation: a cohort study. Ann. Intern. Med. 159, 721–728 (2013).

Diener, H. C. et al. Dabigatran for prevention of stroke after embolic stroke of undetermined source. N. Engl. J. Med. 380, 1906–1917 (2019).

- Feeny, A. K. et al. Machine learning of 12-lead QRS waveforms to identify cardiac resynchronization therapy patients with differential outcomes. Circ. Arrhythm. Electrophysiol. 13, e008210 (2020).

Ferreira, J. P. et al. Abnormalities of potassium in heart failure: JACC state-of-the-art review. J. Am. Coll. Cardiol. 75, 2836–2850 (2020).

- Galloway, C. D. et al. Development and validation of a deep-learning model to screen for hyperkalemia from the electrocardiogram. JAMA Cardiol. 4, 428–436 (2019).

Gottesman, O. et al. Guidelines for reinforcement learning in healthcare. Nat. Med. 25, 16–18 (2019).

- Gruca, T. S., Pyo, T. H. & Nelson, G. C. Providing cardiology care in rural areas through visiting consultant clinics. J. Am. Heart Assoc. 5, e002909 (2016).
- Han, L. et al. Atrial fibrillation burden signature and near-term prediction of stroke: a machine learning analysis. Circ. Cardiovasc. Qual. Outcomes 12, e005595 (2019).
- Hannun, A. Y. et al. Cardiologist-level arrhythmia detection and classification in ambulatory electrocardiograms using a deep neural network. Nat. Med. 25, 65–69 (2019).
- Hart, R. G. et al. Rivaroxaban for stroke prevention after embolic stroke of undetermined source. N. Engl. J. Med. 378, 2191–2201 (2018).
- Inohara, T. et al. Association of of atrial fibrillation clinical phenotypes with treatment patterns and outcomes: a multicenter registry study. JAMA Cardiol. 3, 54–63 (2018).
- Kashou, A. H. et al. A comprehensive artificial intelligence–enabled electrocardiogram interpretation program. Cardiovasc. Digit. Health J. 1, 62–70 (2020).
- Kashou, A. H. et al. Recurrent cryptogenic stroke: a potential role for an artificial intelligence-enabled electrocardiogram? Heart Rhythm. Case Rep. 6, 202–205 (2020).
- Ko, W. Y. et al. Detection of hypertrophic cardiomyopathy using a convolutional neural network-enabled electrocardiogram. J. Am. Coll. Cardiol. 75, 722–733 (2020).
- Krittanawong, C. et al. Integrating blockchain technology with artificial intelligence for cardiovascular medicine. Nat. Rev. Cardiol. 17, 1–3 (2020).
- Krizhevsky, A., Sustskever, I. & Hinton, G. E. ImageNet classification with deep convolutional neural networks. Adv. Neural Inf. Process. Syst. 25, 1106–1114 (2012).
- Kuo, T. T., Gabriel, R. A., Cidambi, K. R. & Ohno-Machado, L. EXpectation Propagation LOgistic REgRession on permissioned blockCHAIN (ExplorerChain): decentralized online healthcare/ genomics predictive model learning. J. Am. Med. Inform. Assoc. 27, 747–756 (2020
- Levy, A. E. et al. Applications of machine learning in decision analysis for dose management for dofetilide. PLoS ONE 14, e0227324 (2019).
- Lip, G. Y., Nieuwlaat, R., Pisters, R., Lane, D. A. & Crijns, H. J. Refining clinical risk stratification for predicting stroke and thromboembolism in atrial fibrillation using a novel risk factor-based approach: the Euro Heart Survey on atrial fibrillation. Chest 137, 263–272 (2010).
- Lopez-Jimenez, F. et al. Artificial intelligence in cardiology: present and future. Mayo Clin. Proc. 95, 1015–1039 (2020).
- Maron, B. J. et al. Assessment of the 12-lead electrocardiogram as a screening test for detection of cardiovascular disease in healthy general populations of young people (12-25 years of age): a scientific statement from the American Heart Association and the American College of Cardiology. J. Am. Coll. Cardiol. 64, 1479–1514 (2014).
- Maron, B. J. et al. Prevalence of hypertrophic cardiomyopathy in a general population of young adults. Echocardiographic analysis of 4111 subjects in the CARDIA study. Circulation 92, 785–789 (1995).
  Maron, B. J., Haas, T. S., Murphy, C. J., Ahluwalia, A. & Rutten-Ramos, S. Incidence and causes of sudden death in U.S. college athletes. J. Am. Coll. Cardiol. 63, 1636–1643 (2014).
- McLeod, C. J. et al. Outcome of patients with hypertrophic cardiomyopathy and a normal electrocardiogram. J. Am. Coll. Cardiol. 54, 229–233 (2009).
- Palano, F. et al. Assessing atrial fibrillation substrates by P wave analysis: a comprehensive review. High Blood Press. Cardiovasc. Prev. 27, 341–347 (2020).
- Perez, M. V. et al. Large-scale assessment of a smartwatch to identify atrial fibrillation. N. Engl. J. Med. 381, 1909–1917 (2019).
- Pipberger, H. V., Freis, E. D., Taback, L. & Mason, H. L. Preparation of electrocardiographic data for analysis by digital electronic computer. Circulation 21, 413–418 (1960).
- Raghunath, S. et al. Prediction of mortality from 12-lead electrocardiogram voltage data using a deep neural network. Nat. Med. 26, 886–891 (2020).
- Redfield, M. M. et al. Burden of systolic and diastolic ventricular dysfunction in the community: appreciating the scope of the heart failure epidemic. JAMA 289, 194–202 (2003).
- Ribeiro, A. H. et al. Automatic diagnosis of the 12-lead ECG using a deep neural network. Nat. Commun. 11, 1760 (2020).
- Rikli, A. E. et al. Computer analysis of electrocardiographic measurements. Circulation 24, 643–649 (1961).
- Rudin, C. Stop explaining black box machine learning models for high stakes decisions and use interpretable models instead. Nat. Mach. Intell. 1, 206–215 (2019).
- Schlapfer, J. & Wellens, H. J. Computer-interpreted electrocardiograms: benefits and limitations. J. Am. Coll. Cardiol. 70, 1183–1192 (2017).
- Semsarian, C., Ingles, J., Maron, M. S. & Maron, B. J. New perspectives on the prevalence of hypertrophic cardiomyopathy. J. Am. Coll. Cardiol. 65, 1249–1254 (2015).
- Siontis, K. C. et al. Typical, atypical, and asymptomatic presentations of new-onset atrial fibrillation in the community: characteristics and prognostic implications. Heart Rhythm. 13, 1418–1424 (2016).
- Smith, S. W. et al. A deep neural network learning algorithm outperforms a conventional algorithm for emergency department electrocardiogram interpretation. J. Electrocardiol. 52, 88–95 (2019)
- Tison, G. H., Zhang, J., Delling, F. N. & Deo, R. C. Automated and interpretable patient ECG profiles for disease detection, tracking, and discovery. Circ. Cardiovasc. Qual. Outcomes 12, e005289 (2019).
- Uberoi, A. et al. Interpretation of the electrocardiogram of young athletes. Circulation 124, 746–757 (2011).
- Vasan, R. S. et al. Plasma natriuretic peptides for community screening for left ventricular hypertrophy and systolic dysfunction: the Framingham Heart Study. JAMA 288, 1252–1259 (2002).
- Vollmer, S. et al. Machine learning and artificial intelligence research for patient benefit: 20 critical questions on transparency, replicability, ethics, and effectiveness. BMJ 368, l6927 (2020).
- Wang, T. J. et al. Natural history of asymptomatic left ventricular systolic dysfunction in the community. Circulation 108, 977–982 (2003).
- Yancy, C. W. et al. 2013 ACCF/AHA guideline for the management of heart failure: a report of the American College of Cardiology Foundation/ American Heart Association Task Force on Practice Guidelines. Circulation 128, e240–e327 (2013).
- Yao, X. et al. ECG AI-Guided Screening for Low Ejection Fraction (EAGLE): rationale and design of a pragmatic cluster randomized trial. Am. Heart J. 219, 31–36 (2020).
- Yasin, O. Z. et al. Noninvasive blood potassium measurement using signal-processed, single-lead ECG acquired from a handheld smartphone.

  J. Electrocardiol. 50, 620–625 (2017).
- Zhu, H. et al. Automatic multilabel electrocardiogram diagnosis of heart rhythm or conduction abnormalities with deep learning: a cohort study. Lancet Digit. Health 2, E348–E357 (2020).

Artificial Intelligence Advances in the World of Cardiovascular Imaging

CHAPTER

3

In this age of technology, there have been numerous inventions created to expand the boundaries of medical treatment and diagnosis beyond their current capabilities. Among the technological advancements, artificial intelligence (AI) serves as a means to improve various technologies already in practice. Specifically, within the medical field, AI provides greater accuracy to help guide a patient's course of treatment. Physicians are able to make clear initial decisions on how to treat patients presenting with specific symptoms. There is also a reduction in human error seen with the greater precision and automaticity capabilities of artificial intelligence. AI is beneficial for patients themselves as well by guiding patients to understand their symptoms through phone applications that detail whether patients need to go to the emergency room or their local doctor's office based on acuity. Furthermore, AI has been used to strengthen the cardiac imaging modalities such as echocardiography, nuclear cardiac imaging, cardiovascular computed tomography, and cardiovascular magnetic resonance imaging. While AI has shown promise, limitations of AI include a lack of standardization and reproducibility of results as well as decision making and selection bias.

Artificial intelligence refers to the all-encompassing ability of mathematical algorithms to train machines to mimic human intelligence. With the use of programmed algorithms, machines are able to complete tasks, execute decisions, and recognize images . Within AI, machine learning is a subset that identifies patterns among big datasets. It has the unique ability to automatically improve analysis over time with more usage of data and experience. Essentially, machine learning works by implementing algorithms to create a model from a sample dataset without directly programming the decisions needed to be made This is particularly useful in fields such as medicine where decisions are not predictable and vary in every individual patient.

Machine learning provides the opportunity to handle complex data with the ability to become more accurate over time. Machine learning itself can be classified as supervised and unsupervised . These two techniques are applied in different situations. Particularly, supervised learning refers to when models are trained to analyze algorithms based on reference data that have already been entered. Thus, as it works from a reference dataset and applies the same pattern to a new dataset, supervised learning is very accurate. Unsupervised learning refers to finding patterns in data on its own without any given reference. This is advantageous in finding hidden patterns that have not already been identified . Despite its advantages, machine learning has its limitations, especially apparent when applied to the field of medicine. Specifically, machine learning can lead to bias when it comes to analyzing the dataset. This is due to the way the algorithms are organized which is to become better with more exposure to previous datasets. Therefore, this decreases the variety of data that machines have to make information other than what was previously represented .

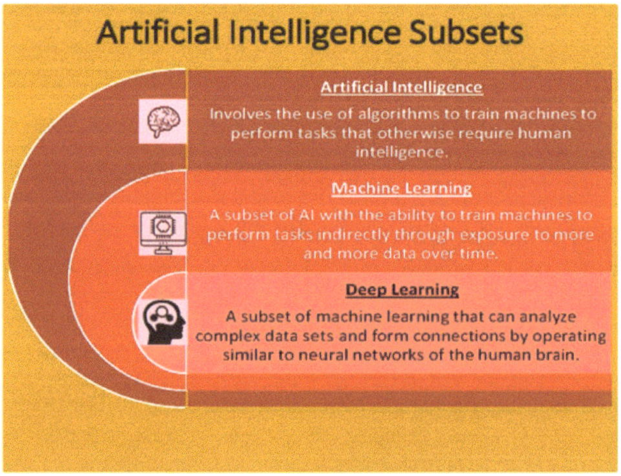

Fig.3.1 Artificial intelligence subsets into which the principles of AI can be divided.

Table 3.1 Methodology of supervised and unsupervised learning within machine learning.

Machine Learning	Classification Types of Problems Each Classification Is Used for
Supervised Learning—Uses reference data to analyze algorithms and apply the algorithms to a similar dataset	**Classification**—Utilizes an algorithm to assign a dataset into specific categories. Specifically, draws conclusions on how specific categories in the dataset should be labeled. **Regression**—Analyzes the relationship between dependent and independent variables, particularly for making projections
Unsupervised Learning—Identifies hidden patterns in data without any given reference	**Clustering**—Organizes unlabeled data based on similarities and differences **Dimension Reduction**—Reduces the number of data inputs while preserving the data integrity; applied when there is an increased number of features or dimensions in a dataset

Furthermore, deep learning is a subset of machine learning. Deep learning uses artificial neural networks to allow machines to train themselves in accomplishing tasks. In other words, it can discover complex relationships that cannot otherwise be analyzed simply by an equation. It works to inspect and analyze an unlimited number of inputs at the same time . A deep convolutional neural network (DCNN) is a specific type of neural network that involves restricted connectivity. Specifically, DCNN is often used for classification tasks as well as detection and localization . DCNNs operate by involving convolutional layers, where each layer combines information from neighboring inputs to have a larger field of view. This is beneficial to finding patterns like visual pieces within an image, such as shapes and lines.

Deep learning is beneficial over traditional machine learning as it requires less data for training and has more accuracy . In particular, deep learning is most valuable with pattern recognition and image identification, particularly when working with large image datasets. Therefore, it is most effective for cardiovascular imaging, such as echocardiography, angiography, and cardiac magnetic resonance. This is especially true as deep learning has the ability to parse through insignificant or noisy data . Although deep learning is useful with image recognition, it is limited insofar as its algorithm cannot be efficiently applied for all types of datasets. For example, simpler machine learning would be easier to use for datasets that are more defined and structured.

AI: General Medical Applications

The field of artificial intelligence allows for advancements to take place that expand the abilities of current technology. The goal of artificial intelligence is to create intelligence that has the ability for computers to solve problems and perform tasks, thus replicating the human mind . AI involves the development of algorithms that can mimic the reasoning skills of humans in solving problems and deducing information in a methodical fashion. Over the years, AI has been applied to many different fields and used for a variety of purposes. Within medicine, AI has been used to improve diagnostic and treatment methods as well as efficiency with healthcare management.For instance, most medical records are a collection of disorganized information hard to rifle through. However, with the application of AI, the information collected can allow physicians to understand a patient's complete medical information prior to making medical decisions in real time. Specifically, algorithms that allow for the ability to search for patients with significant family history or susceptibility of chronic diseases transform the usage of electronic medical records . More efficiently organized electronic medical records ultimately serve as a tool for personalized medicine and early detection of diseases. In addition to programming algorithms, AI has also been applied to physical objects, such as medical devices and robots. For example, robotic-assisted surgeries are more often utilized to operate on patients . The quality of care is drastically improved with the use of robots in surgery as incisions are more minimally invasive. This allows for patients to experience less pain after the surgery and have a shorter recovery time. The robotic surgical tool also serves to dissect, cut, and suture in a more precise fashion. With the addition of AI, surgical robots can identify the movements and patterns of a surgeon performing an operation and convert these into actions for the robot to execute on its own . Additionally, the use of robots eliminates human error from surgeons, such as with hand tremors or accidental cuts . In fact, of the 17 million surgical procedures performed in the United States, it was found that there were 400,000 operations with adverse outcomes attributed to human error . Furthermore, Rajih et al. found robotic surgery error on the da Vinci surgical system in 4.97% of 1228 cases evaluated between 2012 and 2015 . In this case, the use of AI-led robots allows for benefits such as improving the quality of care and providing accuracy and stability to prevent more human error.

AI: Cardiology Imaging Applications

Machine learning is a branch of AI that is particularly useful in the interpretation of cardiovascular imaging because it can combine and correlate information from different sources for a physician to interpret efficiently . Specifically, machine learning has the ability to use a variety of different approaches to analyze a greater quantity of information. Coronary artery disease (CAD) is one of the most prevalent cardiovascular disorders and is responsible for one in every five deaths . Coronary artery disease is generally diagnosed with radionuclide myocardial perfusion imaging (MPI). With the addition of machine learning to supplement the MPI results, the patient-specific risk stratification is improved. A study by Seetharam et al. found evidence that machine learning is greater than parametric statistical models in predicting the presence of obstructive CAD, the need for revascularization, and potential adverse risks . Specifically, Arsajani et al. conducted a study that evaluated the MPI device's accuracy of predicting CAD in 957 patients when used in adjunct with a learning algorithm compared to two experienced imaging readers. The results showed that the machine learning's sensitivity and specificity was significantly superior compared to the experienced readers. Multiple cardiac imaging applications and pertinent publications relating to them are detailed below and lead to generation of data that inform artificial intelligence algorithms to allow for analysis and evaluation.

Echocardiography

Within the field of cardiology, AI has had a tremendous impact on how early and accurately patients are diagnosed as well as receive treatment. Echocardiography is a noninvasive diagnostic test that is performed on patients to detect or monitor the progression of cardiovascular diseases .

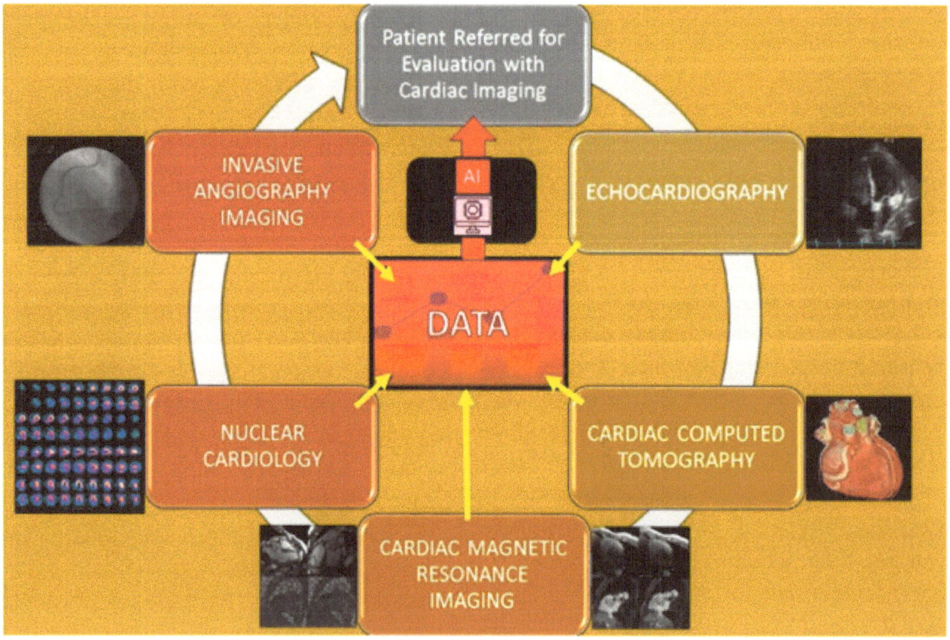

Fig. 3.2 Cardiac imaging modalities that allow for the gathering of data that informs the formation of artificial intelligence that then is used for optimization of the evaluation of patients undergoing cardiac imaging.

It is advantageous in visualizing the structure, function, and hemodynamics of the heart as well as any characteristic abnormalities. Specifically, echocardiography is beneficial as a cost-effective tool and can be performed at bedside rapidly with no known side effects . On the other hand, a limitation of echocardiography is that it relies on a subjective interpretation of the images by the physician. Therefore, although obtaining the images is feasible with echocardiography, there is still a likelihood of an inaccurate diagnosis. To address this limitation, AI provides the ability to produce accurate, consistent, and automated interpretations of echocardiograms . Consequently, this reduces the likelihood of human error and allows physicians to come up with a precise treatment plan. The algorithms of AI also have the ability to accurately identify a wide variety of pathologies such as valvopathies and ischemia with coronary artery disease. In fact, Zhang et al. was able to use AI to accurately identify 96% of parasternal long axis imaging views from echocardiography . The use of AI to improve the diagnostic ability of echocardiograms is still in its early stages and research is still in progress before it becomes more widespread It is often difficult to distinguish between several conditions on echocardiography. Narula et al. states how machine learning can be applied to echocardiography to help differentiate between hypertrophic cardiomyopathy and athlete's heart . Machine learning algorithms are also particularly beneficial to help streamline workflow and prevent errors from physicians reading images after experiencing fatigue and exhaustion. Specifically, Madani et al. applied a CNN algorithm model to 267 echocardiogram images with 15 standard views and trained the algorithm by using labeled images. The results found that the model was immediately able to identify the echocardiogram view with an accuracy of 97.8% as compared to 70.2–84% accuracy with readings by expert echocardiographers

Cardiac Computed Tomography

In addition to echocardiography, computed tomography (CT) is also a valuable imaging tool for cardiovascular diseases. The CT scan produces images of the heart in various planes and allows for 3D image generation.It is particularly applicable for patients with suspected CAD as CT imaging allows physicians to noninvasively assess for calcium and plaque presence in the coronary arteries. This would indicate the presence of a blockage or narrowing in the arteries due to plaque buildup

The amount of calcium in the vessels, also referred to as calcium score, can indicate the extent and prognosis of CAD. A study by Al'Aref et al. used machine learning algorithms to combine the calcium score and clinical factors to predict CAD in 35,281 patients. It was found that machine learning in conjunction with the coronary artery calcium score resulted in the most significantly accurate assessment of obstructive CAD from CT imaging compared to machine learning or calcium score alone . Machine learning has been used to identify a variety of different pathologies on CT with accuracy . Furthermore, machine learning allows for low-dose CT scans to be safer. Low-dose CT imaging brings concerns of increased exposure to radiation for patients that could not be solved by simply decreasing radiation levels as this would decrease the image quality . As a result, to solve this issue, a machine learning framework was developed that allowed for reconstructing image parameters and denoising the quality of the image when low radiation was used. This resulted in improved image quality to equate to the regular-dose CT image quality, thus allowing patients to be exposed to less radiation while still obtaining a diagnostic result

Cardiac Magnetic Resonance Imaging

Cardiac magnetic resonance imaging (MRI) is another noninvasive diagnostic tool for assessing cardiovascular diseases. Specifically, the MRI is considered the gold standard for assessing the ejection fraction and left ventricular volume. In a study by Ruijsink et al., researchers found a high correlation between the deep learning algorithm and manual analysis of the left and right ventricular volumes, filling, and ejection rates . In turn, automated measurements through deep learning were seen to be in strong agreement with the manual interpretation. Particularly, deep learning can be used to reconstruct cardiac images with better 3D visualization to identify disease patterns in association with the right ventricle. This is because the right ventricle is often not easily visualized in 2D with echocardiography. Laser et al. found that reconstruction of the right ventricle with echocardiography and cardiac MRI had incredible accuracy and reproducibility compared to the gold standard direct cardiac MRI . Deep learning also allows for the extraction of specific features to be automated easily, such as identification of the right ventricle and pulmonary artery hypertension A study by Zhang et al. created a deep learning model that created the ability to obtain motion features from the left ventricle and discriminate between ischemic regions on a nonenhanced cardiac MRI. This deep learning framework is beneficial as it allows for confirmation of chronic myocardial infarctions on MRI

Cardiac MRI has increasingly been used as a noninvasive imaging tool over the years. It results in acquiring cross-sectional images aligned with the heart axes. This can pose as an additional challenge when reading MRI results as medical imaging experts require detailed knowledge on cardiac anatomy. Conventionally, the heart is automatically localized to the center of the image, which does not account for the diversity in various patients' anatomy. This assumption leads to lower sensitivity and potential errors in imaging results . Kabani et al. introduced CNN, or deep neural network application, which allows for localizing and detecting a region of interest on an MRI interest. Normally, most localization networks have a bounding box around the region of interest. In this case, the CNN neural network applied a classification task where each pixel in the image was a separate class. Then, the CNN was trained to determine where the object was in the image and classify the pixels as in the background or in the bounding box. Specifically, this neural network considered the problem as a classification task where the pixels were classified as in the background or in a box

Nuclear Cardiology

Nuclear cardiology uses noninvasive techniques to measure blood flow through the heart. This test is particularly applicable when diagnosing coronary artery disease and possible ischemia, or lack of oxygen to the heart due to decreased blood flow. There are two types of nuclear cardiology tests that can be performed, the cardiac SPECT and PET-CT. In both tests, a PET scan is formed following injection of radioactive chemicals into the bloodstream via IV.Artificial intelligence, particularly deep learning, can also be applied to nuclear cardiology in order to address disparities regarding the diagnostic ability of SPECT . Deep learning allows for a greater ability to analyze images by identifying high dimensional patterns. Juarez-Orozco et al. applied deep learning to evaluate perfusion polar maps in ischemia by PET. It was found that deep learning had an area under the receiver-operating curve (AUC) of 0.90, which was better than all comparator models . Additionally, Hu et al. implemented the subset of AI, machine learning, to predict the likelihood of early coronary revascularization within 90 days after SPECT imaging. When comparing the AUC of machine learning with the standard quantitative analysis, it was found that the AUC of early coronary revascularization prediction was higher than and outperformed that of standard quantitative analysis

Angiography Imaging

Another imaging tool used in the field of cardiology is invasive angiography imaging. This is considered the reference standard when diagnosing obstructive coronary artery disease as it provides a detailed outlook on the structure and function of the heart's blood vessels. Despite its benefits, there are risks associated with the invasive angiography procedure including serious complications as well as expensive costs, exposure to high radiation, and discomfort . As such, Wolterink et al. validated a feasible method to obtain reduced radiation dose CT images by training a deep learning model . This shows how deep learning can help improve diagnostic imaging tools as well to make procedures safer for patients while also providing more accurate results.

Furthermore, cardiac computed tomography angiography (CCTA) is another method to diagnose coronary artery disease. Although CCTA can be used to rule out CAD, there are many drawbacks to using this diagnostic tool as it overestimates the amount of stenosis of the vessel and takes a lot of time to yield results. However, with the addition of AI, CCTA can be significantly improved to result in a more accurate evaluation of coronary stenosis, plaque characterization, and degree of myocardial ischemia . For example, van Hamersvelt et al. evaluated the addition of deep learning algorithm to analyze the left ventricular myocardium in CCTA for degree of stenosis. It was found that there was improved diagnosis and identification of patients with functionally significant coronary artery stenosis when using CCTA in combination with deep learning analysis. Specifically, sensitivity and specificity of results were 84.6% and 48.4%, respectively . Motwani et al. applied machine learning to evaluate 5-year all-cause mortality in patients undergoing CCTA . Specifically, 10,030 patients with possible CAD underwent CCTA as part of their standard of care. Machine learning was then applied to predict 5-year mortality of these patients using the CCTA data. After comparison of a 5-year follow-up from these patients via the CCTA international multicenter registry, it was found that ML combined with CCTA data was significantly better at predicting patient prognosis for the next 5 years compared to CCTA metrics alone . ML-based fractional flow reserve-computed tomography (FFR-CT) is increasingly used in diagnosing CAD. Specifically, FFR-CT is a noninvasive procedure that generates a 3D image of the patient's coronary arteries .An FFR measurement refers to identifying the ratio between the maximum blood flow possible in a diseased coronary artery and maximum flow in a normal coronary artery. An FFR of 1.0 is considered normal whereas an FFR of less than 0.75–0.80 is associated with myocardial ischemia . A study by Jiang et al. evaluated the features and severity of coronary calcification by ML-based CCTA-derived FFR, or FFR-CT. In this study, 442 patients went through CCTA, ML-based FFR-CT, and invasive FFR and the results were compared. It was found that ML-based FFR-CT had an accuracy of 0.90 in determining calcification lesions as compared to invasive FFR. Additionally, CT-FFR generally had higher accuracy in diagnosis and differentiating ischemia in blood vessels as compared to CCTA by itself.

A study by Yang et al. analyzed the relation of stenosis and plaque characteristics with myocardial implications. The study analyzed 1013 vessels via fractional flow reserve measurement and CT angiography. Then, Yang et al. incorporated machine learning to identify the features associated with a low FFR and the patient prognosis. In this case, machine learning was beneficial in categorizing characteristics of blood vessels with a low FFR. The six functionally relevant features found included minimum lumen area, percent atheroma volume, fibrofatty and necrotic core volume, plaque volume, proximal left anterior descending coronary artery lesion, and remodeling index.

Intravascular Imaging

Intravascular imaging is performed by using a specialized catheter-based intravascular ultrasound (IVUS) or optical coherence tomography (OCT) that allows for providing a real-time visual of the inside of a coronary artery. Particularly, it shows the degree of narrowing or thickening of an artery and a visual of the lumen of the artery. Intravascular ultrasound is often used to gain a better insight into the nature of the plaque in the artery as well as in the placement of stents. This imaging technique is invasive and involves great expertise to place the catheters inside the coronary arteries. Researchers have incorporated artificial intelligence to increase the speed of diagnosis and interpretation of intravascular imaging in real time. Specifically, the artificial intelligence algorithm is exposed to multiple images and given information on each image, such as the vessel's geometry and distribution of different tissue types. Therefore, as it is exposed to more images, the AI algorithm can easily and quickly interpret the image created by the intravascular imaging and discern a diagnosis.

IVUS imaging creates an image with low resolution but with high tissue penetration while OCT imaging creates an image with higher resolution but limited tissue penetration. As these two intravascular imaging modalities have their differences, artificial intelligence can connect the two results together. Specifically, AI processes data from IVUS and OCT images into a single imaging procedure to allow physicians to review all the data at once . This is beneficial as it allows for a more rapid, comprehensive evaluation of any damaged arteries.

Software Programs in Clinical Practice That Employ AI

Artificial intelligence is already being used in clinical practice by physicians today. There are software programs, such as IBM Watson®, that help organizations automate complex processes to improve efficiency and effectivity. IBM Watson® includes Merge Healthcare®, which provides medical imaging artificial intelligence solutions to help physicians with patient care. Specifically, Merge PACS™ is an artificial-intelligence-ready workflow platform that eases the physician workload of reading and understanding numerous dense images . This is extremely beneficial as physicians have received an increasing number of images to read over the years, including as many as 100,000 images a day [50]. Therefore, artificial intelligence and computer programming offered through Merge Healthcare® serves to provide a more rapid and automated diagnosis for patients.

Limitations of Artificial Intelligence

Overall, AI applications mimic human intelligence with the purpose of solving problems or making decisions. AI has many advantages with its accuracy, cost-effectiveness, and reliability. However, there are still some limitations to AI, especially with its application in the medical field. Specifically, the gold standard for clinical reasoning in decision making should still be at the physicians' discretion. Since AI results in producing automated decisions, this can lead to a decision-making bias as physicians can be more likely to trust diagnostic test results by AI-led machines without intense scrutiny.Consequently, there is a gray area as to with whom the responsibility lies in the case of an error. Data interpretation with AI can be susceptible to selection bias as well . This is because the results AI produces are dependent upon the data entered. Therefore, if there is poor data entry, the results lead to invalid assumptions without a fair, accurate representation. Furthermore, another limitation of newer models of AI is the ability to reproduce and standardize the method . It is difficult to compare diagnostic results from different providers if they are analyzing the data with varying techniques.

Table 3.2 Pertinent publications regarding artificial intelligence.

Pertinent Publications Related to Artificial Intelligence in the Field of Cardiovascular Imaging	Findings in Publication
Improved accuracy of myocardial perfusion single-photon emission computed tomography [SPECT] for the detection of coronary artery disease using a support vector machine algorithm	Arsajani et al. found that the accuracy of predicting CAD with an MPI device improved significantly when in adjunct with a learning algorithm
Fully Automated Echocardiogram Interpretation in Clinical Practice	Zhang et al. determined 96% accuracy in identifying images with echocardiography
Machine learning of clinical variables and coronary artery calcium scoring for the prediction of obstructive coronary artery disease on coronary computed tomography angiography: analysis from the CONFIRM registry	Al'Aref et al.'s results showed a significantly more accurate assessment of obstructive CAD from CT imaging using machine learning with the coronary artery calcium score
Cardiac Imaging on the Cusp of an Artificial Intelligence Revolution	Laser et al. determined that the right ventricle reconstruction with echocardiography and cardiac MRI had more accuracy compared to the gold standard direct cardiac MRI

New AI Can Automatically Detect a Serious Heart Condition

Utilizing intravascular optical coherence tomography images, a new technique made it easier to identify plaque erosion

Researchers have created a brand-new artificial intelligence (AI) technique that uses optical coherence tomography (OCT) images to automatically detect plaque erosion in the arteries of the heart. Monitoring arterial plaque is crucial because, if it disintegrates, it may obstruct blood flow to the heart, triggering a heart attack or other dangerous problems "If cholesterol plaque lining arteries starts to erode it can lead to a sudden reduction in blood flow to the heart known as acute coronary syndrome, which requires urgent treatment," said research team leader Zhao Wang from the University of Electronic Science and Technology of China. "Our new method could help improve the clinical diagnosis of plaque erosion and be used to develop new treatments for patients with heart disease."

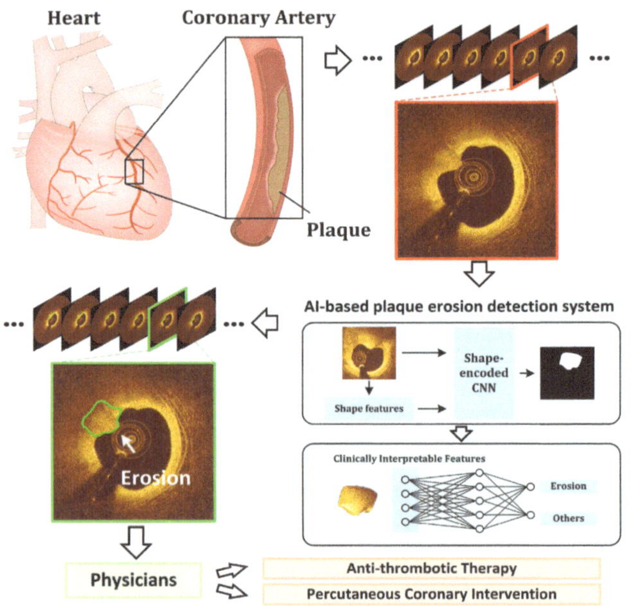

Fig.3.3 Researchers have developed a new AI method that can automatically detect plaque erosion in arteries using OCT images. This type of erosion can block blood flow to the heart, leading to a heart attack or other serious conditions. Credit: Zhao Wang, University of Electronic Science and Technology of China

OCT is an optical imaging technique with micron-scale resolution that may be utilized within blood vessels to produce 3D pictures of the coronary arteries, which carry blood to the heart. Although intravascular OCT is being used by doctors more frequently to check for plaque erosion, there is a substantial level of interobserver variability because of the volume of data generated and the difficulty of visually interpreting the images. In order to address this issue, Wang collaborated with a team of engineers from his institution and medical professionals from The 2nd Affiliated Hospital of Harbin Medical University under the direction of Bo Yu to create an automated, objective method that uses AI to identify plaque erosion based on OCT images. They explain the new method in the Optica Publishing Group journal Biomedical Optics Express and demonstrate that it is accurate enough to possibly serve as the foundation for clinical diagnosis. "Our new AI-based method can automatically detect the presence of plaque erosion using the original OCT images without any additional input," said Wang. "The ability to detect plaque erosion objectively and automatically will reduce the laborious manual assessment associated with diagnosis."

Applying AI

The new method consists of two primary steps. First, an AI model known as a neural network uses the original image and two pieces of shape information to predict regions of possible plaque erosion. The initial prediction is then refined with a post-processing algorithm based on clinically interpretable features that mimic the knowledge professional physicians use to make a diagnosis. "We had to develop a new AI model that incorporates explicit shape information, the key feature used to identify plaque erosion in OCT images," said Wang. "The underlying intravascular OCT imaging technology is also crucial because it is currently the highest resolution imaging modality that can be used to diagnose plaque erosion in living patients."

When OCT is used for intravascular imaging, the imaging probe is automatically pulled backward inside a catheter, producing hundreds of images for each pullback. The researchers tested their method using 16 pullbacks of 5,553 clinical OCT images with plaque erosion and 10 pullbacks of 3,224 images without plaque erosion. The automated method correctly predicted 80 percent of the plaque erosion cases with a positive predictive value of 73 percent. They also found that diagnoses based on the automated method matched well with those from three experienced physicians

"Although further safety validation and regulatory approval are needed for stand-alone clinical use in patients, the technique could be used to facilitate diagnosis of plaque erosion," said Wang. "This would involve physicians making a final check of the algorithm's finding and then determining the cause of acute coronary syndrome and the best treatmentstrategies.

Studying new treatments

The method could also be useful for analyzing the massive amounts of existing OCT data by eliminating the time-consuming and tedious process of manual image analysis. This could help scientists improve the identification and treatment of plaque erosion. For example, a stent is often used to recover reduced blood flow in patients with acute coronary syndrome, but recent studies suggest that some medications might offer a less-invasive alternative.

"Intravascular imaging, accompanied with AI technologies,

It can be an extremely valuable tool for diagnosis of coronary artery disease and treatment planning," said Wang. "In the future, this new approach could help physicians develop individualized treatment strategies for optimal management of patients with acute coronary syndrome."

The researchers are now working to improve their new technique by better incorporating 3D information and incorporating more unlabeled data to improve the AI model's performance. In the future, they also plan to use a larger dataset that includes a global population for training and evaluating the algorithm. They also want to explore how it might be used in various clinical situations to further demonstrate its potential utility and value.

Future Applications of Artificial Intelligence

As newer techniques are emerging, AI is constantly expanding beyond its limits and capabilities. Within the field of medicine, it has the potential to lead to newer advances in drug therapies as well as diagnoses of diseases at an earlier stage . It is anticipated that AI will have the ability in the future to fully automate reading echocardiography images and detecting pathology . Furthermore, it allows treatment plans to become more standardized based on an automated process. With AI completing tasks at a quicker rate, physicians have more time to be free from mundane tasks such as data input and electronic health records to focus on educating the patient and fostering a stronger patient–physician relationship Although AI holds great potential for the future of medicine, physicians should still be responsible for making the final clinical judgment.

Bibliography and Acknowledgement

- Al'Aref S.J., Anchouche K., Singh G., Slomka P.J., Kolli K.K., Kumar A., Pandey M., Maliakal G., van Rosendael A.R., Beecy A.N., et al. Clinical applications of machine learning in cardiovascular disease and its relevance to cardiac imaging. Eur. Heart J. 2019;40:1975–1986.
- Al'Aref S.J., Maliakal G., Singh G., van Rosendael A.R., Ma X., Xu Z., Alawamlh O.A.H., Lee B., Pandey M., Achenbach S., et al. Machine learning of clinical variables and coronary artery calcium scoring for the prediction of obstructive coronary artery disease on coronary computed tomography angiography: Analysis from the CONFIRM registry. Eur. Hear. J. 2019;41:359–367.
- Alsharqi M., Woodward W., Mumith A., Markham D., Upton R., Leeson P. Artificial intelligence and echocardiography. Echo Res. Pract. 2018;5:R115–R125.
- Amisha P.M., Pathania M., Rathaur V.K. Overview of artificial intelligence in medicine. J. Fam. Med. Prim. Care. 2019;8:2328–2331
- Arafati A., Hu P., Finn J.P., Rickers C., Cheng A.L., Jafarkhani H., Kheradvar A. Artificial intelligence in pediatric and adult congenital cardiac MRI: An unmet clinical need. Cardiovasc. Diagn. Ther. 2019;9:S310–S325.
- Arsanjani R., Xu Y., Dey D., Fish M., Dorbala S., Hayes S., Berman D., Germano G., Slomka P. Improved Accuracy of Myocardial Perfusion SPECT for the Detection of Coronary Artery Disease Using a Support Vector Machine Algorithm. J. Nucl. Med. 2013;54:549–555
- Buch V.H., Ahmed I., Maruthappu M. Artificial intelligence in medicine: Current trends and future possibilities. Br. J. Gen. Pr. 2018;68:143–144.
- Di Jiang M., Zhang X.L., Liu H., Tang C.X., Li J.H., Wang Y.N., Xu P.P., Zhou C.S., Zhou F., Lu M.J., et al. The effect of coronary calcification on diagnostic performance of machine learning–based CT-FFR: A Chinese multicenter study. Eur. Radiol. 2020;31:1482–1493.
- Dorado-Díaz P.I., Sampedro-Gómez J., Vicente-Palacios V., Sánchez P.L. Applications of Artificial Intelligence in Cardiology. The Future is Already Here. Rev. Española Cardiol. 2019;72:1065–1075.
- Eiman Jahangir M.D., Fractional Flow Reserve (FFR) Measurement . Medscape; 2021. [(accessed on 9 January 2022)]. Fractional Flow Reserve (FFR) Measurement. Background, Indications, Outcomes. Background, Indications, Outcomes.
- El-Tallawi K.C., Aljizeeri A., Nabi F., Al-Mallah M.H. Myocardial Perfusion Imaging Using Positron Emission Tomography. Methodist DeBakey Cardiovasc. J. 2020;16:114–121. doi: 10.14797/mdcj-16-2-114.
- Fractional Flow Reserve—Computed Tomography: Heart Care in NJ. RWJBarnabas Health. [(accessed on 9 January 2022)].
- Gottdiener J.S., Bednarz J., Devereux R., Gardin J., Klein A., Manning W.J., Morehead A., Kitzman D., Oh J., Quinones M., et al. American Society of Echocardiography recommendations for use of echocardiography in clinical trials. J. Am. Soc. Echocardiogr. 2004;17:1086–1119.
- Hamet P., Tremblay J. Artificial Intelligence in medicine. Metabolism. 2017;69:S36–S40.
- Haoyue Sun, Chen Zhao, Yuhan Qin, Chao Li, Haibo Jia, Bo Yu and Zhao Wang, "In vivo detection of plaque erosion by intravascular optical coherence tomography using artificial intelligence"16 June 2022, Biomedical Optics Express. DOI: 10.1364/BOE.459623
- IBM Supervised vs. Unsupervised Learning: What's the Difference? [(accessed on 9 January 2021)]. Available online: https://www.ibm.com/cloud/blog/supervised-vs-unsupervised-learning
- Immonen E., Wong J., Nieminen M., Kekkonen L., Roine S., Törnroos S., Lanca L., Guan F., Metsälä E. The use of deep learning towards dose optimization in low-dose computed tomography: A scoping review. Radiography. 2021;28:208–214.
- Itchhaporia D. Artificial intelligence in cardiology. Trends Cardiovasc. Med. 2020;32:34–41. doi: 10.1016/j.tcm.2020.11.007
- Kabani A., El-Sakka M.R. Object Detection and Localization Using Deep Convolutional Networks with Softmax Activation and Multi-class Log Loss. In: Campilho A., Karray F., editors. Image Analysis and Recognition. Springer International Publishing; Cham, Switzerland: 2016. pp. 358–366.
- Knaapen P. Computed Tomography to Replace Invasive Coronary Angiography? Circ. Cardiovasc. Imaging. 2019;12:e008710.
- Kuehn B.M. Cardiac Imaging on the Cusp of an Artificial Intelligence Revolution. Circulation. 2020;141:1266–1267.
- Lim L.J., Tison G.H., Delling F.N. Artificial Intelligence in Cardiovascular Imaging. Methodist DeBakey Cardiovasc. J. 2020;16:138–145. doi: 10.14797/mdcj-16-2-138.
- Lin A., Kolossváry M., Motwani M., Išgum I., Maurovich-Horvat P., Slomka P.J., Dey D. Artificial intelligence in cardiovascular CT: Current status and future implications. J. Cardiovasc. Comput. Tomogr. 2021;15:462–469.
- Mathur P., Srivastava S., Xu X., Mehta J.L. Artificial Intelligence, Machine Learning, and Cardiovascular Disease. Clin. Med. Insights Cardiol. 2020;14
- McCollough C., Leng S. Use of artificial intelligence in computed tomography dose optimisation. Ann. ICRP. 2020;49:113–125.
  Merge PACS—Overview. IBM. (n.d.) [(accessed on 14 November 2021)]. Available online: https://www.ibm.com/products/merge-pacs
- Miller R. IBM Buying Merge Healthcare for $1B to Bring Medical Image Analysis to Watson Health. TechCrunch. Aug 6, 2015. [(accessed on 14 November 2021)].
- Momentum Janitorial Ai-Enabled Robotic Surgery: How Collaborative Robots are Assisting Surgeons. Far North Surgery. Oct 18, 2020.
- Motwani M., Dey D., Berman D.S., Germano G., Achenbach S., Al-Mallah M., Andreini D., Budoff M.J., Cademartiri F., Callister T.Q., et al. Machine learning for prediction of all-cause mortality in patients with suspected coronary artery disease: A 5-year multicentre prospective registry analysis. Eur. Hear. J. 2016;38:500–507.
- Muscogiuri G., Van Assen M., Tesche C., De Cecco C.N., Chiesa M., Scafuri S., Guglielmo M., Baggiano A., Fusini L., Guaricci A.I., et al. Artificial Intelligence in Coronary Computed Tomography Angiography: From Anatomy to Prognosis. BioMed Res. Int. 2020;2020:6649410.
- Narula S., Shameer K., Omar A.M.S., Dudley J.T., Sengupta P.P. Machine-Learning Algorithms to Automate Morphological and Functional Assessments in 2D Echocardiography. J. Am. Coll. Cardiol. 2016;68:2287–2295.
  Rajih E., Tholomier C., Cormier B., Samouëlian V., Warkus T.,
- Liberman M., Widmer H., Lattouf J.-B., Alenizi A.M., Meskawi M., et al. Error reporting from the da Vinci surgical system in robotic surgery: A Canadian multispecialty experience at a single academic centre. Can. Urol. Assoc. J. 2017;11:E197–E202.

- Seetharam K., Brito D., Farjo P.D., Sengupta P.P. The Role of Artificial Intelligence in Cardiovascular Imaging: State of the Art Review. Front. Cardiovasc. Med. 2020;7:618849
- Seetharam K., Raina S., Sengupta P.P. The Role of Artificial Intelligence in Echocardiography. Curr. Cardiol. Rep. 2020;22:99
- Seetharam K., Shresthra S., Mills J.D., Sengupta P.P. Artificial Intelligence in Nuclear Cardiology: Adding Value to Prognostication. Curr. Cardiovasc. Imaging Rep. 2019;12:14.
- Shah S.J., Katz D., Selvaraj S., Burke M.A., Yancy C.W., Gheorghiade M., Bonow R.O., Huang C.-C., Deo R.C. Phenomapping for Novel Classification of Heart Failure with Preserved Ejection Fraction. Circulation. 2015;131:269–279.
- Shameer K., Johnson K., Glicksberg B., Dudley J.T., Sengupta P.P. Machine learning in cardiovascular medicine: Are we there yet? Heart. 2018;104:1156–1164. doi: 10.1136/heartjnl-2017-311198.
- Siegersma K., Leiner T., Chew D., Appelman Y., Hofstra L., Verjans J. Artificial intelligence in cardiovascular imaging: State of the art and implications for the imaging cardiologist. Neth. Hear. J. 2019;27:403–413
- Using AI to Facilitate Diagnosis Harvard-MIT Health Sciences and Technology. 2021. [(accessed on 9 January 2022)]. Available online: https://hst.mit.edu/news-events/using-ai-facilitate-diagnosis
- Van Hamersvelt R.W., Zreik M., Voskuil M., Viergever M.A., Išgum I., Leiner T. Deep learning analysis of left ventricular myocardium in CT angiographic intermediate-degree coronary stenosis improves the diagnostic accuracy for identification of functionally significant stenosis. Eur. Radiol. 2018;29:2350–2359.
- West D.M. What is Artificial Intelligence? Brookings Institution. 2019. [(accessed on 28 October 2021
- Yang S., Koo B.-K., Hoshino M., Lee J.M., Murai T., Park J., Zhang J., Hwang D., Shin E.-S., Doh J.-H., et al. CT Angiographic and Plaque Predictors of Functionally Significant Coronary Disease and Outcome Using Machine Learning. JACC Cardiovasc. Imaging. 2020;14:629–641
- Yu A.C., Eng J. One Algorithm May Not Fit All: How Selection Bias Affects Machine Learning Performance. RadioGraphics. 2020;40:1932–1937.
- Zhang J., Gajjala S., Agrawal P., Tison G.H., Hallock L.A., Beussink-Nelson L., Lassen M.H., Fan E., Aras M.A., Jordan C., et al. Fully Automated Echocardiogram Interpretation in Clinical Practice. Circulation. 2018;138:1623–1635.
- Zhang N., Yang G., Gao Z., Xu C., Zhang Y., Shi R., Keegan J., Xu L., Zhang H., Fan Z., et al. Deep learning for diagnosis of chronic myocardial infarction on nonen-hanced cardiac cine MRI. Radiology. 2019;291:606–617.
- Zhang X.-D. A Matrix Algebra Approach to Artificial Intelligence. Springer; Singapore: 2020. Machine learning; pp. 223–440

CHAPTER 4

Artificial Intelligence in Hypertension Management

Arterial hypertension (AH) is a global public health problem, and its treatment is primarily aimed at reducing associated cardiovascular (CV) morbidity and mortality. AH affected more than 1.13 billion individuals in 2015, and the prevalence appears to affect approximately 35–45% of Campo's overall population. Moreover, AH is the most significant contributor to the global burden of CV diseases and represents a heavy socio-economic burden for many countries . indeed, even moderate elevations in arterial blood pressure (BP) are associated with a significant reduction in life expectancy Furthermore, current data suggest that over 14 million people are unaware of their abnormal BP level; consequently, they are not receiving appropriate medication for it, nor do they engage in other interventions to maintain BP in the normal range Regardless of guidelines, BP control in hypertensive patients in treatment is insufficient due to many factors, including poor adherence to therapy . Moreover, the definition of "hypertension" recapitulates several different sub-phenotypes influenced, by multiple variables: gender , BMI ,lifestyle conditions, and so on . Furthermore, the pharmacological therapy used to treat essential AH has remained substantially unchanged in the last 20 years and is mainly focused on regulating vascular resistance Therefore, there is an evident gap in the knowledge required to deepen the multifaced aspects of AH and prompt the research and development of novel approaches.In this scenario, the possibility of collecting, storing, and analyzing multiple pieces of information from a single patient in the form of electronic health records (EHRs) requires revising the conventional healthcare model of AH management using new technologies or monitoring techniques In this context, artificial intelligence (AI) is a technological method that has been in development in recent years, and, if used appropriately, it could have surprising results in developing predictive models of AH, formulating the diagnosis, stratifying patients, and identifying the most effective therapy

Table 4.1. AI application in hypertension management.

	Applications	Benefits
Measuring BP	Estimate BP by analyzing PPG signal with ML and DL algorithms	Self-monitoring BP for hypertension
Predicting AH development	Predict the risk of developing AH by using genetics, medical data, and behavioral, environmental, and socioeconomic factors.	Timely intervention
Diagnosing AH	Accurately diagnosing AH by using CV risk factors, anthropometric data, vital signs, and laboratory data.	Precision diagnosis
Predicting AH treatment success	Identify factors contributing to treatment success	Personalized treatment plan
Predicting AH prognosis	Stratify patients and predict CV outcomes	Treatment plan adjustment

AI: artificial intelligence; BP: blood pressure; PPG: photoplethysmograph; ML: machine learning; DL: deep learning; AH: arterial hypertension; CV: cardiovascular.

Specifically, accurate BP estimation is essential because BP is a risk factor for many clinical CV events, including stroke and dementia, and therefore can be integrated into several models for risk stratification moreover, in the computational simulation of CV disease, BP can influence the value of focal hemodynamic metrics, e.g., fractional flow]; consequently, patient-specific BP values can improve the accuracy of simulation results and have been applied in some recent models .

Therefore, AI-based systems might change clinical practice for AH by identifying patient trajectories for new, personalized care plans and predicting patients' risks and necessary therapy adjustments due to changes in disease progression and/or therapy response. Accordingly, a basic knowledge of this science is essential because AI might change medical practice jobs: tiring and routine tasks could be completed by computers to free up time and allow cardiologists to carry out more difficult and sensitive tasks. Therefore, in this review, we describe multiple applications of AI, encompassing diagnostic, prognostic, and therapeutic issues currently unsolved in managing AH Overall, this manuscript aims to provide a complete picture of the state of the art of AI in AH (primary and secondary) management, analyzing every aspect of the diagnosis, treatment, and patient follow-up, without neglecting the limitations and all of the possible tools to overcome them.

The Principles of AI

AI is a wide-ranging branch of computer science concerned with building smart machines capable of increasing their knowledge through an automatic learning process that typically requires human intelligence . Therefore, AI is an interdisciplinary science with multiple approaches that incorporate reasoning (making inferences using data), natural language processing (ability to read and understand human languages), planning (ability to act autonomously and flexibly to create a sequence of actions to achieve a final goal), and machine learning (ML) (algorithms that develop automatically through experience) . Specifically, AI based on ML techniques is used to perform predictive analyses by examining mechanisms and associations among given variables from training datasets, which may consist of a variety of data inputs, including wearable devices, multi-omics, and standardized EHRs Essentially, in ML, the rules would be learned by algorithms directly from a set of data rather than being encoded by hand ,consequently, by using specific algorithms, ML can establish complex relationships among data, rules governing a system, behavioral patterns, and classification schemes .The classic ML process begins with data acquisition, continues with feature extraction, algorithm selection, and model development, and leads to model evaluation and application Supervised and unsupervised learning are the most popular approaches employed in ML.

Supervised learning is used to predict unknown outputs from a known labeled dataset, hypotheses, and appropriate algorithms, such as an artificial neural network (ANN), support vector machine (SVM), and K-nearest neighbor. The choice of the technique depends on the dataset's features, number of variables, learning curve, training, and computationtime. Specifically, supervised learning provides predictions from big data analytics but requires manually labeled datasets and biases that can arise from the dataset itself or the algorithms .On the other hand, in unsupervised learning techniques, there is no information on the features to be predicted; consequently, these techniques must learn from the relationships among the elements of a dataset and classify them without basing them on categories or labels . Therefore, they look for structures, patterns, or characteristics in the source data that can be reproduced in new datasets ML mainly mimics the nervous system's structure by creating ANNs, which are networks of units called artificial neurons structured into layers .The system learns to generate patterns from data entered in the training session .A specific ANN, consisting of more layers that allow for improved predictions from data, is known as a deep neural network (DNN). Its performance could be enhanced as the dimension of the training dataset rises . Still, it largely depends on the distribution gap between training and test datasets: a highly divergent test dataset would test an ML prediction model on a feature space that it was not trained on, resulting in poor testing and results; additionally, a highly overlapping test dataset would not test the model for its generalization ability .

Specifically, DL employs algorithms such as DNNs and convolutional neural networks (CNNs. Nevertheless, regardless of its capability of using unlabeled datasets, unsupervised learning still has some limitations, such as the generalizability of cluster patterns identified from a cohort of patients, which can lead to overfitting to the training dataset, and the need to be validated in different large datasets . In the real world, AI can provide tools to improve and extend the effectiveness of clinical interventions. For example, incorporating AI into hypertension management could improve every stage of patient care, from diagnosis to therapy; consequently, the clinical practice could become more efficient and effective.

Methods

We conducted a detailed search on AI applications in AH. The research includes topics ranging from big data to complex technology-based interventions. Specifically, the articles reviewed in this paper were obtained by searching journal databases such as PubMed and subject-specific professional websites, including Google Scholar. The search terms included artificial intelligence, artificial neural network, deep learning, machine learning, big data, arterial

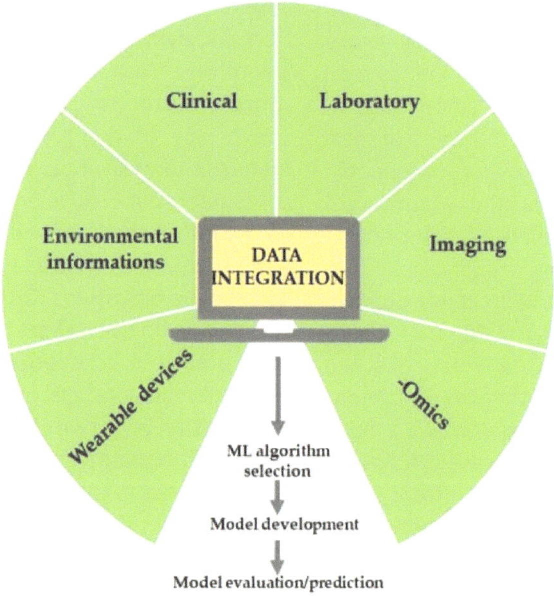

Fig. 4.1. The typical ML workflow in healthcare research.

hypertension, blood pressure, blood pressure measurement, CV disease, and personalized medicine. The inclusion criteria focus on articles directly or indirectly related to the topic of AI and AH. Specifically, both quantitative (measurable data) and qualitative (reasons, opinions, and motivations) reports were reviewed.

The authors independently screened titles and abstracts; subsequently, full texts were sourced for relevant articles. The reference lists of included trials and meta-analyses were also reviewed for significant articles.

AI in the Measurement of Blood Pressure

The commonly used methods for BP monitoring are either non-invasive inflatable cuff-based oscillometric or invasive arterial line manometric measurement. The former takes intermittent measures because a pause of at least 1–2 min between two BP measurements is necessary to avoid errors in the measurement , moreover, the inflation of the cuff may disturb the patient, and the consequences of these disturbances are alterations in BP . On the other hand, invasive arterial line manometric measurement has an elevated risk of complications; consequently, these unsolved issues drive the search for new non-invasive BP monitoring techniques.In this scenario, AI algorithms could help improve precision, accuracy, and reproducibility in diagnosing and managing AH using emerging wearable technologies. Alternatives for monitoring BP are cuff-based devices (such as volume-clamp devices or wrist-worn inflatable cuffs) and cuffless devices that use mechanical and optical sensors to determine features of the blood pulse waveform shape (for example, tonometry, photoplethysmography , andcapacitance. In particular, cuffless blood pressure monitoring has been evaluated using a two-step algorithm with a single-channel photoplethysmograph (PPG). This system achieved an AAMI/ISO standard accuracy in all blood pressure categories except systolic hypotension . Independently of the acquisition method, the received signals are preprocessed and sent for feature extraction and selection. Subsequently, the signals and the gathered data can be used to feed ML to obtain systolic BP (SBP) and diastolic BP (DBP) estimations from the raw signals . Since the volume and distension of arteries can be related to the pressure in the arteries, the PPG signal produces pulse waveforms that are similar to pressure waveforms created by tonometry. PPG offers the added advantage that it can be measured continuously using miniature, inexpensive, and wearable optical electronics . However, PPG signal measurements are not without technical challenges; indeed, they require noise elimination, multisite measurement, multiphotodector development, event detection, event visualization, different models, the accurate positioning of sensors, and the calculation of propagation distances, without neglecting the impact of the variable PEP time on the pulse wave velocity timing . Moreover, there are several PPG-based methods for estimating BP: the PPG signal alone and its derivate, ECG and PPG signals, BCG and PPG signals, and PCG and PPG signals; each has advantages and limitations ,which, however, are beyond this discussion.

ML Algorithms in BP Estimation

To adapt to the nonlinearity of the dataset and to create a relationship between features and estimated BP, there are different ML approaches

1. **Gaussian Process Regression:** A Bayesian regression approach gives a probability distribution over all possible values
2. **Ensemble trees:** The idea is to pull together a set of weak learners to create a strong learner
3. **Multivariate Linear Regression:** It is a method to analyze the correlation, correlation direction, and strength between multiple independent variables and the dependent variable
4. **Support vector regression:** It is a non-parametric algorithm that uses a kernel function (a class of algorithms for pattern analysis, whose general task is to find and study relations in datasets
5. **Random forest, gradient boosting,** and adaptive boosting regression CNN

After hyper-parameter optimization, it is necessary to evaluate the performance of ML algorithms through the correlation between the acquired predicted data and the ground-truth data. The difference between reference and estimated BP could be considered using the following criteria: the mean absolute error, mean squared error, and correlation coefficient.The role of parameter optimization is to lower the value of the predicted error. The mean absolute and standard deviations are the model's predictive performance indicators. Specifically, these AI-based systems could help continuously monitor BP using wearable technologies and improve AH management and outcomes.. Starting from the input (raw signals), we can reach the output (estimated SBP and DBP) through the algorithms of ML . In particular, BP can be estimated from a PPG signal obtained from a smartphone or a smartwatch by using DL Moreover, future studies on AI and wearable devices need to confirm the above results and provide conclusive clinical data to support using a combination of AI and wearable-device-obtained data to correctly perform BP measurements, which may offer an alternative to current oscillometric methods

Use of AI for the Prediction of Undiagnosed Hypertension

AH is generally asymptomatic or variably occurs with symptoms such as headache, dizziness, tinnitus, and nosebleeds in a minority of patients. For this reason, it is not always possible to readily identify and predict this

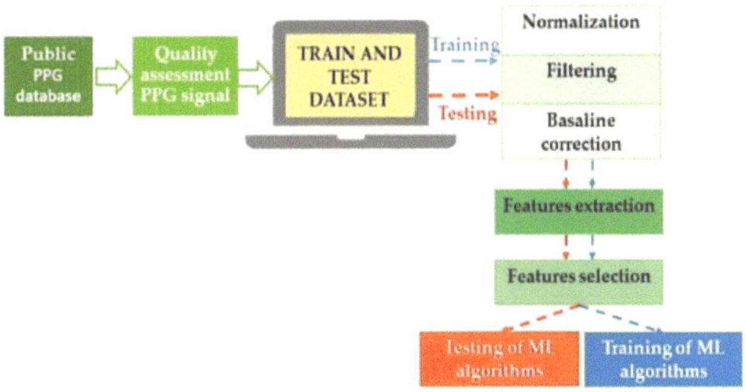

Fig. 4.2. Block diagram of the blood pressure estimation process using ML techniques. In detail, the raw signals are prepared through normalization, the correction of baseline wandering due to respiration, and finally, signal filtration. Specifically, to construct a dataset for BP estimation models, it is necessary to accurately extract the features of the original waveform (and underlying demographic and statistical data) and select effective features, improving the generalization and reducing the risk of overfitting the algorithms. PPG: photoplethysmograph; ML: machine learning.

disease The goal should be to implement primary and secondary prevention methods. This task could greatly benefit AI implementation, featuring the individual identification of each patient's previous and new CV risk factors and treating modifiable risk factors. AI can predict the patient's risk of AH development thanks to different algorithm settings with big sets of data. Predicting AH onset has been attempted in the last decade with progressively greater precision thanks to technological advancements.

Accordingly, risk factors for AH, such as low levels of education, a sedentary job, a family history of AH, demographic data, routine blood tests, BMI, waist and hip circumference and ratio, diet, physical exercise, and salt and alcohol intake, showed effectiveness in predicting elevated SBP using ML techniques, for instance, an ANN . On the other hand, AI techniques are also emerging in gene expression analysis; specifically, it is possible to improve AH predictive models by integrating data from a combination of gene expression and next-generation sequencing in ML analysis . Furthermore, thanks to ML algorithms, it is possible to identify new hypertension genes; accordingly, Li et al, analyzed gene expression in hypertensive patients, thus identifying 177 new hypertension genes thanks to ML algorithm development: this was then integrated with environmental factors in evaluating the risk of AH.Furthermore, health risk prediction using a DL architecture appears suitable for extensive complex datasets, as shown by Maxwell et al. . Using physical examination records of 110,300 patients, it was possible to examine, classify, and learn each risk factor contributing to chronic diseases such as AH, diabetes, and liver steatosis .

With the same principle, Ye et al. validated an accurate 1-year risk prediction model for the incidence of essential AH. In this retrospective and prospective study, risk factors (type 2 diabetes, dyslipidemias, CV diseases, etc.) were calculated, evaluated, and stratified, yielding an accuracy of 91.7% for the prediction of the AH incidence at 1 year, with 87% in the prospective cohort (validation)

Furthermore, the AI risk assessment of AH development can also benefit from cardiorespiratory fitness data obtained from treadmill exercise stress testing. Overall, AI has the potential to increase efficacy by aggregating immense volumes of information, virtually predicting the risk of AH and consequently preventing or delaying the development of this disease by directing early interventions.

Making the AH diagnosis using validated guidelines , is an easy task for AI. Using inputs such as BP, comorbidities, demographic data, and routine blood tests, the accuracy can reach 92.85% with an ANN . With a similar dataset (age, BP, BMI, serum lipoproteins profile, smoking habit, and exercise), using ML, the accuracy is estimated at 82%.. The most common example of AI for AH diagnosis, and probably still the most accurate, is twenty-four-hour ambulatory BP monitoring (ABPM) . Thanks to direct and regular interval BP measurements and a relatively easy algorithm, ABPM software can identify and classify AH. ABPM is particularly useful in correctly evaluating white coats and masked AH. New approaches based on ANNs try to estimate BP for AH diagnosis in healthy individuals using factors such as BMI, age, exercise, smoking, and alcohol consumption, although with limited accuracy and efficacy . An interesting method for SBP prediction is the use of retinal fundus images. This factor was used by Poplin et al. who showed that DL could be used in this case, even if the BP error was 11.23 mmHg, clearly not accurate enough to be of diagnostic use. The ability of AI to diagnose AH is dependent on its accuracy. Further studies will identify more methods of BP prediction for the early diagnosis of AH and complication prevention. Looking at the world around us, AI's future in AH diagnosis and management probably lies in systems that can constantly retrieve vital signs, such as smartphones, smartwatches, and all of the relative accessories .

Targeting AH by AI

Optimizing pharmacological therapy to achieve the optimal control of BP levels represents a tough challenge for physicians. The management of AH is based on evidence-based medicine and expert opinions; BP control rates remain poor worldwide and are far from satisfactory across Europe Specifically, the importance of AI in this field is in the robust identification of modifiable factors that impact the evolution of AH, moreover , this new instrument could supportthe choice of the most appropriate management of AH. Indeed, most hypertensive patients need medication and lifestyle changes to achieve optimal BP control, and AI is helpful due to its better capability of identifying the best combination therapy compared to standard analysis. Several works discussed and analyzed the opportunity of using AI to evaluate the impacts of different factors on BP values. Koren et al. applied ANN and decision trees to identify parameters contributing to Campo's success in his AH drug treatment . Indeed, ML algorithms allow better real-world data analysis, identifying patterns and trends not easily recognized with classical experimental or observational approaches. Randomized trials usually compare the effectiveness of a drug to a placebo or, at best, to an already-approved compound. However, evaluating the differences between and advantages of drug combinations, frequently necessary for AH treatment, is a more complex task,that AI could fulfill. Here, we provide some previous experience and approaches; for example, the computer was presented with a training dataset in the first training phase, and for each instance, it was given the correct classification. Specifically, the appropriate classification of the algorithm was divided into two reference categories: "treatment success", defined as BP lower than 140/90 mmHg within 90 days after starting therapy, and "treatment failure" in any other case. Finally, AI decision trees and ANN compared various classes of antihypertensives in patients: beta-blockers alone or in combination were the most effective In another study, ML methods predicted individual treatment effects of intensive BP therapy notably, the results revealed an improvement in the discrimination and calibration of individualized medications from clinical trial data. Moreover, Ye X. et al. demonstrated the potential of using predictive models to select optimal AH treatment pathways; specifically, along with clinical guidelines and guideline-based CDS systems, the LSTM models show the best prediction for achieving the optimal control of BP with different combinations of treatments. ML can also detect adherence to antihypertensive therapy by analyzing data recorded from a smartphone application to promote patients' awareness, self-monitoring, and treatment compliance . Nonetheless, the exploitation of AI in the healthcare field is still in its early phases, and its potential is not entirely explored. Indeed, AI represents the opportunity for a global evaluation of the patient in his or her complexity because it allows the integration of clinical, demographic, biochemical, and instrumental data to develop models that physicians and healthcare providers could use to improve AH management and test new drug therapies using the multi-omics method.

We are now entering an era in which omics-based technology evolution will start to deliver long-promised elements that may improve the understanding of the complex mechanistic basis of this disease. Accordingly, the key to better disease management will pass through personalized medicine. The key to this is future drug discovery that will be possible thanks to enhanced AI technologies exploiting information integration. Data from sequenced genomes, functional genomics, protein profiling, metabolomics, and bioinformatics may ensure a better comprehensive systems-based analysis for further understanding AH disease's complexities. Integrating AI with omics-based technologies will lead to the definition of the trajectory of the hypertensive patient and the use of the mostappropriatedrug.

In conclusion, AI can improve intelligent healthcare systems that provide personalized recommendations and treatment approaches.

Definition of the Hypertensive Patient's Trajectory: Role of AI in AH Prognosis

According to the recent AHA and ESC guidelines , the evaluation of the prognosis of AH is related to the demographic characteristics, the progression of organ injury, and comorbidities of the patients. Predicting the outcomes of hypertensive patients is significant research work.

There are currently several clinical risk scores Intended for specific populations and risk groups. Nevertheless, most of these scores are based on linear models and might therefore lack specificity and sensitivity in certain subgroups.Moreover, the wide variety of scores may also cause slow adoption in real-world clinical practice The role of AI concerning the prognostic establishment of AH is due to the utility of ML algorithms trained on large datasets to estimate prognoses and potentially guide medical treatments.

The recent focus on AI and ML methods for AH prognosis is related to the critical repercussions of elevated BP for the risk of developing organ damage. Despite commonly used statistical methods, AI systems can process large amounts of complex data. Therefore, AI and ML aim to process a prognostic model that has clinical relevance in managing patients in the real world .The prognostic impact of AH needs the stratification of patients based on their global evaluation with the integration of different parameters, such as the grade and stage of AH, BP control, and concomitant comorbidities. Indeed, AI can stratify patients correctly through the use of classification algorithms (SVM, C4.5 decision tree, random forest (RF), and extreme gradient boosting (XGBoost)); specifically, XGBoost has the best prediction performance .

However, the accuracy of the definition of the individual trajectory can be enhanced by a prolonged follow-up , and an increase in the number of relevant features, such as genomic variants associated with specific hypertensive phenotypes and different outcomes.

Moreover, the prognosis determines the frequency and the type of clinical monitoring. Specifically, AI allows the elaboration of new risk stratification to develop novel prognostic layers in favor of personalized medicine with the prospect of efficiently measuring the grade classification of AH and identifying different outcomes' profiles . In conclusion, the clinical advantages of implementing AI systems and their integration into current prognostic stratification might grant the correct identification of classes of outcomes of patients, improving their clinical management.

AI in Secondary Arterial Hypertension

The causes of hypertension are multiple, and we must not overlook secondary arterial hypertension; indeed, in 10–15% of cases, the specific cause underlying hypertension can be identified . Specifically, to arrive at the diagnosis of essential hypertension, all causes of secondary hypertension must be ruled out, and the accurate history, thorough examination, and performance of all necessary tests based on the data collected always place the physician and his or her knowledge of internal medicine at the basis of the evaluation of each hypertensive patient. Consequently, diagnosis and patient management must be connected to the clinician, who can use AI to speed up and facilitate his or her task. In any case, AI and ML cannot wholly replace the doctor's role, but they represent a useful tool in his hands. Identifying secondary hypertension in its various subtypes is essential to preventing and targeting the treatment of CV complications. However, screening for secondary hypertension can be time-consuming, expensive, and difficult; consequently, simplified diagnostic tests are urgently required to distinguish between primary and secondary hypertension to address the current underdiagnosis of the latter. In children and adolescents, the most common causes of hypertension are renal parenchymal or vascular disease and aortic coarctation in adults, earlier studies identified renal parenchymal and vascular diseases as the most common causes of secondary hypertension. Obstructive sleep apnea (OSA) was recognized as an exceedingly common cause of secondary hypertension . Among endocrine causes, we include primary aldosteronism (the most common), thyroid disease (hypo- or hyperthyroidism),hypercortisolism (Cushing's), and finally, phaeochromocytoma. The application of ML methods to the etiological diagnosis The application of ML methods to the etiological diagnosis of secondary hypertension can be helpful in clinical practice. Accordingly, AI technology should be implemented cautiously; to be a partner of clinicians, there is still a long way to go, but it can serve as a virtual assistant and enable clinicians to promote quality and increase efficiency. Based on EMRs from Fuwai Hospital, five ML prediction models with good performance and applicability to the etiology detection of secondary hypertension were developed by Campo which demonstrated that ML approaches were feasible and effective in diagnosing secondary hypertension. Reel and colleagues showed that the MOmics approach provided better discriminatory power compared to single-omics (monoomics) data analysis and appropriately classified different forms of endocrine hypertension with high sensitivity and specificity, providing potential diagnostic biomarker combinations for diagnosing secondary hypertension subtypes. However, there still needs to be more data in the literature on the application of AI in the field of secondary hypertension; consequently, these innovative and clinically relevant prediction models still require further validation and more clinical tests before being implemented into clinical practice

Limitations of Applying ML in CV Research

Despite the great importance that AI has taken on in the last few years, it is necessary to underline that this system is not free from technical issues and biases . The quality of the algorithms underlying AI technology can be affected by some limitations, such as the inconsistent quality of the studies that form the databases at the heart of AI. Specifically, overfitting is a significant issue common to all ML models: this happens when a model has become overly attuned to the training data, such that it does not generalize to new datasets; this is the opposite of underfitting, where the algorithm cannot wholly capture the predictive power of the data. These two issues (over- and underfitting) could be solved by improving the parameters of the model or making modifications to the training set.Moreover, it is also essential to consider the adversarial robustness of a model (ability to resist being fooled), which could be improved by enlarging the training set.

Furthermore, many clinicians remain wary of ML because of concerns about the "black-box" nature of many ML algorithms. These models are sufficiently complex that they are not directly interpretable to humans. Subsequently, the lack of interpretability of predictive models can undermine trust in those models, especially in the medical field, in which so many decisions are life-and-death issues. To be trusted, users must comprehend the model outputs . Consequently, the "explainability" technique in ML seeks to imbue humans with a high level of understanding of how an algorithm works and makes decisions without carefully considering each step , however, the nature of explanations as approximations may omit important information about how black-box models work and why they make specific predictions.

Another flaw is the lack of discernment of predisposing factors for specific CV diseases from confounding factors. Moreover, it is also possible that, during data analysis processes by specialized clinicians, some may contribute to lowering the accuracy of the databases owing to their biases, thus making their validation even more time-consuming . It would also be necessary for some AI-automated diagnostic CV algorithms to identify CV risk factors that are essential but still not unanimously recognized since, sometimes, there is no consensus among cardiologists. Therefore, it would be desirable to validate data through a clinical consensus before merging them into the AI, though expensive and time-consuming. Another important aspect is the disparity between various racial groups, ethnic minorities, and social classes. Some CV diseases are more represented in some races and/or ethnic minorities and can express themselves with different phenotypes .

Prospectively, it will be necessary to render AI accessible to patients and promote awareness, self-monitoring, healthy behaviors, and therapeutic adherence by integrating new technologies, such as wearable devices that can automatically analyze activity levels and give feedback, such as lifestyle and drug dose changes .

Conclusion

The study of AH needs a revolution, and its future may lie in the favorable convergence of digital data and biotechnological and biomedical sciences and their implementation in healthcare delivery with new delivery models and effective strategies for population health. With AI, we could better understand epigenetic changes relevant to AH onset and progression, potentially classify the risk of AH in individuals, identify the mechanism of poorly controlled AH, and evaluate treatment responses in clinical trials using a multi-omics approach. Furthermore, AI could target healthy individuals who are at higher risk of developing AH and may benefit from lifestyle modifications for the primary prevention of CV disease .

In conclusion, AH prediction and management using a combination of AI and wearable technology could potentially be the first real chance for precision CV medicine . Moreover, future AI-enhanced AH care will encourage patient awareness, self-monitoring, healthy behaviors, and treatment adherence, along with developing digital technologies..Therefore, future research needs to focus on precision AH medicine utilizing AI-based technologies.

Bibliography and Acknowledgement

- Ahuja, A.S. The impact of artificial intelligence in medicine on the future role of the physician. PeerJ 2019, 7, e7702. [Google Scholar] [CrossRef]
- Arar, M.Y.; Hogg, R.J.; Arant, B.S., Jr.; Seikaly, M.G. Etiology of sustained hypertension in children in the southwestern United States. Pediatr. Nephrol. 1994, 8, 186–189. [Google Scholar] [CrossRef]
- Asayama, K.; Thijs, L.; Li, Y.; Gu, Y.M.; Hara, A.; Liu, Y.P.; Zhang, Z.; Wei, F.F.; Lujambio, I.; Mena, L.J.; et al. Setting thresholds to varying blood pressure monitoring intervals differentially affects risk estimates associated with white-coat and masked hypertension in the population. Hypertension 2014, 64, 935–942. [Google Scholar] [CrossRef]
- Banerjee, R.; Choudhury, A.D.; Sinha, A.; Visvanathan, A. HeartSense: Smart phones to estimate blood pressure from photoplethysmography. In Proceedings of the 12th ACM Conference on Embedded Network Sensor Systems, Memphis, TN, USA, 3–6 November 2014. [Google Scholar]
- Bonderman, D. Artificial intelligence in cardiology. Wien. Klin. Wochenschr. 2017, 129, 866–868. [Google Scholar] [CrossRef]
- Bzdok, D.; Krzywinski, M.; Altman, N. Machine learning: Supervised methods. Nat. Methods 2018, 15, 5–6. [Google Scholar] [CrossRef]
- Campbell, N.R.; Chockalingam, A.; Fodor, J.G.; McKay, D.W. Accurate, reproducible measurement of blood pressure. CMAJ 1990, 143, 19–24. [Google Scholar]
- Chaikijurajai, T.; Laffin, L.J.; Tang, W.H.W. Artificial Intelligence and Hypertension: Recent Advances and Future Outlook. Am. J. Hypertens. 2020, 33, 967–974. [Google Scholar] [CrossRef]
- Chang, W.; Liu, Y.; Xiao, Y.; Yuan, X.; Xu, X.; Zhang, S.; Zhou, S. A Machine-Learning-Based Prediction Method for Hypertension Outcomes Based on Medical Data. Diagnostics 2019, 9, 178. [Google Scholar] [CrossRef]
- Chen, J.; Qian, L.; Urakov, T.; Gu, W.; Liang, L. Adversarial Robustness Study of Convolutional Neural Network for Lumbar Disk Shape Reconstruction from MR images. SPIE Med. Imaging Image Process. 2021, 11596, 1159615. [Google Scholar]
- Chen, S.; Ji, Z.; Wu, H.; Xu, Y. A Non-Invasive Continuous Blood Pressure Estimation Approach Based on Machine Learning. Sensors 2019, 19, 2585. [Google Scholar] [CrossRef][Green Version]
- Chowdhury, M.H.; Shuzan, M.N.I.; Chowdhury, M.E.H.; Mahbub, Z.B.; Uddin, M.M.; Khandakar, A.; Reaz, M.B.I. Estimating Blood Pressure from the Photoplethysmogram Signal and Demographic Features Using Machine Learning Techniques. Sensors 2020, 20, 3127. [Google Scholar] [CrossRef]
- Conroy, R.M.; Pyorala, K.; Fitzgerald, A.P.; Sans, S.; Menotti, A.; De Backer, G.; De Bacquer, D.; Ducimetiere, P.; Jousilahti, P.; Keil, U.; et al. Estimation of ten-year risk of fatal cardiovascular disease in Europe: The SCORE project. Eur. Heart J. 2003, 24, 987–1003. [Google Scholar] [CrossRef][Green Version]
- Crea, F. The new SCORE2 risk prediction algorithms and the growing challenge of risk factors not captured by traditional risk scores. Eur. Heart J. 2021, 42, 2403–2407. [Google Scholar] [CrossRef]
- D'Angelo, G.; Della-Morte, D.; Pastore, D.; Donadel, G.; De Stefano, A.; Palmieri, F. Identifying patterns in multiple biomarkers to diagnose diabetic foot using an explainable genetic programming-based approach. Future Gener. Comput. Syst. 2023, 140, 138–150. [Google Scholar] [CrossRef]
- da Silva, V.J.; da Silva Souza, V.; Guimaraes da Cruz, R.; Mesquita Vidal Martinez de Lucena, J.; Jazdi, N.; Ferreira de Lucena Junior, V.Commercial Devices-Based System Designed to Improve the Treatment Adherence of Hypertensive Patients. Sensors 2019, 19, 4539. [Google Scholar] [CrossRef]
- De Luca, V.; Tramontano, G.; Riccio, L.; Trama, U.; Buono, P.; Losasso, M.; Bracale, U.M.; Annuzzi, G.; Zampetti, R.; Cacciatore, F.; et al. "One Health" Approach for Health Innovation and Active Aging in Campania (Italy). Front. Public Health 2021, 9, 658959. [Google Scholar][CrossRef]
- Diciolla, M.; Binetti, G.; Di Noia, T.; Pesce, F.; Schena, F.P.; Vagane, A.M.; Bjorneklett, R.; Suzuki, H.; Tomino, Y.; Naso, D. Patient classification and outcome prediction in IgA nephropathy. Comput. Biol. Med. 2015, 66, 278–286. [Google Scholar] [CrossRef]
- Diller, G.P.; Kempny, A.; Babu-Narayan, S.V.; Henrichs, M.; Brida, M.; Uebing, A.; Lammers, A.E.; Baumgartner, H.; Li, W.; Wort, S.J.; et al. Machine learning algorithms estimating prognosis and guiding therapy in adult congenital heart disease: Data from a single tertiary centre including 10 019 patients. Eur. Heart J. 2019, 40, 1069–1077. [Google Scholar] [CrossRef]
- Dorado-Diaz, P.I.; Sampedro-Gomez, J.; Vicente-Palacios, V.; Sanchez, P.L. Applications of Artificial Intelligence in Cardiology.
- The Future is Already Here. Rev. Esp. Cardiol. Engl. Ed. 2019, 72, 1065–1075. [Google Scholar] [CrossRef]
- Duan, T.; Rajpurkar, P.; Laird, D.; Ng, A.Y.; Basu, S. Clinical Value of Predicting Individual Treatment Effects for Intensive Blood Pressure Therapy. Circ. Cardiovasc. Qual. Outcomes 2019, 12, e005010. [Google Scholar] [CrossRef]
- Dzau, V.J.; Balatbat, C.A. Future of Hypertension. Hypertension 2019, 74, 450–457. [Google Scholar] [CrossRef]
- Elgendi, M.; Fletcher, R.; Liang, Y.; Howard, N.; Lovell, N.H.; Abbott, D.; Lim, K.; Ward, R. The use of photoplethysmography for assessing hypertension. NPJ Digit. Med. 2019, 2, 60. [Google Scholar] [CrossRef]
- Fernandes, M.; Olde Rikkert, M.G.M. The new US and European guidelines in hypertension: A multi-dimensional analysis. Contemp. Clin. Trials 2019, 81, 44–54. [Google Scholar] [CrossRef]
- Gesche, H.; Grosskurth, D.; Kuchler, G.; Patzak, A. Continuous blood pressure measurement by using the pulse transit time: Comparison to a cuff-based method. Eur. J. Appl. Physiol. 2012, 112, 309–315. [Google Scholar] [CrossRef]
- Goldstein, A.; Kapelner, A.; Bleich, J.; Pitkin, E. Peeking inside the black box: Visualizing statistical learning with plots of individual conditional expectation. J. Comput. Graph. Stat. 2015, 24, 44–65. [Google Scholar] [CrossRef]
- Golino, H.F.; Amaral, L.S.; Duarte, S.F.; Gomes, C.M.; Soares Tde, J.; Dos Reis, L.A.; Santos, J. Predicting increased blood pressure using machine learning. J. Obes. 2014, 2014, 637635. [Google Scholar] [CrossRef]
- Hare, A.J.; Chokshi, N.; Adusumalli, S. Novel Digital Technologies for Blood Pressure Monitoring and Hypertension Management. Curr. Cardiovasc. Risk Rep. 2021, 15, 11. [Google Scholar] [CrossRef]
- Held, E.; Cape, J.; Tintle, N. Comparing machine learning and logistic regression methods for predicting hypertension using a combination of gene expression and next-generation sequencing data. BMC Proc. 2016, 10, 141–145. [Google Scholar] [CrossRef]
- Hermida, R.C.; Smolensky, M.H.; Ayala, D.E.; Portaluppi, F. Ambulatory Blood Pressure Monitoring (ABPM) as the

reference standard for diagnosis of hypertension and assessment of vascular risk in adults. Chronobiol. Int. 2015, 32, 1329–1342. [GoogleScholar][CrossRef]

- Huan, T.; Meng, Q.; Saleh, M.A.; Norlander, A.E.; Joehanes, R.; Zhu, J.; Chen, B.H.; Zhang, B.; Johnson, A.D.; Ying, S.; et al. Integrative network analysis reveals molecular mechanisms of blood pressure regulation. Mol. Syst. Biol. 2015, 11, 799. [Google Scholar] [CrossRef]
- Izzo, C.; Vitillo, P.; Di Pietro, P.; Visco, V.; Strianese, A.; Virtuoso, N.; Ciccarelli, M.; Galasso, G.; Carrizzo, A.; Vecchione, C. The Role of Oxidative Stress in Cardiovascular Aging and Cardiovascular Diseases. Life 2021, 11, 60. [Google Scholar] [CrossRef]
- Johnson, K.W.; Torres Soto, J.; Glicksberg, B.S.; Shameer, K.; Miotto, R.; Ali, M.; Ashley, E.; Dudley, J.T. Artificial Intelligence in Cardiology. J. Am. Coll. Cardiol. 2018, 71, 2668–2679. [Google Scholar] [CrossRef]
- Kachuee, M.; Kiani, M.M.; Mohammadzade, H.; Shabany, M. Cuffless Blood Pressure Estimation Algorithms for Continuous Health-Care Monitoring. IEEE Trans. Biomed. Eng. 2017, 64, 859–869.[GoogleScholar][CrossRef]
- Krittanawong, C.; Bomback, A.S.; Baber, U.; Bangalore, S.; Messerli, F.H.; Wilson Tang, W.H. Future Direction for Using Artificial Intelligence to Predict and Manage Hypertension. Curr. Hypertens. Rep. 2018, 20, 75. [Google Scholar] [CrossRef]
- Kumar, P.S.; Rai, P.; Ramasamy, M.; Varadan, V.K.; Varadan, V.K. Multiparametric cloth-based wearable, SimpleSense, estimates blood pressure. Sci. Rep. 2022, 12, 13059.[Google Scholar] [CrossRef]
- Lafrenière, D.; Zulkernine, F.H.; Barber, D.; Martin, K. Using machine learning to predict hypertension from a clinical dataset. In Proceedings of the IEEE Symposium Series on Computational Intelligence (SSCI), Athens, Greece, 6–9 December 2016; pp. 1–7. [GoogleScholar]
- Leng, X.; Lan, L.; Ip, V.H.L.; Liu, H.; Abrigo, J.; Liebeskind, D.S.; Wong, L.K.S.; Leung, T.W. Noninvasive fractional flow in intracranial atherosclerotic stenosis: Reproducibility, limitations, and perspectives. J. Neurol. Sci. 2017, 381, 150–152.
- Li, Y.H.; Zhang, G.G.; Wang, N. Systematic Characterization and Prediction of Human Hypertension Genes. Hypertension 2017, 69, 349–355.[GoogleScholar][CrossRef]
- Mase, M.; Mattei, W.; Cucino, R.; Faes, L.; Nollo, G. Feasibility of cuff-free measurement of systolic and diastolic arterial blood pressure.J.Electrocardiol.2011,44,201–207.
- Miller, D.D. Machine Intelligence in Cardiovascular Medicine. Cardiol. Rev. 2020, 28, 53–64. [Google Scholar] [CrossRef] NCD Risk Factor Collaboration. Worldwide trends in blood pressure from 1975 to 2015: A pooled analysis of 1479 population-based measurement studies with 19.1 million participants. Lancet 2017, 389,37–55.[GoogleScholar][CrossRef]
- O'Brien, E.; Asmar, R.; Beilin, L.; Imai, Y.; Mancia, G.; Mengden, T.; Myers, M.; Padfield, P.; Palatini, P.; Parati, G.; et al. Practice guidelines of the European Society of Hypertension for clinic, ambulatory and self blood pressure measurement. J. Hypertens. 2005,23,697–701.[GoogleScholar][CrossRef]
- Padmanabhan, S.; Tran, T.Q.B.; Dominiczak, A.F. Artificial Intelligence in Hypertension: Seeing Through a Glass Darkly. Circ. Res. 2021, 128, 1100–1118. [Google Scholar] [CrossRef] Wall, H.K.; Ritchey, M.D.; Gillespie, C.; Omura, J.D.; Jamal, A.; George, M.G. Vital Signs: Prevalence of Key Cardiovascular Disease Risk Factors for Million Hearts 2022—United States, 2011–2016. MMWR Morb. Mortal Wkly. Rep. 2018, 67, 983–991.
- Wang, X.; Liu, H.; Xu, M.; Chen, C.; Ma, L.; Dai, F. Efficacy assessment of superficial temporal artery-middle cerebral artery bypass surgery in treating moyamoya disease from a hemodynamic perspective: A pilot study using computational modeling and perfusion imaging. Acta Neurochir. 2023. [Google Scholar] [CrossRef]
- Whitworth, J.A.; World Health Organization; International Society of Hypertension Writing Group. 2003 World Health Organization (WHO)/International Society of Hypertension (ISH) statement on management of hypertension. J. Hypertens. 2003, 21, 1983–1992. [GoogleScholar][CrossRef]
- Williams, B.; Mancia, G.; Spiering, W.; Agabiti Rosei, E.; Azizi, M.; Burnier, M.; Clement, D.L.; Coca, A.; de Simone, G.; Dominiczak, A.; et al. 2018 ESC/ESH Guidelines for the management of arterial hypertension. Eur. Heart J. 2018, 39, 3021–3104. [Google Scholar] [CrossRef]
- Wang, X.; Liu, H.; Xu, M.; Chen, C.; Ma, L.; Dai, F. Efficacy assessment of superficial temporal artery-middle cerebral artery bypass surgery in treating moyamoya disease from a hemodynamic perspective: A pilot study using computational modeling and perfusion imaging. Acta Neurochir. 2023. [Google Scholar] [CrossRef]
- Whitworth, J.A.; World Health Organization; International Society of Hypertension Writing Group. 2003 World Health Organization (WHO)/International Society of Hypertension (ISH) statement on management of hypertension. J. Hypertens. 2003, 21, 1983–1992. [GoogleScholar][CrossRef]
- Williams, B.; Mancia, G.; Spiering, W.; Agabiti Rosei, E.; Azizi, M.; Burnier, M.; Clement, D.L.; Coca, A.; de Simone, G.; Dominiczak, A.; et al. 2018 ESC/ESH Guidelines for the management of arterial hypertension. Eur. Heart J. 2018, 39, 3021–3104. [Google Scholar] [CrossRef]
- Wu, X.; Yuan, X.; Wang, W.; Liu, K.; Qin, Y.; Sun, X.; Ma, W.; Zou, Y.; Zhang, H.; Zhou, X.; et al. Value of a Machine Learning Approach for Predicting Clinical Outcomes in Young Patients With Hypertension. Hypertension 2020, 75, 1271–1278. [Google Scholar] [CrossRef] Yan, C.; Li, Z.; Zhao, W.; Hu, J.; Jia, D.;
- Wang, H.; You, T. Novel Deep Convolutional Neural Network for Cuff-less Blood Pressure Measurement Using ECG and PPG Signals. Annu. Int. Conf. IEEE Eng. Med. Biol. Soc. 2019, 2019, 1917–1920. [GoogleScholar][CrossRef]
- Ye, X.; Zeng, Q.T.; Facelli, J.C.; Brixner, D.I.; Conway, M.; Bray, B.E. Predicting Optimal Hypertension Treatment Pathways Using Recurrent Neural Networks. Int. J. Med. Inform. 2020, 139, 104122.
- Zhang, Q.; Zhou, D.; Zeng, X. Highly wearable cuff-less blood pressure and heart rate monitoring with single-arm electrocardiogram and photoplethysmogram signals. Biomed. Eng. Online 2017, 16, 23. [Google Scholar] [CrossRef]
- Zheng, Y.; Poon, C.C.; Yan, B.P.; Lau, J.Y. Pulse Arrival Time Based Cuff-Less and 24-H Wearable Blood Pressure Monitoring and its Diagnostic Value in Hypertension. J. Med. Syst. 2016, 40, 195.
- Zhong, L.; Zhang, J.M.; Su, B.; Tan, R.S.; Allen, J.C.; Kassab, G.S. Application of Patient-Specific Computational Fluid Dynamics in Coronary and Intra-Cardiac Flow Simulations: Challenges and Opportunities. Front. Physiol. 2018, 9, 742. [Google Scholar] [CrossRef]
- Zhou, J.; Lee, S.; Wong, W.T.; Waleed, K.B.; Leung, K.S.K.; Lee, T.T.L.; Wai, A.K.C.; Liu, T.; Chang, C.; Cheung, B.M.Y.; et al. Gender-specific clinical risk scores incorporating blood pressure variability for predicting incident dementia. J. Am. Med. Inform. Assoc. 2022, 29, 335–347. [Google Scholar] [CrossRef]

Artificial Intelligence In Atherosclerotic Cardiovascular Disease

CHAPTER 5

Atherosclerotic cardiovascular disease (ASCVD) affects the coronary, cerebral and peripheral arteries and remains the most common cause of death globally . Over the last 60 years, numerous clinical trials, registries and prospective studies along with advances in basic science and biomedicine have formed our current understanding of the pathogenesis of ASCVD and have established the current clinical standards regarding diagnosis, prevention and treatment .With the advent of digitalization and information era, large amounts of heterogenous ASCVD data, such as clinical, imaging, biosensing, administrative and basic science data, are now available . Big data analytics, artificial intelligence (AI) and particularly their computational branch of machine learning (ML) bear the promise of incorporating and utilizing these large amounts of heterogenous information to enhance our armament against ASCVD .

Specifically, ML applications have already been employed, or are currently being researched, to improve ASCVD detection, assist with diagnosis, advance our understanding of ASCVD phenotypes in order to promote precision cardiovascular medicine, and to improve outcome prediction . Experts in the field of ASCVD anticipate significant advancements and changes in the next 10 years .The broad spectrum of ML applications in ASCVD in combination with the lack of familiarity with ML methodologies for most cardiovascular physicians may create boundaries in the understanding and potential use of this technology in clinical practice.Several reviews have been published to address this issue in ASCVD. In fact, the majority of existing reviews focus on coronary artery (CAD) and cardiac disease, in general or, more specifically, on imaging applications in CAD . For this reason, a separate category of reviews concentrates solely on non-cardiac ASCVD . Also, complementary to the above-mentioned works, other studies provide more "technical" aspects by describing specific AI concepts and methods within the field of ASCVD

In this chapter attempt has been done to provide not only a "clinical" aspect via an overview of AI applications in four forms of ASCVD

1. Peripheral arterial disease(PAD)
2. Crotid artery disease
3. Coronary arterial disease (CAD)
4. 4..Aortic aneurysm (AA)

but also "technical" insights about the specific AI concepts and algorithms. Thus, our focused overview of key AI concepts for the ASCVD specialist enriches the description of the use of AI in ASCVD clinical practice/research and the discussion about the future insights of AI as a tool to improve the personalized care in patients with ASCVD.

Key concepts

The term "big data" was coined to describe large quantities of information that is typically derived from different sources, in different formats and are produced at a high rate. AI is a broad term and refers to how human intelligence can be approached by artificial systems .The term includes theoretical approaches of what constitutes Intellgence, as well as practical aspects such as computational methods. ML and pattern recognition constitute a computational branch of AI that aims to develop and apply algorithms for the purpose of recognizing patterns/regularities in data. ML algorithms require training, typically with the use of big data which are large and highly diverse datasets. For example, ML algorithms could be trained to recognize atherosclerotic plaques in cardiac computed tomography angiographies (CTAs). Training of such Machine learning algorithms would require supervision, so that the algorithm would be given previously labeled CTA images as an input, and its training would entail optimization of its parameters to a forced output (whether an atherosclerotic plaque is present or not). Accuracy of such ML algorithms would be then judged by their ability to correctly recognize the presence or absence of plaques in new CTA pictures. In another example, supervised ML may aim at predicting clinical outcomes.

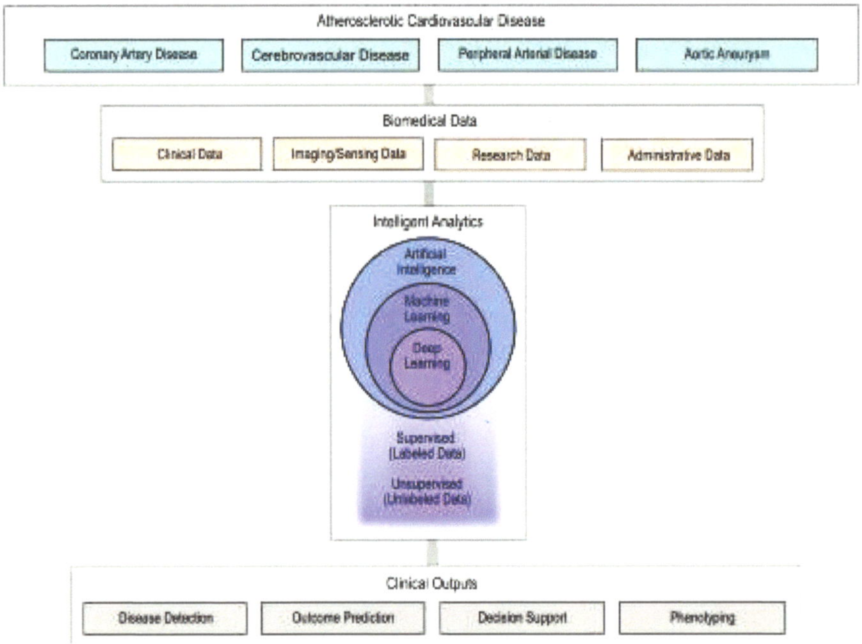

Fig 5.1 Usual workflow of AI approaches in ASCVD. Highly diverse biomedical data from patients with ASCVD are collected and used as input in AI algorithms to provide intelligent analytics. The developed AI algorithms (ML and DL) undergo supervised or unsupervised training to enable disease detection, outcome prediction, clinical decision support, and phenotyping. AI, artificial intelligence; ASCD, atherosclerotic cardiovascular disease; ML, machine learning; DL, deep learning.

In this case, ML models are trained by forcing a known clinical outcome, e.g., long-term survival or death, to corresponding patient (e.g., cardiovascular) profiles . Machine learning algorithms can be also trained without supervision (non-labeled data). Such an option is particularly helpful when the inherent structure of the available dataset, e.g., patient demographics/ biometrics, medical images, or biosignals, is not known a priority

Moreover, there is often a need to perform phenotyping where groups of patients (clinical phenotypes) or images (imaging phenotypes) with similar characteristics are automatically identified within an initial population/dataset. ML can offer unparalleled ways for the identification of unknown phenotypes in "big data." Most importantly, the identification of new, unknown phenotypes that are closer to individual patient characteristics, essentially promotes personalized medicine and its integration in everyday clinical practice

The main representatives of commonly used ML algorithms include, but are not limited to neural networks, naive Bayes models, decision making trees, clustering algorithms, k nearest neighbor, and SVM. Deep learning (DL) essentially refers to neural networks with complex computational architectures and the use of additional layers of neurons to enhance performance

Regardless of the data or algorithms used, one can recognize four broad categories of clinical ML applications:

1. Detection of disease,
2. Outcome prediction and risk assessment,
3. Phenotyping for better understanding of disease and precision medicine, and
4. Clinical decision support. Of tentimes, applications may serve more than one purpose,

e.g., phenotyping may assist outcome prediction. In addition, many AI applications fall into the preclinical setting and are mostly the subject of engineers or data scientists who collaborate with ASCVD experts. In this work, we focus on AI applications that are mostly clinical or describe the clinical aspect of preclinical applications.

Coronary Artery Disease

1.Disease detection via medical recordings

Several studies have already focused on applying a wide variety of ML models to diagnose CAD using clinical recordings, or else patient demographics, symptoms and examination reports, electrocardiographic (EKG) and imaging data along with laboratory tests . For example, Alizadehsani et al. employed different ML algorithms/methods, such as the Sequential Minimal Optimization (SMO), Naïve Bayes, Bagging SMO, and neural networks to diagnose CAD. The best predictive performance with an accuracy of 94.08% was achieved by the SMO models trained on the features selected using SVM weights .

In another study, the same group proposed a hybrid ML method based on combining genetic algorithms to put forward the initial weights of the shallow neural network approach. The hybrid model outperformed the neural network model by 10% improvement in CAD diagnosis accuracy by achieving 93.85% . Similarly, Alizadehsani et al. applied the C4.5, Adaboost, SMO, and Naïve Bayes algorithms on more comprehensive recordings of laboratory and echocardiographic information. In this case, the SMO reported the best predictive capability with 82.16 ± 5.45% accuracy . Furthermore, Alizadehsani et al. explored the effect of adding a MetaCost algorithm to improve the efficacy of the ML models to detect/ diagnose CAD. The authors implemented different ML models: Naïve Bayes, SMO, K-Nearest Neighbors (KNN), SVM, and C4.5. The study concluded that the combination of the SMO and MetaCost algorithms yielded very high sensitivity 97.22% and accuracy 92.09% in comparison to other models . In another notable attempt by Nasarian et al. additional stress-, work-related and environmental features enriched an initial traditional clinical dataset in order to improve performance. The authors proposed a novel hybrid feature selection algorithm named heterogeneous hybrid feature selection (2HFS). The study trained different algorithms: Decision tree, Gaussian Naive Bayes, RF, and XG Boost classifiers

Outcome showed that the XGBoost classifier achieved a classification accuracy of 81.23% by employing the additional features . Moreover, Hassannataj Joloudari et al. proposed a novel hybrid ML model called "Genetic Support Vector Machine ANOVA" (GSVMA) method. The study combined a genetic optimization algorithm for feature selection and SVM with ANOVA kernel. The model achieved 89.45% accuracy in CAD prediction . Finally, Khozeimeh et al. employed cardiac magnetic resonance (CMR) image data for CAD detection. The newly developed ML model was based on a RF, trained on a new image features representation extracted from a convolutional neural network (CNN). The novel model achieved a 99.18% accuracy compared to the 93.91% of the CNN .Apart from simply diagnosing CAD, several studies focused on detecting the location of stenosis in the coronary tree. For example, Alizadehsani et al. applied C4.5, Naïve Bayes, and KNN with the C4.5 model reporting the best performance for stenosis diagnosis by achieving 74.20 ± 5.51% for the LAD, 63.76 ± 9.73% for the LCX, and 68.33 ± 6.90% for the RCA . The later work was extended in Alizadehsani et al..where the Bagging algorithm was employed for the same tasks and achieved 79.54, 61.46, and 68.96% for the LAD-, LCX-, and RCA-stenosis, respectively. Another study used SVM, which outperformed the reported results in the literature by achieving accuracy rates of 86.14% (LAD), 83.17% (LCX), and 83.50% (RCA), respectively. Alizadehsani et al. further elaborated on their previous work by training several SVM machines with different kernel methods: polynomial, linear, sigmoid, and radial basis functions to quantify the uncertainty in the RCA-, LCX-, and LAD-stenosis diagnosis based on the sample distance from the hyperplane. The SVM highest accuracies achieved were: 82.67±2.3% (linear kernel), 83.67±2.1% (sigmoid kernel), and 86.43±2.1% (linear kernel) for RCA, LCX, and LAD prediction, respectively . Recently, Alizadehsani et al. proposed a novel and improved feature selection method named "assurance feature selection." Extracted features were again used to train SVM with different kernel methods achieving accuracies of 86.64% (LAD), 83.47% (LCX), and 82.85% (RCA) .In another approach, Alizadehsani et al. developed and proposed a two-stage ML model to improve the accuracy of CAD prediction. In the first stage, three classifiers were trained on weighted SVM extracted features to detect the stenosis in the three coronary arteries and a fourth classifier was built to predict/ detect CAD cases. In the second stage, a new classifier was trained on the outcomes of the four first-stage classifiers to diagnose CAD. The proposed pipeline achieved a high accuracy rate of 96.40% in predicting CAD . Finally, Alizadehsani et al. introduced a comprehensive database to encapsulate all previous work in CAD diagnosis using ML techniques . Such an approach might facilitate the development of meta-databases and give a further boost to the use of ML in the management of future patients with CAD in order to improve prognosis and optimize outcomes.

Non-invasive imaging

1.Automated plaque detection and coronary artery calcium calculation

Cardiac CTA is a widely used non-invasive modality for the diagnosis of coronary artery disease (CAD) . Several studies have reported AI algorithms for the automatic detection of atherosclerotic plaques from CTA images . For example, Kang et al. developed a ML algorithm that identified coronary stenosis of 25% or more with an accuracy of 94% compared to visual identification of lesions with stenosis by expert readers using consensus reading . Yoneyama et al. developed a neural network for the detection of coronary stenoses from CTA images that cause perfusion defects on single-photon emission CT, achieving comparable results with physician experts.Several studies have reported neural networks that automatically grade CAD severity from CTA images according to the Coronary Artery Disease Reporting and Data System (CAD-RADS),with satisfactory results .Such approaches could reduce the physician workload, time needed for diagnosis and the diagnostic accuracy . Coronary artery calcium score (CACS) as assessed by computed tomography (CT) correlates with clinical ASCVD events and is used for risk stratification of asymptomatic individuals .CACS is typically calculated via a time-consuming semi-automatic methodology by physicians with the help of a software based on the Agatston score . Fully automated software assessing coronary calcification has been developed using AI algorithms with satisfactory reliability and agreement when compared to manual scores . Automated quantification of CACS can reduce the time of assessment without additional costs or exposure to radiation . In a recent study, van Velzen et al. developed and validated a DL method for automatic calcium scoring using different types of CT examinations that included the heart (e.g., diagnostic CT of the chest, PET attenuation correction CT, CAC scoring CT). The performance of the ML algorithm was evaluated against manual Agatson score and the results showed that the DL calcium scoring algorithm was robust, regardless of differences in CT protocol and subject population. Nevertheless, training of the algorithm with dedicated, protocol-specific images further augmented algorithm performance .

2.Plaque characterization and detection of high-risk features

Machine learning algorithms have been developed to assist with atherosclerotic coronary plaque evaluation beyond the degree of stenosis. Masuda et al. for instance, developed a ML algorithm for identification of fatty vs. fibro-fatty atherosclerotic plaques from cardiac CTA with an area under the curve (AUC) of 0.92. ML could also be used to automatically identify high-risk features in coronary plaques, such as the napkin-ring sign.The latter identification has an additional importance, since the napkin-ring sign is a qualitative finding, thus automated identification could decrease inter-reader variability. Another interesting approach is ability of ML models to process hundreds of imaging features in order to identify known or discover new high-risk patterns in non-invasive studies. For example, a study showed that a large number of features are different between plaques with vs. without napkin-ring sign and exhibit remarkable discriminatory value, superior to conventional quantitative CT metrics .

3.Derivation of functional indices

Machine learning can also assist with automatic evaluation of CT-derived functional indices such as fractional flow reserve (FFR) . FFR is a coronary physiology index that is considered the gold standard for ruling out obstructive CAD and assessing lesion severity of intermediate stenosis in patients with chronic CAD . FFR is derived during invasive coronary angiography with the insertion of a pressure-wire catheter, and it is defined as the ratio between maximal achievable blood flow in the presence of coronary artery stenosis and maximal blood flow in the absence of that stenosis. Notably, based on the results of several studies including the FFR vs. Angiography for Multivessel Evaluation (FAME I) trial, have suggested that an FFR below 0.8 corresponds to a hemodynamically significant stenosis that requires PCI, whereas an FFR above 0.8 suggests that optimal medical therapy is sufficient .Several methods have been developed to estimate FFR based on computational flow dynamics (CFD) techniques applied to three-dimensional modeling of the coronary artery derived from angiogram or CT images without the use of invasive intracoronary wires. Example of software applications that have been developed and validated include Quantitative Flow Ratio (QFR), Vessel Fractional Flow Reserve (vFFR), and Fractional Flow Reserve Derived from Coronary Angiography (FFRangio). A number of studies have also developed methods to derive CT-FFR based on CFD techniques, and CT-FFR has been reported to have good diagnostic accuracy, prognostic value and therefore potential for clinical utility. Nevertheless, commercially available CFD software platforms to derive angiography-based or CT-based FFR have been restricted due to their low availability as they require remote and computationally demanding analyses significantly increasing the cost and delaying the diagnostic process

Thus, ML algorithms have been used as an alternative to calculate FFR with less computational requirements. ML models have been trained using geometrical and flow data from 3D coronary models derived from coronary angiograms or CT images. Importantly, ML-based software can be used on-site by standard configuration personal computers . Preliminary results show that ML-based CT-FFR performs equally well compared to CFD-based CT-FFR at decreased cost. To illustrate, a non-commercial software that uses DL to evaluate CT-FFR has been developed and tested by Rother et al. Compared to invasive FFR, CT-FFR showed high accuracy in detecting ischemia and a significant reduction in calculation time when compared to existing CFD models that calculate FFR from CT images. More recently, the accuracy of the software was also tested using previous generation CT scanners to assess whether the imaging quality could potentially affect the results . However, the results showed good diagnostic performance for detection of flow-limiting obstructive coronary lesions. ML-based software that estimate FFR can enable a wider implementation of this promising coronary physiology index that has proven to be an important indicator of coronary ischemia and predictor of adverse coronary events.

Invasive imaging

1.Automated lesion detection and characterization

Similar to non-invasive coronary imaging, ML algorithms can enhance the efficacy of invasive coronary angiography by enabling the automated detection of stenoses and their types, as well as the conduction of quantitative coronary angiography (QCA). For example, Du et al. trained a deep neural network using over 6,000 coronary angiograms to automatically identify stenoses and characterize them as dissections, thrombotic or calcified lesions . Apart from assistance in detection of disease, ML algorithms could also assist with quantitative angiography, which removes the subjective interpretation of lesions, however, is not widely used today. A significant number of researchers have focused on applying ML algorithms to intravascular imaging such as intravascular ultrasound and optical coherence tomography(OCT),which are used today complementary to angiography for plaque characterization and importantly, optimization of percutaneous coronary intervention (PCI). Specifically for OCT, ML algorithms can achieve high accuracy in identifying lesion composition . Recently, the FDA approved Abbotts' Ultreon™ 1.0 Software for automated and assisted OCT use (Abbott, Abbott Park, IL). ML algorithms are also being investigated to further improve functional indices of coronary lesions, such as FFR, or calculate them via alternative means. For example, a ML algorithm was developed to measure FFR from OCT-derived data showing high correlation ($r = 0.85$, $P < 0.001$) with invasive FFR .

2.Assistance with clinical decision-making regarding revascularization

The incorporation of angiographic data and functional indices could be used to offer an overall assessment of a coronary lesion with regards to the decision for revascularization or not, essentially mimicking human expertise. CEREBRIA-1 study was a representative study multinational study (ML vs. Expert Human Opinion to Determine Physiologically Optimized Coronary Revascularization Strategies), where DL was used to approach the clinical decision making of world experts in this matter . The study aimed to evaluate the predictive accuracy of a ML model developed based on computational interpretation of pressure wire pull back data. The ML algorithm was compared to expert human interpretation in determining the need for PCI as well as for the decision of PCI strategy in patients with stable CAD. The results showed that the ML program was non-inferior to expert opinion. The notable benefit of this approach is that the ML algorithm essentially couldprovide an expert recommendation to the interventional cardiologist of every catheterization laboratory.

3.Image quality improvement via ML

In addition to automated lesion characterization and clinical decision-making regarding revascularization, AI may further assist the interventional cardiologist by detecting artifacts or poor image quality and correct it appropriately and automatically . Such an option might have essential clinical impact, by improving the accuracy of calculated functional indices, which frequently drive decision making, especially taking into account that almost 30% of the functional indices derived intraoperatively in catheterization laboratories cannot be reliably used for clinical decision-making .

Assisted diagnosis of myocardial infarction

Physicians are extremely capable in diagnosing and treating myocardial infarction (MI) in symptomatic patients seeking medical care. A systematic review has reported low rates of missed MIs in the hospital setting, ranging between 1 and 2% . Hospitals in rural areas and those with a low proportion of classical chest pain patients were at greater risk for missing an MI. ML models to enhance automated detection of MIs from 12-lead EKGs have been developed with accuracy comparable to that of cardiologist . EKG machines equipped with this ML software could therefore decrease the rates of in-hospital missed MIs even further or could help emergency medical services enhance their response times in patients with MIs. The most significant contribution of ML technology, however, would be the detection of MIs and their complications in the community. In patients suffering from ST elevation MI (STEMI), delay to reperfusion translates into more extensive myocardial injury and increased mortality: every minute counts and hospital systems have adopted internationally accepted response times referred to as door to balloon time . However, a critically important time is frequently lost before patients seek medical care. Smartwatch technology is already being used for the screening and detection of atrial fibrillation in the community setting ,and an expansion of its use for the detection of MIs is very appealing. However, the problem is more complex, as atrial fibrillation screening can be performed with analysis of pulse or a single EKG lead, whereas EKG detection of MI requires multiple EKG leads. Spaccarotella et al. showed in a pilot study that a 9-lead EKG obtained asynchronously from a single smart watch device could be used to detect STEMI and non-STEMI with good accuracy compared to a standard 12-lead EKG . This technology could be coupled with ML algorithms to enable the early detection of MIs in the outpatient setting, and in fact, studies toward that goal are already being conducted . Importantly, as in the case of atrial fibrillation, prospective studies will be required to prove the clinical validity and benefit of such new technologies.

Phenotyping and precision medicine

Machine learning methodologies have been applied in CAD datasets with the purpose of discovering new clinical phenotypes that can improve our understanding of the disease and/or our ability to better predict outcomes. In general, as the number of phenotypes increases, prediction comes closer to the individual level and ML facilitates precision medicine. However, there is no strict definition as to what constitutes precision medicine. A classic example of imaging phenotyping in CAD is a ML algorithm developed by Yoon et al. where unsupervised training led to the creation of four different groups of plaques based on their imaging characteristics from the PARADIGM registry .Patients from cluster 1 had plaques that consisted of a necrotic core surrounded by mainly fibrotic and lipid tissue. In cluster 2, plaques were mainly fibrotic and fatty, in cluster 3, the plaques had mainly fibrotic and calcified tissue, and in cluster 4 plaques were mostly calcified. Patients with plaques classified to clusters 2 and 3 had the highest risk for major adverse cardiovascular events, whereas cluster 1 had the lowest risk. These results can assist our understanding of what constitutes a high-risk plaque and how it can be used to predict outcomes. Furthermore, ML models have the ability to process hundreds of imaging features and discover new important characteristics .A characteristic example of clinical phenotyping and precision medicine in CAD was recently published by Puchner et al., where a phenomapping-derived tool was developed and validated with the aim to personalize the selection of anatomical (cardiac CT) vs. functional testing (stress testing) in individuals with suspected CAD.The investigators included participants from PROMISE trial (Clinical Trials.gov identifier: NCT01174550) where individuals presenting with stable chest pain were randomized to either anatomical (CTCA) or functional testing (exercise electrocardiography, nuclear stress testing, or stress echocardiography). Utilizing baseline characteristics including,among others,demographics, anthropometrics, cardiovascularriskfactors,and laboratory measurements, the investigators first broke down the trial cohort to numerous, distinct phenotypes based on a data similarity index. For each phenotype, they then estimated the hazard ratio of major adverse cardiac events with stress test vs. cardiac CTA. Training of an extreme gradient boosting algorithm was then performed to identify patient features that were strongly associated with improved outcomes. Feature performance was evaluated using SHAP (Shapley Additive Explanations) values which identify a predictor contribution, either positively or negatively, to the prediction. Finally, internal validation of the algorithm was performed in a subset of patients from PROMISE trial, while external validation of the chosen method was also performed using the Scottish Computed Tomography of the Heart (SCOT-HEART) trial (ClinicalTrials.gov identifier: NCT01149590) and showed a reduction in the composite clinical endpoint In another study by the same group, researchers developed a ML algorithm based on > 1,000 cardiac CTA perivascular adipose tissue features to predict the probability of major adverse cardiac events within 5 years in patients with stable CAD, defining it as the "fat radiomic profile" . They further examined the correlation of CTA features with genes expressing inflammation, fibrosis, and vascularity. A "fat radiomic profile" above 0.63 was linked with a 10-fold increase in the risk of MACE, even after adjustment for all pertinent covariates. In the same study, the authors point out that lack of standardization in coronary CTs and image post-processing remains a problem that can hinder the robustness of these methods—namely, the ability to obtain comparable CTA features results from a wide variety of hardware, scan settings and software configurations .

Risk assessment and outcome prediction

Risk assessment is important for different subgroups of CAD patients and guides patient management. In people without known CAD, several tools have been developed and are currently used for the risk assessment and prediction of future cardiovascular events, including the Framingham score, SCORE and SCORE2, as well as the American College of Cardiology/American Heart Association (ACC/AHA) risk tool .These tools were derived using traditional statistical methods and show only moderate to good discrimination in predicting ASCVD outcomes .ML models have been developed with the goal of improving the predictive accuracy of these tools. In a recent study, Ambale-Venkatesh et al. combined deep phenotyping with ML to train an algorithm for cardiovascular disease prediction . Using over 700 clinical, imaging, laboratory, and biomarker variables from the Multi-Ethnic Study of Atherosclerosis (MESA) study ,a prospective study of over 6,000 asymptomatic individuals with serial ASCVD evaluation and long term follow up, the authors developed a ML algorithm to predict cardiovascular outcomes, including all-cause mortality, coronary heart disease, and stroke, over 12 years of follow-up. Specifically, a random survival forests ML technique was used to identify the 20 most important predictors of cardiovascular outcomes and the final ML model achieved better predictive accuracy compared to established risk scores . showed improved predictive accuracy . As an example of the clinical importance of improved predictive accuracy achieved by ML algorithms, application of an ML model developed based on data from the MESA and the Flemish Study of Environment, Genes and Health Outcomes (FLEMENGHO) would have reduced statin prescriptions by 68% while simultaneously increasing the statin use of true high-risk patients (patients that went on to experience a CVD event) by 52% . Besides improving prognostication, ML analyses can improve our understanding of ASCVD by showing the important role of biomarkers; tissue necrosis factor-alpha, C-reactive protein, fibrinogen, interleukin-2, and interleukin-6 were top predictors of outcomes in the abovementioned ML models. In contrast, established risk assessment tools do not incorporate such biomarkers. In patients with known or suspected CAD, estimation of CAD progression can also be clinically helpful. Along these lines, an ML model developed using clinical and imagine data of patients that underwent serial cardiac CTA from the PARADIGM study, demonstrated reasonably good predictive value for progression of coronary plaque (area under the curve 0.83.In patients with CAD undergoing PCI, assessment of bleeding risk remains challenging. The American College of Cardiology has developed a bleeding risk score using data from over 1 million PCIs from the CathPCI registry . Although ML techniques have not proven to outperform the CathPCI risk score in a head-to-head comparison, results of a ML study have been promising.Lastly, ML-based models may in the future have a role in clinical decision-making beyond risk assessment, as in assisting with revascularization strategy .

Peripheral arterial disease (PAD)

1.Detection of disease

Peripheral arterial disease refers to the narrowing of the arteries that supply the upper and lower limbs, most commonly due to atherosclerosis . Although it is estimated that more than 200 million patients worldwide suffer from PAD , more than 50% of these patients are asymptomatic and often remain undiagnosed and untreated . Advanced tools, such as AI, have been used for facilitating not only the detection, but also the management and outcome prediction in PAD .For example, an ML algorithm, which employs clinical variables (e.g., history of hypertension) and serum biomarkers, was used to create a unique score and predict the presence of PAD in a sub-population of CASABLANCA registry's including patients referred for diagnostic peripheral and/or coronary angiography . The novel score achieved a sensitivity of only 65% but a specificity of 88% with a positive predictive value of 76% with the cut-off having been optimally set . In another study targeting elderly patients, a random forest (RF) approach provided better results in diagnosing PAD compared to simple logistic regression and the traditional ankle-brachial index (ABI) .In fact, the seven most important features of the developed RF model were the: (i) ABI, (ii) creatinine level in blood, (iii) fasting blood glucose, (iv) age, (v) presence of CAD, (vi) presence of diabetes, and (vii) presence of hypertension.

In another approach the clinical narrative notes of 1,569 patients were processed using an AI natural language processing (NLP) algorithm . Results were compared to algorithms employing the International Classification of Diseases (ICD) codes, as well as the ABI measurements of the patients. The NLP outperformed its competitors ($P < 0.001$) yielding 91.8% accuracy, 92.5% sensitivity, and 92.9% positive predictive value . In a follow-up study, the same team assessed the efficacy of the NLP approach to diagnose critical ischemia of lower extremities . As previously, they compared the knowledge-driven NLP algorithm to an ICD-based one. Despite having no statistically significant difference in specificity, the NLP method had better positive predictive value, specificity and F1-scores ($P < 0.001$) compared to the ICD model , indicating the superiority of AI-based NLP in diagnosing PAD, compared to other traditional approaches. Moreover, Weissler et al. performed a comparison between the NLP of medical notes and the least absolute shrinkage and selection operator (LASSO) ML methodology, which is based on administrative data . The NLP algorithm led to an AUC of 0.888, whereas the LASSO's AUC was 0.801 ($P < 0.0001$ according to DeLong test) . Above mentioned studies highlight the capability of NLP in PAD detection with great implications for initial PAD screening in everyday clinical practice Furthermore, Ghanzouri et al. used electronic health records (EHRs) to detect undiagnosed PAD in a cohort of 3,168 patients. The authors compared the developed DL-based approach to traditional models showing a clear superiority of the DL model (average AUC of 0.96) over RF (average AUC of 0.91), and logistic regression approaches (average AUC of 0.8). Another significant point of that study is the demonstration, via a corresponding analysis, that clinicians are generally receptive to automated EHR-based models for PAD detection .Moreover, apart from clinical and EHR data, AI may well be applied on other data types to achieve PAD detection. McBane et al. applied DL for the detection of PAD via arterial (posterior tibial artery) Doppler waveform data.

In specific, the proposed DL algorithm predicted normal (>0.9) or pathological (≤0.9) post-exercise ABI based on posterior tibial artery Doppler waveforms recorded at the resting state. The model included 1,941 patients with PAD and 1,491 control subjects and detected PAD with an AUC of 0.94 (CI=0.92–0.96) The heterogeneity of the datasets included in the above-described studies demonstrates the importance of employing diverse datasets in detecting PAD.

2.Severity stratification and outcome prediction

The option to accurately assess disease severity facilitates not only the patient management process, but also the objectification of applied therapies. Qutrio Baloch et al. investigated the relationship between disease severity and patient functional impairment . In total, administrative data from 703 patients were analyzed with supervised ML. Quality of life, 6-min walk test scores, calf circumference, toe-branchial index, and basic demographics constituted the feature set .the not striking results of the applied ML method, compared to conventional statistical methods, the study highlighted the non-linear relationship between disease severity and mobility restriction , showing that AI interventions provide results if not better at least as accurate as conventional statistics do.In another study, Sonnenschein et al. developed a ML approach with the use of a multi-dimensional set of clinical features (demographics, biometrics, blood tests) to calculate an AI-based PAD score (AI-PAD). The calculated score (range 0–100) categorized the patients with PAD (n = 46) into two groups (stable PAD, sPAD, Fontaine stages I–II and unstable PAD, unPAD, Fontaine stages III–IV) based on a cut-off value of 50 AI-PAD units (AI-PAD < 50 for sPAD and AI-PAD > 50 for unPAD) and showed good correlation with the measured ABI values and severity of disease . Outcome prediction in PAD is a pivotal step to be taken after diagnosis, as it sets the strategy for the patient management to be followed. A study conducted by Davis et al. aimed to reveal predictive indices of infection of the surgical wounds in patients undergoing open surgical revascularization (via bypass) of the lower limbs . The authors utilized an ML technique (Super Learner algorithm) to develop a prediction model for surgical wound infection. The study population included 3,033 patients in total. Major predictors of postoperative infection were dialysis-requiring renal failure (OR 4.35, P < 0.001) and hypertension (OR 4.29 P < 0.001) . In another study, 81.930 patients were analyzed using the LASSO ML methodology to select variables and define a score (OAC3-PAD Risk Score) which can effectively predict the major bleeding events after the hospitalization for PAD . Independent predictors were oral anticoagulation therapy, age > 80, presence of chronic limb threatening ischemia, congestive heart failure and severe chronic kidney disease, previous bleeding event, anemia, and dementia. The novel score displayed good calibration and discrimination among four risk groups (c = 0.69, 95% confidence interval 0.67–0.71) ranging from low (1.3%) to high bleeding risk (6.4%) in the first year after the hospitalization for PAD

Finally, Ross et al. developed several tailored ML models which included clinical, demographic, imaging and genomic data to predict future mortality in patients with PAD . The newly designed ML models outperformed (AUC 0.76 vs. 0.65, respectively, P = 0.1) traditional approaches (logistic regression models) for the task-at-hand: the prediction of future mortality. The studies described above demonstrate the wide range of applicability for AI in the management of patients suffering from PAD.

Abdominal aortic aneurysm

Abdominal aortic aneurysm (AAA) is one of the most severe complications of ASCVD conveying significant mortality risk due to rupture . Its size and growth rate determine the risk of rupture and, thus, the necessity for operative therapy . AI has been already employed in the management of AAA, mainly in setting the diagnosis, predicting its growth and risk of rupture or in the preoperative planning and postoperative outcome prediction .

Computed tomography angiography is the gold-standard technique for the diagnosis, as well, as the preoperative planning and postoperative outcome assessment in AAA. For this reason, the majority of AI techniques in AAA management are CTA-based. Adam et al. employed a DL approach (Augmented Radiology for Vascular Aneurysm—ARVA) to detect an AAA and measure its maximal diameter in 489 CTA scans . ARVA outcomes were compared to a reference expert, demonstrating a median absolute difference of 1.2 mm, while the median absolute differences of another six experts compared to the same reference expert were 1–2 mm. Lareyre at al. combined a supervised DL algorithm with a feature-based expert system to improve the accuracy of the automatic segmentation of the abdominal aorta and its major branches . Such AI-powered approaches could facilitate preoperative planning of endovascular AAA interventions, especially in complex anatomies.

In another application, the prediction of AAA growth, Hirata et al. used as an input to an ML algorithm 9 CTA-extracted anatomic features of small AAAs (38.5 ± 6.2 mm).ML achieved an AUC of 0.86 in predicting expansions of more than 4 mm per year outperforming traditional features, such as the AAA major axis (AUC of 0.78) .Along the same lines, Kontopodis et al. developed an AI-based approach that could stratify AAAs into high and low growth rate groups. Using a diverse set of 29 different variables (clinical, biological, morphometric, and biomechanical), a gradient boosting (XGboost) and a support vector machines (SVM) model were trained in order to predict which AAA would reach a growth rate higher than the cohort median. XGboost achieved the highest AUC 81.2% in predicting high growth rate AAAs compared to low growth rate ones. The study included a small cohort of 40 patients with small AAAs (maximum diameter 32–53 mm)

Nevertheless, in order to precisely predict the growth of AAAs, usually larger longitudinal datasets are required. Jiang et al. tried to tackle the usual problem of lack of such datasets by employing a two-step computational approach to generate an expanded in silico dataset of AAA growth and structural features . Then, they employed a DL algorithm to combine both in silico and real CTA patient data to predict the evolution of the AAA in 20 patients. The DL method outperformed a conventional mixed-effect model by 65% in predicting the size increase of AAAs, showcasing an average relative error of 3.1%.The issue of the need for large datasets in order to apply AI in the management of AAA is also discussed in a study by Fujiwara et al. where the authors evaluate the accuracy of AI to detect and measure AAA using limited-size CT datasets. The authors employ label-free CTs, avoiding possible complications associated with the intravenous use of contrast, such as renal failure or allergic reactions. In a dataset of 145 label-free CT scans (n = 111 with AAA), the proposed approach achieved a sensitivity of 94.6% for AAA detection and a good estimation of the AAA size (42.5 ± 8.8 mm) compared to those of diagnostic reports (44.6 ± 8.4 mm) . Even if endovascular aortic repair (EVAR) is generally characterized by good outcomes , it can be still be followed by complications, such as the endoleak (EL). Korzadeh et al. applied AI to predict not only the presence, but also the severity of EL (I–III). The model was fed with 26 non-imaging clinical attributes (e.g., biometrics, demographics, blood values) recorded preoperatively and achieved an overall accuracy of more than 86% . The authors notice that the model may well be further enhanced with imaging data, highlighting the adaptability of AI in different and diverse datasets and its high potential to provide even more powerful tools for the clinical management of AAA in the future.Finally, in an attempt to provide insights into the risk for rupture—the most serious complication of AAA, Chung et al. used AI to predict wall stress in AAAs: a feature that is associated with the risk for rupture. The novel AI-based framework was compared to traditional analysis in terms of AAA automatic segmentation, 3D geometry reconstruction and aortic wall stress calculation. The trained U-NET was found to perform in a statistically similar way compared to traditional analysis but in a significantly smaller amount of time (20 s vs. 4 h) . Although the role of AI in the management of AAA seems promising, the aforementioned results are still preliminary and remain to be evaluated in large-scale clinical trials.

Carotid artery disease

Imaging plays a pivotal role in the management of carotid artery disease. For example, CTA is frequently performed to set the diagnosis and plan the surgical treatment of a patient (e.g., open vs. endovascular). The decision to operate is typically based on the degree of carotid stenosis and the presence of symptoms. However, patients often have transient ischemic attacks or stroke with only mild to moderate carotid luminal stenosis . Moreover, studies show that a more detailed plaque characterization expanding beyond luminal stenosis could provide additional value in predicting future events .

In a recent study, radiomic features were extracted from carotid CT scans of patients with cerebrovascular events to investigate their robustness and reliability, and whether they could provide incremental prognostic value in identifying high-risk culprit carotid arteries from non-culprit carotid arteries . Using feature extraction hyperparameters, the researchers ended up with 93 radiomic-derived variables, more than half of whom displayed high robustness to simulated inter-observer variability in region of interest (ROI) demarcation. Using only the top 10 informative and robust radiomics variables, the authors trained an ElasticNet logistic regression model that outperformed the calcium score alone in pinpointing culprit lesions. When both modalities were combined, an AUC of 0.73 was achieved

Radiomic features have also been extracted from carotid MRI scans to construct a high-risk plaque model for differentiating symptomatic from asymptomatic carotid plaques . In a recent study by Zhang et al. 162 patients with carotid stenosis were randomly divided into training and test cohorts. Multi-contrast and contrast enhanced MRI images were obtained and radiological features of carotid plaques were recorded to build a traditional model. Additionally, radiomic features on these images were derived to construct a high-risk MRI based model with least absolute shrinkage and selection operation algorithm in the training cohort. The performance of the model was evaluated in the test cohort. Finally, a combined model was developed using both the traditional and the radiomics model and a comparison between the traditional, the radiomics and the combined models was performed. The radiomics model could accurately distinguish symptomatic from asymptomatic carotid stenosis and was found to be superior to the traditional model in the differentiation of high-risk plaques while the combined model did not provide any additional benefit compared to the radiomics model . Carotid plaque morphology as recorded by high-resolution ultrasound images can also have prognostic implications and assist in identifying asymptomatic individuals with carotid stenosis at risk for stroke .Stable plaques are assumed to present as echogenic, smooth, and homogeneous, while vulnerable plaques typically are echolucent, irregular, and heterogeneous . Kordzadeh et al. applied AI in the detection of carotid artery disease via static grayscale duplex ultrasound images. A dataset of 156 ultrasound images (with and without carotid artery stenosis) was used to train a geometry group network based on CNN architecture. The algorithm detected carotid artery stenosis of any grade with a sensitivity, specificity, and accuracy of 87, 82, and 90%, respectively . Jain et al. used an Attention-UNet DL model to identify/segment carotid plaques in complex ultrasound images with bright and fuzzy plaques of the internal (ICA) and common carotid artery (CCA). The study included 970 ICA and 679 CCA images from three different centers. The performance of Attention-UNet model was benchmarked against UNet, UNet++, and UNet3P models yielding an AUC value of 0.97, compared to 0.964, 0.966, and 0.965 AUC values for the three other models, respectively . Along similar lines, Latha et al. classified 361 carotid ultrasound images into normal or pathologic by means of several different ML methods, such as the CART decision tree, RF, logistic regression, CNN, Mobilenet, and Capsulenet. The latter was characterized by a superior classification performance, as reported by a 12.91, 8.33, 5.47, 43.12, and 1.75% improvement in accuracy compared to the CART decision tree, logistic regression, RF, CNN, and Mobilenet, respectively . Finally, in another study, a computer-aided system could provide a more standardized and accurate classification of carotid plaques. As an early example of such an approach, a computer-aided classification system was developed using multi-feature texture analysis, neural network classifiers, and statistical pattern recognition techniques. The system managed to automatically characterize carotid plaques imaged with high-resolution ultrasound, achieving an AUC of 0.75 at predicting which patients would develop stroke .Studies described above demonstrate how AI can facilitate the management of carotid artery disease by providing effective and automated image-based tissue characterization and patient classification

Challenges and limitations in the application of AI in ASCVD

Although the applications of AI in ASCVD are promising, several challenges and limitations remain. First, overtraining may lead to overfitting of the applied ML model and, thus, poor generalization with limited performance using real-world data. This challenge can be overcome by using large, trustworthy datasets that are representative of the target population as well as appropriate ML algorithms. Second, in contrast to classic statistical approaches, many ML implementations are characterized as "black-box" or else "non-explainable," because the patterns that are created cannot be easily interpreted. As a result, ML models cannot be easily trusted by expert users, which is particularly true for ASCVD physicians. The development of explainable AI (xAI) approaches is an answer to this limitation. For example, SHAP (Sharpley Additive Explanations) explainability analysis approximates any complex, generalized ML prediction model with local, linear models that explain individual predictions using a game theory approach . Third, AI requires the collection and pre-processing of large and diverse datasets, which can be time-consuming. The development of international database collaborations for the availability of data to researchers globally could overcome some of these challenges . Fourth, the development and application of AI in ASCVD requires not only high computational power but also specialized AI skills and steady collaboration between data scientists and physicians. To this end, tailored AI frameworks and ASCVD-AI laboratories are under development. Finally, although ML algorithms are clearly superior in automated detection of disease and phenotyping, one has to recognize that results in risk assessment and prognostication have often been inferior to traditional statistics.

Conclusion and future directions

As presented herein, AI methodologies, in combination with the growing availability of "big data" have already started enhancing disease detection, risk assessment, phenotyping, and providing clinical decision support in ASCVD. Over the past two decades, there is a growing interest in ML and AI especially in the field of ASCVD . Applications empowered by AI algorithms are becoming daily practice, particularly in the field of cardiovascular imaging. For this reason, there is a significant interest for the development of community-based ML applications that can be embedded in smart portable or wearable devices for different purposes (e.g., detection of acute coronary syndromes). Researchers are now

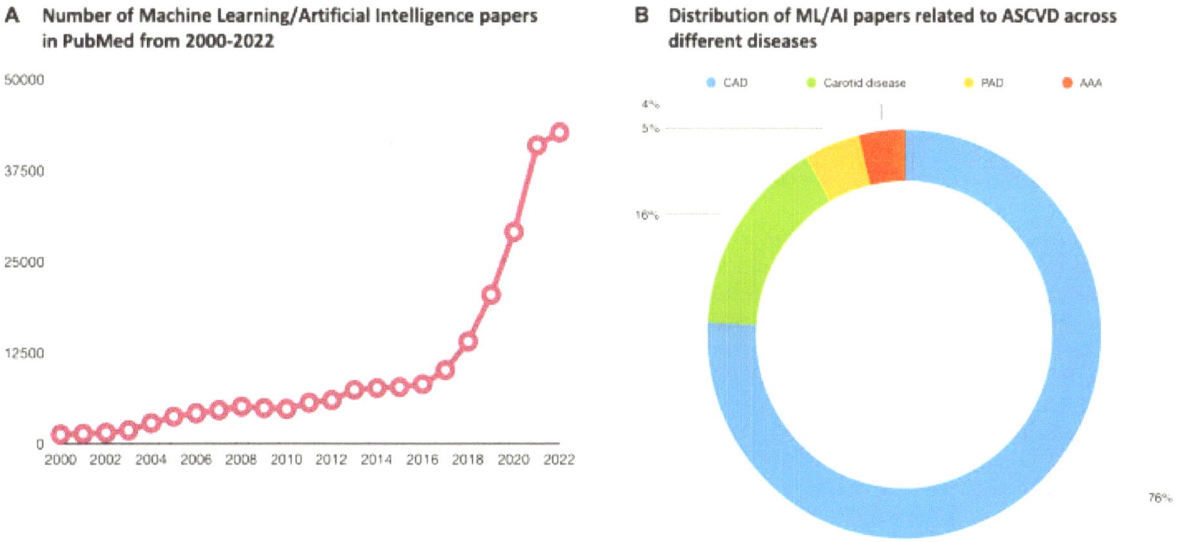

Fig 5.2 Current body of evidence related to ML/AI in the field of ASCVD. (A) Demonstrates how the number of papers in PubMed related to ML/AI has increased dramatically over the past two decades. (B) Shows how the ML/AI papers related to ASCVD specifically are distributed across the different diseases under the umbrella of ASCVD. In PubMed, the vast majority of ASCVD ML/AI papers are related to CAD. ML, machine learning; AI, atherosclerosis artificial intelligence; ASCVD, atherosclerotic cardiovascular disease; CAD, coronary artery disease; PAD, peripheral artery disease; AAA, abdominal aortic aneurysm.

applying ML algorithms to uncover previously unknown or neglected associations, such as the role of image- or signal-based biomarkers in predicting cardiovascular events. In parallel, the application of ML in large datasets bears the promise of leading to a more precision medicine approach in the risk assessment and therapy of patients with ASCVD.However, current ML models in the ASCVD field are still in their infancy, focusing mainly on the classification and regression models for a single task-at-hand. Nevertheless, available AI models can go beyond those basic tasks, for example toward generating more realistic medical images using generative models such as Variational Auto-Encoders (VAEs) and Generative Adversarial Networks (GANs). One of the major challenges in the medical domain is the limited number and size of patient datasets for training ML or AI models. A promising AI field called meta-learning aims at solving this problem by building models that can learn from limited-sized datasets with only few data points. Several algorithms are listed in this domain, so far, such as: Siamese Networks, Prototypical Networks, and Relation Networks. Finally, another trending AL approach is deep multimodal learning that focuses on linking patient information such as EHRs, genomics, and imaging with multiple techniques to improve the final regression/classification performances.As different needs and applications arise in the ASCVD field, an even more disseminated use of AI approaches in managing and studying ASCVD is expected to be established in the near future. On the one hand, the ASCVD physician should seek a stronger and stable collaboration with AI experts in order to increase familiarity and understanding with this exciting technology. On the other hand, the AI expert should focus on tailoring developed approaches to real-world ASCVD physician needs. In any case, the future ASCVD patient is going to benefit from a more effective, precise, and personalized management of disease in daily practice.

Bibliography and Acknowledgement

- Adam C, Fabre D, Mougin J, Zins M, Azarine A, Ardon R, et al. Pre-surgical and post-surgical aortic aneurysm maximum diameter measurement: full automation by artificial intelligence. Eur J Vasc Endovasc Surg. (2021) 62:869–77. 10.1016/j.ejvs.2021.07.013 [PubMed] [CrossRef] [Google Scholar]
- Alizadehsani R, Alizadehsani R, Hosseini M, Sani ZA, Ghandeharioun A, Boghrati R, et al. Diagnosis of coronary artery disease using cost-sensitive algorithms. Proceedings of the 2012 IEEE 12th International Conference on Data Mining Workshops. Brussels: (2012). p. 9–16. 10.1109/ICDMW.2012.29 [CrossRef] [Google Scholar]]
- Alizadehsani R, Roshanzamir M, Abdar M, Beykikhoshk A, Khosravi A, Nahavandi S, et al. Hybrid genetic-discretized algorithm to handle data uncertainty in diagnosing stenosis of coronary arteries. Exp Syst. (2022) 39:e12573. 10.1111/exsy.12573 [CrossRef] [Google Scholar]
- Ambale-Venkatesh B, Yang X, Wu C, Liu K, Hundley W, McClelland R, et al. Cardiovascular event prediction by machine learning: the multi-ethnic study of atherosclerosis. Circ Res. (2017) 121:1092–101. 10.1161/CIRCRESAHA.117.311312 [PMC free article] [PubMed] [CrossRef] [Google Scholar]
- Arabasadi Z, Alizadehsani R, Roshanzamir M, Moosaei H, Yarifard AA. Computer aided decision making for heart disease detection using hybrid neural network-Genetic algorithm. Comput Methods Programs Biomed. (2017) 141:19–26. 10.1016/j.cmpb.2017.01.004 [PubMed] [CrossRef] [Google Scholar]
- Badillo S, Banfai B, Birzele F, Davydov I, Hutchinson L, Kam-Thong T, et al. An introduction to machine learning. Clin Pharmacol Ther. (2020) 107:871–85. 10.1002/cpt.1796 [PMC free article] [PubMed] [CrossRef] [Google Scholar]
- Blaha M, Mortensen M, Kianoush S, Tota-Maharaj R, Cainzos-Achirica M. Coronary artery calcium scoring: is it time for a change in methodology? JACC Cardiovasc Imaging. (2017) 10:923–37. 10.1016/j.jcmg.2017.05.007 [PubMed] [CrossRef] [Google Scholar]
- Bourgeois FT, Gutiérrez-Sacristán A, Keller M, Liu M, Hong C, Bonzel C, et al. International analysis of electronic health records of children and youth hospitalized With COVID-19 infection in 6 countries. JAMA Netw Open. (2021) 4:e2112596. [PMC free article] [PubMed] [Google Scholar]
- Buzaev IV, Plechev V, Nikolaeva I, Galimova R. Artificial intelligence: neural network model as the multidisciplinary team member in clinical decision support to avoid medical mistakes. Chronic Dis Transl Med. (2016) 2:166–72. 10.1016/j.cdtm.2016.09.007 [PMC free article] [PubMed]
- Cha JJ, Son TD, Ha J, Kim J, Hong S, Ahn C, et al. Optical coherence tomography-based machine learning for predicting fractional flow reserve in intermediate coronary stenosis: a feasibility study. Sci Rep. (2020) 10:20421. 10.1038/s41598-020-77507-y [PMC free article] [PubMed] [
- Christodoulou CI, Pattichis C, Pantziaris M, Nicolaides A. Texture-based classification of atherosclerotic carotid plaques. IEEE Trans Med Imaging. (2003) 22:902–12. 10.1109/TMI.2003.815066 [PubMed] [CrossRef] [Google Scholar]
- Coenen A, Kim Y, Kruk M, Tesche C, De Geer J, Kurata A, et al. Diagnostic accuracy of a machine-learning approach to coronary computed tomographic angiography-based fractional flow reserve: result from the MACHINE consortium. Circ Cardiovasc Imaging. (2018) 11:e007217. 10.1161/CIRCIMAGING.117.007217 [PubMed] [CrossRef] [Google Scholar]
- Covas P, De Guzman E, Barrows I, Bradley A, Choi B, Krepp J, et al. Artificial intelligence advancements in the cardiovascular imaging of coronary atherosclerosis. Front Cardiovasc Med. (2022) 9:839400. 10.3389/fcvm.2022.839400 [PMC free article] [PubMed] [CrossRef] [Google Scholar]
- Cury RC, Abbara S, Achenbach S, Agatston A, Berman D, Budoff M, et al. CAD-RADS(TM) coronary artery disease - reporting and data system. an expert consensus document of the Society of
- cardiovascular computed tomography (SCCT), the American college of radiology (ACR) and the North American society for cardiovascular imaging (NASCI). endorsed by the American college of cardiology. J Cardiovasc Comput Tomogr. (2016) 10:269–81. 10.1016/j.jcct.2016.04.005 [PubMed] [CrossRef] [Google Scholar]
- Davies J. CEREBRIA-1: machine learning vs expert human opinion to determine physiologically optimized coronary revascularization strategies. Paper Presented at Transcatheter Cardiovascular Therapeutics Symposium (TCT) 18. San Diego, CA: (2018). [Google Scholar]
- Davis FM, Sutzko D, Grey S, Mansour M, Jain K, Nypaver T, et al. Predictors of surgical site infection after open lower extremity revascularization. J Vasc Surg. (2017) 65:1769–78.e3. 10.1016/j.jvs.2016.11.053 [PubMed] [CrossRef] [Google Scholar]
- Dey D, Slomka P, Leeson P, Comaniciu D, Shrestha S, Sengupta P, et al. Artificial intelligence in cardiovascular imaging: JACC state-of-the-art review. J Am Coll Cardiol. (2019) 73:1317–35. 10.1016/j.jacc.2018.12.054 [PMCfreearticle] [PubMed][CrossRef] [Google Scholar]
- Discharge Trial Group, Maurovich-Horvat P, Bosserdt M, Kofoed K, Rieckmann N, Benedek T, et al. CT or invasive coronary angiography in stable chest pain. N Engl J Med. (2022) 386:1591–602. [PubMed] [Google Scholar]
- Elatrozy T, Nicolaides A, Tegos T, Griffin M. The objective characterisation of ultrasonic carotid plaque features. Eur J Vasc Endovasc Surg. (1998) 16:223–30. 10.1016/S1078-5884(98)80224-4 [PubMed] [CrossRef] [Google Scholar]
- Fairbairn TA, Nieman K, Akasaka T, Nørgaard B, Berman D, Raff G, et al. Real-world clinical utility and impact on clinical decision-making of coronary computed tomography angiography-derived fractional flow reserve: lessons from the ADVANCE registry. Eur Heart J. (2018) 39:3701–11. 10.1093/eurheartj/ehy530 [PMC free article] [PubMed] [CrossRef] [Google Scholar]]
- Fujiwara JF, Orii O, Araki KA, Ogura MO, Ito TI, Oyamada KO, et al. Fully automatic detection and measurement of abdominal aortic aneurysm using artificial intelligence. Eu Heart J. (2021) 42(Supplement_1):ehab724.3070. 10.1093/eurheartj/ehab724.3070 [CrossRef] [Google Scholar]
- Gao JM, Ren Z, Pan X, Chen Y, Zhu W, Li W, et al. Identifying peripheral arterial disease in the elderly patients using machine-learning algorithms. Aging Clin Exp Res. (2022) 34:679–85. 10.1007/s40520-021-01985-x [PubMed]

- Gautam N, Saluja P, Malkawi A, Rabbat M, Al-Mallah M, Pontone G, et al. Current and future applications of artificial intelligence in coronary artery disease. Healthcare. (2022) 10:232. 10.3390/healthcare10020232 [PMC free article] [PubMed] [CrossRef] [Google Scholar]
- Han C, Song Y, Lim H, Tae Y, Jang J, Lee B, et al. Automated detection of acute myocardial infarction using asynchronous electrocardiogram signals-preview of implementing artificial intelligence with multichannel electrocardiographs obtained from smartwatches: retrospective study. J Med Internet Res. (2021) 23:e31129. 10.2196/31129 [PMC free article] [PubMed] [CrossRef] [Google Scholar]
- Hassannataj Joloudari J, Azizi F, Nematollahi M, Alizadehsani R, Hassannatajjeloudari E, Nodehi I, et al. GSVMA: a genetic support vector machine ANOVA method for CAD diagnosis. Front Cardiovasc Med. (2022) 8:760178. 10.3389/fcvm.2021.760178 [PMC free article] [PubMed] [CrossRef] [Google Scholar]
- Hathaway QA, Yanamala N, Budoff M, Sengupta P, Zeb I. Deep neural survival networks for cardiovascular risk prediction: the multi-ethnic study of atherosclerosis (MESA). Comput Biol Med. (2021) 139:104983. 10.1016/j.compbiomed.2021.104983 [PubMed] [CrossRef] [Google Scholar]]]
- Hoyer C, Sandermann J, Petersen LJ. The toe-brachial index in the diagnosis of peripheral arterial disease. J Vasc Surg. (2013) 58:231–8. 10.1016/j.jvs.2013.03.044 [PubMed] [CrossRef] [Google Scholar]
- Iannuzzi A, Wilcosky T, Mercuri M, Rubba P, Bryan F, Bond M, et al. Ultrasonographic correlates of carotid atherosclerosis in transient ischemic attack and stroke. Stroke. (1995) 26:614–9. 10.1161/01.STR.26.4.614 [PubMed] [CrossRef] [Google Scholar]
- Ino Y, Kubo T, Matsuo Y, Yamaguchi T, Shiono Y, Shimamura K, et al. Optical coherence tomography predictors for edge restenosis after everolimus-eluting stent implantation. Circ Cardiovasc Interv. (2016) 9:e004231. 10.1161/CIRCINTERVENTIONS.116.00423[PubMed] [CrossRef] [Google Scholar]
- Jeremias A, Maehara A, Généreux P, Asrress K, Berry C, De Bruyne B, et al. Multicenter core laboratory comparison of the instantaneous wave-free ratio and resting Pd/Pa with fractional flow reserve: the RESOLVE study. J Am Coll Cardiol. (2014) 63:1253–61. 10.1016/j.jacc.2013.09.060 [PubMed] [CrossRef] [Google Scholar]
- Jiang Z, Do H, Choi J, Lee W, Baek S. A deep learning approach to predict abdominal aortic aneurysm expansion using longitudinal data. Front Phys. (2020) 7:235. 10.3389/fphy.2019.00235 [CrossRef] [Google Scholar]
- Johnson KW, Torres Soto J, Glicksberg B, Shameer K, Miotto R, Ali M, et al. Artificial intelligence in cardiology. J Am Coll Cardiol. (2018) 71:2668–79. 10.1016/j.jacc.2018.03.521 [PubMed] [CrossRef] [Google Scholar]
- Kakadiaris IA, Vrigkas M, Yen A, Kuznetsova T, Budoff M, Naghavi M, et al. Machine learning outperforms ACC/AHA CVD Risk calculator in MESA. J Am Heart Assoc. (2018) 7:e009476. 10.1161/JAHA.118.009476 [PMC free article] [PubMed] [CrossRef] [Google Scholar]
- Kamtchum-Tatuene J, Wilman A, Saqqur M, Shuaib A, Jickling G. Carotid plaque with high-risk features in embolic stroke of undetermined source: systematic review and meta-analysis. Stroke. (2020) 51:311–4. 10.1161/STROKEAHA.119.027272 [PMC free article] [PubMed] [CrossRef] [Google Scholar]
- Karlsson L, Kangefjärd E, Hermansson S, Strömberg S, Österberg K, Nordanstig A, et al. Risk of recurrent stroke in patients with symptomatic mild (20-49% NASCET) carotid artery stenosis. Eur J Vasc Endovasc Surg. (2016) 52:287–94. 10.1016/j.ejvs.2016.05.014 [PubMed] [CrossRef] [Google Scholar]
- Kavousi M, Leening M, Nanchen D, Greenland P, Graham I, Steyerberg E, et al. Comparison of application of the ACC/AHA guidelines, adult treatment panel III guidelines, and European society of cardiology guidelines for cardiovascular disease prevention in a European cohort. JAMA. (2014) 311:1416–23. 10.1001/jama.2014.2632 [PubMed] [CrossRef] [Google Scholar]]
- Kolossvary M, Karády J, Szilveszter B, Kitslaar P, Hoffmann U, Merkely B, et al. Radiomic features are superior to conventional quantitative computed tomographic metrics to identify coronary plaques with napkin-ring sign. Circ Cardiovasc Imaging. (2017) 10:e006843. 10.1161/CIRCIMAGING.117.006843 [PMC free article] [PubMed] [CrossRef] [Google Scholar]
- Kolossvary M, Kellermayer M, Merkely B, Maurovich-Horvat P. Cardiac computed tomography radiomics: a comprehensive review on radiomic techniques. J Thorac Imaging. (2018) 33:26–34. 10.1097/RTI.0000000000000268 [PubMed] [CrossRef] [Google Scholar]
- Kontopodis N, Klontzas M, Tzirakis K, Charalambous S, Marias K, Tsetis D, et al. Prediction of abdominal aortic aneurysm growth by artificial intelligence taking into account clinical, biologic, morphologic, and biomechanical variables. Vascular. (2022) [Epub ahead of print]. 10.1177/17085381221077821 [PubMed] [CrossRef] [Google Scholar]
- Kordzadeh A, Askari A, Abbassi O, Sanoudos N, Mohaghegh V, Shirvani H, et al. Artificial intelligence and duplex ultrasound for detection of carotid artery disease. Vascular. (2022) [Epub ahead of print]. 10.1177/17085381221107465 [PubMed] [CrossRef] [Google Scholar]
- Krittanawong C, Zhang H, Wang Z, Aydar M, Kitai T. Artificial intelligence in precision cardiovascular medicine. J Am Coll Cardiol. (2017) 69:2657–64. 10.1016/j.jacc.2017.03.571 [PubMed] [CrossRef] [Google Scholar]
- Kwok CS, Bennett S, Azam Z, Welsh V, Potluri R, Loke Y, et al. Misdiagnosis of acute myocardial infarction: a systematic review of the literature. Crit Pathw Cardiol. (2021) 20:155–62. 10.1097/HPC.0000000000000256 [PubMed] [CrossRef] [Google Scholar]
- Lareyre F, Lê C, Ballaith A, Adam C, Carrier M, Amrani S, et al. Applications of artificial intelligence in non-cardiac vascular diseases: a bibliographic analysis. Angiology. (2022) 73:606–14. 10.1177/00033197211062280 [PubMed] [CrossRef] [Google Scholar]
- Le EPV, Rundo L, Tarkin J, Evans N, Chowdhury M, Coughlin P, et al. Assessing robustness of carotid artery CT angiography radiomics in the identification of culprit lesions in cerebrovascular events. Sci Rep. (2021) 11:3499. 10.1038/s41598-021-82760-w [PMC free article] [PubMed] [CrossRef] [Google Scholar]
- Lederle F, Kyriakides T, Stroupe K, Freischlag J, Padberg F, Jr., Matsumura J, et al. Open versus endovascular repair of abdominal aortic aneurysm. N Engl J Med. (2019) 380:2126–35. 10.1056/NEJMoa1715955 [PubMed] [CrossRef] [Google Scholar]
- Lundberg S, Lee S-I. A unified approach to interpreting model predictions. In: Guyon I, Luxburg UV, Bengio S, Wallach H, Fergus R, Vishwanathan S, et al. editors. Advances in Neural Information Processing Systems. Red Hook, NY: Curran Associates, Inc; (2017).
- Martin SS, Mastrodicasa D, van Assen M, De Cecco C, Bayer R, Tesche C, et al. Value of machine learning-based coronary CT Fractional flow reserve applied to triple-rule-out CT angiography in acute chest pain. Radiol Cardiothorac Imaging. (2020) 2:e190137. 10.1148/ryct.2020190137 [PMC free article] [PubMed] [CrossRef]

- Masuda T, Nakaura T, Funama Y, Okimoto T, Sato T, Higaki T, et al. Machine-learning integration of CT histogram analysis to evaluate the composition of atherosclerotic plaques: validation with IB-IVUS. J Cardiovasc Comput Tomogr. (2019) 13:163–9. 10.1016/j.jcct.2018.10.018 [PubMed] [CrossRef] [Google Scholar]
- McBane RD, II, Murphree D, Liedl D, Lopez-Jimenez F, Attia I, Arruda-Olson A, et al. Artificial intelligence for the evaluation of peripheral artery disease using arterial doppler waveforms to predict abnormal ankle-brachial index. Vasc Med. (2022) 27:333–42. 10.1177/1358863X221094082 [PubMed] [CrossRef] [Google Scholar]
- Mortazavi BJ, Bucholz E, Desai N, Huang C, Curtis J, Masoudi F, et al. Comparison of machine learning methods with national cardiovascular data registry models for prediction of risk of bleeding after percutaneous coronary intervention. JAMA Netw Open. (2019) 2:e196835.10.1001/jamanetworkopen.2019.6835 [PMC free article] [PubMed] [CrossRef] [Google Scholar]]
- Motwani M, Dey D, Berman DS, Germano G, Achenbach S, Al-Mallah MH, et al. Machine learning for prediction of all-cause mortality in patients with suspected coronary artery disease: a 5-year multicentre prospective registry analysis. Eur Heart J. (2017) 38:500-7.10.1093/eurheartj/ehw188 [PMC free article] [PubMed] [CrossRef] [Google Scholar]
- Muntner P, Colantonio L, Cushman M, Goff D, Jr., Howard G, Howard V, et al. Validation of the atherosclerotic cardiovascular disease Pooled Cohort risk equations. JAMA. (2014) 311:1406–15. 10.1001/jama.2014.2630 [PMC free article] [PubMed] [CrossRef] [Google Scholar]
- Muscogiuri G, Van Assen M, Tesche C, De Cecco C, Chiesa M, Scafuri S, et al. Artificial intelligence in coronary computed tomography angiography: from anatomy to prognosis. Biomed Res Int. (2020) 2020:6649410. 10.1155/2020/6649410 [PMC free article] [PubMed] [CrossRef] [Google Scholar]
- Nasarian E, Abdar M, Fahami MA, Alizadehsani R, Hussain S, Basiri ME, et al. Association between work-related features and coronary artery disease: a heterogeneous hybrid feature selection integrated with balancing approach. Pattern Recogn Lett. (2020) 133:33–40. 10.1016/j.patrec.2020.02.010 [CrossRef]
- Oikonomou EK, Siddique M, Antoniades C. Artificial intelligence in medical imaging: a radiomic guide to precision phenotyping of cardiovascular disease. Cardiovasc Res. (2020) 116:2040–54. 10.1093/cvr/cvaa021 [PMC free article] [PubMed] [CrossRef] [Google Scholar]
- Oikonomou EK, Williams M, Kotanidis C, Desai M, Marwan M, Antonopoulos A, et al. A novel machine learning-derived radiotranscriptomic signature of perivascular fat improves cardiac risk prediction using coronary CT angiography. Eur Heart J. (2019) 40:3529–43. 10.1093/eurheartj/ehz592 [PMC free article]
- Perez MV, Mahaffey K, Hedlin H, Rumsfeld J, Garcia A, Ferris T, et al. Large-scale assessment of a smartwatch to identify atrial fibrillation. N Engl J Med. (2019) 381:1909–17. 10.1056/NEJMoa1901183 [PMC free article] [PubMed] [CrossRef] [Google Scholar]
- Peters F, Behrendt CA. External validation of the OAC3-PAD risk score to predict major bleeding events using the prospective germanvasc cohort study. Eur J Vasc Endovasc Surg. (2022) 64:429–30. 10.1016/j.ejvs.2022.07.055 [PubMed] [CrossRef]
- Puchner SB, Liu T, Mayrhofer T, Truong Q, Lee H, Fleg J, et al. High-risk plaque detected on coronary CT angiography predicts acute coronary syndromes independent of significant stenosis in acute chest pain: results from the ROMICAT-II trial. J Am Coll Cardiol. (2014) 64:684–92. 10.1016/j.jacc.2014.05.039 [PMC free article] [PubMed] [CrossRef] [Google Scholar]
- Qutrio Baloch Z, Ali Raza S, Pathak R, Marone L, Ali A. Machine learning confirms nonlinear relationship between severity of peripheral arterial disease, functional limitation and symptom severity. Diagnostics. (2020) 10:515. 10.3390/diagnostics10080515 [PMC free article] [PubMed] [CrossRef] [Google Scholar]
- Raffort J, Adam C, Carrier M, Ballaith A, Coscas R, Jean-Baptiste E, et al. Artificial intelligence in abdominal aortic aneurysm. J Vasc Surg. (2020) 72:321–33.e1. 10.1016/j.jvs.2019.12.026 [PubMed] [CrossRef] [Google Scholar]
- Rao SV, McCoy L, Spertus J, Krone R, Singh M, Fitzgerald S, et al. An updated bleeding model to predict the risk of post-procedure bleeding among patients undergoing percutaneous coronary intervention: a report using an expanded bleeding definition from the national cardiovascular data registry CathPCI registry. JACC Cardiovasc Interv. (2013) 6:897–904. 10.1016/j.jcin.2013.04.016 [PubMed] [CrossRef] [Google Scholar]
- Rowe M. An introduction to machine learning for clinicians. Acad Med. (2019) 94:1433–6. 10.1097/ACM.0000000000002792 [PubMed] [CrossRef] [Google Scholar]
- Sakalihasan N, Michel J, Katsargyris A, Kuivaniemi H, Defraigne J, Nchimi A, et al. Abdominal aortic aneurysms. Nat Rev Dis Primers. (2018) 4:34. 10.1038/s41572-018-0030-7 [PubMed] [CrossRef] [Google Scholar]
- Singh TP, Moxon J, Gasser T, Golledge J. Systematic review and meta-analysis of peak wall stress and peak wall rupture index in ruptured and asymptomatic intact abdominal aortic aneurysms. J AmHeartAssoc. (2021) 10:e019772.10.1161/JAHA.120.019772 [PMC free article] [PubMed] [CrossRef] [Google Scholar]
- Takx RA, de Jong P, Leiner T, Oudkerk M, de Koning H, Mol C, et al. Automated coronary artery calcification scoring in non-gated chest CT: agreement and reliability. PLoS One. (2014) 9:e91239. 10.1371/journal.pone.0091239 [PMC free article] [PubMed] [CrossRef] [Google Scholar
- van Nunen LX, Zimmermann F, Tonino P, Barbato E, Baumbach A, Engstrøm T, et al. Fractional flow reserve versus angiography for guidance of PCI in patients with multivessel coronary artery disease (FAME): 5-year follow-up of a randomised controlled trial. Lancet. (2015) 386:1853–60. 10.1016/S0140-6736(15)00057-4 [PubMed] [CrossRef] [Google Scholar]
- Ward A, Sarraju A, Chung S, Li J, Harrington R, Heidenreich P, et al. Machine learning and atherosclerotic cardiovascular disease risk prediction in a multi-ethnic population. NPJ Digit Med. (2020) 3:125. 10.1038/s41746-020-00331-1 [PMC free article] [PubMed] [CrossRef]
- Yin Y, He C, Xu B, Li Z. Coronary plaque characterization from optical coherence tomography imaging with a two-pathway cascade convolutional neural network architecture. Front Cardiovasc Med. (2021) 8:670502. 10.3389/fcvm.2021.670502 [PMC free article] [PubMed] [CrossRef] [Google Scholar]
- Zreik M, van Hamersvelt R, Wolterink J, Leiner T, Viergever M, Isgum I, et al. A recurrent CNN for automatic detection and classification of coronary artery plaque and stenosis in coronary CT angiography. IEEE Trans Med Imaging. (2019) 38:1588–98. 10.1109/

CHAPTER

6

AI In Cardiovascular Imaging for Risk Stratification In CAD

Artificial intelligence (AI) describes the use of computational techniques to perform tasks that normally require human cognition. Machine learning and deep learning are subfields of AI that are increasingly being applied to cardiovascular imaging for risk stratification. Deep learning algorithms can accurately quantify prognostic biomarkers from image data. Additionally, conventional or AI-based imaging parameters can be combined with clinical data using machine learning models for individualized risk prediction. The aim of this review is to provide a comprehensive review of state-of-the-art AI applications across various noninvasive imaging modalities (coronary artery calcium scoring CT, coronary CT angiography, and nuclear myocardial perfusion imaging) for the quantification of cardiovascular risk in coronary artery disease

- Artificial intelligence (AI) is increasingly being applied to noninvasive cardiovascular imaging modalities for risk stratification in coronary artery disease.
- Deep learning algorithms can perform automated measurements of prognostic biomarkers directly from image data.
- Conventional or AI-based imaging parameters can be integrated with clinical data using machine learning models for per-patient risk prediction.
- The objective ranking of variables in individualized machine learning prediction models increases the explainability of AI findings.

Various Techniques used for Risk Stratification In CAD

AI is a field of computer science that aims to mimic human cognition in performing tasks such as object or pattern recognition, planning, and problem-solving.

The term big data refers to large and heterogeneous data sets that require computational techniques such as AI for their analysis and interpretation In health care, this includes data from the omics fields (eg, genomics, metabolomics, proteomics, lipidomics), tabular data from electronic health records, and imaging data. Within big data exist individual measurable characteristics or datapoints known as features. In imaging, this could be represented by voxel intensity, the spatial distribution of voxels, a vector of motion, or conventional metrics used in clinical practice. The quality, accuracy, and richness of features in data are key determinants of AI model performance.

Machine learning (ML), a subfield of AI, enables computer algorithms to automatically learn and improve from experience through exposure to vast amounts of data While many different algorithmic approaches—or models—exist within ML, they all aim to achieve one of two tasks. The first is supervised learning, in which a labeled data set is used to predict a known outcome. This involves the iterative selection and weighting of individual features to learn the underlying patterns within the data that best fit the outcome.Examples of supervised learning algorithms include linear regression, support vector machines, and random forest. The second task is unsupervised learning, whereby unlabeled data are used to predict unknown associations. These models attempt to capture relationships inherent to the structure of the features themselves; examples include clustering and principal component analysis Deep learning (DL) is a specific form of ML that uses multilayered artificial neural networks to make predictions directly from input data. The most commonly used DL networks for image analysis are convolutional neural networks (CNNs). These contain many layers stacked on top of each other,

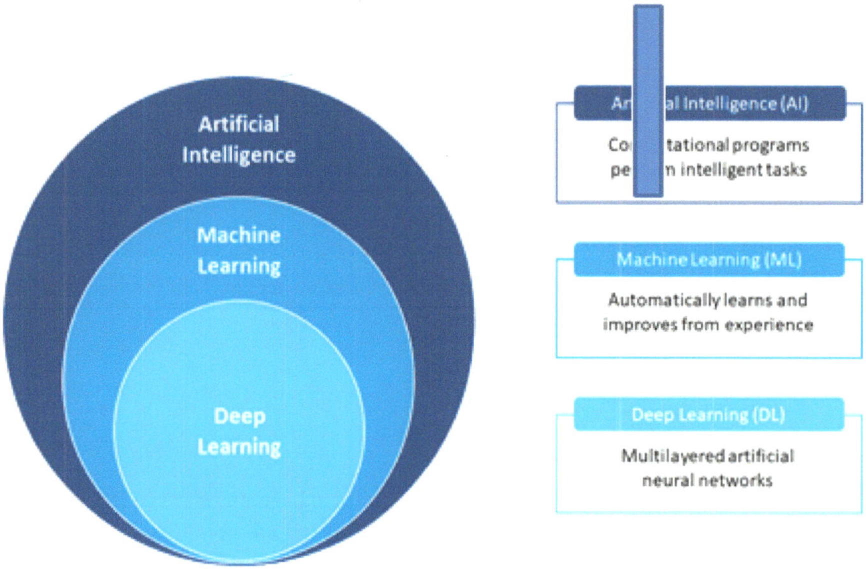

Fig.6.1 Basics of artificial intelligence (AI), machine learning (ML), and deep learning. Artificial intelligence describes the use of computational techniques to perform tasks characteristic of human intelligence. ML is a subfield of AI that enables computers to automatically learn by being exposed to large amounts of data. Deep learning is a specific form of ML that uses multilayered artificial neural networks to make predictions directly from input data.

including one or more convolutional layers that create a feature map summarizing the presence of detected features in the input (6). In health care, some of the greatest successes of DL have been in the field of computer vision, which handles tasks such as object classification, detection, and segmentation from digital images or videos .Raw image data are typically transformed to features prior to input into the CNNs. Another emerging application of DL has been for processing of tabular data contained in electronic health records for per-patient predictions. This includes structured data such as laboratory results, diagnostic codes, and demographics, as well as unstructured data that requires standardization and sequencing. Radiomics is the process of extracting thousands of computational quantitative features (most of which are invisible to the human eye) from medical images. These features capture the complex spatial relationship between voxels by describing textural patterns or geometric properties within a given imaging region of interest. ML techniques can then be applied to these data sets to identify imaging biomarkers of significant clinical value.In cardiovascular imaging, AI algorithms can be used to both identify new imaging biomarkers and integrate data from many different sources to provide patient-tailored risk prediction.

1.Noncontrast Cardiac CT

Coronary Artery Calcium Scoring

Coronary artery calcium (CAC), a specific marker of coronary atherosclerosis, is a powerful predictor of angiographically significant obstructive CAD (26) and incident cardiovascular events . Incremental prognostic value over standard clinical risk scores has also been consistently reported . In current clinical practice, CAC scoring from noncontrast electrocardiographically gated cardiac CT requires manual interaction by a human operator. Using commercially available software, the reader identifies and labels all voxels above a threshold of 130 HU to quantify the Agatston score (30) or volume score . This approach can be labor-intensive and time-consuming; thus, a more automated workflow that reduces the need for human interaction is highly desirable. ML approaches for the rapid and automated quantification of CAC from dedicated noncontrast cardiac CT have shown promising results. Wolterink et al trained a random forest classifier comprising numerous individual decision trees to distinguish between true calcifications and other candidate calcifications based on size, shape, position, and intensity features. The resultant per-patient Agatston and volume scores demonstrated a strong correlation (r = 0.94) with expert manual measurements

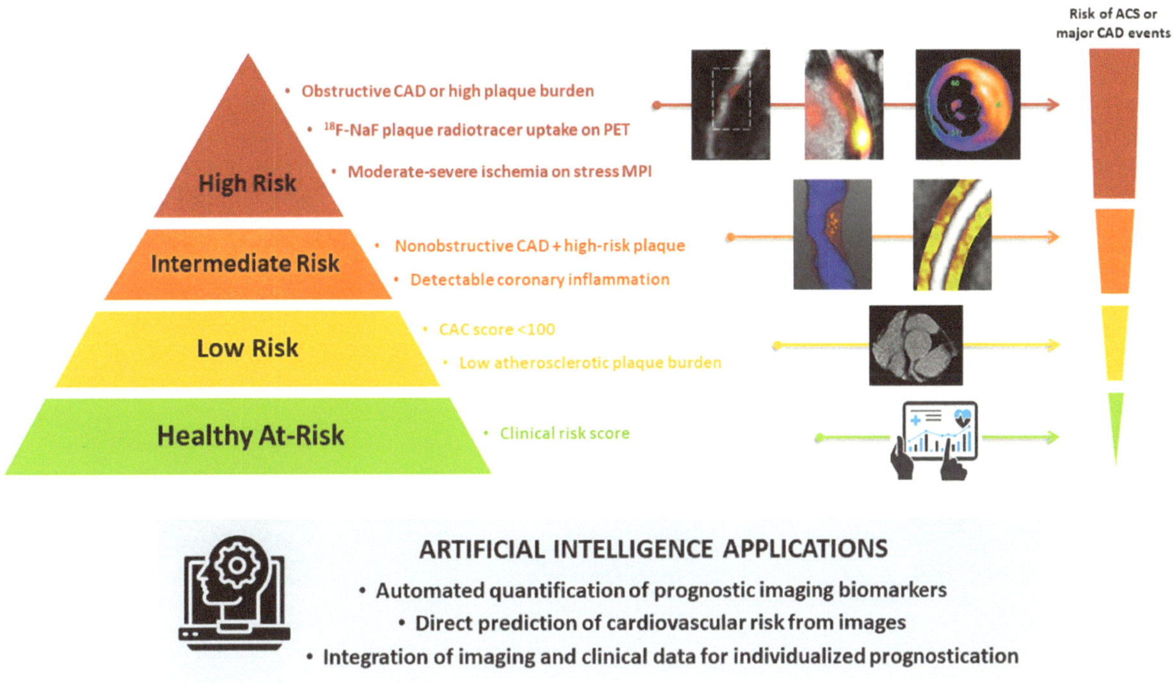

Fig.6.2 Artificial intelligence (AI) in cardiovascular imaging for risk stratification. Clinical risk stratification based on anatomic and functional imaging assessment of coronary artery disease (CAD). The image case examples (from left to right) correspond to the descriptions (from top to bottom) adjacent to the risk pyramid. AI algorithms can perform automated measurements of prognostic biomarkers from image data. Additionally, conventional or AI-based imaging parameters can be combined with clinical data using machine learning models for individualized risk prediction. ACS = acute coronary syndrome, CAC = coronary artery calcium, 18F-NaF = fluorine 18 sodium fluoride, MPI = myocardial perfusion imaging. Overview of AI Applications for Risk Stratification in Cardiovascular Imaging Studies

In an extension of this work, the authors introduced a multiclass classification of candidate coronary calcifications to detect CAC per artery, along with an ambiguity detection system that flagged difficult cases for expert review. Intraclass correlation coefficients between automatic and fully manual CAC volume scores improved with expert review of difficult cases that had been flagged by the algorithm: left anterior descending artery (0.98 vs 1.00), left circumflex artery (0.69 vs 0.95), and right coronary artery (0.95 vs 0.99). No ambiguous candidates were identified in close to half of all CT scans. Automatic scoring combined with expert review led to a faster processing time of 45 seconds, compared with 128 seconds per scan for fully manual scoring.CAC scores can also be derived from chest CT performed for other indications, such as lung cancer screening, thus paving the way for application of AI algorithms in large sets of screening data. Fully automated ML- and DL-based quantification of CAC has been evaluated in large data sets of low-dose, ungated CT scans from national lung cancer screening trials in Europe and the United States, demonstrating feasibility and high reliability compared with manual measurements. Similar results were observed for a CAC scoring DL algorithm trained using radiation therapy–planning CT scans of patients with breast cancer acquired during free breathing Recently, van Velzen et al sought to validate a DL method for automated CAC scoring using multiple cardiac and chest CT protocols. In 7240 patients who underwent various types of noncontrast chest CT scans, the investigators used two consecutive CNNs to quantify the Agatston score. The first CNN detected candidate calcifications on each image and assigned them to a coronary artery, and the second CNN classified these calcifications as true positive or false positive . The DL algorithm was trained and tested on three separate data sets stratified by scan type

Compared with manual CAC scoring, the DL algorithm produced reliable measurements, with intraclass correlation coefficients of 0.79–0.97 across the range of scan types. In cardiovascular risk categorization according to the Agatston score, DL had excellent agreement with manual CAC scoring (κ = 0.90 for all test scans). These findings lend support to the use of such a DL method to aid clinicians in CAC scoring across a wide range of noncontrast chest CT images.While AI enables direct computation of CAC measures from CT images, the Agatston score quantified by conventional methods can also be used as an input into AI models for risk prediction.Al'Aref et al trained an ML algorithm with extreme gradient boosting (XGBoost; https://xgboost.ai/) using clinical data from 35 281 patientseither suspected of having CAD or with established CAD. An ML model incorporating clinical variables (age, sex, risk factors, and cholesterol levels) yielded an area under the receiver operating characteristic curve (AUC) of 0.77 for predicting the presence of obstructive CAD at CCTA. The addition of CAC score to the ML model resulted in a significantly higher AUC (0.88), which also outperformed a statistical model containing the CAC score and CAD consortiumclinical score (AUC, 0.86) and the CAD consortium clinical score alone (AUC, 0.73; P < .05 for all comparisons). Hence, integration of the CAC score and clinical data with ML could potentially be adopted in clinical practice to enhance risk stratification and inform referral for downstream testing such as CCTA

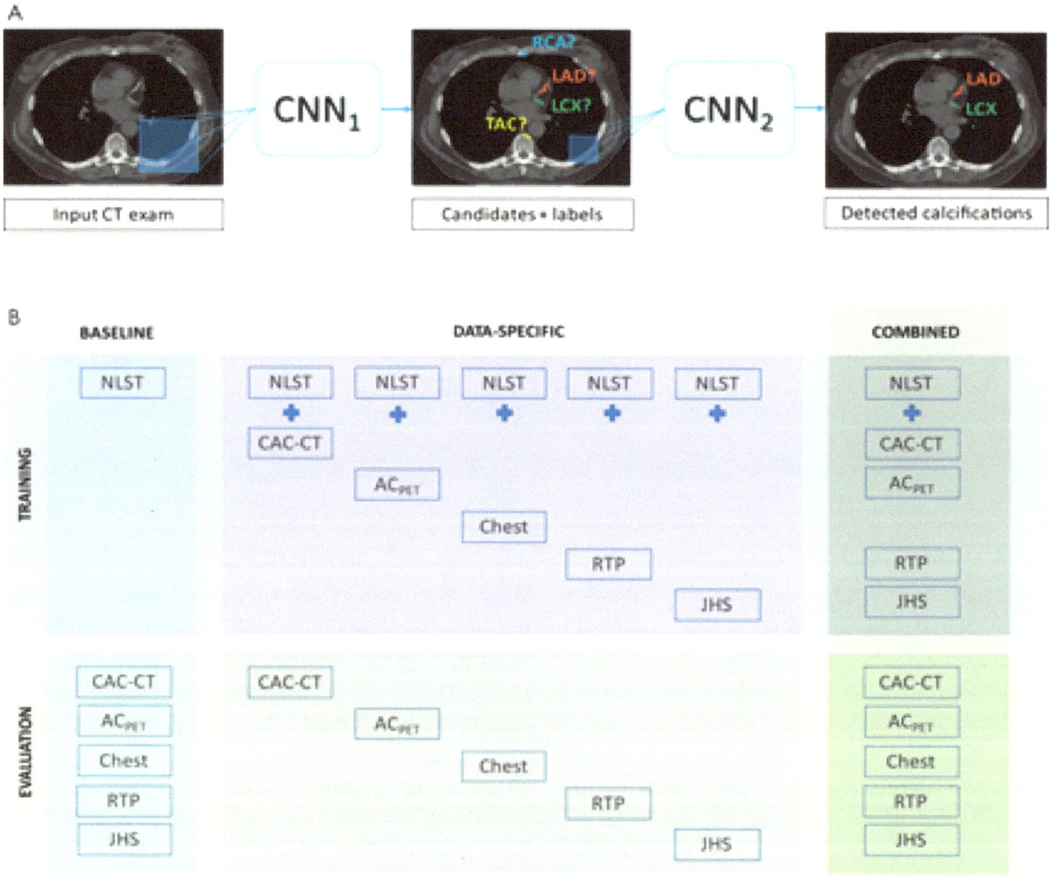

Fig.6.3 Automatic coronary artery calcium scoring. A, The deep learning algorithm consists of two convolutional neural networks (CNNs). The first CNN (CNN1) detects candidate calcifications (voxels) with attenuation of greater than 130 HU and assigns them to a coronary artery, and the second CNN (CNN2) detects true calcified voxels among candidates detected by the first CNN. B, The baseline algorithm was trained with National Lung Screening Trial (NLST) scans, and its performance was evaluated in each CT protocol type. Five data-specific algorithms were trained, according to CT protocol type, and evaluated in the respective CT type. The combined algorithm was trained and evaluated using all available CT protocol types. CT types used for training were NLST CT scans, coronary artery calcium scoring CT (CAC-CT), PET attenuation correction CT (ACPET), diagnostic chest (Chest) CT, radiation therapy treatment planning (RTP) CT, and Jackson Heart Study (JHS) CT scans. exam = examination, LAD = left anterior descending artery, LCX = left circumflex artery, RCA = right coronary artery, TAC = thoracic aorta calcification. (Reprinted, with permission)

In 66 636 asymptomatic individuals from the CAC Consortium, Nakanishi et al developed a LogitBoost-based ML model incorporating 20 CAC measures (total and per-vessel Agatston, volume, and density scores), non-CAC metrics (including thoracic and aortic calcium scores), and 46 clinical variables for the prediction of CAD-related death at 10-year follow-up. The ML model (AUC, 0.86) provided superior risk prediction compared with either the atherosclerotic cardiovascular disease (ASCVD) risk score (AUC, 0.83) or the CAC score (AUC, 0.82; P < .001 for both). This comprehensive ML approach also outperformed ML with clinical data alone or CT data alone. Hence, an ML model that can use all available information has the potential to become a routine risk assessment tool, especially as electronic health records are widely adopted in clinical practice and their platforms enable increasingly seamless integration of clinical and imaging data.

2.Epicardial Adipose Tissue Quantification

Epicardial adipose tissue is a metabolically active fat depot located between the myocardium and visceral pericardium that modulates coronary arterial function.Epicardial adipose tissue volume, which traditionally has been quantified from routine CAC scoring CT using manual or semiautomated techniques , has been shown to associate with coronary atherosclerosis and incident cardiac events.Recently, Commandeur et al developed a fully automated DL-based method for epicardial adipose tissue quantification., which was tested in a large multicenter study and showed a strong correlation with expert manual measurements (r = 0.97; P < .001). DL computation was rapid, with a time of approximately 6 seconds per case, compared with a time of 15 minutes per case for experts. Epicardial adipose tissue measures derived using this DL algorithm were subsequently used for prognostication in 2068 asymptomatic participants from the Early Identification of Subclinical Atherosclerosis by Noninvasive Imaging Research (EISNER) trial . In that study, DL-based epicardial adipose tissue volume was independently associated with increased risk of major adverse cardiovascular events (MACEs) (hazard ratio, 1.35 [95% CI: 1.07, 1.68] per case for experts. Epicardial adipose tissue measures derived using this DL algorithmwere subsequently used for prognostication. in 2068 asymptomatic participants from the Early Identification of Subclinical Atherosclerosis by Noninvasive Imaging Research (EISNER) trial . In that study, DL-based epicardial adipose tissue volume was independently associated with increased risk of major adverse cardiovascular events (MACEs)(hazard ratio, 1.35 [95% CI: 1.07, 1.68] per doubling; P = .009), following adjustment for ASCVD risk score and CAC score

Epicardial adipose tissue attenuation by this method was inversely associated with MACE risk (hazard ratio, 0.83 [95% CI: 0.72, 0.96] per 5 HU increase; P = .01). Such rapid, automated measurements of epicardial adipose tissue have the potential for integration into routine reporting of calcium scoring CT, providing real-time, complementary information on cardiovascular risk In addition, Commandeur et al combined DL-based epicardial adipose tissue metrics with clinical variables and the CAC score using an XGBoost algorithm for risk stratification in a separate EISNER substudy. The ML risk score (AUC, 0.82) outperformed the ASCVD risk score or CAC score alone (AUC, 0.77 for both; P < .05) for long-term prediction of MACE. A major advantage of this ML approach is its ability to explicitly describe the influence of each variable for individualized prediction and provide so-called explainable AI.

This is particularly important given that many ML algorithms are considered "black boxes" with no clear justification for their decision-making. Further, such stratification of significant clinical and imaging parameters could potentially guide therapy targeted at the specific factors affecting cardiovascular outcomes.

3.Coronary CT Angiography

Coronary Artery Stenosis Detection and Grading

The prognostic value of anatomic assessment of CAD with CCTA is well established, with coronary stenosis detection and quantification being the cornerstone of routine clinical reporting. Currently, these tasks rely on visual assessment and are therefore subject to substantial interobserver variability A number of AI approaches have been able to automatically

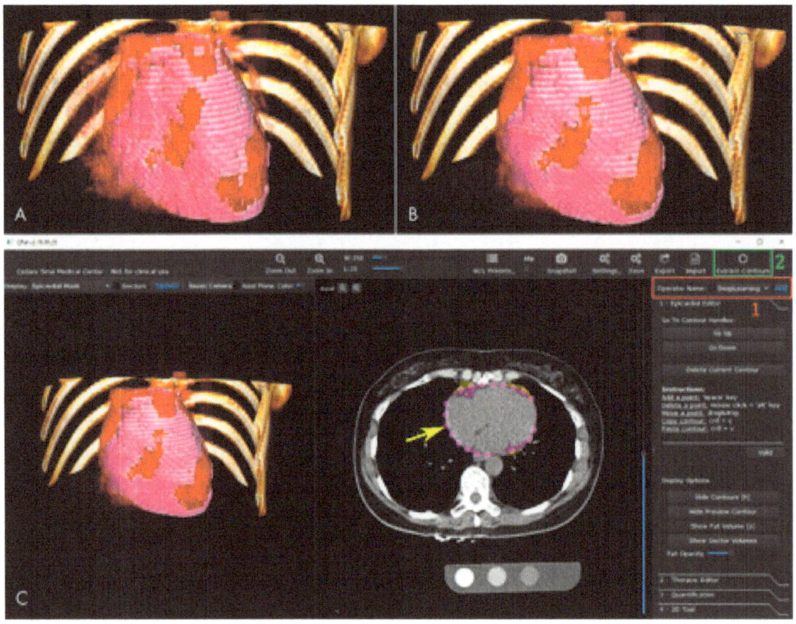

Fig.6.4 Deep learning–based quantification of epicardial adipose tissue. A, Three-dimensional rendering of epicardial adipose tissue (pink overlay) derived from coronary artery calcium scoring CT, B, as manually measured by an expert, and C, as automatically quantified by a deep learning algorithm embedded in research software (QFAT [version 2.0; Cedars-Sinai Medical Center]). (Reprinted, with permission)

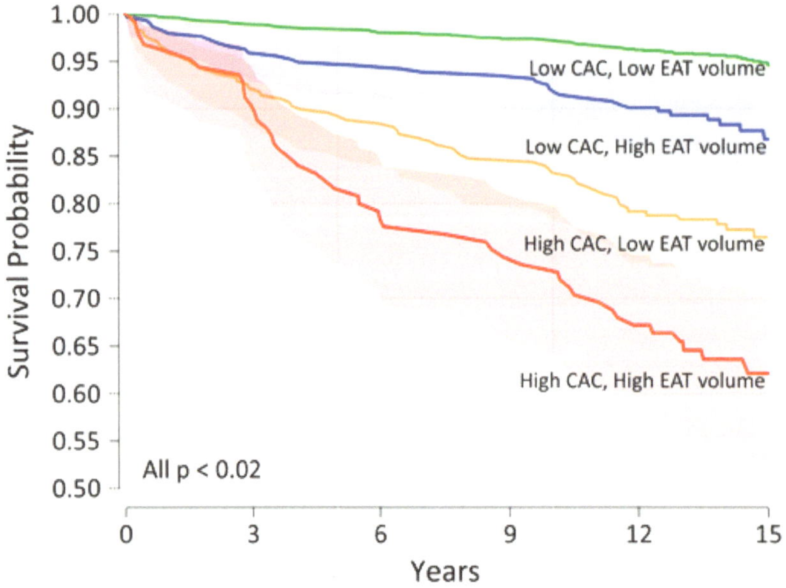

Fig.6.5 Risk stratification by coronary artery calcium (CAC) score and deep learning–based epicardial adipose tissue (EAT) volume. Kaplan-Meier curves of MACE-free survival in asymptomatic individuals from the Early Identification of Subclinical Atherosclerosis by Noninvasive Imaging Research trial stratified by low (< 100) versus high (≥ 100) CAC score and low (< 113 cm3) versus high (≥ 113 cm3) EAT volume. Risk was highest in individuals with a high CAC score and high EAT volume. (Reprinted, with permission)

determine the degree of coronary stenosis directly from image data. Kang et al used a support vector machine incorporating geometric and plaque features to detect coronary artery lesions with at least 25% stenosis in a data set of 42 patients, yielding high sensitivity (93%) and specificity (95%) compared with expert visual assessment. Kelm et al trained a random forest ML algorithm to automatically estimate luminal cross-sectional area and detect obstructive (> 50%) stenosis, achieving a sensitivity of 95% and specificity of 67% compared with experts, at an average speed of 1.8 seconds per case. Hong et al used a CNN to automatically quantify the percentage diameter stenosis and minimal luminal area, with DL measures correlating strongly with expert manual annotations (r = 0.957 for stenosis, r = 0.984 for minimal luminal area; P < .001 for both).

CCTA-derived measures of coronary stenosis have also been integrated into ML models for outcome prediction. In 10 030 patients, Motwani et al trained a Logit. Boost algorithm using 25 clinical variables and 44 visually determined CCTA parameters of CAD extent and severity for the prediction of 5-year all-cause mortality. The resultant ML score (AUC, 0.79) outperformed traditional CCTA-based segment scores (AUC, 0.64 for both segment stenosis score and segment involvement score) and the Framingham risk score (AUC, 0.61; P < .001 for all) . Among the highest ranked variables in the ML model were the number of noncalcified segments and number of vessels with diameter stenosis less than 50%.

Coronary Plaque Characterization and Quantification

CCTA also enables assessment of plaque morphology, which previously could only be evaluated using invasive intracoronary imaging. Qualitative "high-risk plaque" features (positive remodeling, low attenuation plaque, spotty calcification, and napkin-ring sign) derived from CCTA have predictive value for acute coronary syndrome . Of these features, identification of the napkin-ring sign is most prone to interreader variability as it relies exclusively on visual assessment .Kolossváry et al sought to use CCTA-based radiomics to improve the detection of napkin-ring sign. Of 4400 radiomic features analyzed in this study, 440 (9.9%) exhibited high diagnostic accuracy (AUC > 0.80). Most of these features were textural or geometric, describing the complex spatial distribution of voxels. In another study, radiomic analysis was shown to outperform qualitative features at CCTA for the identification of vulnerable plaques determined by using intracoronary imaging. Finally, Kolossváry et al combined CCTA-based radiomic analysis with ML for the identification of histologically determined advanced atherosclerotic lesions. After using 1919 radiomic features to train eight independent ML models, a test model based on least angle regression and fitted with the 13 most predictive parameters was able to outperform visual CCTA assessment (AUC, 0.73 vs 0.65; P = .04).In a study by Motoyama et al , the presence of qualitative high-risk plaque at CCTA (defined by positive remodeling and/or low attenuation plaque) was an independent predictor of future acute coronary syndrome. Importantly, however, the cumulative number of events was similar among patients with and without high-risk plaques; this was primarily attributed to the diffuse nature of coronary atherosclerosis. In more recent studies, CCTA-based quantification of plaque volume and burden in the entire coronary tree using software applications has demonstrated independent prognostic value . In a landmark post hoc analysis of the multicenter Scottish COmputed Tomography of the HEART (SCOT-HEART) trial with 5-year follow-up, Williams et al showed that patients with a high >4%) low-attenuation noncalcified plaque burden were five times more likely to develop myocardial infarction than patients with a low (≤4%) plaque burden, independent of risk factors, stenosis severity, or CAC score. CCTA-derived quantitative plaque measures have been incorporated into ML models to enhance outcome prediction. In a lesion-level analysis of a matched cohort of patients with and without acute coronary syndrome, Al'Aref et al input qualitative and quantitative plaque features measured by conventional methods into an XGBoost algorithm for the prediction of culprit lesions associated with acute coronary syndrome. The ML model provided superior performance (AUC, 0.77) compared with quantitative plaque features or qualitative high-risk plaque features alone.Lesion-specific ischemia by invasive fractional flow reserve, which has a well-established association with adverse cardiac events , has been used as the outcome for training AI algorithms. Dey et al combined conventional quantitative plaque and vessel-based metrics in an ML model that provided superior prediction for lesion-specific ischemia (AUC, 0.84) compared with stenosis severity (AUC, 0.76) or pretest probability of CAD (AUC, 0.63). The burdens of noncalcified plaque and low-attenuation noncalcified plaque provided the highest ML information gain Noninvasive fractional flow reserve measurement derived from CCTA can also be performed with the assistance of DL techniques that identify lumen boundaries and thus enable assessment of computational fluid dynamics. In a real-world study, this method (AUC, 0.94) outperformed conventional CCTA stenosis assessment (AUC, 0.83) and PET (AUC, 0.87; P < .01 for both) for the detection of per-vessel ischemia when compared with invasive angiography as the reference standard .An ML framework has also demonstrated promising results in predicting the risk of rapid plaque progression. In patients undergoing serial CCTA over a median interval of 3.3 years, Han et al showed a Logit Boost-based model incorporating baseline clinical variables as well as qualitative and quantitative plaque parameters to have greater discriminatory value in identifying patients with rapid plaque progression compared with ML models with clinical variables or qualitative plaque features alone, and also compared with traditional risk scores. Quantitative plaque parameters provided the highest information gain for ML, followed by qualitative plaque parameters and clinical variables.

Detecting Coronary Inflammation

Beyond coronary assessment, CCTA imaging of pericoronary adipose tissue (PCAT) enables detection of coronary inflammation and several AI techniques have recently been applied to PCAT quantification. Oikonomou et al input radiomic features extracted from PCAT into a random forest ML model to develop a patient-level "fat radiomic profile." When tested in 1575 participants from the SCOT-HEART trial, this metric had incremental value for MACE prediction beyond traditional CCTA-based risk stratification (AUC, 0.88 vs 0.75; P < .001).In a prospective case-control study, Lin et al (56) examined 1103 radiomic features of PCAT

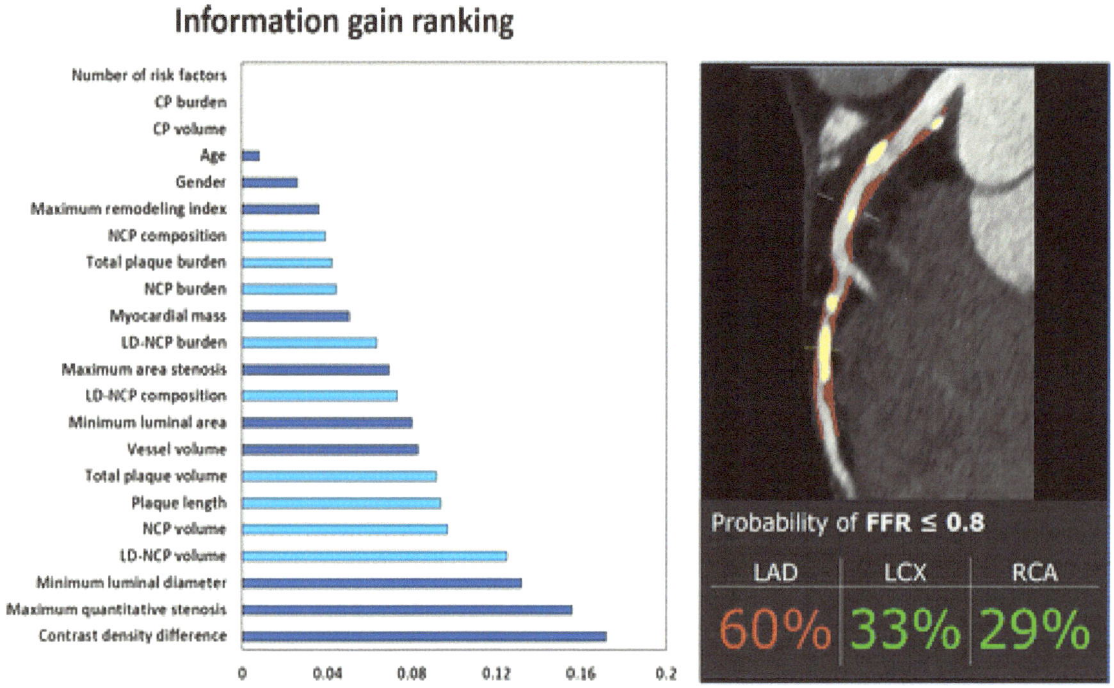

Fig.6.6 Machine learning (ML) prediction of lesion-specific ischemia. The left panel shows information gain ranking of variables in a coronary CT angiography (CCTA)–based ML model used to predict lesion-specific ischemia by invasive fractional flow reserve. Quantitative plaque measures are shown in light blue, and other CCTA and clinical variables are shown in dark blue. The right panel is a case example of the ML prediction applied to a symptomatic patient undergoing CCTA, with noncalcified plaque (NCP) and calcified plaque (CP) shown in red and yellow overlay, respectively. Invasive fractional flow reserve (FFR) of the left anterior descending artery (LAD) was positive (0.73). LCX = left circumflex artery, LD-NCP = low-density noncalcified plaque, RCA = right coronary artery. (Reprinted, with permission)

in patients with and without acute myocardial infarction. Using XGBoost, an ML model integrating clinical data, the average CT attenuation of PCAT, and PCAT radiomic features (AUC, 0.87) outperformed a model with clinical data and PCAT attenuation (AUC, 0.77; P = .001) and clinical data alone (AUC, 0.87 vs 0.76; P < .001) in identifying patients with myocardial infarction . Textural features of PCAT provided the greatest variable importance in the radiomics-based ML model . Together, these studies show how combining advanced CCTA-based quantification of PCAT with ML can identify new imaging biomarkers of the so-called vulnerable patient.

4.Nuclear Cardiology

Early studies of AI in nuclear cardiology used quantitative and functional parameters from SPECT myocardial perfusion imaging (MPI) for the prediction of obstructive CAD at invasive angiography.Arsanjani et al combined imaging measures (including stress total perfusion deficit and inducible ischemic and ejection fraction changes) with clinical data and stress electrocardiogram changes using LogitBoost. The integrated ML model provided superior accuracy for detecting obstructive CAD compared with not only total perfusion deficit alone or visual analysis, butalso with an ML model without clinical data. Recently, Betancur et al used 1638 MPI scansfrom REgistry of Fast Myocardial Perfusion Imaging with NExt generation SPECT (REFINE SPECT) for training of a DL algorithm to directly analyze polar map images and detect obstructive CAD . This model outperformed standard total perfusion deficit assessment (AUC, 0.80 vs 0.78; P < .01), with a computation time of less than 0.5 second per patient.MPI data have also been input into ML models for outcome prediction. In another REFINE SPECT substudy, Hu et al used LogitBoost to combine measures of regional perfusion deficits with stress test and clinical variables to predict early revascularization. The per-vessel and per-patient prediction by ML was higher than that of standard quantitative analysis using total perfusion deficit or expert visual analysis. In a subsequent report, Hu et al used clinical and stress perfusion parameters from all 20 414 patients from the REFINE SPECT registry to develop an ML model for automatic rest scan cancellation based on prognostic safety. An XGBoost algorithm was trained on the data to predict MACE, and the resultant ML score was used to select patients for simulated cancellation of their rest scans. This resulted in lower annualized MACE rates

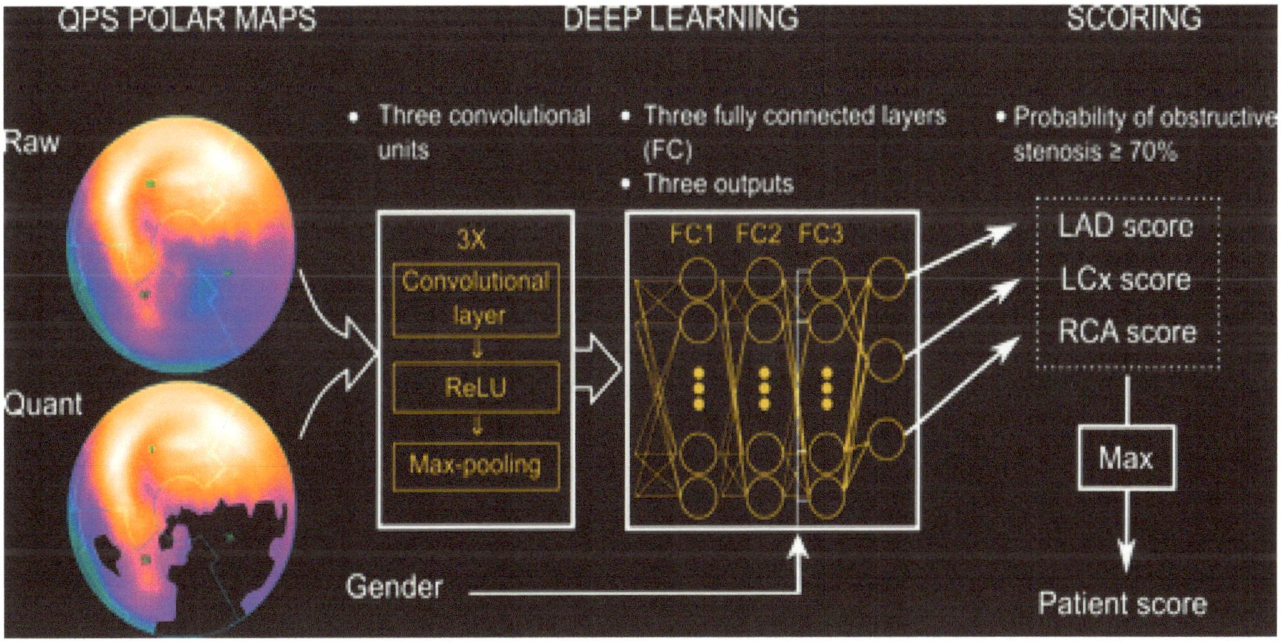

Fig.6.7 Deep learning prediction of obstructive coronary artery disease (CAD) from myocardial perfusion imaging. SPECT polar map images are directly connected to the convolutional neural network, and patterns of perfusion defects are identified by feature extraction (left). These image features then pass through three fully connected layers (FC) in a deep learning process (center), which predicts the probability of obstructive CAD in each vascular territory (right). LAD = left anterior descending artery, LCx = left circumflex artery, Max = maximum probability of obstructive CAD, QPS = quantitative perfusion SPECT, ReLU = rectified linear unit (linear function mapping input to output values), RCA = right coronary artery. (Reprinted, with permission)

compared with rest scan cancellation by conventional clinical criteria. For example, the algorithm could potentially cancel 60% of the rest scans, and in these patients the annual MACE risk would be 1.4%; the same cancellation rate based on visual scoring would result in an annual 2.1% MACE rate. These findings lend support to the clinical adoption of such an ML approach, which could reduce radiation exposure and health care costs while ensuring prognostic safety. Betancur et al applied a LogitBoost algorithm for the prediction of 3-year MACE risk in 2619 patients undergoing clinically indicated exercise or pharmacologic MPI. They showed a comprehensive ML model integrating imaging, stress test, and clinical variables to outperform expert visual interpretation, automated measures of total perfusion deficit, or ML with only imaging variables (AUC, 0.81 vs 0.73, 0.71, and 0.65, respectively; $P < .01$ for all). Further, the combined ML model provided a 26% ($P < .001$) risk reclassification for MACE compared with visual analysis. Different ML algorithms using MPI and clinical data have been tested in parallel against traditional statistical methods for the prediction of cardiac death. In an analysis by Haro Alonso et al , a support vector machine model with 49 features had the highest accuracy compared with a baseline logistic regression model with 122 features (AUC, 0.83 vs 0.76; $P < .0001$). A least absolute shrinkage and selection operator approach minimized the number of predictive features to six, while providing slightly better accuracy than logistic regression (AUC, 0.77; $P = .045$). These findings highlight the role of ML in selecting the most important predictive variables, enabling the relevance of risk factors to be readily appreciated within the time constraints of clinical practice.Automated cardiovascular risk assessment can also be performed using a hybrid imaging approach. In patients undergoing 82Rb PET/CT, Išgum et al applied an ML method of automated CAC scoring to low-dose CT attenuation correction images, which are routinely acquired after the PET studies. There was excellent agreement between automated CT attenuation correction scoring and the reference standard of dedicated CAC scoring CT with manual quantification (κ =0.79–0.82).

Hence, this AI approach is not only highly feasible but may enable clinical cardiovascular risk assessment using the CT attenuation correction component of PET/CT MPI without the need for any additional protocols or radiation exposure.

Challenges to AI Implementation

Although the described AI applications hold great promise for cardiovascular risk stratification, there are several barriers to their clinical implementation. First, the accuracy of ML models will always be limited by the availability and quality of data used for training. Hence, ML algorithms may not perform as well in areas of cardiovascular imaging that do not generate large data sets, such as with rare diseases, uncommon presentations of common diseases, or historic archived images. Further, standardization of image acquisition protocols and formats is required before data from different institutions can be input into a standard AI model. Second, running AI algorithms to handle vast data sets can be computationally expensive, thereby limiting their widespread availability. However, advances in increasingly affordable hardware (eg, graphics processing units) and software (eg, cloud-based computing services) solutions will facilitate the integration and storage of imaging big data. Finally, AI algorithms trained and tested at a single institution may not be generalizable to different cohorts. Thus, all models will require external validation across multiple centers and imaging vendors before their widespread clinical adoption. Moreover, as patient characteristics, disease patterns, and image acquisition and reconstruction techniques change over time, AI models may benefit from continuous updating using large and dynamic data sets.

Summary

Noninvasive cardiovascular imaging is data-rich and primed for AI-powered solutions. AI can be used to quantify cardiovascular risk by two main methods: (a) through the direct application of DL algorithms to image data for automated quantification of prognostic biomarkers; or (b) through integration of conventional or AI-based imaging metrics with tabular data in ML models for individualized outcome prediction. For all the potential applications, however, high-quality data and model validation on unseen data sets are key to success. real-time prognostication and guide personalized therapy.

Bibliography And Acknowledgement

- Agatston AS, Janowitz WR, Hildner FJ, Zusmer NR, Viamonte M Jr, Detrano R. Quantification of coronary artery calcium using ultrafast computed tomography. J Am Coll Cardiol 1990;15(4):827–832
- Al'Aref SJ, Maliakal G, Singh G, et al.. Machine learning of clinical variables and coronary artery calcium scoring for the prediction of obstructive coronary artery disease on coronary computed tomography angiography: analysis from the CONFIRM registry. Eur Heart J 2020;41(3):359–367
- Al'Aref SJ, Singh G, Choi JW, et al.. A Boosted Ensemble Algorithm for Determination of Plaque Stability in High-Risk Patients on Coronary CTA. JACC Cardiovasc Imaging 2020;13(10):2162–2173
- Antonopoulos AS, Sanna F, Sabharwal N, et al.. Detecting human coronary inflammation by imaging perivascular fat. SciTranslMed2017;9(398):eaal2658.
- Arbab-Zadeh A, Hoe J. Quantification of coronary arterial stenoses by multidetector CT angiography in comparison with conventional angiography methods, caveats, and implications. JACCCardiovascImaging2011;4(2):191–202.
- Arsanjani R, Xu Y, Dey D, et al.. Improved accuracy of myocardial perfusion SPECT for detection of coronary artery disease by machine learning in a large population. J Nucl Cardiol 2013;20(4):553–562.
- Betancur J, Commandeur F, Motlagh M, et al.. Deep Learning for Prediction of Obstructive Disease From Fast Myocardial Perfusion SPECT: A Multicenter Study. JACC Cardiovasc Imaging2018;11(11):1654–1663.
- Betancur J, Otaki Y, Motwani M, et al.. Prognostic Value of Combined Clinical and Myocardial Perfusion Imaging Data Using Machine Learning. JACC Cardiovasc Imaging 2018;11(7):1000–1009.
- Budoff MJ, Diamond GA, Raggi P, et al.. Continuous probabilistic prediction of angiographically significant coronary artery disease using electron beam tomography. Circulation 2002;105(15):1791–1796.
- Budoff MJ, Shaw LJ, Liu ST, et al.. Long-term prognosis associated with coronary calcification: observations from a registry of 25,253 patients. J Am Coll Cardiol 2007;49(18):1860–1870
- Callister TQ, Cooil B, Raya SP, Lippolis NJ, Russo DJ, Raggi P. Coronary artery disease: improved reproducibility of calcium scoring with an electron-beam CT volumetric method. Radiology 1998;208(3):807–814.
- Chang HJ, Lin FY, Lee SE, et al.. Coronary Atherosclerotic Precursors of Acute Coronary Syndromes. J Am Coll Cardiol 2018;71(22):2511–2522.
- Commandeur F, Goeller M, Razipour A, et al.. Fully Automated CT Quantification of Epicardial Adipose Tissue by Deep Learning: A Multicenter Study. Radiol Artif Intell 2019;1(6):e190045
- Commandeur F, Slomka PJ, Goeller M, et al.. Machine learning to predict the long-term risk of myocardial infarction and cardiac death based on clinical risk, coronary calcium, and epicardial adiposetissue:aprospectivestudy.CardiovascRes 2020;116(14):2216–2225.
- De Mauro A, Greco M, Grimaldi M.A formal definition of BigData basedon its essential features.LibraryRev2016;65(3):122–135.
- DeoRC.MachineLearninginMedicine.Circulation2015;132(20):1920–1930.
- Dey D, Gaur S, Ovrehus KA, et al.. Integrated prediction of lesion-specific ischaemia from quantitative coronary CT angiography using machine learning: a multicentre study. EurRadiol2018;28(6):2655–2664
- Dey D, Slomka PJ, Leeson P, et al.. Artificial Intelligence in Cardiovascular Imaging: JACC State-of-the-Art Review. JAmCollCardiol2019;73(11):1317–1335.
- Dey D, Wong ND, Tamarappoo B, et al.. Computer-aided non-contrast CT-based quantification of pericardial and thoracic fat and their associations with coronary calcium and MetabolicSyndrome.Atherosclerosis2010;209(1):136–141.
- Driessen RS, Danad I, Stuijfzand WJ, et al.. Comparison of Coronary Computed Tomography Angiography, Fractional Flow Reserve, and Perfusion Imaging for Ischemia Diagnosis.JAmCollCardiol2019;73(2):161–173
- Eisenberg E, McElhinney PA, Commandeur F, et al.. Deep Learning-Based Quantification of Epicardial Adipose Tissue Volume and Attenuation Predicts Major Adverse Cardiovascular Events in Asymptomatic Subjects. Circ CardiovascImaging2020;13(2):e009829.
- Erbel R, Möhlenkamp S, Moebus S, et al.. Coronary risk stratification, discrimination, and reclassification improvement based on quantification of subclinical coronary atherosclerosis: the Heinz Nixdorf Recall study. J Am CollCardiol2010;56(17):1397–1406.
- Esteva A, Robicquet A, Ramsundar B, et al.. A guide to deep learning in healthcare. Nat Med 2019;25(1):24–29. Friedman J, Hastie T, Tibshirani R. Additive logistic regression: a statistical view of boosting (with discussion and a rejoinder by the authors).AnnStat2000;28:337–407
- Gernaat SAM, van Velzen SGM, Koh V, et al.. Automatic quantification of calcifications in the coronary arteries and thoracic aorta on radiotherapy planning CT scans of Western and Asian breast cancer patients.
- RadiotherOncol2018;127(3):487–492. Gorter PM, de Vos AM, van der Graaf Y, et al.. Relation of epicardialand pericoronary fat to coronary atherosclerosis andcoronaryarterycalciuminpatientsundergoing coronaryangiography.AmJCardiol2008;102(4):380–385.
- HanD,Kolli KK, Al'Aref SJ, et al.. Machine Learning Framework to Identify Individuals at Risk of Rapid Progression of Coronary Atherosclerosis: From the PARADIGM Registry.JAmHeartAssoc2020;9(5):e013958
- Haro Alonso D, Wernick MN, Yang Y, Germano G, Berman DS, SlomkaP. Prediction of cardiac death after adenosine myocardial perfusion SPECT based on machine learning. JNuclCardiol2019;26(5):1746–1754
- Hong Y, Commandeur F, Cadet S, et al.. Deep learning-based stenosis quantification from coronary CT Angiography.ProcSPIEIntSocOptEng2019;10949:109492I
- Hu LH, Betancur J, Sharir T, et al.. Machine learning predicts per-vesselearlycoronaryrevascularizationafterfastmyocardial perfusion SPECT: results from multicentre REFINE SPECTregistry.EurHeartJ Cardiovasc Imaging 2020;21(5):549–559.

- vHu LH, Miller RJH, Sharir T, et al.. Prognostically safe stress-only single-photon emission computed tomography myocardial perfusion imaging guided by machine learning: report from REFINE SPECT. Eur Heart J Cardiovasc Imaging doi:10.1093/ehjci/jeaa134.Published online June 12, 2020. AccessedNovember21,2020 .
- Išgum I, de Vos BD, Wolterink JM, et al.. Automatic determination of cardiovascular risk by CT attenuation correction maps in Rb-82 PET/CT. J Nucl Cardiol 2018;25(6):2133–2142 [Published correction appears in J Nucl Cardiol 2018;25(6):2143.].
- Johnson NP, Tóth GG, Lai D, et al.. Prognostic value of fractional flow reserve: linking physiologic severity to clinical outcomes. JAmCollCardiol2014;64(16):1641–1654.
- Kang D, Dey D, Slomka PJ, et al.. Structured learning algorithm for detection of nonobstructive and obstructive coronary plaque lesions from computed tomography angiography. J Med Imaging (Bellingham)2015;2(1):014003.
- Kelm BM, Mittal S, Zheng Y, et al.. Detection, grading and classification of coronary stenoses in computed tomography angiography. Med Image Comput Comput Assist Interv 2011;14(Pt3):25–32
- Kolossváry M, Karády J, Kikuchi Y, et al.. Radiomics versus Visual and Histogram-based Assessment to Identify Atheromatous Lesions at Coronary CT Angiography: An ex Vivo Study.Radiology2019;293(1):89–96.
- Kolossváry M, Karády J, Szilveszter B, et al.. Radiomic Features Are Superior to Conventional Quantitative Computed Tomographic Metrics to Identify Coronary Plaques With Napkin-Ring Sign. Circ Cardiovasc Imaging 2017;10(12):e006843
- Kolossváry M, Kellermayer M, Merkely B, Maurovich-Horvat P. Cardiac Computed Tomography Radiomics: A Comprehensive Review on Radiomic Techniques. J Thorac Imaging 2018;33(1):26–34
- Kolossváry M, Park J, Bang JI, et al.. Identification of invasive and radionuclide imaging markers of coronary plaque vulnerability using radiomic analysis of coronary computed tomography angiography. Eur Heart J Cardiovasc Imaging 2019;20(11):1250–1258.
- Krittanawong C, Zhang H, Wang Z, Aydar M, Kitai T. Artificial Intelligence in Precision Cardiovascular Medicine. J Am CollCardiol2017;69(21):2657–2664.
- Lessmann N, van Ginneken B, Zreik M, et al.. Automatic Calcium Scoring in Low-Dose Chest CT Using Deep Neural Networks With Dilated Convolutions. IEEE Trans Med Imaging 2018;37(2):615–625.
- Lin A, Dey D, Wong DTL, Nerlekar N. Perivascular Adipose Tissue and Coronary Atherosclerosis: from Biology to Imaging Phenotyping. Curr Atheroscler Rep 2019;21(12):47
- Lin A, Kolossváry M, Išgum I, Maurovich-Horvat P, Slomka PJ, Dey D. Artificial intelligence: improving the efficiency of cardiovascular imaging. Expert Rev Med Devices 2020;17(6):565–577
- Lin A, Kolossváry M, Yuvaraj J, et al..Myocardial Infarction Associates With a DistinctPericoronary Adipose Tissue Radiomic Phenotype: A Prospective Case-Control Study. JACC Cardiovasc Imaging 2020;13(11):2371–2383.
- Maurovich-Horvat P, Hoffmann U, Vorpahl M, Nakano M, Virmani R, Alkadhi H. The napkin-ring sign: CT signature of high-risk coronary plaques? JACC Cardiovasc Imaging2010;3(4):440–444
- Min JK, Dunning A, Lin FY, et al.. Age- and sex-related differences in all-cause mortality risk based on coronary computed tomography angiography findings: results from the International Multicenter CONFIRM (Coronary CT Angiography Evaluation for Clinical Outcomes: An International Multicenter Registry) of 23,854 patients without known coronary artery disease. J Am Coll Cardiol 2011;58(8):849–860
- Motoyama S, Ito H, Sarai M, et al.. Plaque Characterization by Coronary Computed Tomography Angiography and the Likelihood of Acute Coronary Events in Mid-Term Follow-Up. J AmCollCardiol2015;66(4):337–346.
- Motoyama S, Sarai M, Harigaya H, et al.. Computed tomographic angiography characteristics of atherosclerotic plaques subsequently resultinginacutecoronary syndrome. J AmCollCardiol2009;54(1):49–57.
- Motwani M, Dey D, Berman DS, et al.. Machine learning for prediction of all-cause mortality in patients with suspected coronary artery disease: a 5-year multicentre prospective registryanalysis.EurHeartJ2017;38(7):500–507
- Nakanishi R, Slomka P, Rios R, et al.. Machine Learning Adds to Clinical and CAC Assessments in Predicting 10-Year CHD and CVD Deaths. JACC Cardiovasc Imaging doi:10.1016/j.jcmg.2020.08.024. Published online October 28, 2020. AccessedNovember21,2020.
- Oikonomou EK, Williams MC, Kotanidis CP, et al.. A novel machine learning-derived radiotranscriptomic signature of perivascular fat improves cardiac risk prediction using coronary CTangiography.EurHeartJ2019;40(43):3529–3543
- Otsuka K, Fukuda S, Tanaka A, et al.. Napkin-ring sign on coronary CT angiography for the prediction of acute coronary syndrome. JACC Cardiovasc Imaging 2013;6(4):448–457. Takx RAP, de Jong PA, Leiner T, et al.. Automated coronary artery calcification scoring innon-gated chest CT: agreemeand reliability. PLoSOne2014;9(3):e91239.
- van Velzen SGM, Lessmann N, Velthuis BK, et al.. Deep Learning for Automatic Calcium Scoring in CT: Validation Using Multiple Cardiac CT and Chest CT Protocols. Radiology 2020;295(1):66–79.
- Williams MC, Kwiecinski J, Doris M, et al.. Low-Attenuation Noncalcified Plaque on Coronary Computed Tomography Angiography Predicts Myocardial Infarction: Results From the Multicenter SCOT-HEART Trial (Scottish Computed Tomography of the HEART). Circulation 2020;141(18):1452–1462.
- Wolterink JM, Leiner T, Takx RAP, Viergever MA, Isgum I. Automatic Coronary Calcium Scoring in Non-Contrast-Enhanced ECG-Triggered Cardiac CT With Ambiguity Detection. IEEE Trans MedImaging2015;34(9):1867–1878.
- Yeboah J, McClelland RL, Polonsky TS, et al.. Comparison of novel risk markers for improvement in cardiovascular risk assessment in intermediate-risk individuals. JAMA 2012;308(8):788–79

CHAPTER 7

Current and Future Applications of Artificial Intelligence in Coronary Artery Disease

Clinically significant atherosclerosis of the coronary arteries, known as coronary artery disease (CAD), is an endemic condition that is associated with significant morbidity and mortality. For instance, CAD is reported to have affected 20.1 million American adults between 2015 and 2018 .Current societal guidelines emphasize the importance of early detection and risk stratification in the appropriate age and risk groups, with the goal of implementation of goal-directed medical therapies that can alter the natural trajectory of CAD to a less morbid course. Traditional population-derived primary and secondary prevention cardiovascular risk assessment tools (e.g., Framingham risk score, ASCVD, TIMI score, GRACE score, etc.) have historically relied on patient-level data that are easily retrievable and practical to utilize in the clinical setting. Despite their importance, such tools are inherently limited by design due to relying on regression models that make many mathematical assumptions that often do not hold in a real-world setting, such as collinearity between variables and homogeneity of effects. The complex nature and multifactorial pathology of CAD make such regression-based tools less generalizable across different populations. Recently, the digitization of health records has improved access to large repositories of clinical and imaging datasets for clinical care and research purposes. This is coupled with advances in diagnostic tools that are available for the detection and quantification of CAD. To that end, recent studies have highlighted the usefulness of these tools in enhancing risk assessment and decision making through incorporation of different yet complementary findings from these imaging modalities (e.g., quantitative and qualitative plaque features on computed tomographic imaging of the coronary circulation coupled with functional and physiologic findings on stress-test imaging). In addition, there has been an increasing interest in using the plethora of data in electronic health records and genomic data for better risk assessment .Such tools are being integrated in practice as complementary methods to traditional tools.Yet, despite the ever-increasing amounts of data, risk-prediction methodshave been historically limited by whatwas possible with traditional statistical tools. The concept of Artificial Intelligence (AI) was introduced to mankind as early as the 1950s, with its employment in medical sciences commencing in the 1970s . AI has gained momentum recently, fueled by an improvement in computational power, accumulation of data, and cloud processing. With the attempt to transfer a significant portion of human intelligence to machines, there has been a concerted effort aimed at harnessing the power of AI for biomedical applications in the past two decades Machine learning (ML) is a subfield of AI that involves the creation of algorithms that analyze large datasets without prior assumptions and learn rules and patterns between variables to make predictions and classifications On the other hand, deep learning (DL) is a subset of ML geared towards image analysis and utilizes more intricate algorithms known as neural networks with multiple deep, hidden layers. Specifically, while ML usually relies on structured data with handcrafted features often in tabular form, DL algorithms can input both structured and raw, unstructured data (e.g., images, video, and text) and extract their own feature

ML algorithms can incorporate a larger number of variables from different modalities, including both patient-level clinical parameters as well as two- and three-dimensional imaging data that take into account the multidimensional nonlinear interactions between variables Implementing such techniques in healthcare mainly aims to improve the accuracy of risk prediction and customize clinical decisions to each individual, which is the overarching theme in the goal of achieving precision medicine. In this paper, we summarize the recent advances in ML and current attempts at improving predictive analytics with relevance to CAD. We also elucidate on the role of AI in genetics, the incremental role of AI in improving post-procedure risk prediction and long-term mortality. Lastly, we discuss the limitations and potential near-future applications of AI within cardiovascular medicine.

Integration of Genetics and AI in Cardiovascular Diseases

Over the last two decades, the emergence of technologies able to measure biological processes at a large scale have resulted in an enormous influx of data. For instance, the completion of the Human Genome Project has paved the way to design single-nucleotide polymorphism (SNP) and mRNA microarrays, which can broadly test for millions of genetic variants in a simple point-of-care test. This has paved the way for the emergence of modern data-driven sciences such as genomics and other "omics" .Genome-wide association studies (GWASs) operate by simultaneous comparison of millions of SNPs between diseased individuals and disease-free controls to detect a statistically significant association between an SNP locus and a particular condition. Erdmann et al. reported that up until the year 2018, GWASs have successfully identified 163 distinct genetic loci for SNPs that are associated with CAD. The risk for expressing a complex trait like CAD can be represented by a mathematical model that assumes a normal distribution of a binary outcome (i.e., CAD or no CAD) and captures the aggregate influence of multiple genetic variants that are predisposed to disease. Such a model is referred to as a polygenic risk score (PRS). PRSs were proposed early on to improve risk stratification in CAD risk models, especially when combined with traditional cardiovascular risk factors. However, the complex genetic architecture along with the multifactorial nature of CAD have been major challenges in CAD risk prediction. For instance, Kathiresan et al. built a genetic risk score to predict major adverse cardiovascular events based on nine different dyslipidemia-related SNPs previously identified in GWASs. Adding the genetic score to a Cox proportional hazard model along with traditional risk factors did not improve predictive accuracy as measured by the C statistic model; however, there was a significant improvement in the net reclassification index, which accounts for correct movement of categories (assigning high-risk for patients who developed the disease, and low-risk for those who were disease-free. Brautbar et al. also suggested a genetic risk score to predict coronary heart disease based on SNPs. Adding the genetic risk score to traditional risk factors in a Cox proportional hazard model only modestly improved the area under the curve (AUC) for prediction of coronary heart disease from 0.742 to 0.749 (Δ = 0.007; 95% CI, 0.004–0.013). ML and particularly DL algorithms are inherently designed to extract patterns and associations from large-scale data, including clinical and genomic data. Giventhe complexity and multifaceted nature of cardiovascular diseases in general, and CAD in particular, an approach that integrates all these factors into a risk-stratification model would be expected to better predict incident events than existent models

Multiple studies have emphasized the role of ML in identifying genetic variants and expression patterns associated with CAD from mRNA arrays using differential expression analysis and protein–protein interaction networks . For example, Zhang et al. used ML to perform differential expression analysis on mRNA profiles from CAD patients and healthy controls to identify a set of differentially expressed genes between the two groups, then built a network representation of functional protein–protein interaction. The top 20 genes in the network were identified using a maximal clique centrality (MCC) algorithm. Finally, to test the performance, a logistic regression model was built using the top five predictor genes to classify individuals into the presence or absence of CAD. The model achieved an AUC of 0.9295 and 0.8674 in the training and internal validation setsrespectively Dogan et al. built an ensemble model of eight random-forest (RF) classifiers to predict the risk of symptomatic CAD using genetic and epigenetic variables along with clinical risk factors. The model was trained on a cohort derived from the Framingham heart study (n = 1545) and utilized variables derived from genome-wide array chips to extract epigenetic (DNA methylation loci) and genetic (SNP) profiles. The initial number of available variables were 876,014 SNP and DNA methylation (CpG) loci, which required multiple reduction steps, ending up with 4 CpG and 2 SNP predictors fed into the model along with age and gender. The model predicted symptomatic CAD with an accuracy, sensitivity, and specificity of 0.78, 0.75, and 0.80, respectively, in the internal validation cohort (n = 142). For comparison, a similar ensemble model was built using clinical risk factors only as predictor variables and had an accuracy, sensitivity, and specificity of 0.65, 0.42, and 0.89, respectively . Pattarabanjird et al. tested multiple ML models to predict anatomical CAD severity (extent of diameter stenosis) in a binary fashion using clinical variables along with SNP loci. Quantitative coronary angiography and the Gensini score, which is a summation score that quantifies the severity of CAD by accounting for the segment-based most severe stenosis and the location of the stenosis within the coronary arteries, were used to assess model performance. The best-performing model (Sequential Neural Network; training set n = 325 and internal validation set n = 82) accurately classified CAD severity with AUC of 0.84 in the validation set . Similarly, Naushad et al. trained ML models to predict the presence of CAD and the percentage of coronary diameter stenosis using clinical and genetic variables. The best-performing model (an ensemble model; training set n = 648) accurately predicted CAD using 11 variables (clinical and genetic variants) with an AUC of 0.96 in the training set. The model also predicted the percentage of diameter stenosis with a correlation of 82.5% with the actual stenosis assessed using the gold-standard invasive angiography. However, these models were not internally nor externally validated. Finally, the coronary artery calcium (CAC) score, calculated using the Agatston method on noncontrast ECG-gated cardiac computed tomography, is an established strong predictor of major adverse cardiovascular events in asymptomatic individuals. Genomic studies have previously focused on identifying genetic loci linked to CAC . Oguz et al. suggested the use of ML algorithms to predict advanced CAC from SNP arrays and clinical variables. They identified a set of SNPs that ranked the highest in predictive importance and correlated with advanced CAC scores, defined as the 89th–99th percentile CAC scores in the derivation and replication cohorts, and trained different RF models to predict advanced CAC scores using clinical and genetic variables. Adding SNPs to clinical variables significantly improved AUC from 0.61 ± 0.02 to 0.83 ± 0.01; ($p < 0.001$) [26] for prediction of advanced CAC scores.

Risk Prediction Models and Imaging Modalities for Estimating Pretest Probability of CAD

Traditionally, stratifying patients presenting with stable chest pain using pretest probability (PTP) estimates of CAD has been commonly used to help with decision-making regarding downstream testing and the choice of an appropriate diagnostic modality. Historically, the Diamond–Forrester model—developed using age, sex, and chest pain characteristics—was used as a clinician's risk stratification tool in predicting the PTP of CAD . However, numerous studies showed its limitation in overestimating PTP by approximately threefold, especially in women This led to the development of the updated Diamond–Forrester model (UDF) and the CAD consortium score.These scores, incorporating demographic and clinical risk factors, have been proven to be better at predicting the risk of CAD.Therefore, improving the ability to predict CAD using more accurate risk-assessment modeling is imperative, given the potential to reduce downstream testing and associated costs. Using clinical and demographic features, ML models have been employed to estimate the PTP of CAD.In a recent multicenter cross-sectional study, a deep neural network algorithm based on the facial profile of individuals was able to achieve a higher performance than traditional risk scores in predicting PTP of CAD (AUC for the ML model 0.730 vs. 0.623 for Diamond –Forrester and 0.652 for the CAD consortium, p , $p < 0.001$) . Though the study is limited by the lack of external validity and low specificity (54%), such approaches can potentially lead to a paradigm change in CAD management by facilitating earlier detection and initiation of primary prevention using readily available parameters, such as an individual's facial profile.When available, a CAC score has been shown to add to the PTP of CAD, with a CAC score of zero identifying low-risk patients who might not need additional testing . ML models, combining clinical and imaging parameters, have been shown to have higher predictive power than traditional risk scores when predicting the PTP of obstructive CAD . Al'Aref et al. included 25 clinical and demographic features to devise a ML model which, when combined with the Agatston CAC score, fared better than the ML model or CAD consortium score alone or in combination with the CAC score (AUC 0.881 for ML + CAC as compared to 0.866, 0.773, and 0.734 for the CAD consortium + CAC, ML model, and CAD consortium respectively, $p < 0.05$) . As expected, CAC, age, and gender were the highest-ranked features in the mode. Various ML algorithms based on stress imaging, particularly single-photon emission computed tomography (SPECT), have been devised to facilitate the prediction of CAD. These models combined the clinical and demographic characteristics with the quantitative variables, as evaluated via SPECT to better predict CAD compared with the visual interpretation or quantitative variables alone . Cardiac phase-space analysis is a novel noninvasive diagnostic platform that combines advanced disciplines of mathematics and physics with ML . Thoracic orthogonal voltage gradient (OVG) signals from a patient are evaluated by cardiac phase-space analysis to quantify physiological and mathematical features associated with CAD. The analysis is performed at the point of care without the need for a change in physiologic status or radiation. Initial multicenter results suggest that resting cardiac phase-space analysis may have comparable diagnostic utility to functional tests currently used to assess CAD Finally, the assessment of regional wall motion abnormalities (RWMAs) on echocardiography has been associated with the presence of obstructive CAD, and as such can be useful in helping clinicians with downstream decision-making. Recently, a deep-learning model developed by Kusunose et al.

achieved performance similar to that of experienced cardiologists in the assessment of RWMAs on echocardiography (AUC of 0.99 vs. 0.98, $p = 0.15$) . Other than the assessment of obstructive CAD, machine learning has found its wide applicability in echocardiography to predict ventricular capacities, abnormal valvular function, as well as cardiac hemodynamics.

Artificial Intelligence in Management of CAD in the Emergency Department

Chest pain is a common emergency department presentation, and distinguishing cardiac from noncardiac pain causes is crucial for optimal management. Modalities such as electrocardiography (ECG) serve as a quick way to recognize patterns associated with unstable CAD, and in particular acute coronary syndromes (ACSs). Deep neural networks have shown a consistent performance in image recognition, and models have hence been devised to identify patterns related to CAD and myocardial infarction (MI) .By reducing interobserver variability and providing accurate results efficiently, this approach holds the promise of improving workflow across healthcare systems, while helping patients in areas of limited medical infrastructure and specialized care.

Cardiac biomarkers, such as high-sensitivity troponin, have been well-validated as markers of myocardial ischemia and damage. High-sensitivity troponin I (hs-cTnI) assay forms the core of the 'rule in and rule out' clinical decision pathway as per ESC 2020 chest pain guidelines and 2021 ACC/AHA chest pain guidelines . For instance, a very low hs-cTnI at hospital admission or a negative one-hour delta troponin (in the background of a low hs-cTnI value at admission) has a high negative predictive value (>99%) for ACS . On the other hand, a high admission hs-cTnI value or a significant increase in values in an hour portends a high positive-predictive value (70–75%), warranting additional downstream testing. Using the strategy mentioned above, approximately one-third of the patients fall in the 'indeterminate' zone. Diagnosis and management of this group is challenging, necessitating an approach based on clinical history, pre-existing risk factors, serial hs-cTnI trends, and further imaging. A recent ML model based on three clinical (age, sex, and prior percutaneous coronary intervention) as well as levels of three biomarkers (hs-cTnI, KIM-1, and adiponectin) demonstrated excellence in predicting obstructive CAD in the validation cohort (AUC 0.86 for prediction of >50%diameter stenosis). Notably, the model performed remarkably well in patients in the 'indeterminate' zone, with AUC of 0.88 and a positive predictive value of 93%, hence identifying patients who will benefit from further testing.

The 2021 American College of Cardiology/American Heart Association (ACC/AHA) chest pain guidelines advocate for the use of coronary CT angiography (CCTA) in intermediate-risk patients presenting with acute chest pain who either have no known history or a history of nonobstructive CAD (defined ascoronary artery disease with less than 50% diameter stenosis). Given the ability of CCTA toaccurately define coronary anatomy and extent/distribution of atherosclerotic plaque, it has been consistently shownnoninvasive imaging modality for patient selection, particularly for those who might require further invasive evaluation. However, interpretation of CCTA scans requires expertise and is time-intensive. Therefore, automatic interpretation of CCTA, which can lead to a significant reduction in the processing times, is highly desirable. ML algorithms have recently been developed, achieving a 70–75% reduction in reading time compared to that required for human interpretation (2.3 min for AI vs. 7.6–9.6 min for human readers). Though the model described performed slightly lower than highly experienced readers in interpreting CCTA (AUC 0.93 vs. 0.90 for human vs. AI, $p < 0.05$), when combined with low-experience human readers, it augmented the reader's ability to correctly reclassify obstructive CAD (per-vessel net reclassification index (NRI) 0.07, $p < 0.001$) . In addition, ML has been applied for various segmentation and classification tasks on cardiac CT imaging, from automatic segmentation of calcified and noncalcified plaque to automated calculation of the Agatston CAC score, and finally quantification of cardiac structures on CT imaging Therefore, the application of ML could provide reliable results in real time, while bridging the dearth of experts in low-resource settings. Stress testing, which provides an estimate of myocardial perfusion and viability, has been recommended as an alternative to CCTA in intermediate-risk chest pain patients.Myocardial perfusion imaging, particularly SPECT, has been employed to recognize patients who might need an invasive evaluation, with a diagnostic sensitivity of 75–88% and specificity of 60–79% .SPECT can be evaluated qualitatively in terms of size, severity, location, and reversibility of perfusion defect, and quantitatively, in terms of total perfusion deficit (TPD), summed stress score (SSS), summed rest score (SRS), as well as stress and rest volumes . Automatically generated polar maps (representing radiotracer distribution in a two-dimensional plane) after three-dimensional segmentation of the left ventricle (LV) have been used as raw data for quantitative analysis. After the LV polar map is divided into 17 segments, each of the segments is graded on a scale of 0–4 based on the severity of ischemia. The scores are then summated to generate SSS and SRS. Polar maps also provide information about the overall extent and magnitude of ischemia, in terms of TPD

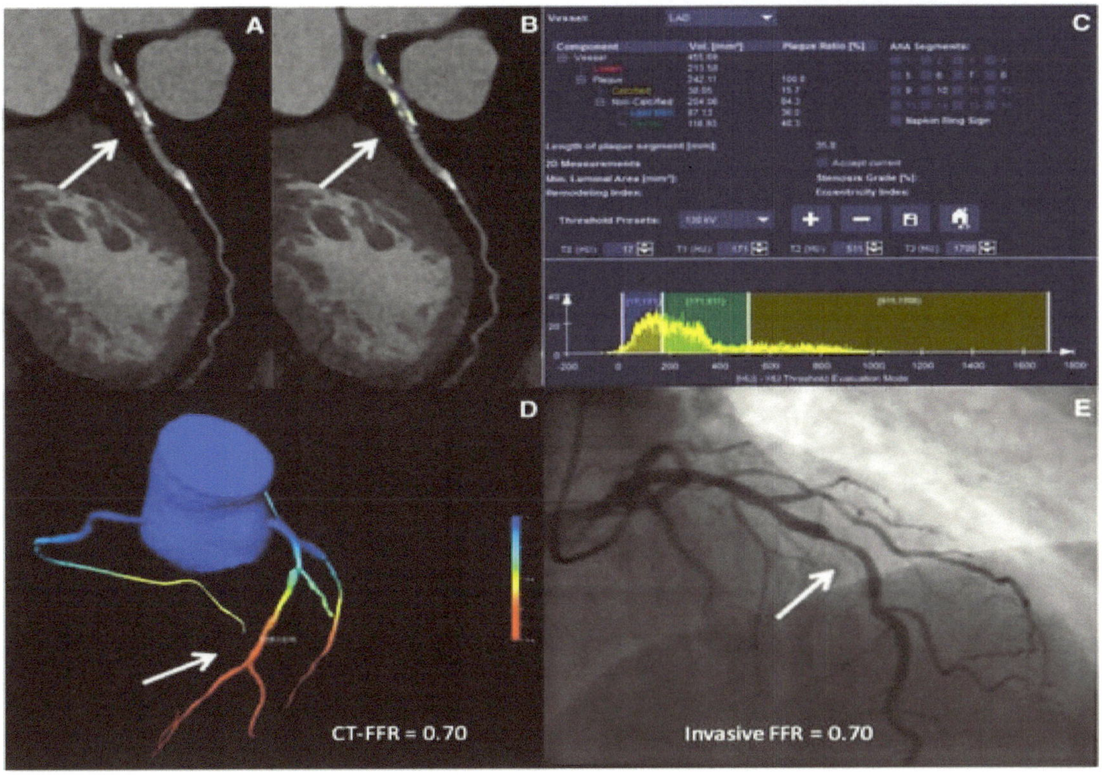

Fig.7.1 ML-based fractional flow reserve from cardiac CT (CT-FFRML). Machine-learning-based coronary plaque analysis quantifies atherosclerotic plaque into calcified and noncalcified components (A,B). This is further integrated with other quantitative parameters (C) and transformed into 3-D images of the vessels to give CT-FFRML (D), which has been shown to have a good correlation with invasive fractional flow reserve (FFR—E). Adapted with permission from Von Knebel Doeberitz et al.

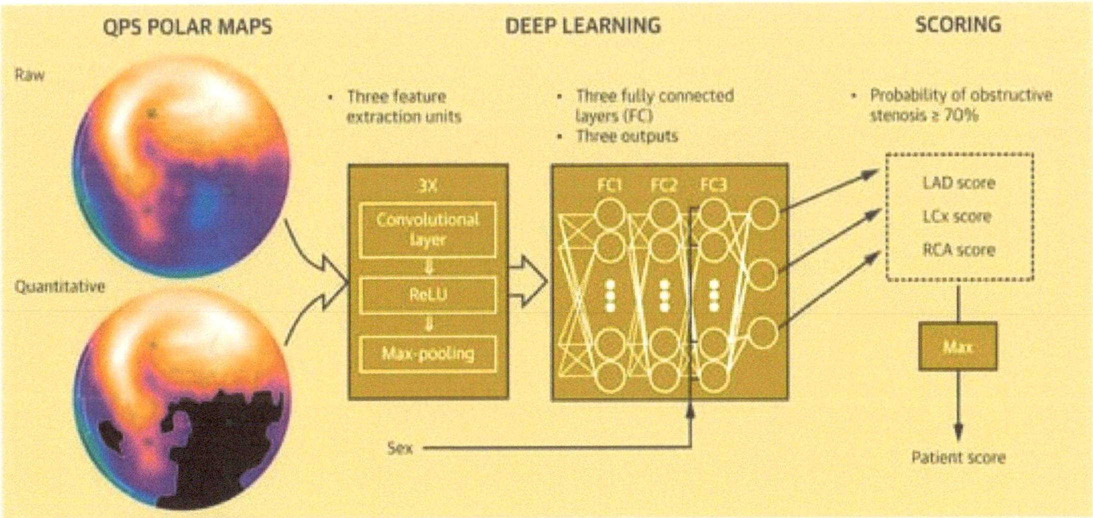

Fig.7.2 Deep-learning model to predict obstructive CAD from polar maps. Raw polar maps and extent polar maps (maps with abnormal pixels representing ischemia blackened out) are fed into deep neural networks, with the extracted data used to calculate scores for individual vessels to predict the probability of CAD. Adapted with permission from Betancur et al. Elsevier.

Artificial Intelligence to Predict Functionally Obstructive CAD and Lesion-Specific Ischemia as a Gatekeeper to the Catheterization Laboratory

One of the inherent limitations of CCTA is its limited ability to predict the functional significance of coronary stenosis. To overcome this shortcoming, CT-derived fractional flow reserve (FFRCT) was developed based on the critical concept of computational fluid dynamics (CFD), with numerous trials demonstrating its strong correlation with invasive fractional flow reserve (FFR) as determined by invasive coronary angiography (ICA) . Rabbat et al. demonstrated that FFRCT added to CCTA safely deferred ICA in patients with CAD of indeterminate hemodynamic significance. In addition, a high proportion of those who underwent ICA were revascularized . These studies and others led to FFRCT being incorporated in the 2021 ACC/AHA chest pain guidelines in intermediate-risk patients to detect lesion-specific ischemia in proximal or middle segments of the coronary arteries and determined to have atherosclerotic plaque with 40% to 90% diameter stenosis.Despite its excellent correlation, the off-site computation of FFRCT hampers its use in real time, owing to the need for longer processing times To overcome this limitation and to allow for quick computation of a value for the functional significance of a particular lesion, novel ML approaches based on artery lumen segmentation. left ventricular myocardial segmentation and artery centerline tracking have been proposed.

A .ML-Based CT-FFR Estimation and Diagnostic Accuracy

Based on the concept of artery lumen segmentation, the ML-based FFR estimation (CT-FFRML) has generated significant interest in the past few years. The CT-FFRML model was trained on 12,000 synthetically generated coronary geometric datasets and used deep neural networks, allowing for automatic computation of FFR in real-time [93]. Coenen et al. performed a multicenter, prospective study to evaluate the diagnostic performance of CT-FFRML to predict lesion-specific ischemia, comparing it with traditional CCTA parameters, with invasive FFR being the gold standard . They demonstrated an excellent correlation between CT-FFRML and FFRCT ($r = 0.997$) and a superior performance of CT-FFRML over traditional CCTA in predicting lesion-specific ischemia (AUC: 0.84 vs. 0.69, $p < 0.001$ on a per-vessel level). Since then, multiple retrospective studies have been performed to evaluate the diagnostic accuracy of CT-FFRML, validated against the gold-standard invasive FFR.

They have further demonstrated superior diagnostic performance of CT-FFRML over CTA stenosis severity and quantitative atherosclerotic plaque features derived from CCTA. To further highlight the incremental diagnostic value of CT-FFRML over anatomic plaque features derived from CCTA in vessels with intermediate stenosis, several other studies have been performed [99,102,103,106]. Tang et al. evaluated the diagnostic value of CT-FFRML in predicting lesion-specific ischemia [103]. Based on a study sample of 122 vessels in 101 patients, CT-FFRML performed better than anatomic CCTA parameters (AUC 0.96 for CT-FFRML vs. 0.63 for CCTA on a per-vessel basis $p < 0.05$).

B. Impact of Calcification Burden on the Performance of CT-FFRML

The impact of coronary calcification on the diagnostic performance of CCTA has been well-established, with more extensive calcification limiting the ability of CCTA to evaluate for the presence of obstructive CAD]. Multiple indices have been devised to compute a CAC score, with the Agatston score, calcium volume, calcification remodeling index (CRI), and segmental arc calcification method being common examples . The Agatston Score (AS) is the most widely validated approach, which summates the calcium score (function of peak density and area of the lesion) of the individual lesions across all coronary artery segments . CRI provides a lesion-specific calcium estimate and is calculated as a ratio of the cross-sectional luminal area of the most severely calcified site to the proximal luminal area. The segmental arc calcification method estimates lesion-specific calcium burden by measuring the greatest circumferential extent of coronary calcium, grading as nil (noncalcified), mild (0–90°), moderate (90–180°), and severe >180°) calcification.

Recent studies have evaluated the performance of CT-FFRML with varying calcification burden as assessed by the parameters mentioned above. Tesche et al. did a retrospective analysis using 482 vessels in 314 patients to evaluate the impact of calcifications on the performance of CT-FFRML .They showed a statistically significant decrease in discriminatory power of CT-FFRML, measured in terms of AUC with increasing Agatston scores (AUC for CT-FFRML 0.85 and 0.81 in low–intermediate Agatston score (1–400) and high Agatston score (>400) ranges respectively, $p = 0.04$).

Di Jiang et al. evaluated the impact of calcification arc and CRI on the performance of CT-FFRML No statistically significant difference was found in the discriminatory power of CT-

FFRML with increasing calcification burden. In the proportion of patients where the Agatston score was available, there was no difference in the diagnostic performance of CT-FFRML across severity of calcification. The difference from Tesche et al. can be explained by a lower mean Agatston score (288 vs. 492 and 138 vs. 187 at a per-patient and per-vessel level, respectively) and smaller sample size (n = 150) for whom the Agatston score was available, resulting in low power to detect a difference.Furthermore, Koo et al. carried out a similar study and found no impact of increasing Agatston score on the performance of CT-FFRML. Interestingly, a sizeable proportion of the sample had higher coronary calcification (mean Agatston score of 311 on a per-vessel basis). More research in this area is needed in order to further validate the diagnostic performance of CT-FFRML across varying degrees of coronary calcification.

C. CT-FFRML in Predicting Revascularization Events

CT-FFRML has been shown to be a better predictor than plaque features derived from CCTA for the determination of the presence of lesion-specific ischemia, but whether CT-FFRML influences the eventual treatment plan and outcomes (as guided by ICA-FFR) remains an active area of investigation. Qiao et al. demonstrated the added benefit of CT-FFRML compared to relying on an anatomy-based strategy in patients with stable chest pain (reduction rate of ICA by 54.5% and 4.4% fewer revascularizations). Additionally, this study demonstrated that adding CT-FFRML to CCTA can decrease the rate of unnecessary ICA by 35.2% (thereby increasing the proportion of revascularizations when ICA is undertaken), truly acting as a gatekeeper to ICA. Furthermore, lower CT-FFRML was associated with higher major adverse cardiovascular event (MACE) risk when compared to diameter stenosis on CCTA (HR, 6.84 vs. 1.47) or ICA (HR, 6.84 vs. 1.84). Liu et al. found a similar rate of MACE (2.9%) after revascularization based on either combining CCTA stenosis ≥ 50% and CT-FFRML ≤ 0.8 or ICA stenosis ≥ 75% in a 2-year follow-up . This study further highlighted the use of CT-FFRML as a gatekeeper to ICA with a positive impact on lower health care costs

CT-FFRML comes with its own set of shortcomings. The diagnostic performance of the CT-FFRML model is lower, with the invasive FFR closely approaching the diagnostic threshold of 0.8 . Traditional statistical and DL approaches have shown that stenosis severity; plaque characteristics, such as low-density, noncalcified plaque; and remodeling index are independent predictors of lesion-specific ischemia that are not related to CT-FFRML.An integrated DL approach in the future that combines clinical features, anatomical plaque characteristics, vessel features, and functional assessment could potentially overcome this limitation.

Artificial Intelligence in the Field of Intracoronary Imaging

During ICA, intravascular ultrasound (IVUS) and optical coherence tomography (OCT) have been widely adopted for coronary luminal imaging, and some of the main applications involve assessment of plaque burden and optimization of stent placement . IVUS uses ultrasound waves to generate cross-sectional images of coronary vessels with axial and lateral resolution ranging from 70–200 microns and 200–400 microns, respectively The penetration depth of IVUS is 10 mm, which allows for a complete cross-sectional analysis of the coronary vessel walls . IVUS can help describe plaque characteristics, with high-risk plaques (plaques with large necrotic cores) appearing as areas of echo-attenuation . On the other hand, calcifications in the IVUS frame indicate a calcified plaque, with heavily calcified plaque increasing the risk of stent underexpansion during percutaneous coronary intervention (PCI) .Virtual histology IVUS (VH-IVUS) is another technique derived from radiofrequency data from IVUS, allowing for in vivo assessment of plaque composition .

By characterizing plaque features and vessel dimensions, IVUS has found its pre-procedural role in the quantitative and qualitative assessment of atherosclerotic plaque as well as interventional planning, ranging from vessel dimension assessment and evaluation of stent placement. Post-procedurally, IVUS can be employed to visualize stent expansion, identify stent edge dissection, stent mal-apposition, and confirm the presence of in-stent thrombosis in the right clinical context.Given the benefits, IVUS has been shown to optimize stent implantation and improve outcomes, including revascularization, MACE, and mortality when used routinely in the cardiac catheterization laboratory . On the other hand, OCT works on the principle of near-infrared light waves, generating cross-sectional images with a much higher axial and lateral resolution of 10 microns and 20–40 microns, respectively This allows for a detailed view of the lumen–plaque interface, providing accurate dimensions of the luminal area and better plaque characterization.

The vulnerability of a plaque is a function of the thickness of its fibrous cap, the size of the necrotic core, and the presence of macrophages. A thin, fibrous cap; sizeable necrotic core; and increased macrophages increase the risk of plaque rupture and subsequent ACS . Given the high resolution provided by OCT, it is considered a gold-standard invasive imaging modality for detecting thin-cap fibroatheroma (TCFA), which, pathologically, is a precursor of vulnerable plaque and clinically proven to be an independent predictor of MACE . A significant drawback of OCT is its inherent low penetration depth (1–2 mm), which makes IVUS a better modality for a full-thickness analysis of vessel wall.Though fascinating, IVUS and OCT have a low adoption rate in the US, being employed only at tertiary-care centers owing to cost, need for additional procedural time, and the associated technical complexities . By using deep-learning algorithms to optimize the workflow associated with image acquisition and interpretation, ML has the potential to reduce procedural costs and time required, which are the two major hindrances to the widespread use of IVUS and OCT.

A. Artificial Intelligence to Optimize Peri-Intervention Workflow

To predict OCT-derived TCFA on IVUS images, Bae et al. created a ML model, enrolling 517 patients who underwent ICA . A total of 40,908 IVUS-OCT co-registered sections in 517 coronary arteries were divided into training and testing sets in a ratio of 4:1. An artificial-neural-network-based model using 17 features achieved the highest performance with a sensitivity and specificity of 85 ± 4% and 79 ± 6%, respectively, and good discriminatory power (AUC of 0.80 ± 0.08). Larger plaque burden, minimal diameter, decreased lumen area, and increased lumen eccentricity were seen to be strongly associated with OCT-derived TCFAs. Min et al. utilized a deep learning algorithm (densely connected convolutional neural network) on 35,678 OCT frames to automatically detect TCFAs from OCT images . After the frames were interpreted for the presence/absence of TCFA, data was fed into the algorithm to devise a deep-learning model. By achieving high sensitivity and specificity of 88.7 ± 3.4%and 91.8 ± 2.0% on the test data, such deep-learning models can significantly reduce processing times and allow for easy interpretation when it comes to identifying a vulnerable high-risk plaque

As mentioned earlier, IVUS can help characterize high-risk plaques, which appear as areas of attenuation on IVUS frames due to the presence of a large necrotic core. Identifying such lesions becomes imperative to reduce the incidence of complications such as periprocedural MI. To accurately classify plaque characteristics and tofacilitate detection of high-risk lesions, Cho et al. described a deep-learning algorithm to accurately differentiate IVUS segments as attenuated or calcified, or plaque without attenuation or calcification. A total 598 vessels in 598 patients were evaluated, and a DL model with five-fold cross-validation was developed. The deep-learning model closely correlated with the expert read, and correlation coefficients for calcification, attenuation, and no attenuation or calcification respectively. Stent underexpansion is a frequently encountered entity that has been associated with an increased risk of in-stent restenosis. Studies have demonstrated the postprocedural minimum stent area (MSA) and IVUS-measured stent length to be independent predictors for in-stent restenosis Min et al. devised a deep-learning model to predict stent underexpansion based on pre-PCI IVUS frames. They evaluated 618 coronary lesions from 618 patients undergoing pre- and postprocedural IVUS and divided them into training and testing sets in stent area. Features extracted from the CNN a 5:1 ratio. A convolutional neural network (CNN)model was used to predict the poststenting stent area. Features extracted from the CNN were combined with additional image-derived features via a boosted ensemble algorithm, which yielded sensitivity and specificity of 68% and 98%, respectively, and an AUC of 0.95 to predict stent underexpansion. The stent areas and volumes predicted via the CNN correlated well with poststenting IVUS (r for stent area and volume 0.832 and 0.958, respectively). The most important features predicting stent underexpansion were luminal area, external elastic membrane (EEM) area (both at the reference and the target), and plaque area of the region of interest.

To predict OCT-derived TCFA on IVUS images, Bae et al. created a ML model, enrolling 517 patients who underwent ICA . A total of 40,908 IVUS-OCT co-registered sections in 517 coronary arteries were divided into training and testing sets in a ratioa 5:1 ratio. A convolutional neural network (CNN)model was used to predict the poststenting of 4:1. An artificial-neural-network-based model using 17 features achieved the highest performance with a sensitivity and specificity of 85 ± 4% and 79 ± 6%, respectively, and good discriminatory power (AUC of 0.80 ± 0.08). Larger plaque burden, minimal diameter, decreased lumen area, and increased lumen eccentricity were seen to be strongly associated with OCT-derived TCFAs

Min et al. utilized a deep learning algorithm (densely connected convolutional neural network) on 35,678 OCT frames to automatically detect TCFAs from OCT images .After the frames were interpreted for the presence/absence of TCFA, data was fed into the algorithm to devise a deep-learning model.

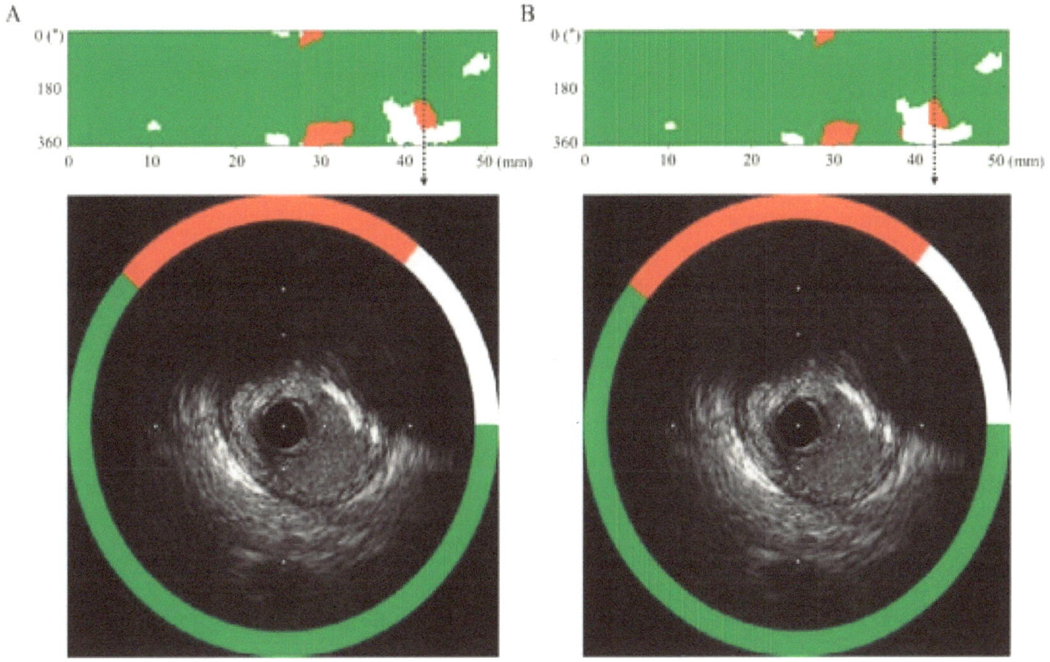

Fig.7.3 ML(A) vs. human (B) interpretations for plaque characterization for IVUS images. The upper panel shows representation of plaque features along the long axis of the vessel (x-axis represents the distance from ROI (region of interest) and y-axis represents the angular position (0–360°) of the plaque. The lower panel shows the plaque characterization on a cross-sectional view of the IVUS frame. Attenuation, calcification, and regions without attenuation or calcification are represented by red, white, and green respectively. Adapted with permission from Cho et al.

By achieving high sensitivity and specificity of 88.7 ± 3.4% and 91.8 ± 2.0% on the test data, such deep-learning models can significantly reduce processing times and allow for easy interpretation when it comes to identifying a vulnerable high-risk plaque As mentioned earlier, IVUS can help characterize high-risk plaques, which appear as areas of attenuation on IVUS frames due to the presence of a large necrotic core. Identifying such lesions becomes imperative to reduce the incidence of complications such as periprocedural MI. To accurately classify plaque characteristics and to facilitate detection of high-risk lesions, Cho et al. described a deep-learning algorithm to accurately differentiate IVUS segments as attenuated or calcified, or plaque without attenuation or calcification. A total 598 vessels in 598 patients were evaluated, and a DL model with five-fold cross-validation was developed. The deep-learning model closely correlated with the expert read, and correlation coefficients for calcification, attenuation, and no attenuation or calcification were 0.79, 0.74, and 0.99, respectively The most important features predicting stent underexpansion were luminal area, external elastic membrane (EEM) area (both at the reference and the target), and plaque area of the region of interest.

B.Applications of Artificial Intelligence in Intra and Post-InterventionWorkflow

Optimal stent expansion is vital to successful outcomes, with stent underexpansion predisposing to stent restenosis and a greater stent expansion exposing the procedure to a risk of stent edge dissection .IVUS, by allowing direct visualization of vessel architecture, can help in the earlier identification and management of these complications. Nishi et al. developed a ML model to compute the luminal area and the vessel area accurately, as well as the stent area, which exhibited an excellent correlation between ML-derived and expert-derived dimensions while dramatically reducing the time required for segmentation of IVUS images (37s) compared with expert analysis Virtual histology IVUS (VH-IVUS) is a well-studied intracoronary imaging modality used for in vivo visualization of high-risk plaques .

Zhang et al. devised a deep-learning model to predict the location of high-risk plaques in nonculprit vessels in patients who underwent IVUS at baseline and after one year . Though large-scale validation is required, the model predicted the occurrence of TCFAs, plaque burden >70%, and minimal luminal area ≤4 mm2 reasonably well at a one-year follow-up on a per-lesion level.

C. Artificial Intelligence-Based Post-Procedure Risk Prediction Models

In addition to early detection and the institution of guideline-directed therapy in the appropriate risk strata, accurate prediction of unheralded adverse events forms the cornerstone for managing CAD. Identifying the high-risk target population can potentially provide a window for aggressive risk factor modulation, thereby reducing mortality and contributing towards better health at a population level. Multiple risk-prediction models have been developed to predict in-hospital mortality and the long-term risk of MACE in high-risk cohorts PCI is a relatively safe procedure, with a reported overall in-hospital mortality rate of 1–2% . The risk of complications increases with increasing patient morbidity, with an incidence of technical difficulties and periprocedural complications 2.2 times higher than in the average population . The Mayo clinic risk score (MCRS) and New York State risk score (NYSRS) were developed to predict in-hospital and 30-day mortality in patients undergoing PCI. Both scores performed equivalently well, showing an excellent discriminative ability to identify patients at a higher risk for in-hospital and 30-day mortality. They employed regression-based models, assuming a linear interplay between patient variables and mortality outcomes. ML models have been recently developed to potentially uncover complex and nonlinear relationships between multiple factors, hence improving diagnostic accuracy over current models.

Zack et al. evaluated 11,709 patients to train two RF regression models—one using 52 demographic and clinical parameters to predict in-hospital mortality and the second model also incorporating 358 discharge variables in addition to the 52 admission parameters to predict 180-day cardiovascular mortality and 30-day heart failure rehospitalization.They compared the model performances against logistic regression models trained using the same variables. No significant difference was found between the RF model and logistic regression in predicting in-hospital mortality (AUC 0.923 vs. 0.925, $p = 0.84$). The ML model performed significantly better than the logistic regression model for prediction of 30-day heart failure hospitalizations (AUC 0.899 vs. 0.846, $p = 0.003$) and 180-day cardiovascular death (AUC 0.881 vs. 0.812, $p = 0.02$).Al'Aref et al. developed a supervised machine learning approach to predict in-hospital mortality among patients undergoing PCI. Utilizing 479,804 patients from the New York state registry, they utilized 49 clinical, angiographic, and periprocedural event characteristics to create a ML model via adaptive boosting. It performed better than the logistic regression model (AUC 0.927 for ML vs. 0.908 for logistic regression, $p < 0.01$). Age and ejection fraction emerged as the most important variables predicting mortality.Periprocedural bleeding is one of the most common complications of PCI and has been linked to adverse in-hospital outcomes. Current risk scores such as the NCDR bleeding risk-prediction model and the simplified NCDR bleeding-risk score have performed modestly well in identifying patients at a high risk of periprocedural bleeding . To improve the performance of the existing risk model, an ML-based model was developed on 3,316,465 patients enrolled in the CathPCI registry. In addition to the 31 variables used in the existing model, 28 new variables were incorporated to devise an integrated model via the gradient-boosting approach. The blended model using ML had a higher discriminatory power than the existing model (C statistic 0.82 vs. 0.78, $p < 0.05$) and improved the positive predictive value to 26.6%, compared with 21.5% for the existent model.

One of the primary challenges faced in the PCI era is in-stent restenosis, which is linked to neointimal proliferation due to vascular wall damage . The incidence of ISR has been estimated to be 20–40% for bare metallic stents and 10–15% for drug-eluting stents .Smaller vessel size, increasing stent length, complex lesion morphology, diabetes mellitus, and prior bypass surgery are risk factors for stent restenosis . These factors have been incorporated with other variables to devise risk models such as PRESTO 1, PRESTO 2, and EVENT scores to provide an estimated risk of ISR . These models have a modest discriminatory power in predicting ISR, leaving room for improvement.

A big-data approach incorporated 68 variables relating to clinical, demographic, and angiographic characteristics to devise a risk prediction model for ISR.The ML model, when applied post-PCI, achieved a higher discriminatory power (AUC for the precision recall curve was 0.45 vs. 0.31, 0.27, and 0.18 for PRESTO-1, PRESTO-2, and EVENT, respectively, $p < 0.05$) to predict ISR at 12 months. Interestingly, post-PCI TIMI flow was one of the prominent predictors of ISR, alongside diabetes mellitus and the presence of ≥2 vessel CAD. Though the model requires external validation, given the small sample size of the population ($n = 263$), the study yet again underscores the merit of ML in identifying crucial parameters from a vast dataset to predict outcomes

D.Artificial Intelligence-Based Long-Term Mortality and MACE Prediction Models

Prognostic modeling via ML has been validated with the use of electronic health records (EHRs) integrated with clinical scores and imaging modalities to predict MACE .

Utilizing the array of data available in EMR and identifying patterns based on clinical course, ML models have been used to create a personalized treatment algorithm (ML4CAD) for every patient, based on risk factors,past medical history, time present in the EMR system, and medications. The illustrated model makes clinical decisions for patients based on these factors and suggests a decision with an aim to increase prescription effectiveness, evaluated in the terms of time from initial diagnosis to the first potential adverse event (time to adverse event, TAE). The model had superior performance when compared to standard of care, increasing the time to adverse event (TAE) from 4.56 to 5.66 years (24.3% increase), hence furthering the idea of precision medicine . Imaging findings, such as CAC score quantified from cardiac computed tomography, are an independent risk factor adding to the traditional clinical risk factors in predicting long-term risk of cardiovascular events Noncontrast CT imaging, other than providing information on the CAC score, provides valuable measures such as epicardial adipose tissue (EAT) volume, and EAT attenuation, all of which have been shown to provide additional information regarding the long-term risk of cardiovascular disease Extracting these pieces of data can be tedious and labor-intensive, and automated techniques can result in more standardized evaluations in a more time-efficient manner. Multiple ML techniques have been proposed to automatically evaluate CAC score from dedicated cardiac and non-EKG gated chest CT scans ML techniques incorporating CAC score and other imaging parameters have been shown to be a better predictor than the traditional risk scores employed for cardiovascular disease risk stratification. An ensemble-boosting model developed by Nakanishi et al. incorporating a total of 77 clinical and imaging variables had a superior discriminatory power for predicting coronary heart disease deaths than imaging and clinical data alone (AUC for ML model: 0.845 compared to 0.821 and 0.781 for clinical data and CAC respectively, $p < 0.001$) Apart from CAC scoring and traditional CT metrics, the role of EAT volume and attenuation in the prediction of future cardiovascular risk has been an active area of research. Deep-learning approaches to automatically compute EAT volume and EAT attenuation from CT have been developed,significantly reducing generation time from 15 min to 2 s . Eisenberg et al. demonstrated an independent association between deep-learning-derived EAT volume and attenuation with the risk of future MACE, defined as myocardial infarction, late (>180 days) revascularization, and cardiac death (HR:1.35, $p < 0.01$ and 0.83, $p = 0.01$,demonstrating a direct correlation with EAT volume and an inverse correlation with EAT attenuation respectively) .Subsequently, these parameter have been combined with other physiologic and radiology variables to develop new deep-learning approaches, which have further been shown tohave a higher predictive value than the traditional risk scores.Apart from its role in CAD diagnosis, CCTA has been shown to have an incremental prognostic value in terms of short- and long-term risk prediction. Results from the CONFIRM registry validated two CCTA parameters, namely the number of proximal segments with stenosis > 50% and the number of proximal segments with mixed or calcified plaque as important prognostic markers above the predictive value of the Framingham risk score (FRS) A multitude of ML approaches have been described, combining imaging parameters with clinical and demographic parameters for better prognostication of cardiovascular outcomes Including 10,030 patients with suspected CAD from the CONFIRM registry, Motwani et al. utilized a boosting ensemble algorithm using 25 clinical and 44 CCTA parameters . The ML algorithm performed better in predicting 5-year all-cause mortality than CCTA segment stenosis score or FRS (AUC 0.79 for ML vs. 0.664 for segment stenosis score and 0.61 for FRS, respectively, $p < 0.001$). More recently, models incorporating high-risk plaque features with the traditional imaging and clinical parameters have performed better than either of the parameters in isolation Although anatomical CT scores and plaque features provide useful diagnostic and prognostic data, the complex interplay of factors at the molecular level, in addition to patient-level characteristics leading to specific phenotypic manifestations in terms of plaque burden and features, is not well-elucidated and remains an area of active research. In particular, elucidating important factors that "drive" the process of atherosclerotic plaque formation and progression is not only vital from a therapeutic perspective, but it can also improve risk-assessment strategies. Recent studies have demonstrated that coronary artery inflammation inhibits lipid accumulation in the perivascular adipose tissue [200]. This results in a higher attenuation of the affected perivascular area, identified on CCTA as the fat attenuation index (FAI). FAI has been shown to be a sensitive marker of coronary inflammation, with higher FAI values (≥−70.1 HU) independently predicting cardiovascular mortality A posthoc analysis of the CRISP-CT study showed an incremental value of adding FAI to high-risk plaque characteristics, pointing towards a more significant role of these precursor lesions in predicting patient outcomes. A more recent ML approach created a pericoronary fat 'radiomic' profile (FRP), identifying radiomic variables predicting tissue inflammation, fibrosis, and vascularity on

CCTA.The incorporation of FRP significantly improved the MACE predictive ability of the traditional model (AUC for traditional + FRP 0.88 vs. 0.754 for the traditional model, $p < 0.001$). Using a cut-off of 0.63, individuals in the high FRP group were at a higher risk of MACE (HR = 10.84, $p < 0.001$). Importantly, Kaplan–Meir analysis showed an additional value of FRP over high-risk plaque (HRP) characteristics in predicting long-term survival (HR for the FRP-/HRP+ subgroup 5.97, p = 0.03 compared to 43.33 for the FRP+/HRP+ subgroup). Such 'radiotranscriptomic' approaches incorporating molecular biology and radiology and evaluating their interaction via artificial intelligence can help uncover deeper relationships between metabolic pathways and clinical outcomes, helping to better understand the pathophysiology and elements involved in the clinical progression of cardiovascular disease.With significant developments occurring in the last decade in terms of data processing and analytics, AI can provide new and sophisticated tools that could help us to better understand disease processes, which ultimately should translate into better patient care and outcomes . Nevertheless, AI comes with its own set of limitations. ML models lack interpretability and suffer from the 'black box' problem . ML models based on neural networks and ensemble methods are inherently complex and are derived from complicated mathematical algorithms. 'Explainable (interpretable) machine learning', whereby simple approximations of the model are devised to make it more understandable, is being developed to overcome the black box problem. Another limitation of ML encountered at the model-development phase is sampling bias and lack of external validation [207,208]. ML learning models usually derive their weights from large datasets. Datasets, particularly those derived from EHRs, might be skewed and not representative of the entire population, leading to significant sampling bias and limited generalizability. A few models have tried to address this problem by stratifying the datasets at the model-development phase to ensure not to lose representation of any subgroup and preserve the model's generalizability. Nevertheless, randomized controlled trials are needed to potentially overcome this bias and establish the model performance against the standard clinical parameters. In addition, imputation methods such as MICE have been used to address the missing data issue Furthermore, the creation of bigger datasets by pooling data from multiple hospital systems has led to a lack of standardization of datasets, potentially compromising the quality of analysis. Datasets might internally differ from each other because of the different mechanisms used to generate them. For instance, one dataset might define the presence of diabetes mellitus through ICD-10 codes, while another dataset might define it using glycemic indices, such as the hemoglobin A1c. On a similar theme, ML models developed by using imaging modalities deserve a special mention. For instance, differences can exist at the level of image scanning (different scanner characteristics and vendors), image quality (radiation dose, motion artifacts), and image processing (reconstruction filters, post-processing) which can potentially lead to significant variability and differences of the assimilated data. A prerequisite to the development of any ML model is the centralization of data, which is tedious given the different image processing algorithms employed at various institutions. This lack of standardization needs to be addressed before AI can be fully integrated into clinical practice. Verfitting is another concern encountered during ML model development, which occurs when the algorithm learns the data 'too well' and interprets the signal noise as concepts . This usually happens with smaller datasets and can lead to a lack of external validity, despite high performance in the training and internal validation datasets. A definite solution is k-fold cross-validation, whereby data is randomly divided into an arbitrary k number of partitions. The model is trained using $k - 1$ number of data subsets and tested on the remaining subset. This process is repeated k total number of times, using different combinations of training and testing datasets to select the best model hyper-parameters to yield the final model. This can potentially reduce noise and lead to better generalizability of the model in the overall population.Apart from the problems encountered at the model development and training phase, there are a few noteworthy practical limitations to the implementation of ML within healthcare workflows. Firstly, unauthorized data access is an issue, as handling such large amounts of data also poses a risk of leaking sensitive patient information, thereby violating patient confidentiality and privacy Furthermore, comparisons between various machine-learning methods are difficult, given the different combinations of model parameters and different population characteristics used for in model development.Hence, it becomes difficult for physicians to compare and choose one model over the other. Prospective future trials, comparing these models on the same dataset, are needed to select the best algorithm fit for integration into routine clinical decision-making. Proper integration of AI can only be achieved once these models are embedded within EHRs. However, the full implementation and assimilation of developed AI models into EHRs can be a complex issue, as it depends on organizational resources and patient-privacy policies. Furthermore, available algorithms may be limited to off-the-shelf ML models, rather than more intricate and complex neural networks, whichis easier to implement in a real clinical setting.

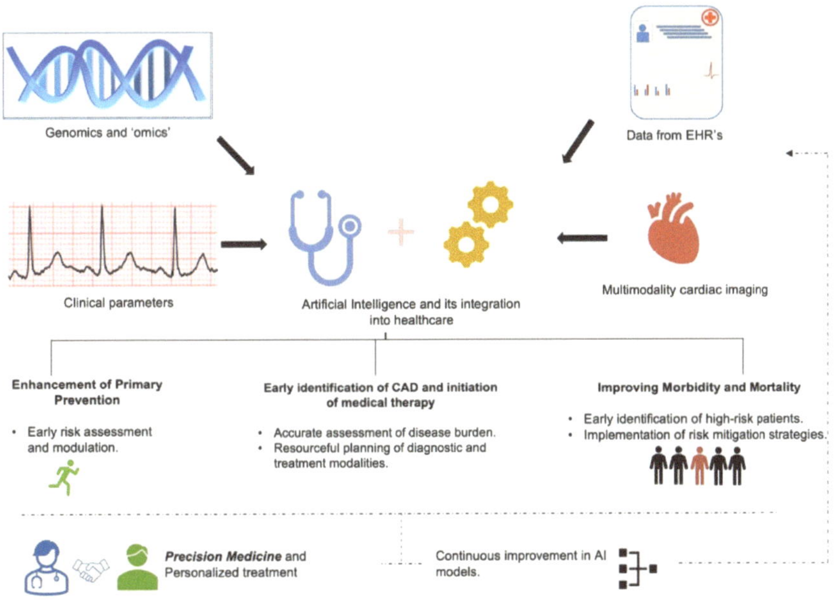

Fig.7.4 Current applicability and future directions for AI in coronary artery disease.

Bibliography And Acknowledgement

- Arnett, D.K.; Blumenthal, R.S.; Albert, M.A.; Buroker, A.B.; Goldberger, Z.D.; Hahn, E.J.; Himmelfarb, C.D.; Khera, A.; Lloyd-Jones, D.; McEvoy, J.W.; et al. 2019 ACC/AHA Guideline on the Primary Prevention of Cardiovascular Disease: A Report of the American College of Cardiology/American Heart Association Task Force on Clinical Practice Guidelines. Circulation 2019
- Benjamin, E.J.; Muntner, P.; Alonso, A.; Bittencourt, M.S.; Callaway, C.W.; Carson, A.P.; Chamberlain, A.M.; Chang, A.R.; Cheng, S.; Das, S.R.; et al. Heart Disease and Stroke Statistics—2019 Update: A Report From the American Heart Association. Circulation 2019,
- Gaur, S.; Ovrehus, K.A.; Dey, D.; Leipsic, J.; Botker, H.E.; Jensen, J.M.; Narula, J.; Ahmadi, A.; Achenbach, S.; Ko, B.S.; et al. Coronary plaque quantification and fractional flow reserve by coronary computed tomography angiography identify ischaemia-causing lesions. Eur. Heart J. 2016,
- Kumamaru, K.K.; Fujimoto, S.; Otsuka, Y.; Kawasaki, T.; Kawaguchi, Y.; Kato, E.; Takamura, K.; Aoshima, C.; Kamo, Y.; Kogure, Y.; et al. Diagnostic accuracy of 3D deep-learning-based fully automated estimation of patient-level minimum fractional flow reserve from coronary computed tomography angiography. Eur. Heart J. Cardiovasc. Imaging 2020, 21, 437–445.
- Sekimoto, T.; Akutsu, Y.; Hamazaki, Y.; Sakai, K.; Kosaki, R.; Yokota, H.; Tsujita, H.; Tsukamoto, S.; Kaneko, K.; Sakurai, M.; et al. Regional calcified plaque score evaluated by multidetector computed tomography for predicting the addition of rotational atherectomy during percutaneous coronary intervention. J. Cardiovasc. Comput. Tomogr. 2016, 10, 221–228
- Taylor, A.J.; Bindeman, J.; Feuerstein, I.; Cao, F.; Brazaitis, M.; O'Malley, P.G. Coronary calcium independently predicts incident premature coronary heart disease over measured cardiovascular risk factors: Mean three-year outcomes in the Prospective Army Coronary Calcium (PACC) project. J. Am. Coll. Cardiol. 2005, 46, 807–814.
- Li, D.; Xiong, G.; Zeng, H.; Zhou, Q.; Jiang, J.; Guo, X. Machine learning-aided risk stratification system for the prediction of coronary artery disease. Int. J. Cardiol. 2021, 326, 30–34
- Muhammad, L.J.; Al-Shourbaji, I.; Haruna, A.A.; Mohammed, I.A.; Ahmad, A.; Jibrin, M.B. Machine Learning Predictive Models for Coronary Artery Disease. SN Comput. Sci. 2021, 2, 350.
- Noll, D.R.; Ginsberg, T.; Elahi, A.; Cavalieri, T.A. Effective Patient-Physician Communication Based on Osteopathic Philosophy in Caring for Elderly Patients. J. Osteopath. Med. 2016, 116, 42–47.
- Pu, J.; Mintz, G.S.; Biro, S.; Lee, J.-B.; Sum, S.T.; Madden, S.P.; Burke, A.P.; Zhang, P.; He, B.; Goldstein, J.A.; et al. Insights Into Echo-Attenuated Plaques, Echolucent Plaques, and Plaques With Spotty Calcification: Novel Findings From Comparisons Among Intravascular Ultrasound, Near-Infrared Spectroscopy, and Pathological Histology in 2294 Human Coronary Artery Segments. J. Am. Coll. Cardiol. 2014, 63, 2220–2233.
- Slomka, P.; Xu, Y.; Berman, D.; Germano, G. Quantitative analysis of perfusion studies: Strengths and pitfalls. J. Nucl. Cardiol. Off. Publ. Am. Soc. Nucl. Cardiol. 2012, 19, 338–346.
- van Velzen, S.G.M.; Lessmann, N.; Velthuis, B.K.; Bank, I.E.M.; van den Bongard, D.; Leiner, T.; de Jong, P.A.; Veldhuis, W.B.; Correa, A.; Terry, J.G.; et al. Deep Learning for Automatic Calcium Scoring in CT: Validation Using Multiple Cardiac CT and Chest CT Protocols. Radiology 2020, 295, 6
- Wang, W.; Wang, H.; Chen, Q.; Zhou, Z.; Wang, R.; Wang, H.; Zhang, N.; Chen, Y.; Sun, Z.; Xu, L. Coronary artery calcium score quantification using a deep-learning algorithm. Clin. Radiol. 2020, 75, 237.e11–237.e16
- Zack, C.J.; Senecal, C.; Kinar, Y.; Metzger, Y.; Bar-Sinai, Y.; Widmer, R.J.; Lennon, R.; Singh, M.; Bell, M.R.; Lerman, A.; et al. Leveraging Machine Learning Techniques to Forecast Patient Prognosis After Percutaneous Coronary Intervention. JACC Cardiovasc. Interv. 2019, 12, 1304–1311

Machine Learning and Artificial Intelligence to Improve Peripheral Artery Disease Management

CHAPTER 8

Peripheral artery disease is an atherosclerotic disorder which, when present, portends poor patient outcomes. Low diagnosis rates perpetuate poor management, leading to limb loss and excess rates of cardiovascular morbidity and death. Machine learning algorithms and artificially intelligent systems have shown great promise in application to many areas in health care, such as accurately detecting disease, predicting patient outcomes, and automating image interpretation. Although the application of these technologies to peripheral artery disease are in their infancy, their promises are tremendous. In this review, we provide an introduction to important concepts in the fields of machine learning and artificial intelligence, detail the current state of how these technologies have been applied to peripheral artery disease, and discuss potential areas for future care enhancement with advanced analytics.

The first Circulation Research Compendium on Peripheral Artery Disease (PAD) was assembled in 2015, powerfully noting that many with PAD are dying of neglect. Despite being a major atherosclerotic disease with a global prevalence of >200 million,2 physicians often fail to diagnose PAD, due in part to conflicting screening recommendations, low patient and provider awareness, and the high prevalence of asymptomatic or atypical symptoms. Even once recognized by clinicians, rates of initiation of evidence-based therapies lag that of other atherosclerotic diseases, such as coronary artery disease.The large amount of undiagnosed PAD cases is unfortunate because preventive therapies, such as statins and antithrombotic agents, can save both life and limb. Recent years have seen a major investment in identifying effective treatments for PAD, including several randomized clinical trials of both medical and revascularization approaches. At the same time, health care is at major crossroads—with the generation of massive amounts of data from sources such as electronic health records (EHRs), medical imaging, wearables, and large-scale genetic sequencing. The high volume of data provide opportunities to revolutionize how care for vascular patients is delivered. Since the publication of the original Compendium, multiple medical specialties have sought to leverage "Big Data" and advanced analytics, but the real-world integration of artificially intelligent systems and medicine remains in its infancy. When applied to PAD, advanced analytics promise to identify latent disease, refine disease and risk phenotyping, and aid treatment choices with consideration of the full breadth of demographic, biological, and clinical data . Artificial intelligence (AI)-based vascular imaging tools will also provide support for diagnostic, prognostic, and intraoperative settings. Given that PAD care is often fragmented across different locations and specialties, AI can also aid with integrating care data points, thereby promoting the holistic, interdisciplinary care that is critical to optimizing management and outcomes. This chapter reviews contributions of AI and machine learning (ML) to PAD care and explores what integration of AI and PAD care can mean for patients, internists, surgeons, and the multidisciplinary care team as a whole. In some instances, we draw from developments in other vascular diseases such as carotid and aortic aneurysm disease, highlighting the need to develop AI for PAD specifically to help rescue patients from dying of neglect.

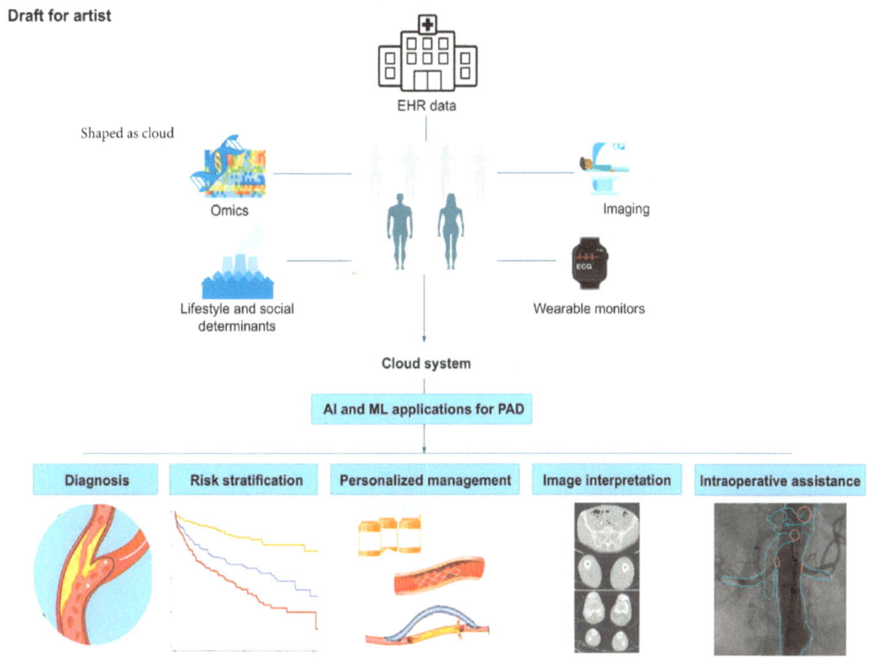

Fig.8.1 Applications of AI and ML across the spectrum of peripheral artery disease care, spanning diagnosis, risk stratification, management, and intraoperative guidance.AI, artificial intelligence. EHR, electronic health record. ML, machine learning. PAD, peripheral artery disease. (Illustration credit: Ben Smith)

What we know about AI and ML?

AI can be defined as the use of computer algorithms to automate a specific task with the goal of mimicking human thought processes and learning. For example, digital assistants such as Apple's Siri and Amazon's Alexa are powered by a range of AI technologies that enable each system to understand, parse, and respond to speech in a manner similar to a human's response. These digital assistants also "learn" over time to improve the accuracy of their responses. And while AI encompasses task automation, AI is powered by computational algorithms, broadly known as ML algorithms, which enable this automation.There are many types of ML algorithms that are broadly classified by the way in which each algorithm "learns". Learning, as it applies to ML algorithms, involves applying a mathematical formula or series of formulas to data such that relationships between features (or variables) can be summarized mathematically. The final result of this application is a model that represents the mathematical summary. This model can then be applied to new data to estimate expected values (eg, predict laboratory values or yes/no patient outcomes).

When algorithms are provided data where the outcome or class (disease, nondiseased) are labeled this is considered supervised learning—supervised because the ground truth is known and provided to the algorithm. In unsupervised learning, there is no ground truth label and the algorithm finds structure within the data. we summarize different ML algorithms based on the type of learning methods employed. Key terms for interpreting ML model development are listed

Vascular Disease Diagnosis

Disease Detection Using Supervised Learning Approaches

ML models can enable automated disease detection. One of the first studies to demonstrate the utility of using ML to identify undiagnosed PAD was published in 2016 (Online Dataset I).26 Data were derived from a clinical trial of patients presenting for elective coronary angiography. Of all patients included in the study, 17% had PAD and 68% of these patients were undiagnosed at study enrollment, confirming that PAD is underrecognized.

Integrating disparate data variables spanning sociodemographics, medical history, genetic, and coronary angiography findings, our group developed a classification model that was trained in a hypothesis-free fashion to identify cases of patients with PAD who were previously undiagnosed. The most accurate PAD prediction model was based on a random forest algorithm . Supervised Learning). The final model included over 120 baseline characteristics and achieved an area under the receiver operating curve (AUC) of 0.84 for PAD classification, notably outperforming classifications made on the basis of traditional linear models using the same data (AUC=0.60). Additionally, the ML model achieved a sensitivity of 76% compared with 57% from a traditional linear model. Such improvements in sensitivity can significantly improve detection of undiagnosed patients with PAD.Other efforts to apply ML algorithms have attempted to predict angiographically significant or advanced disease based on proteomics and functional metrics, respectively. In a study using data from patients referred for diagnostic coronary or peripheral angiography, a least absolute selection and shrinkage operator regression model combined >50 clinical variables and 109 biomarkers to predict obstructive PAD, defined as

>50% stenosis in at least 1 peripheral vessel. The final model incorporated hypertension and 6 biomarkers and had an AUC of 0.85 for obstructive PAD. Authors concluded that the tool may be used as a gatekeeper for invasive angiography and predict need for revascularization. Another study sought to identify patients at risk of critical limb ischemia in a cohort with critical limb ischemia (cases) and no PAD (controls)(defined as toe-brachial index <0.7 and >0.7, respectively). Authors developed an ML model using data on demographics, 6-minute walk test distance, symptom scores derived from vascular quality of life questionnaire, and calf circumference. Their random forest and generalized linear algorithms resulted in similar AUCs of 0.69 and 0.68 for identifying cases of critical limb ischemia, respectively.

Disease Detection Using Natural Language Processing

Because of the large amount of text data in the EHR, natural language processing (NLP) methods have been analyzed as a tool to identify cases of PAD. For example Afzal et al applied a rule-based NLP Natural Language Processing) to notes retrieved from the Mayo clinical data warehouse with the goal of automating detection of prevalent PAD. First, in analyzing 300 364 notes from a community-based cohort, the NLP model was built using PAD-related concepts and keywords (eg, “lower extremity, occlusive disease”) to ascertain PAD status (defined as Ankle Brachial Index ≤0.9 or >1.4). Authors optimized the NLP model by reviewing and sequentially excluding select note types that led to the most false positives to maximize accuracy. Compared with a disease detection model based on International Classification of Diseases and Current Procedural Terminology codes, the NLP model was more accurate (92% versus 82%), had a higher PPV (93%versus 74%), and greater specificity (93% versus 64%) for identifying true PAD cases.29 Similarly, to identify severity of PAD, Afzal et al30 refined their NLP models and established the superiority of using NLP algorithms to classify patients with critical limb ischemia relative to billing codes (F1 Scores: NLP 90% versus billing code 76%, P<0.001) Recently, Weissler et al31 also leveraged NLP methodology to query Duke University Medical Center’s EHR system to identify patients with PAD. In comparison to Afzal et al, rather than using rule-based algorithms applied to predefined note types or sections, Weissler and colleagues trained an embedding-based NLP algorithm using notes from all clinical encounters and evaluated model performance on a broader PAD cohort adjudicated by imaging reports, surgical/intervention documentation, and ABIs. Clinical notes were analyzed using an algorithm known as hierarchical Label-Embedding Attention Model that considered the frequency of individuals words, their learned representations, and the aggregate implication of numerous notes from each patient.

Word embeddings were aggregated from all notes for a given patient and served as input to a neural network that generated a classification probability for PAD status. The NLP model applied to free-text outperformed a PAD classification strategy based on structured billing and procedure codes, with an AUC of 0.888 versus 0.801 (P<0.0001), respectively

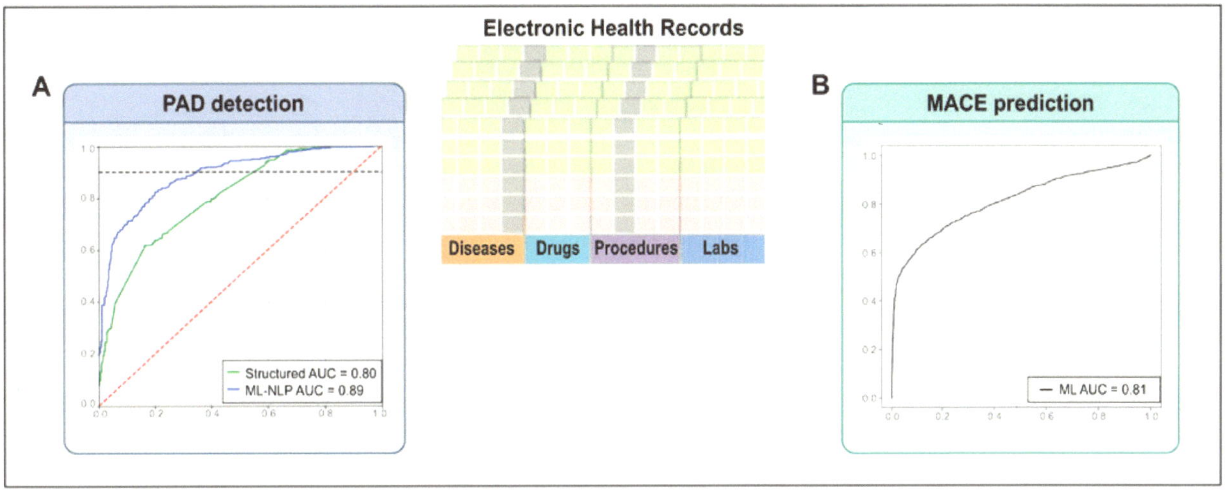

Fig.8.2 When applied to the EHR, machine learning models reliably identify PAD and predict future cardiovascular events. A, ML-based natural language processing (ML-NLP) of clinical notes identifies patients with PAD more accurately than structured data based on administrative diagnosis codes. B, By incorporating structured and unstructured EHR data, ML algorithms accurately risk stratify PAD patients at high risk for major adverse cardiovascular events (MACE). AUC, area under the receiver operating curve. EHR, electronic health record. MACE, major adverse cardiovascular event. PAD, peripheral artery disease. X-axis represents 1-specificity. Y-axis represents sensitivity. A, modified from Weissler et al.31 B, modified from Ross et al.

Disease Detection Using Complementary Clinical and Genetic Data

Although not yet applied to PAD detection, investigators have sought to combine the rich data from the EHR with genetic information, paving the way for the development and deployment of personalized health applications For example, Li et al developed an ML model to combine whole-genome sequencing and EHR data to automate identification of those with abdominal aortic aneurysms (AAAs). Their ML algorithm examined the clinical relevance of > 23 million genetic variants—agnostically identified genes with disease-distinct mutational patterns—and incorporated EHR data to complement predictions from individual genomes. EHR data utilized in the model included lifestyle and physiological measurements such as fasting glucose, lipid profiles, waist-to-hip ratios, and more. Compared with a genome-only model (AUC=0.69) or an EHR-only model (AUC=0.78), integrating both data sources resulted in a significant increase in the ML model's predictive power for AAA development (AUC=0.80, P<1×10 Efforts to combine EHR data with genetic risk assessment of other vascular disease processes such as PAD have been hampered by lack of large enough sample sizes to identify unique genetic risks. However, with the recent landmark genome-wide association study on PAD in the large-scale biobank, the Million Veteran Program, we now have the ability to combine genetic susceptibility with EHR data. Such data could potentially be combined to create a precision health screening platform for vascular disease. These platforms would enable health care systems to identify individuals with high pretest probability of having or developing highly morbid diseases. Targeted early diagnosis and treatment may subsequently reduce disease complications, improve patient outcomes, and decrease health care costs

Vascular Disease Phenotyping and Management

Identifying Unique Disease Subtypes With Unsupervised Clustering

PAD shares many risk factors with coronary artery disease, including hypertension, smoking, and hyperlipidemia. However, there is growing evidence that suggests PAD is a more distinct atherosclerotic disorder. For example, unlike in the coronary and carotid vasculature, the presence of unstable plaques that lead to acute events is relatively uncommon in PAD. These findings suggest that their shared risk factors may contribute differently to disease pathogenesis, in addition to having unique pathophysiologic mechanisms. Further, within the PAD population, there is broad heterogeneity in clinical profiles and outcomes To help resolve disease heterogeneity, ML approaches can be applied for deep phenotyping of PAD. Unsupervised cluster analysis has emerged as a promising approach to discovering clinically unique phenotypes in complex diseases Unsupervised Learning Rather than being limited to a known handful of risk factors, clustering algorithms can group patients based on robust, multidimensional patient data. Unsupervised clustering holds a number of advantages: it can generate novel disease subgroups, reveal population health patterns, and generate actionable information to tailor therapies. Such approaches have been applied to identify distinct phenotypes, reveal differences in population practice patterns, and detect subgroup heterogeneity in responses to common and new therapies.A more nuanced understanding of the unique characteristics of PAD and risk factors specific to individual patients can generate insights on the remaining curious distinctions that impact PAD severity, as well as differences between PAD and other atherosclerotic disorders like coronary artery disease or cerebrovascular disease. While prior cluster analyses have relied on analysis of one type of data with complete observations, advances in unsupervised algorithms are now enabling discovery of patient phenotypes using mixed categories of data and even missing data entries.These clustering frameworks are particularly suited for the data present in the EHR and will enable us to resolve phenotypic heterogeneity and personalize PAD management.

Identifying Appropriate Medical Treatment for Vascular Disease

The current approach to medical management of PAD is largely based on a reductionist methods—where patients with largely similar symptoms and broad diagnoses are given the same treatments. However, with the growing evidence base of therapies for PAD, there are now more options to consider beyond aspirin, high-intensity statins, and smoking. Even so, the increased costs of newer treatments and their attendant risks must be considered when selecting an appropriate treatment strategy and prescribing newer agents. ML models can assist with matching preventative efforts to patients who may most benefit from new or existing drugs, and achieve appropriate polypharmacy, which is especially prevalent in the highly comorbid PAD population. For example, Hansen et al used random forest to investigate warfarin-drug interactions with 220 drug groups from >61 000 prescriptions of patients with atrial fibrillation. ML approaches have also been developed to model polypharmacy side effects with networks of drug-protein interactions, drug-drug interactions, and protein-protein interactions. With numerous treatment guidelines for PAD and its frequent comorbid conditions, training such algorithms on patients with PAD can help develop plans that synchronize therapy and limit interactions leading to side effects. AI tools that can automate identification of PAD subgroups and integrate data such as polypharmacy interactomes and even pharmacogenetics will advance us from the conventional reductionist approach to personalized PAD care.In addition, advanced data science methods may be used to characterize long-term treatment safety in a real-world setting, including questions that are not likely to be addressed in clinical trials. For instance, in trials of cilostazol for the treatment of claudication, patients with congestive heart failure (CHF) were excluded largely based on theoretical safety concerns of a drug from a similar class. To conduct safety surveillance, Leeper and colleagues used NLP to mine clinical notes from patients with PAD and identify a subset of patients with CHF who were prescribed cilostazol. They found no adverse impact of cilostazol on cardiovascular events or mortality on patients with PAD, including in patients with CHF.

Novel Approaches to Risk Prediction

Predicting Cardiovascular Outcomes

PAD confers increased cardiovascular morbidity and mortality, including MI, stroke, and cardiovascular death.44 Unlike conventional risk models that incorporate a handful of risk factors, ML approaches have the advantage of being able to consider 100s of different risk factors and identify risk factors for which complex relationships amplify or attenuate risk. There has been significant interest in using EHR data for risk stratification. A major challenge in this application is to coerce enough structure into EHR data with processing pipelines that are reproducible and portable across multiple health care settings (eg, institutions, geographic locations). Through an analysis of a clinical trial database, ML models have been developed to predict mortality risk in patients with PAD.26 Advancing efforts into the real-world EHR from 2 different medical institutions, our group recently built a risk stratification model that accurately identifies which patients with PAD are most likely to go on to have a major adverse cardiovascular event (MACE) before event occurrence . EHR data were coded using the Observational Medical Outcomes Partnership Common Data Model, which enables transformation of disparate date types present in the EHR into a cohesive database structure In our specific models, data included patient prescriptions, laboratory values, International Classification of Diseases and Current Procedural Terminology codes, and annotated text from clinical notes. A random forest algorithm was then applied to the EHR data from both institutions. Interestingly, clinical text was vital for optimal model performance, where removal resulted in a significant decline in model AUC. The final predictive model was able to accurately discriminate between patients with PAD at high versus low risk of MACE occurrence (AUC=0.81) and showed good calibration (Brier score=0.10

Predicting Limb Outcomes

Vascular specialists are also keenly interested in limb-related outcomes. One study by Davis et al applied a combination of regularized linear regression algorithms Supervised Learning) to predict surgical site infections after lower extremity revascularization. Combining elastic net and random forest algorithms, their model had an AUC of 0.66 for post-bypass surgical site infections and identified a number of patient and procedure risk factors, including modifiable factors such as iodine-only skin preparation.To continue to advance applications of ML and AI for PAD, evidence supporting reliable model prediction of amputation and acute limb ischemia are needed.

Major adverse limb events (MALEs) are associated with a dire prognosis for patients with PAD, including MACE, prolonged hospitalization, and downstream impairments in quality of life.Even so, there are no well-vetted ML-based MALE prognostication tools. Such developments would be welcome given the far-reaching implications of MALE on PAD outcomes and care. Considerations of what type of data to utilize for MALE prognostication are important. Data from noninvasive studies based on velocity and stenosis criteria are abundant but can be unreliable and underestimate disease severity.EHR data can be considered given its depth and breadth; however, EHR data may miss important physiological markers. More than likely, a multimodal data approach will be needed where clinical data in the EHR or elsewhere are merged with imaging data (eg, hemodynamic noninvasive studies or computed tomography) to develop the most accurate MALE prognostic tools.

Computer Vision for Image Interpretation and Diagnosis

Carotid Atherosclerosis Imaging

Computer vision is a branch of AI in which deep learning algorithms are applied to automate analysis of images and videos. Computer vision for medical image analysis has shown great promise in multiple use cases including use cases specific to vascular disease. Successes in the application of computer vision have particularly begun to shape interpretation of carotid ultrasound images identifying features that correlate with stroke risk, such as the lipid core, fibrous cap and vessel-wall volume.

One AI solution was developed by See-Mode AVA (See-ModeAugmented Vascular Analysis, Singapore). Their software can perform automated carotid vessel segmentation and measure intima-media thickness. The software was developed using a convolutional neural network. The model accurately estimated carotid intima-media thickness and achieved a correlation of 0.93 with experts, which was greater than the correlation between experts. See-Mode AVA's deep learning software received premarket FDA clearance in late 2020 for analysis of carotid and lower extremity ultrasounds and generation of reports including carotid intima-media thickness, velocities, and waveform type. This software is exciting as

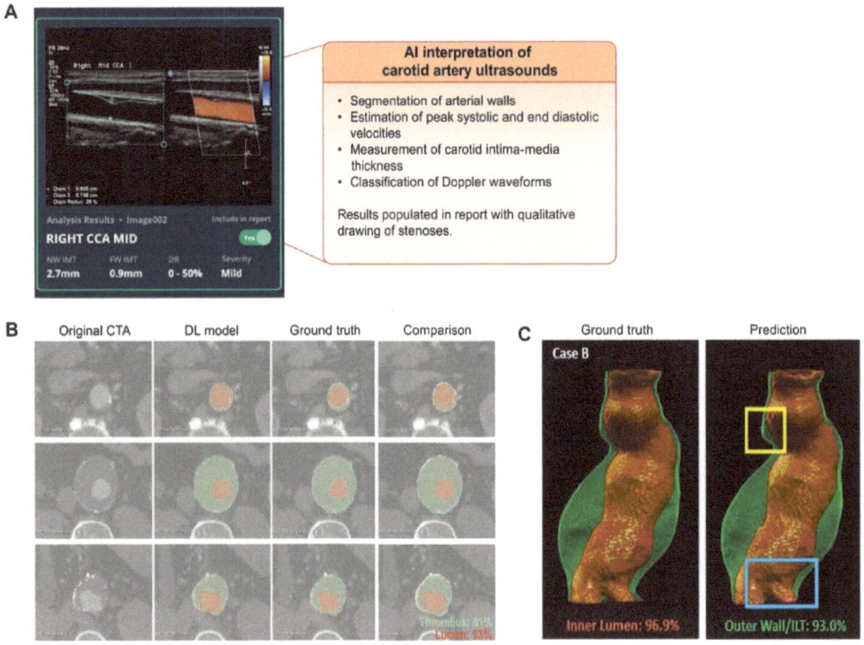

Fig.8.3 Imaging assessment of carotid atherosclerosis and AAA disease using deep learning A, AI software enables automated analysis and reporting of carotid ultrasounds. B,C, Deep learning pipelines have also been developed for fully automated volumetric analysis of AAA disease from CT images. B, Representative axial CTA slices are shown for automated segmentation of the aortic lumen (red) and thrombus (green) and the manually extracted ground truth. Key for comparison image: true positive lumen and thrombus (green and yellow, respectively), false negatives (red), false positives (blue). C, 3D U-Net output for the inner wall and outer wall/ILT (intraluminal thrombus) along with its respective ground truth. Points of discrepancy are boxed. Percentages in B-C represent the Dice coefficient. AAA, abdominal aortic aneurysm. AI, artificial intelligence. CTA, computed topography angiography. DL, deep learning. A, modified from See-Mode AVA user interface.63 B, modified from Caradu et al.68 C, modified from Chandrashekar et al.

Box 8.1: Key terms for ML model development.

Terms for Model Development:

Features: variables from a dataset used to train a model

- Training dataset: data sample used for fitting a model and learning parameters
- Validation dataset: data sample used for fine-tuning the model hyperparameters
- Test dataset: data sample used for evaluation of model performance, independent of the training data
- Overfitting: model can be too customized to the training data and generalizes poorly
- Cross validation: resampling procedure that involves a variety of approaches for partitioning a dataset into training and test subsamples, thereby providing checks on generalizability to unseen data through training and testing
  - o k-fold cross validation: commonly used cross validation technique in which a dataset is randomly partitioned into k-1 subsamples for training and one subsample for testing (often k = 5 or 10)
- Bootstrapping: another resampling procedure, involving random sampling with or without replacement

widespread adoption can lead to more timely diagnosis and easier postoperative surveillance. In addition, AI vascular ultrasoundtools can assist with obtaining high-quality images, which would be especially impactful in resource-poor settings where experienced sonographers may not be available. For example, AI software can provide real-time guidance during localization and interrogation of vascular structures (Caption Health, Brisbane, CA) and automate image enhancement for optimized quality (ContextVision, Sweden).

Additional automated methods for carotid plaque characterization have been achieved using MRI data. Wu et al report a deep neural network that diagnoses carotid atherosclerosis after being trained on manually labeled vessel-wall MRI images to learn visual features separately from the lumen and outer wall areas. Their model included use of a pretrained CNN developed specifically for biomedical imaging segmentation known as U-Net. This segmentation process involves labeling specific parts of images and with this labeled data deep learning algorithms learn important features that are predictive of predefined outcomes. In Wu et al's work, performance of the trained modified U-Net CNN was evaluated in 2 test datasets and could successfully diagnose carotid atherosclerosis (AUC, 0.92–0.95).

Aortic Aneurysm Imaging

While most computer vision algorithms such as CNNs are trained on 2-dimensional images, 3-dimensional (3D) CNNs provide the opportunity to automate characterization of lesions for which additional measurements are of great importance. The clinical significance of aneurysm disease, for example, is better characterized by capturing 3-dimensional features such as volume, rather than just length and/ or width. Applying a 3D CNN for post-endovascular aneurysm repair (EVAR) endoleak detection, Hahn et al demonstrate that these deep learning algorithms are able to identify multiple types of post-EVAR endoleaks with high performance (AUC=0.94). Using a 3D U-Net CNN, they also automate detection of AAA diameter and other key features such as AAA and endograft volumes. Other groups have applied U-Net CNNs for preoperative assessment of patients with AAAs, extracting aortic and thrombus volumes from computed tomography angiograms (CTAs) and noncontrast images. Application areas for automated AAA diagnosis and characterization are many, such as aiding vascular surgeons with surveillance and providing volumetric measurements that may be of greater prognostic value than diameter.Tools that can identify patients who may benefit from different endovascular repair approaches could also be helpful to vascular surgical practice.

PAD Imaging

Applications of computer vision algorithms to PAD-specific imaging are just starting to be reported and have the possibility to inform approaches to revascularization and potentially reduce the number of invasive diagnostic studies. Ara et al developed a computer vision model to automate classification of Doppler waveforms and detect aortoiliac, femoral-popliteal, and tibial trifurcation disease. Their model classified waveforms using a CNN, followed by a hierarchical neural network that integrated waveform classifications at each segment to classify normal versus diseased segments. In one model, CNN had an accuracy of 0.69, 1, and 0.86 for classifying mono-, bi-, and triphasic waveforms, respectively. In detecting disease, the hierarchical model achieved high F1 scores of 0.98 in normal arteries, 0.91 on aortoiliac disease, 0.93 on femoral-popliteal disease, and 0.85 on tibial trifurcation disease.Another important imaging modality for PAD is CTA, where automatic peripheral vessel identification may be used for localizing and quantifying disease, defining runoff, and helping define surgical or endovascular targets. A recent study by Dai et al developed a CNN to interpret lower extremity CTAs and classify disease in above-knee and below-knee arteries. They used 17 050 axial images from 265 patients to develop a CNN that classifies above-knee artery stenosis into 5 classes (0, 1%–50%, 51%–69%, 70–99%, 100%) and below-knee artery stenosis into 3 classes (0%–50%, 51%–99%, and 100%). Using digital subtraction angiography as the reference standard, their model achieved an accuracy of >90% in the majority of stenosis classes. The lowest accuracies were 79% for 51-69% stenosis in above-knee segments and 88% for 51-99% stenosis in below-knee segments. For both above and below-knee segments, CNN classifications had similar accuracies (P=0.27 and P=0.81) and specificities (P=0.12 and P=0.97) as radiologist reads, but had significantly lower sensitivities (P<0.001 and P=0.02).

Innovative studies in MRI analysis have also been recently reported and may reduce the time and labor-intensive processing of MRI images. Zhang et al developed a computer vision model to accelerate mapping of calf muscle perfusion from dynamic contrast-enhanced MRIs. Their feedforward neural network was developed using MRI scans, including pre- and post-exercise scans from healthy subjects and patients withPAD.The model had comparable exercise-stimulated perfusion estimates as the reference standard based on tracer kinetic analysis (correlation efficient=0.95) and generated the calf muscle perfusion maps much faster (<1 second versus 80 minutes). The Yuan group has also reported an efficient and accurate deep learning approach developed to evaluate atherosclerosis in the popliteal arteries Using knee MRI scans from an osteoarthritis cohort study, their CNN reduced vessel wall segmentation times from 4 hours to 8 minutes and performed similarly as human readers (Dice coefficient: 0.79). Following segmentation, their model was trained to quantify vessel features including mean wall thickness, maximum wall thickness, wall area, and lumen area, for which correlation coefficients were 0.73, 0.78, 0.90, and 0.99

Vascular Image-Based Prognostication

Extending from disease characterization and detection to prediction and prognosis, ML-aided image interpretation offers an opportunity to improve risk stratification. A seminal example of this is predicting the presence, progression, and development of diabetic retinopathy. Following demonstration of accurate diagnosis, AI software for retinal evaluation

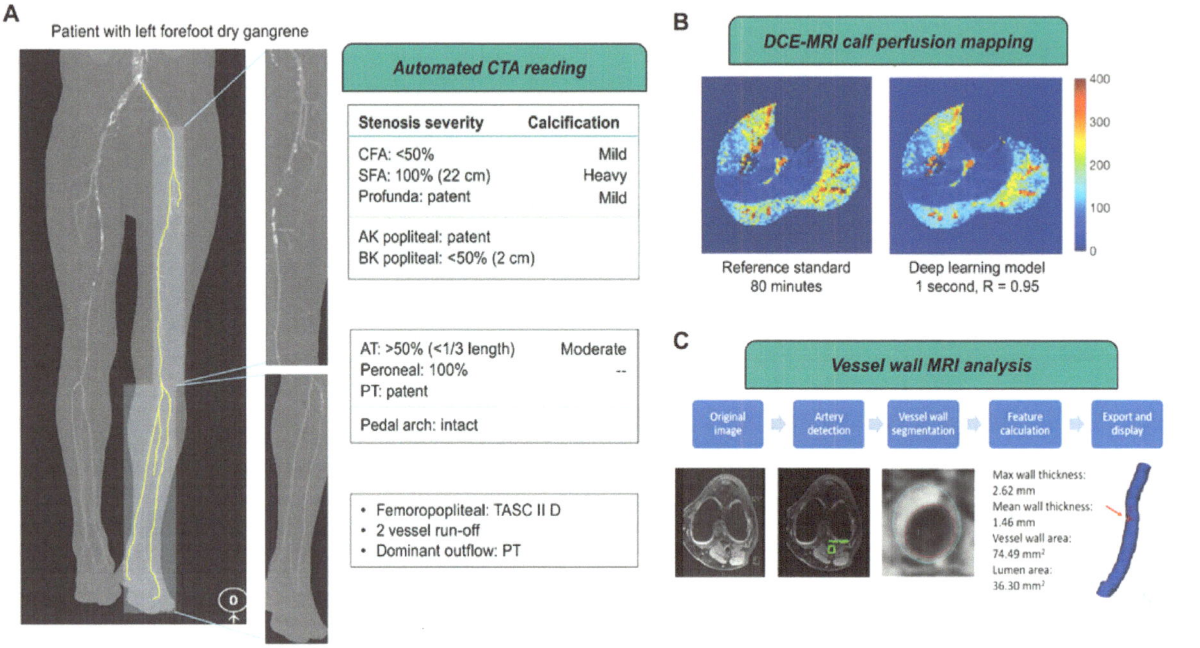

Fig.8.4 Computer vision for PAD imaging interpretation.

A, AI systems may automate interpretation of CTAs and generate reports based on TASC II classification. B,C, Computer vision algorithms may also enable more efficient processing of MRI images without compromising accuracy. Computer vision models generate accurate calf muscle perfusion maps in less than 1 second, compared to 180 minutes by standard modeling (B, modified from Zhang et al.73). Using standardized knee MRIs, fully automated pipelines for assessing atherosclerosis burden in the popliteal arteries have also been reported (C, modified from Chen et al.75). AI, artificial intelligence. AK, above knee. AT, anterior tibial. BK, below knee. CFA, common femoral artery. CTA, computed topography angiography. DCE-MRI, dynamic contrast-enhanced magnetic resonance imaging. R, correlation coefficient. PT, posterior tibial. SFA, superficial femoral artery. TASC II, Trans-Atlantic Intersociety Consensus II.

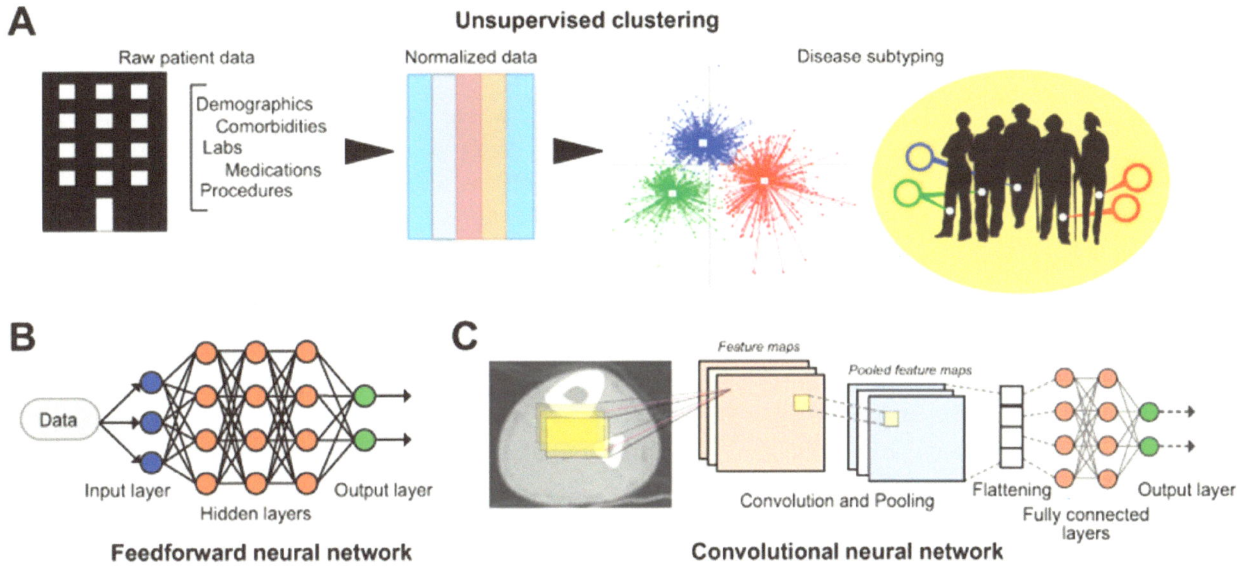

Fig.8.5. Framework for unsupervised cluster analysis and types of deep neural networks

A, Unsupervised cluster analysis can reveal clinically relevant patterns in data in a process where raw high-dimensional data is mathematically summarized and clustered. This general framework may be used to derive unique disease subtypes from patient data elements in a clinical database or the electronic health record. B, Feedforward neural network, composed of an input layer, multiple hidden layers, and an output layer. C, Convolutional neural networks capture local image features which are down-sampled in pooling layers to retain the most valuable features. Many pooled feature maps then pass through a flatten layer to form a single linear vector, thereby enabling input to fully connected layers that perform image classification. A, modified from Ross et al.

subsequently moved to prospective studies and one company received FDA approval in 2018 (IDx-DR, Iowa City, IA Beyond disease-specific screening, the developments by Google Health and multiple academic research teams exemplify the broader capabilities of deep learning models for prognostication and their ability to discover hidden associations. For example, one AI-system is able to predict sex, smoking status, systolic blood pressure, and risk of MACE based solely on retinal image analysis

Computer-Aided Prediction of Stroke

Automatically incorporating image-derived features into a vascular risk stratification tool has shown earlypotential in AI software developed by Suri and colleagues (Online Dataset II) Investigators developed a 3D CNN for characterization of carotid ultrasounds and detection of symptomatic or asymptomatic carotid stenosis.The network was trained and tested on ultrasounds from 150 asymptomatic patients and 196 with symptomatic disease. The 3D CNN framework was benchmarked against 2 types of deep learning models that were developed using a process known as transfer learning .Rather than training a network from scratch, transfer learning fine-tunes a CNN that is pretrained on a large dataset of natural images (eg, of scenes, animals, and plants) for medical image tasks.Compared with the two fine-tuned pretrained models, the de novo 3D CNN model better discriminated between symptomatic and asymptomatic plaques (AUC=0.79, 0.83, and 0.96, respectively). The authors note that an AI platform could be used by vascular surgeons to guide patient selection for intervention, and they highlight the need for external model validation beyond their single-center. With 100 000 carotid ultrasounds planned for public release by the UK Biobank study there is a major opportunity to train more ML models using this robust imaging and associated longitudinal data, potentially improving prediction of stroke based on earlier stage disease and uncovering new features predictive of adverse outcomes.

Computer-Aided Prediction of Aneurysm Growth and Rupture

There has also been special interest in image-derived prediction models for aneurysm growth and rupture. One group combined a deep learning and a computational model of growth and remodeling to predict AAA sac expansion. To overcome the need for a large volume of longitudinal data, investigators pretrained a deep neural network known as a deep belief network on 32 900 computer generated samples, then fine-tuned the network on longitudinal CT scans from 20 patients. At 9 months, their model produced accurate predictions of maximum AAA diameter with a root mean square error of 1.8 millimeters Another intriguing study predicted AAA growth based on 3 automated geometric features, including maximum diameter, radius of curvature, and undulation index (a measure of surface concavity). This model predicted annual AAA growth with a root mean square error of 1.3 mm and had AUCs of 0.80 for slow growth (<2.5 mm/year) and 0.79 for fast growth (>5 mm/year). In a study using follow-up CTAs from 22 patients treated with EVAR, López-Linarez et al extracted biomechanical features to predict ongoing aneurysm evolution. CNNs were used for AAA segmentation, followed by principal components analysis of the aneurysm strain fields that were then used as input for a support vector machine algorithm. Their ML model demonstrated a good correlation between the principal components of biomechanical strain and long-term prognosis, achieving an AUC of 0.89 for post-EVAR sac expansion or rupture.

Computer Vision-Aided Prediction of MACE and MALE

In prediction of MACE, one study by Pickhardt and colleagues evaluated the prognostic value of a panelof automated biometric measures from abdominal CTs. The burden of abdominal aortic calcification was quantified using a CNN and was found to predict MACE in 9223 generally healthy asymptomatic adults, outperforming the Framingham risk score.89 In particular, all AUC values (2-, 5-, and 10-year) for abdominal aortic calcification were significantly greater than Framingham risk score and further improved when combined with other automated measures such as visceral-to-subcutaneous fat and muscle density. For example, the 5-year AUC of 3 imaging biomarkers and Framingham risk score was 0.74 versus 0.69 for MACE ($P<0.05$), respectively. Building off prior work quantifying the burden of popliteal atherosclerosis from knee MRIs,74 Chen et al75 recently investigated whether the fully automated vessel wall features correlate with cardiovascular risk. High cardiovascular risk was defined as individuals ≥65 years old with a history of smoking, hypertension, BMI≥25 kg/m2, and one of the following: lower extremity revascularization, stroke/TIA, MI, diabetes, current smoking, BMI≥30 kg/m2, or age ≥75 years. A number of automated vessel measures discriminated between high and low-risk groups, with the greatest discrimination achieved by the ratio of maximum/minimum vessel wall thickness (AUC=0.79) and maximum wall thickness (AUC=0.73; Online Dataset II). Given that these studies were performed on commonly obtained scans from low-risk asymptomatic individuals, their findings highlight the potential utility of ML models that harnesses the readily available information embedded in imaging for improved cardiovascular risk assessment.

Automated derivation of imaging features that specifically predict hard MALE events such as major amputation or need for peripheral reintervention would be a major advance, especially given that what we have interpreted as abnormal from standard noninvasive studies has been inconsistently shown to correlate with clinical outcomes or success. By simultaneously assessing and integrating focal and diffuse disease patterns, ML models may be trained to learn the relationship between CTA images and clinically significant restenosis that occurs with recurrent symptoms or delayed wound healing. Deep learning algorithms have indeed shown progress in predicting functionally significant coronary lesions from coronary CTA, achieving similar accuracies as invasive fractional flow reserve measurements

Optimizing Behavior and Lifestyle Modifications

There have been growing applications of AI and ML in behavioral science to study, recommend, and influence human behaviors. By developing tailored interventions, ML-based decision support systems can help prioritize lifestyle changes for patients in a personally meaningful way. Chi et al used data from the Atherosclerosis Risk in Communities study to develop an ML model that identifies lifestyle changes that maximally reduce an individual's 10-year cardiovascular risk (defined as coronary artery disease event or stroke). This model then formed the basis for a decision support "ML expert system" that made optimized lifestyle recommendations adjusting for patient preferences and limitations (eg, time, food). When comparing the original and optimized recommendations in a clinical trial simulation, the optimized recommendations resulted in a relative risk reduction of 8.6% in patients with single lifestyle changes and 9.9% in patients with multiple lifestyle changes.

AI and ML systems have also been effective in increasing adherence to anticoagulation therapy and incentivizing regular physical activity These developments were each enabled by smartphones and created opportunities for continuous monitoring, enhanced communication, and personalized feedback. Labovitz et al used an AI mobile application (AiCure, New York, NY) that uses computer vision and neural networks to visually confirm medication ingestion and provide reminders within the hour and before the end of a missed dosing window. In a randomized trial of 28 patients with recent ischemic strokes, the AI platform improved adherence to anticoagulation (100% in AI group, 50% in patients without daily monitoring), including a 67% improvement with compliance in patients taking direct oral anticoagulantsIn another study of 27 sedentary patients with type 2 diabetes, individuals received a smartphone-based pedometer, a personal plan for physical activity, and personalized reinforcement messages that encouraged adherence.Investigators used reinforcement learning (RL), a type of algorithm that learns by observing the result of an action taken . The algorithm thus gradually improves in predicting the types and frequency of feedback that effectively encourage physical activity. Compared with individuals who received identical once-weekly reminders, patients in the RL group increased physical activity levels and experienced a superior reduction in HbA1c compared with the control group, with an average improvement of 0.28%. RL could similarly promote supervised exercise therapy for patients with PAD, which is increasingly being delivered through mobile health technologies. RL algorithms could potentially be combined with the Society for Vascular Surgery supervised exercise therapy mobile application, which began pilot study in early 2021. The app implements a provider-prescribed 12-week program of exercise and live health and wellness coaching. Combined with the engagement from mobile health technologies, RL algorithms could add an important component of adaptive messaging to better incentivize exercise and automate certain coaching elements to expand the availability of an exercise therapy coaching program to a broader patient population.

Guiding Vascular Surgical Care

Open versus endovascular revascularization is an age old question for vascular surgeons and specialists. While there have been thousands of studies published on optimal surgical strategies, many are small and underpowered. Although clinical trials offer "gold standard" evidence, costs, struggles with enrollment, patient disease heterogeneity, and potential ethical concerns of withholding surgical treatments can limit their impact on vascular surgical care. Bringing personalized guidance to aid in the choice of surgical approach based on an individual's unique data remains an ideal. Potential solutions include drawing from the large experience of previous patients and surgical outcomes to predict a patient's likely response to open and/or surgical treatments. Initiative's such as Stanford Medicine's "green button service" utilize EHRs to compile real-world evidence and support treatment decisions at the point-of-care (Atropos Health, Palo Alto, CA) The service has helped clinicians across a variety of medical specialties, and drawing from surgical cohorts would enable use by vascular surgeons and specialists. For vascular specialists, this could add an additional dimension of data to the decision-making process by incorporating evidence based on collective real-world practices. Intraoperatively, AI companies are using advanced algorithms to improve the success of

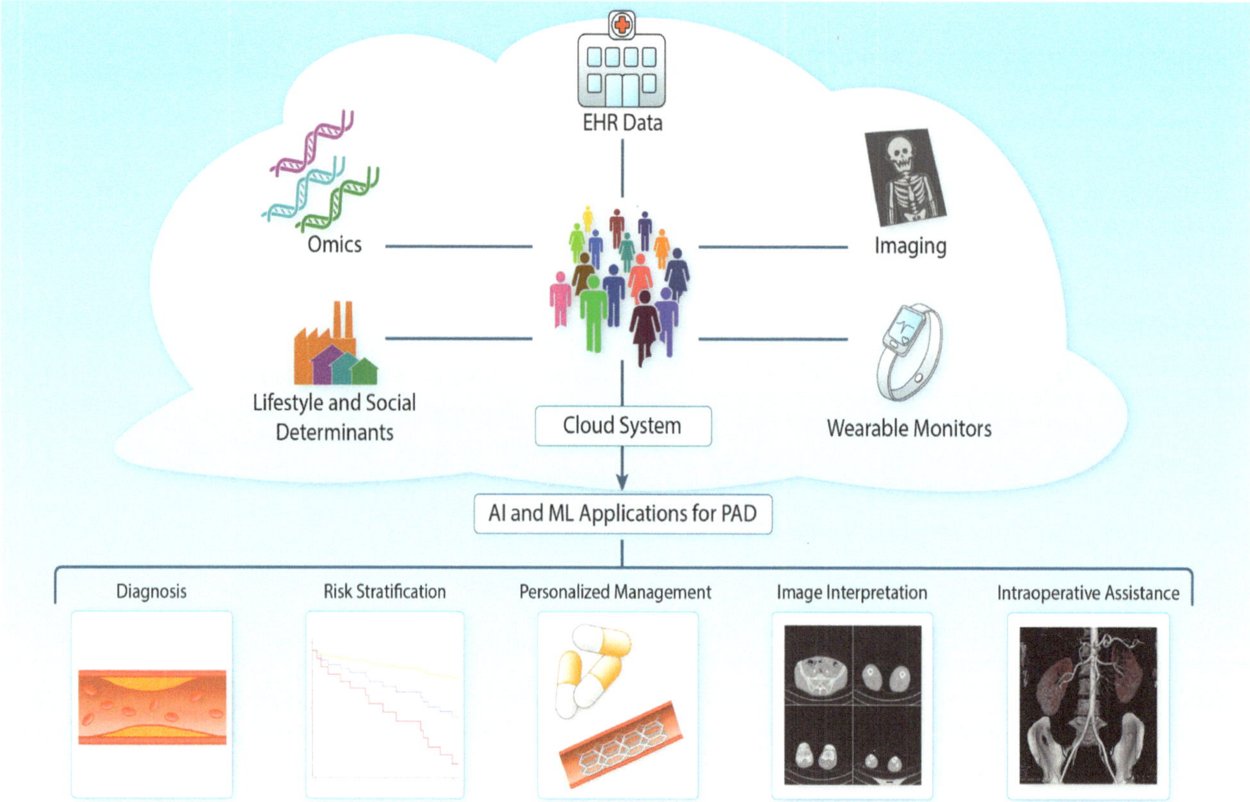

Fig.8.6 Applications of artificial intelligence (AI) and machine learning (ML) across the spectrum of peripheral artery diseasecare, spanning diagnosis, risk stratification, management, and intraoperative guidance. EHR indicates electronic health record; and PAD, peripheral artery disease (Illustration credit: Ben Smith).

image-guided interventions.In one example, AI software is used to provide fully automated 3D overlays onto live fluoroscopic images and continuously adjust to patient movement and deformations due to wires and other devices (Cydar Medical, United Kingdom). This cloud-based AI system has been applied to standard and fenestrated EVAR and has preliminarily been shown to reduce radiation exposure and optimize operative workflow without the need for additional equipment to be installed.

Challenges and Future Considerations

Although the majority of developments around ML and AI are in their early days with regards to vascular disease, the studies highlighted in this review

demonstrate that the practice of medicine and surgery for the vascular patient is on the brink of evolution To date, promising predictive capabilities have been harnessed primarily from retrospective data modeling. Moving forward, prospective validation in real-world settings will enable our ability to truly assess their clinical utility. It will be necessary to demonstrate meaningful end points when compared with standard-of-care to ensure that the technology developed will help move the needle forward. For example EHR-enabled identification of latent PAD and enhanced diagnostic accuracy could be associated with greater adherence to guideline-directed therapy. Subsequent demonstration of improved clinical outcomes will be important as there are many historical examples of screening programs that led to overdiagnosis of early but benign disease and overtreatment.

Bibliography And Acknowledgement

- Ata R, Gandhi N, Rasmussen H, El-Gabalawy O, Gutierrez S, Ahmad A, Suresh S, Ravi R, Rothenberg K, Aalami O. Clinical validation of smartphone-based activity tracking in peripheral artery disease patients.NPJ Digit Med. 2018; 1:66.
- Berger JS, Ladapo JA. Underuse of prevention and lifestyle counseling in patients with peripheral artery disease.J Am Coll Cardiol.2017;69:2293–2300.
- Bhatt DL, Peterson ED, Harrington RA, Ou FS, Cannon CP, Gibson CM, Kleiman NS, Brindis RG, Peacock WF, Brener SJ, et al; CRUSADE Investigators. Prior polyvascular disease: risk factor for adverse ischaemic outcomes in acute coronary syndromes.EurHeartJ.2009;30:1195–1202.
- Bora A, Balasubramanian S, Babenko B, Virmani S, Venugopalan S, Mitani A, de Oliveira Marinho G, Cuadros J, Ruamviboonsuk P, Corrado GS, et al. Predicting the risk of developing diabetic retinopathy using deep learning.Lancet Digit Health.2021.
- Brass EP, Lewis RJ, Lipicky R, Murphy J, Hiatt WR. Risk assessment in drug development for symptomatic indications: a framework for the prospective exclusion of unacceptable cardiovascular risk.Clin Pharmacol Ther. 2006; 79:165–172.
- Caradu C, Spampinato B, Vrancianu AM, Berard X, Ducasse E. Fully automatic volume segmentation of infra-renal abdominal aortic aneurysm CT images with deep learning approaches versus physician controlled manual segmentation [published online ahead of print December 9, 2020]. J Vasc Surg Castelli WP. Epidemiology of coronary heart disease: the Framinghamstudy.AmJMed.1984;76:4–12.
- Chandrashekar A, Handa A, Lapolla P, Shivakumar N, Ngetich E, Grau V, Lee R. Prediction of abdominal aortic aneurysm growth using geometric assessment of computerised tomography images acquired during the aneurysm surveillance period [published online ahead of print December 29, 2020 Ann Surg.
- Chandrashekar A, Handa A, Shivakumar N, Lapolla P, Uberoi R, Grau V, Lee R. A deep learning pipeline to automate high-resolution arterial segmentation with or without intravenous contrast [published online ahead of print November23,2020].AnnSurg
- Chen L, Canton G, Liu W, Hippe DS, Balu N, Watase H, Hatsukami TS, Waterton JC, Hwang JN, Yuan C. Fully automated and robust analysis technique for popliteal artery vessel wall evaluation (FRAPPE) using neural network models from standardized knee MRI.Magn Reson Med. 2020; 84:2147–2160.
- Chi CL, Nick Street W, Robinson JG, Crawford MA. Individualized patient-centered lifestyle recommendations: an expert system for communicating patient specific cardiovascular risk information and prioritizing lifestyle options.J Biomed Inform.2012;45:1164–1174.
- Coenen A, Kim YH, Kruk M, Tesche C, De Geer J, Kurata A, Lubbers ML, Daemen J, Itu L, Rapaka S, et al. Diagnostic accuracy of a machine-learning approach to coronary computed tomographic angiography-based fractional flow reserve: result from the MACHINE consortium.Circ Cardiovasc Imaging. 2018;11:e007217.
- Connell A, Black G, Montgomery H, Martin P, Nightingale C, King D, Karthikesalingam A, Hughes C, Back T, Ayoub K, et al. Implementation of a digitally enabled care pathway (Part 2):qualitative analysis of experiences of health care professionals.J Med Internet Res. 2019; 21:
- Cooke JP, Chen Z. A compendium on peripheral arterial disease.Circ Res.2015;116:1505–1508.
- Criqui MH, Aboyans V. Epidemiology of peripheral artery disease.Circ Res. 2015; 116:1509–1526. doi: 10.1161/CIRCRESAHA.116.303849
- Dai L, Zhou Q, Zhou H, Zhang H, Cheng P, Ding M, Xu X, Zhang X. Deep learning-based classification of lower extremity arterial stenosis in computed tomography angiography.Eur J Radiol. 2021; 136:109528
- Davis FM, Sutzko DC, Grey SF, Mansour MA, Jain KM, Nypaver TJ, Gaborek G, Henke PK. Predictors of surgical site infection after open lower extremity revascularization.J Vasc Surg. 2017; 65:1769–1778
- Dennis BM, Stonko DP, Callcut RA, Sidwell RA, Stassen NA, Cohen MJ, Cotton BA, Guillamondegui OD. Artificial neural networks can predict trauma volume and acuity regardless of center size and geography: a multicenter study.J Trauma Acute Care Surg. 2019;87:181–187.
- Duff S, Mafilios MS, Bhounsule P, Hasegawa JT. The burden of critical limb ischemia: a review of recent literature.Vasc Health Risk Manag. 2019; 15:187–208 Duscha BD, Piner LW, Patel MP, Crawford LE, Jones WS, Patel MR, Kraus WE. Effects of a 12-week mHealth program on functionalcapacity and physical activity in patients with peripheralartery disease.Am J Cardiol. 2018; 122:879–884.
- Esserman LJ, Thompson IM, Reid B, Nelson P, Ransohoff DF, Welch HG, Hwang S, Berry DA, Kinzler KW, Black WC, et al. Addressing overdiagnosis and overtreatment in cancer: a prescription forchange.LancetOncol.2014;15:e234–
- Esteva A, Kuprel B, Novoa RA, Ko J, Swetter SM, Blau HM, Thrun S. Dermatologist-level classification of skin cancer with deep neural networks.Nature.2017;542:115–118.
- Fenton JJ, Weyrich MS, Durbin S, Liu Y, Bang H, Melnikow J. Prostate-Specific Antigen-Based Screening for Prostate Cancer: A Systematic Evidence Review for the US Preventive Services Task Force. 2018; 319:1914–1931. Ferket BS, Spronk S, Colkesen EB, Hunink MG. Systematic review of guidelines on peripheral artery diseasescreening.AmJMed.2012;125:198–208.
- Gerhard-Herman MD, Gornik HL, Barrett C, Barshes NR, Corriere MA, Drachman DE, Fleisher LA, Fowkes FG, Hamburg NM, Kinlay S, et al. 2016 AHA/ACC guideline on the management of patients with lower extremity peripheral artery disease: executive summary: a report of the American College of Cardiology/American Heart Association Task Force on Clinical Practice Guidelines.Circulation. 2017;135:e686
- Ghorbani A, Ouyang D, Abid A, He B, Chen JH, Harrington RA, Liang DH, Ashley EA, Zou JY. Deep learning interpretation of echocardiograms.NPJDigitMed.2020;3:10.
- Gianfrancesco MA, Tamang S, Yazdany J, Schmajuk G. Potential biases in machine learning algorithms using electronic health record data.JAMAInternMed.2018;178:1544–1547.
- Gombar S, Callahan A, Califf R, Harrington R, Shah NH. It is time to learn from patients like mine.NPJ Digit Med. 2019; 2:16
- Gulshan V, Peng L, Coram M, Stumpe MC, Wu D, Narayanaswamy A, Venugopalan S, Widner K, Madams T, Cuadros J, et al. Development and validation of a deep learning algorithm for detection of diabetic retinopathy in retinal fundus photographs.JAMA. 2016; 316:2402–2410.

- Hahn S, Perry M, Morris CS, Wshah S, Bertges DJ. Machine deep learning accurately detects endoleak after endovascular abdominal aortic aneurysm repair.JVS: Vascular Science. 2020; 1:5–12.
- Hannun AY, Rajpurkar P, Haghpanahi M, Tison GH, Bourn C, Turakhia MP, Ng AY. Cardiologist-level arrhythmia detection and classification in ambulatory electrocardiograms using a deep neuralnetwork.NatMed.2019;25:65–69.
- Hansen PW, Clemmensen L, Sehested TS, Fosbøl EL, Torp-Pedersen C, Køber L, Gislason GH, Andersson C. Identifying drug-drug interactions by data mining: a Pilot Study of Warfarin-Associated Drug Interactions.Circ Cardiovasc Qual Outcomes. 2016;9:621–628.
- Hess CN, Bonaca MP. Contemporary review of antithrombotic therapy in peripheral artery disease.Circ Cardiovasc Interv. 2020; 13:e009584.
- Hinton GE, Osindero S, Teh YW. A fast learning algorithm for deep belief nets.Neural Comput. 2006; 18:1527–1554
- Hippe DS, Balu N, Chen L, Canton G, Liu W, Watase H, Waterton JC, Hatsukami TS, Hwang JN, Yuan C. Confidence weighting for robust automated measurements of popliteal vessel wall magnetic resonance imaging.Circ Genom Precis Med. 2020; 13:e002870.
- Hirsch AT, Criqui MH, Treat-Jacobson D, Regensteiner JG, Creager MA, Olin JW, Krook SH, Hunninghake DB, Comerota AJ, Walsh ME, et al. Peripheral arterial disease detection, awareness, and treatment in primary care.JAMA. 2001; 286:1317–1324.
- Jiang Z, Do HN, Choi J, Lee W, Baek S. A deep learning approach to predict abdominal aortic aneurysm expansion using longitudinaldata.FrontiersinPhysics.2020;7.
- Jung K, Covington S, Sen CK, Januszyk M, Kirsner RS, Gurtner GC, Shah NH. Rapid identification of slow healing wounds.Wound Repair Regen. 2016; 24:181–188.
- Kinlay S. Outcomes for clinical studies assessing drug and revascularization therapies for claudication and critical limb ischemia in peripheral artery disease.Circulation. 2013; 127:1241–1250.
- Klarin D, Lynch J, Aragam K, Chaffin M, Assimes TL, Huang J, Lee KM, Shao Q, Huffman JE, Natarajan P, et al; VA Million Veteran Program. Genome-wide association study of peripheral artery disease in the Million Veteran Program.Nat Med. 2019; 25:1274–1279
- Kullo IJ, Leeper NJ. The genetic basis of peripheral arterial disease: current knowledge, challenges, and future directions.Circ Res.2015;116:1551–1560.
- Labovitz DL, Shafner L, Reyes Gil M, Virmani D, Hanina A. Using artificial intelligence to reduce the risk of nonadherence in patients on anticoagulation therapy.Stroke. 2017; 48:1416–1419.
- Leeper NJ, Bauer-Mehren A, Iyer SV, Lependu P, Olson C, Shah NH. Practice-based evidence: profiling the safety of cilostazol by text-mining of clinical notes.PLoS One. 013; 8:
- Li J, Pan C, Zhang S, Spin JM, Deng A, Leung LLK, Dalman RL, Tsao PS, Snyder M. Decoding the genomics of abdominal aortic aneurysm.Cell. 2018; 174:1361–1372.e10.
- Li RC, Asch SM, Shah NH. Developing a delivery science for artificial intelligence in healthcare.NPJ Digit Med. 2020; 3:107
- Littlejohns TJ, Holliday J, Gibson LM, Garratt S, Oesingmann N, Alfaro-Almagro F, Bell JD, Boultwood C, Collins R, Conroy MC, et al. The UK Biobank imaging enhancement of 100,000 participants: rationale, data collection, management and future directions.NatCommun.2020;11:2624
- López-Linares K, García I, García A, Cortes C, Piella G, Macía I, Noailly J, González Ballester MA. Image-based 3D characterization of abdominal aortic aneurysm deformation after endovascular aneurysm repair.Front Bioeng Biotechnol. 2019; 7:267.
- Lyell D, Coiera E. Automation bias and verification complexity: a systematic review.J Am Med Inform Assoc. 2017; 24:423–431.
- Mandel JC, Kreda DA, Mandl KD, Kohane IS, Ramoni RB. SMART on FHIR: a standards-based, interoperable apps platform for electronic health records.J Am Med Inform Assoc. 2016;23:899–908.doi:10.1093/jamia/ocv189
- Maurel B, Martin-Gonzalez T, Chong D, Irwin A, Guimbretière G, Davis M, Mastracci TM. A prospective observational trial of fusion imaging in infrarenal aneurysms.J Vasc Surg. 2018; 68:1706.e1–1713.e1.
- McCarthy CP, Ibrahim NE, van Kimmenade RRJ, Gaggin HK, Simon ML, Gandhi P, Kelly N, Motiwala SR, Mukai R, Magaret CA, et al. A clinical and proteomics approach to predict the presence of obstructive peripheral arterial disease: from the Catheter Sampled Blood Archive in Cardiovascular Diseases (CASABLANCA) Study.Clin Cardiol. 2018; 41:903–909.
- McDermott MM. Lower extremity manifestations of peripheral artery disease: the pathophysiologic and functional implications oflegischemia.CircRes.2015;116:1540–1550.
- McNair D, Price WN. Health Care AI: Law, Regulation, Policy.Artificial Intelligence in Health Care: The Hope, the Hype,thePromise,thePeril.2020.
- Menard MT, Farber A, Assmann SF, Choudhry NK, Conte MS, Creager MA, Dake MD, Jaff MR, Kaufman JA, Powell RJ, et al. Design and rationale of the best endovascular versus best surgical therapy for patients with critical limb ischemia (BEST-CLI)trial.JAmHeartAssoc.2016;5
- Misra S, Shishehbor MH, Takahashi EA, Aronow HD, Brewster LP, Bunte MC, Kim ESH, Lindner JR, Rich K; American Heart Association Council on Peripheral Vascular Disease; Council on Clinical Cardiology; and Council on Cardiovascular and Stroke
- Nursing. Perfusion assessment in critical limb ischemia: principles for understanding and the development of evidence and evaluation of devices: a scientific statement from the American Heart Association.Circulation. 2019; 140:e657–e672.
- Myers KD, Knowles JW, Staszak D, Shapiro MD, Howard W, Yadava M, Zuzick D, Williamson L, Shah NH, Banda JM, et al. Precision screening for familial hypercholesterolaemia: a machine learning study applied to electronic health encounter data.Lancet DigitHealth.2019;
- Nam JG, Park S, Hwang EJ, Lee JH, Jin KN, Lim KY, Vu TH, Sohn JH, Hwang S, Goo JM, et al. Development and validation of deep learning-based automatic detection algorithm for malignant pulmonary nodules on chest radiographs.Radiology. 2019;290:218–228. Observational Health Data Sciences and Informatics. The BookofOHDSI.2019.AccessedMarch18,2021
- Ouyang D, He B, Ghorbani A, Yuan N, Ebinger J, Langlotz CP, Heidenreich PA, Harrington RA, Liang DH, Ashley EA, et al. Video-based AI for beat-to-beat assessment of cardiac function.Nature.2020;580:252–256.
- Patel MR, Conte MS, Cutlip DE, Dib N, Geraghty P, Gray W, Hiatt WR, Ho M, Ikeda K, Ikeno F, et al. Evaluation and treatment of patients with lower extremity peripheral artery disease: consensus definitions from Peripheral Academic Research Consortium (PARC).J Am Coll Cardiol. 2015; 65:931–941.

- Pickhardt PJ, Graffy PM, Zea R, Lee SJ, Liu J, Sandfort V, Summers RM. Automated CT biomarkers for opportunistic prediction of future cardiovascular events and mortality in an asymptomaticscreeningpopulation: a retrospectivecohortstudy.LancetDigitHealth.2020;2:e192–e200
- Poplin R, Varadarajan AV, Blumer K, Liu Y, McConnell MV, Corrado GS, Peng L, Webster DR. Prediction of cardiovascular risk factors from retinal fundus photographs via deep learning.Nat Biomed Eng. 2018; 2:158–164.
- Popplewell MA, Davies H, Jarrett H, Bate G, Grant M, Patel S, Mehta S, Andronis L, Roberts T, Deeks J, et al; BASIL-2 Trial Investigators. Bypass versus angioplastyinsevereischaemiaoftheleg -2(BASIL-2)trial:studyprotocolforarandomisedcontrolled trial.Trials.2016;17:11.
- Qutrio Baloch Z, Raza SA, Pathak R, Marone L, Ali A. Machine learning confirms nonlinear relationship between severity of peripheral arterial disease, functional limitation and symptomseverity.Diagnostics(Basel)2020;10:515.
- Rolls AE, Maurel B, Davis M, Constantinou J, Hamilton G, Mastracci TM. A comparison of accuracy of image- versus hardware-based tracking technologies in 3D fusion in aortic endografting.Eur J Vasc Endovasc Surg. 2016; 52:323–331
- Ronneberger O, Fischer P, Brox T. U-Net: ConvolutionalNetworks for Biomedical Image Segmentation.arXiv. 2015.
- Ross EG, Jung K, Dudley JT, Li L, Leeper NJ, Shah NH. Predicting future cardiovascular events in patients with peripheral artery disease using electronic health record data.Circ Cardiovasc Qual Outcomes. 2019; 12:e004741.
- Ross EG, Shah N, Leeper N. Statin intensity or achieved LDL? practice-based evidence for the evaluation of new cholesterol treatmentguidelines.PLoSOne.2016;11
- Ross EG, Shah NH, Dalman RL, Nead KT, Cooke JP, Leeper NJ. The use of machine 26. learning for the identification of peripheral artery disease and future mortality risk.J Vasc Surg. 2016; 64:1515–1522.
- Saba L, Biswas M, Suri HS, Viskovic K, Laird JR, Cuadrado-Godia E, Nicolaides A, Khanna NN, Viswanathan V, Suri JS. Ultrasound-based carotid stenosis measurement and risk stratification in diabetic cohort: a deep learning paradigm.Cardiovasc Diagn Ther. 2019; 9:439–461.
- Sarikaya R. The Technology Behind Personal Digital Assistants: an overview of the system architecture and key components.IEEE Signal Processing Magazine. 2017; 34:67.
- Talebi S, Madani MH, Madani A, Chien A, Shen J, Mastrodicasa D, Fleischmann D, Chan FP, Mofrad MRK. Machine learning for endoleak detection after endovascular aortic repair.Sci Rep. 2020; 10:18343.doi:10.1038/s41598-020-74936-7
- Udell M, Horn C, Zadeh R, Boyd S. Generalized low rank models.arXiv. 2014. Preprint posted online 5 May 2015 Wanhainen A, Mani K, Golledge J. Surrogate markers of abdominal aortic aneurysm progression.Arterioscler Thromb Vasc Biol. 2016; 36:236–244.
- Ward A, Sarraju A, Chung S, Li J, Harrington R, Heidenreich P, Palaniappan L, Scheinker D, Rodriguez F. Machine learning and atherosclerotic cardiovascular disease risk prediction in a multi-ethnic population.NPJ Digit Med. 2020; 3:125
- Weissler EH, Zhang J, Lippmann S, Rusincovitch S, Henao R, Jones WS. Use of natural language processing to improve identification of patients with peripheral artery disease.Circ CardiovascInterv.2020;13:
- Wolterink JM, Leiner T, de Vos BD, van Hamersvelt RW, Viergever MA, Išgum I. Automatic coronary artery calcium scoring in cardiac CT angiography using paired convolutional neural networks.Med Image Anal. 2016; 34:123–136.
- Wu J, Xin J, Yang X, Sun J, Xu D, Zheng N, Yuan C. Deep morphology aided diagnosis network for segmentation of carotid artery vessel wall and diagnosis of carotid atherosclerosis on black-blood vessel wall MRI.Med Phys. 2019;46:5544–5561.
- Yasaka K, Akai H, Abe O, Kiryu S. Deep learning with convolutional neural network for differentiation of liver masses at dynamiccontrast-enhanced CT: apreliminary study.Radiology. 2018;286:887–896.
- YeoLL and Sharma VK. Automatic Detection and Measurement of Atherosclerotic Plaques in Carotid Ultrasound Using Deep Learning.International Stroke Conference. 2020.
- Yom-Tov E, Feraru G, Kozdoba M, Mannor S, Tennenholtz M, Hochberg I. Encouraging physical activity in patients with diabetes: intervention using a reinforcement learning system.J MedInternetRes.2017;19:e338.
- Zhang JL, Conlin CC, Li X, Layec G, Chang K, Kalpathy-Cramer J, Lee VS. Exercise-induced calf muscle hyperemia: rapid mapping of magnetic resonance imaging using deep learning approach.Physiol Rep. 2020; 8:e14563.
- Zhou R, Fenster A, Xia Y, Spence JD, Ding M. Deep learning-based carotid media-adventitia and lumen-intima boundary segmentation from three-dimensional ultrasound images.Med Phys.2019;46:3180–3193.
- Zierler RE, Jordan WD, Lal BK, Mussa F, Leers S, Fulton J, Pevec W, Hill A, Murad MH. The Society for Vascular Surgery practice guidelines on follow-up after vascular surgery arterial procedures.J Vasc Surg. 2018; 68:256–284
- Zitnik M, Agrawal M, Leskovec J. Modeling polypharmacy side effects with graph convolutional networks.Bioinformatics. 2018;34:i457–i466
- Zreik M, Lessmann N, van Hamersvelt RW, Wolterink JM, Voskuil M, Viergever MA, Leiner T, Išgum I. Deep learning analysis of the myocardium in coronary CT angiography for identification of patients with functionally significant coronary artery stenosis.Med Image Anal. 2018; 44:72–85.

Artificial Intelligence And Automation In Valvular Heart Diseases

CHAPTER

9

Artificial intelligence (AI), which is a branch of computer science that attempts to create machines that perform tasks as though they possessed hu-man brainpower, and this is gradually changing the landscape of the healthcare industry. Clinical procedures that were supposed to, and could only be performed by human experts previously can now been carried out by machines in a more accurate and efficient way. Recently, cardiologists and radiologists have cooperated with computer scientists and have developed a fully automated echocardiography interpretation system for clini-cal practice. Cardiovascular diseases affect 48% of the population (≥ 20 years old) and is the leading cause of death. Echocardiography is an effective method to monitor the state of the heart and allows early diagnosis before the onset of symptoms. However, in primary care clinics and poorer regions, there are inadequately experienced radiologists for echocardiography interpretation, let alone patient follow-up. There is group of researchers who trained AI systems using over 14,000 echocardiograms for multiple tasks including view classification and quantification of chamber volume, ejection fraction and longitudinal strain. The AI system validated its accuracy in diagnosing several cardiac diseases after testing on over 8000 cardiograms obtained from routine clinical flow . Such an AI system holds great potential for the transformation of current clinical practice models as well as the popularization of quality healthcare. The above example is only the tip of the ice-berg in the application of AI in medicine for over half a century. Since "AI" was first proposed by John MacCarthy at the Dartmouth College Conference in 1956, great efforts have been made for apply-ing AI to almost all phases of clinical practice. In 1960s, the concept of "computer-assisted diagnosis" emerged with attemptsemerged with attempts to use mathematical formalism tointerpret clinical problems, although they have little practical value, it has paved the way for subsequent expert systems .In 1970s,researchers began to shift attention to studying the reasoning process of clinicians and simulate it on computer systems, which gave birth to the first generation of medical AI products, i.e. MYCIN. It attempts to diagnose infectious diseases and provide appropriate medication therapies based on over 200 rules that in the form of "if (precon-dition), then (conclusion or action)". Although MYCIN showed reliability in 63% of the cases of bacteremia .it is more like an advanced version of a textbook which has the function of automatic retrievals with little "intelligence". Moreover, the interactions between each rule should be defined by human experts which is extremely arduous with increasingly new knowledge added to the system. However, automatic interpretation of electrocar-diograms has gained great benefits from the rule--based AI system. During the same period, a new model, i.e. the probabilistic reasoning was used to simulate the process of expert decision making . Unlike the categorical mode of reasoning utilized by MYCIN, the probabilistic model assign weight to every symptom and clinical finding to indicate its possibility of occurrence for a certain disease. Based on this, new systems including the present illness program, INTERNIST, CASNET were developed.

With the introduction of "artificial neural network" in 1980s, machine learning began to flourish. Machine learning endows computers with the ability to learn patterns from data and perform tasks without explicit programming It has showed great power in developing robust risk prediction models, redefining patient classes and other tasks with the popularization of electronic health records and digital imaging systems.In 2006, the introduction of deep learning by LeCun et al.

achieved unprecedented progress in im-age recognition and other domains, which brought a new renaissance to the development of AI and made automated medical imaging interpretation one of the hottest topics in AI. AI can generally be classified as either weak AI or strong AI. Strong AI is an intelligence construct that has the ability to understand and think as a human being. Weak AI is limited to a specific or narrow area, which is often designed to perform time-consuming tasks and analyze data in ways that humans sometimes cannot. In this review, a brief introduction to AI is provided and highlights its application in the clinical flow of diagnosing and treating valvular heart diseases, including heart sound auscultation, medical image analysis (echocardiography, cardiac computed tomography [CT] and cardiac magnetic resonance [CMR]), risk factor identification, mor-tality prediction and robotic surgery.

Fundamental concepts in AI

Machine learning

In essence, machine learning is an extension to traditional statistical methods for dealing with large data sets and variables. It enables computers to learn rules and even uncover new patterns from data through a series of algorithms. Most impor-tantly, machine learning can gradually optimize the "reasoning process" between inputs and outputs. Machine learning can be broadly classified into three classes: supervised learning, unsupervised learning and reinforcement learning.

In supervised learning, machines learn the mapping relations between input variables and labeled outcomes and are able to predict outcomes according to inputs. For example, after training with echocardiograms that are labeled with given disease categories, machines are able to assign these disease labels to new echocardiograms. Common computational approaches in supervised learning include artificial neural network (ANN), support vector machine, k-nearest neighbor, naive Bayesian model and decision tree model, among others. Unsupervised learning aims to uncover hid-den structures in unlabeled data and classify it into separate categories, which means machines are only trained with input variables and automatically find potential classification rules.For example, with unsupervised learning, machines uncovered three cardiac phenotypes in patients diagnosed with type 2 diabetes mellitus according to their echocardio-grams Common computational approaches include hierarchical clustering, k-means clustering and principle component analysis. Reinforcement learning signifies that machines learn strategies which can obtain the maximum reward through interaction with the environment or outcomes. Unlike the static mode of supervised or unsuper-vised learning, it is a dynamic learning process. Q-learning, an example of reinforcement learning, has been utilized in clinical trials of lung cancer to find the optimal individualized therapies

Artificial neural network and deep learning

Artificial neural network is composed of multiple interconnected artificial neurons which mimic the biological brain. As mentioned above, ANN is actually a computational model. ANN learns from large amounts of data and continuously optimizes the weight of each connection between neurons. Figure 1B shows a typical ANN, which is also called multilayer perceptron, is composed of three layers: input layer, hidden layer and output layer. Each layer contains multiple neurons that are re-sponsible for different functions. The input layer receives numerical variables from data, each value in first layer neurons combines with the weight of the connection, which is then propagated to a hid-den layer where the values are integrated, while an output layer generates the final value which represents an outcome. Each neuron in the hid-den layer can also set up a threshold to determine whether the information should propagate to the next layer. Now suppose that a database that in-cludes patient data (such as age, body mass index, laboratory results and images results) prior to car-diac surgery and operation results (alive or dead), a mortality prediction model can be built with ANN. Patient variables are input into the neurons in the first layer, the outputs are set as 1 for alive and 0 for dead. The weight of each connection and the excitation threshold of each neuron in the hidden layer are gradually optimized by learning from the data. In this way, after trained with sufficient cases,the ANN model can be accurate enough to predict surgical outcome in new patients.

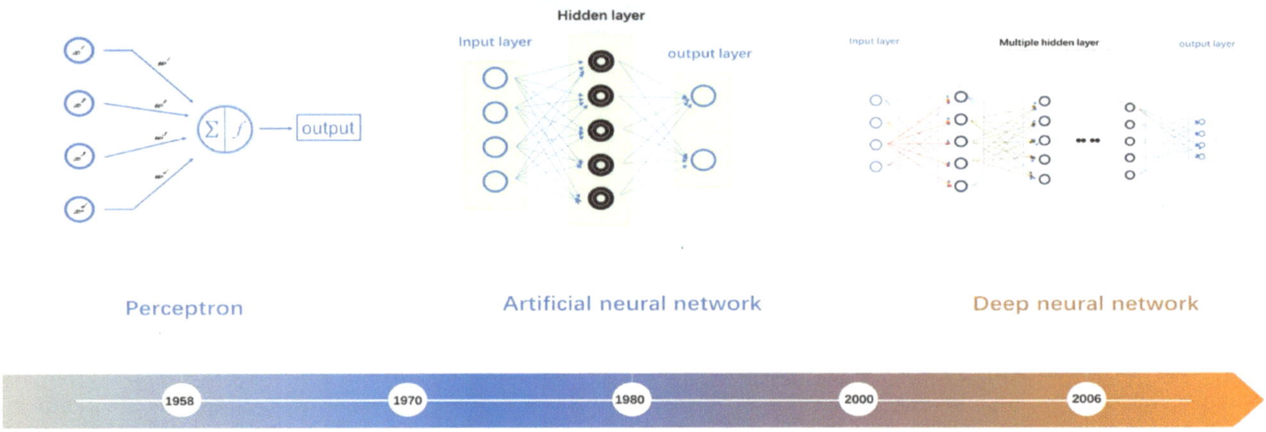

Fig. 9.1 Schematic diagram of the evolvement of artificial neural network. Perceptron, also called single layer neural network, was proposed by Rosenblatt in 1958 (A), classic artificial neural network, also known as double layer neural network or multilayer perceptron (B), deep neural network (C).

It can be imagined that, with more hidden layers, the computational results will be more ac-curate, but this meanwhile requires greater com-putational power using more training data. Thanks to the rapid development of computer processors and arrival of the era of big data, and also the in-troduction of "pre-training process", "fine-tuning technique" by Hinton et al. which decreases the training time substantially, multilayer ANN which is also known as "deep learning" becomes a reality. It now represents the most advanced AI technology. The biggest advantage of deep neural network is that it allows the computing model to automatically extract the features of the data by abstracting the data layer by layer and learning the representative and discriminant features.

Computer vision

Computer vision is a main research field in AI, which simulates the human vision with imaging systems and computers. The main tasks involved in computer vision can be divided into three levels. The basic level includes image acquiring and processing techniques such as noise filtering, image enhancement, image segmentation, pattern recognition. For middle level computer vision, computers should be able to draw conclusions and make decisions based on the information obtained from the basic level. For the top level, computersrecognition. For middle level computer vision, computers should be able to draw conclusions and make decisions based on the information obtained from the basic level. For the top level, computershave the capability to "think" and can understand images like humans do. For now, the first two levels of computer vision are mostly applied to the analy-sis of medical images and assist in diagnosis. As described below, many algorithms and commercial software have been developed for automating the analysis of medical images, which are more accu-rate and efficient compared to human endeavour.

Expert system

Expert systems are in their earliest application of AI in medicine, and will keep playing an impor-tant role in healthcare. In brief, expert systems are a computer program that simulates human experts in solving problems.It is also called a knowl-edge-based system because it contains a large amount of knowledge and experience from experts.

A typical medical expert system is composed of two modules: knowledge base and control system, the latter can be further divided into a human-computerinteractive component, an explanation component, a knowledge acquisition component and an infer-ence engine. The knowledge base is composed of medical knowledge from experts, case-specific knowledge from patients and intermediate results from the reasoning process

Application of AI and automation in diagnosis of valvular heart diseases

AI-assisted "cardiac auscultation"

In spite of the diverse alternatives of imaging tools being the major diagnostic approach to valvu-lar heart diseases (VHDs), physical examination, is the cornerstone of clinical diagnosis and should be the primary screening method for VHDs. Common physical examinations for VHDs include general inspection, pulse palpation, percussion of heart boarder and heart sound auscultation, etc. Among these, auscultation plays a key role of diagnosing VHDs. Valvular heart diseases manifest as heart murmurs or/and extra heart sound before the stress of hemodynamic changes causing other signs and symptoms including dyspnea, fatigue, angina, cough and hemoptysis. While cardiac auscultation provides significant diagnostic and prognostic information for cardiac disease, it is not an easy skill to master, especially when innocent murmurs are confronted. Although experienced clinicians have reached an accuracy over 90% in identifying innocent murmurs from pathologic murmurs, less-experienced residents and primary care physicians perform less than satisfactorily . In addition, auscultation is a highly subjective process which may cause bias when evaluating the intensity, location and shape of murmurs. For over a century, tools for cardiac auscultation is a mechanical stethoscope, however, it can neither store nor play back sounds . Thanks to the invention . Thanks to the invention of electronic (digital) stethoscope, the forgoing problems have been well solved, more than that, it provides clinicians with a handy way of "seeing" the heart sound through phonocardiogram. AI-assisted cardiac auscultation in practice refers to the auto-interpretation of phonocardiogram, which belongs to the domain of signal processing. Key steps involved in heart sound analysis could besummarized as segmentation, feature extraction and classification . Each step is fulfilled through a multitude of algorithms with the ultimate goal of precisely identifying the pathological events underlying heart sounds.

Heart sounds segmentation.

Segmentation aims to locate the fundamental elements includ-ing the first heart sound (S1), systolic period, the second heart sound (S2) and diastolic period in each cardiac cycle. Training machines to think like human so as to solve problems is to mimic the thinking process of human brain to a certain extent. When interpreting heart sounds, A human expert would firstly locate the two fundamental heart sounds then discriminate S1 from S2 by its pitch, intensity and duration, finally the systolic and diastolic regions are determined, as is the process with computational analysis, but in a more logical and mathematical way. In the early exploration of heart sound seg-mentation, electrocardiograph or/and carotid pulse was/ were obtained concurrently with phonocardiogram.
Transformation equation g(n) was used to compute the smooth energy curve of electrocardiograph signal, then the peaks in g(n) was determined as the beginning of S1 and the systolic period, the dicrotic notch of carotid pulse curve was recognized as the beginning of S2 .This approach apparently is impractical in routine clinical work. Envelop-based (or amplitude threshold-based) segmentation algorithm was first introduced by Liang et al. to locate S1 and S2. Envelop of a signal signifies the smooth curves outlining its upper or lower extremes The envelop of the original heart sound waveform was first extracted using specific transformation equations, then a threshold value was selected to filter noise and low intensity signals, the peaks exceed the threshold value were recognized as the S1 and S2, S1 was differentiated form S2 based on an as-sumption that the systolic period was shorter than the diastolic period. A well-fitted extraction equation would allow only two peaks to exceed the threshold when interpreting the normal heart sound, therefore identification accuracy depends largely on an envelope extraction equation. Diverse methods are used to calculate the envelopewere created including normalized Shan-non energy , single-DOF analytical model , wavelet decomposition method, Viola integral approach and others.
However, the envelope-based segmentation method often leads to problems like weak peaks or extra peaks which reduce accuracy of the results. The application of machine learning algorithms to heart sound segmentation based on

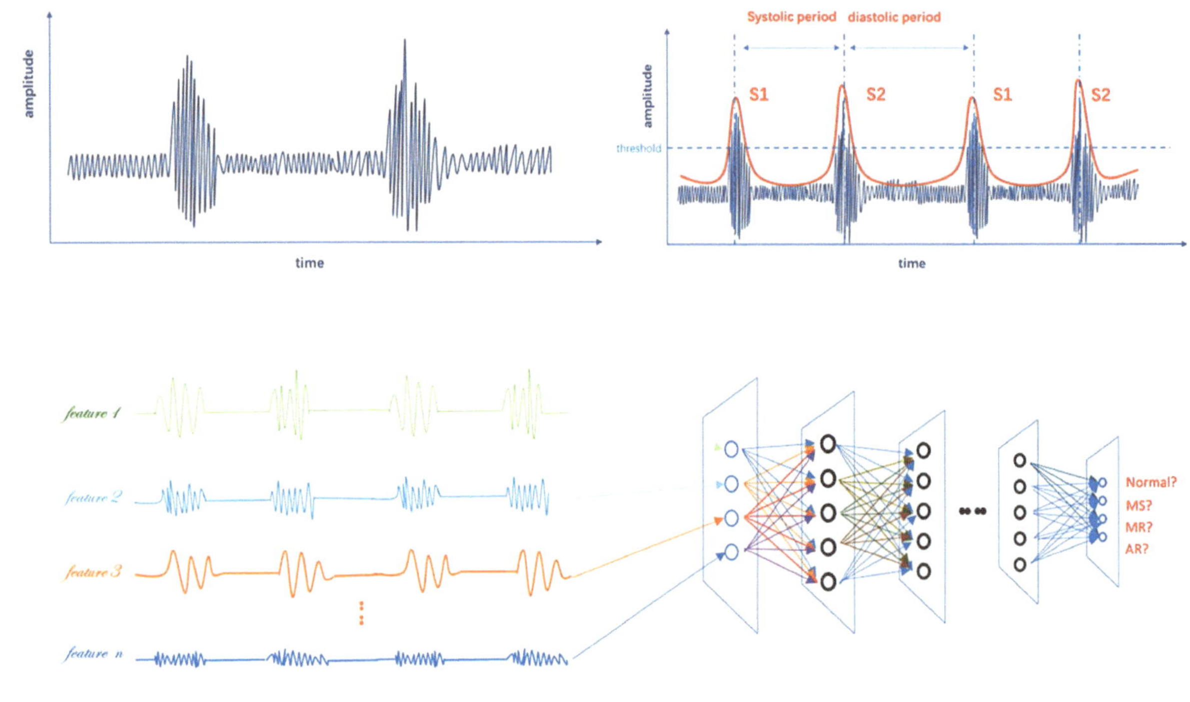

Fig.9.2 Process of artificial intelligence-assisted auscultation. A normal phonocardiogram (A), heart sound segmen-tation (B), feature extraction (C), heart sound classification by deep neural network (D).

features substantially improves the segmentation results (see feature extraction below). Hidden Markov Model (HMM) is the most widely used in the task .To train the HMM, adequate samples pre-labeled with the accurate location of S1, S2, systolic and diastolic period are required at the output end; sequences of feature vectors extracted from original phonocardiogram or transformed envelope are used as the observation end of HMM. Recently, utilization of deep learning achieves even higher precision compared to other classification methods in heart sound segmentation

Feature extraction and feature selection.

This step aims to select and extract discriminative features either for more precise segmentation of heart sound or for following the disease classification step. Feature means the characteristic of an object by which the human brain recognizes and distinguishes it automatically. The concept of feature is similar to "variable" in regression analysis. Features that can be recognized by machines tend to be presented in the form of numbers or symbols.

A human expert draws physiological or pathological information from heart sound through features including heart rate, heart rhythm, timing and shape of the murmur, pitch of the heart sound, and extra heart sound among others. As for phonocardiogram, the features are based on time-domain, frequency-domain, and time-frequency complex domain.Time-domain features include intervals (interval of S1 and S2, systolic intervals, diastolic intervals, the ratio of each component to the cardiac cycle etc.) and amplitude (mean absolute amplitude of S1 and S2 interval). Frequency-domain features refer to the power spectrum of each heart sound component across frequency bands. Theoreti-cally the more input of features into machine train-ing, the better the classification performance it will achieve.

In practice, with the number of training samples being set, the classification performance will drop off when the number of feature inputs exceeds a certain value. In order to exclude the redundant features and improve the classification efficiency, feature selection is often required

Classification and detection of VHDs.

This step aims to classify the phonocardiograms into cardiac disease categories using suitable classi-fiers. Classifier in machine learning refers to the algorithm that learns to assign labels to testing data from training data. This learning process can be supervised or unsupervised. Briefly speaking, supervised learning assigns given labels to data while unsupervised learning seeks labels that could be assigned to data. In the present case, labels are given disease categories like mitral stenosis, mitral regurgitation, aortic stenosis, etc. therefore, supervised learning algorithms/classifiers are uti-lized. The common classifiers used in heart sound classification include a support vector machine , neural networks , HMM , etc. After a careful combination of algorithms used in segmentation, feature extraction and classification, previous studies showed promising and inspiring results in detecting VHDs from phonocardiograms. For instance, an intelligent diagnostic system developed by Sun could discriminate aortic regurgitation, mitral regurgitation, pulmo-nary stenosis with accuracy of 98.9%, 98.4% and 98.7%, respectively. Thompson et al. utilized a murmur detection algorithm developed by CSD labs to distinguish no murmurs and innocent mur-murs from pathologic murmurs. 3180 phonocar-diograms recorded at five different chest location from 603 cases were tested, the algorithm had good sensitivity, specificity and accuracy in detecting a pathologic murmur, which are 93%, 81% and 88%, respectively. The algorithm showed the highest ac-curacy (90%) using recordings from the left upper and lower sternal boarder. However, it was unable to analyze the recordings with precision which had a high heart rate and low signal quality

AI-assisted interpretation of echocardiography

Although heart sounds auscultation is con-venient, cost-effective and a quick way to diagnose VHDs, it only provides qualitative diagnostic information. To further confirm the diagnosis of VHDs as well as to assess the etiology, severity, ventricular responses and prognosis, imaging tools including echocardiography, CMR, multi-slice CT (MSCT) or even cardiac catheterization are indispensable. Echocardiography is the "heart" of cardiology. It is the preferred method of diagnosing and guid-ing the treatment of VHDs as well as other cardiac diseases. However, echocardiographic examination is a time-consuming process which usually takes hours from inspection, analysis to formal report which make it impractical in emergency settings. Moreover, typical echocardiographic examination produces large amounts of data including images from multiple views and up to 70 videos which would cause cognitive overload and be prone to error. In addition, due to the characteristic of multiple views in examination, the problems of intra-observer and inter-observer variability inevi-tably arise. The application of AI and automation in echocardiography would a allow consistent, quick and accurate measurement which promises a more accurate diagnosis and improved patient care.

Image segmentation-valve leaflet detection and tracking.

Segmentation and recognition of anatomical structures from original medical images are preprocessing steps for subsequent quantitative analysis and diagnosis. Morphologi-cal characteristics and motion pattern of the heart valves are key information to diagnose VHDs and to assist surgical valve repair or percutaneous intervention. While many studies have sought the approaches to segment heart chambers and detect endocardial boarder which were reviewed by Noble and Boukerroui , relatively few studies of the segmentation of heart valves and annulus have been published. The reasons for difficulty in segmenting and tracking the heart valves in echocardiographic sequences can be summarized as follows: poor image quality due to low frame rate, speckle noise and artifact which may resultin missing boundaries; (2) lack of features to dis-criminate heart valve from adjacent myocardium for those structures have similar intensity and texture; (3) fast and irregular valve motion making it hard to establish correspondence between frames. Re-ported approaches for valve segmentation including active contour models , thin tissue detector combined with graph cut outlier detection method , J-spline method multi-atlas joint label fusion , trajectory spectrum learning algorithm and neural network

Active contour models (ACM) is the first and most widely used segmentation algorithm for the heart valve. The segmentation process is based on ACM and is initiated by manual placement of contour close to the target, which means it is not fully automated. Zhou et al. formulated the problems of valve detection and tracking as outliner detection in the low-rank representation based on different motion patterns between leaflets and the heart wall, which is fully automated requiring no user interaction. Recently, there is a growing trend of applying machine learning to valve seg-mentation. This approach shifts the manual input to a training phase which makes segmentation fully automated .Ionasec et al. utilized spec-trum learning algorithm and boundary detectors to locate and refine mitral leaflets based on anatomical landmarks in four-dimensional (4D) transesopha-geal echocardiograms and CT which allows precise morphological and functional quantification, and a large amount of data as well as high computational power were required to train the model. Recently, a novel UNet architecture based on a convolutional neural network was utilized by Costa et al. to segment mitral valves in PLAX and A4C views. The biggest strength of UNet architecture is that it does not require a large training dataset to produce accurate results.

Automated quantitative analysis.

Precise and reliable quantitative analysis of stenosis and regurgitation is crucial to severity assessment, prognosis prediction and to evaluate whether sur-gery or intervention is needed. Proximal isoveloc-ity surface area (PISA) method is widely used in measuring mitral valve orifice area and calculating the regurgitant volume.Conventional PISA method of two-dimensional echocardiography is based on the assumption that the shape of the proximal flow convergence region is hemispheric, which is not quite true . The development of three-dimensional (3D) color Doppler echocar-diography enables direct measurement of PISA without assumptions, thereby reducing errors . However, it is not indicated for routine clinical use because it is a time-consuming procedure, thus in desperate need of an automated algorithm. Grady et al. proposed the first automated PISA measurement system based on a random walker algorithm. The system was initiated by the manual input of two points (one at the valve annulus and one at the coaptation site), followed by automated segmentation of valve annulus and the isovelocity region. The segmentation results were then used to generate 3D meshes for computing PISA. In vitro experiments validated its accuracy in measuring PISA, effective regurgitant surface area (EROA) and regurgitant volume. Further in vivo experi-ments showed that measurement of EROA on pa-tients with magnetic resonance (MR) by automated algorithm was significantly correlated with manual measurement of vena contracta . Cobey et al. proposed another novel automated method based on Halcon H Develop Machine Vision. 3D images of PISA were first sliced into 2 mm-thick sequential cuts, the algorithm traced the boundary of each slice and the arc lengths between each slice from which the 3D surface area was generated and computed. Another method of quantitatively assessing MR is to use regurgitant fraction which is calculated from mitral inflow and stroke volume . Wang et al. proposed a novel automated system for estimating mitral inflow and aortic out-flow. The system first detected the left ventricular wall, mitral annulus and left ventricular outflow tract using marginal space learning and placed the measurement plane. The 3D motions of these structures were tracked through a whole cardiac circle to construct and adjust the measurement plane, then the volume of mitral inflow and left ventricular outflow was computed by aggregating color flow values in the 3D space In addition to these pioneering studies,

several commercial software have been developed including Mitral Valve Quantification (Philips Medical Imaging, Andover, MA) eSie Valve (Siemens Healthcare, Mountain View, CA, USA) Mitral Valve Navigator (Philips Medical Systems).Auto Valve Analysis (Siemens; California, USA) , eSie PISA Volume Analysis (Siemens Medi-cal Solutions USA, Inc., Mountain View, CA) which aim to automate the quantitative analysis of 3D echocardiography.These approaches can reduce the measurement time substantially and provide more accurate and reproducible results.The aforementioned automated algorithms and commercial software have validated their reliability in quantitatively measuring aortic and mitral valve apparatus parameters and regurgitation volume

AI-assisted interpretation of cardiac CT images

Computed tomography is not employed as the preferred diagnostic method of VHD. It generally serves as a complementary role when echocardiography is insufficient or inclusive. Nevertheless, cardiac CT has prominent advantages in the evaluation of valve calcification and annulus geometry. It is the golden standard for annulus sizing and an indispensable tool in preoperative planning of transcatheter aortic valve replacement (TAVR). Reliable measurement of aortic valve annulus size, aortic root dimension and the height of coronary ostia are crucial for appropriate transcatheter valve prosthesis selection and intraprocedural valve po-sitioning which may improve success rate and re-duce postoperative complications. In recent years, advances in 3D image techniques have enabled reconstruction of patient-specific models of aortic valve apparatus. Several automated algorithms and commercial software for aortic valve segmentation and quantification have been developed for pre-operative planning of transcathether aortic valve implantation (TAVI).

Patient-specific 3D modeling of aortic valve.

Ionasec et al. proposed the first dy-namic patient-specific aortic valve model from 4D CT images. A generic physiological model which can represent aortic valve and its pathological variations was constructed first, patient-specific parameters of the model were estimated from volu-metric sequences by trajectory spectrum learning, marginal space learning and discriminative learn-ing. Their study was further improved with shape forest to constrain the classical statistical shape model Waechter et al. extracted the aortic valve geometry from CT images using model-based segmentation and applies pattern search method to detect the coronary ostia. The whole heart geom-etry (including heart chambers and great vessels) was first roughly modeled, a generic aortic mesh model was established and boundary detector were trained by annotated images aiming to build more detailed models of the aortic valve and root, the coronary ostia was then detected on the surface of the aortic root. Segmentation results allowed a series of clinical measurements including the di-ameters of annulus and the distance between ostia and aortic valve, etc. Considering that VHDs often involve multivalvular lesion which require joint as-sessment, Grbic et al. proposed an integrated model for quantification of all heart valves from 4D CT images based on marginal space learning and multi-linear shape models. Another study of Grbic et al. [69] extracted both the volumetric model of the aortic valve and calcification, which is closely correlated with postoperative regurgitation

Landmarks detection and quantitative measurement.

A number of parameters should be measured with precision for surgical planning before TAVI. These include annulus diameter, an-nulus area, angulation of annulus plane and the distance from annulus to coronary ostia to name a few. The annulus diameter is crucial for selection of the appropriate valve prosthesis. Size mismatching may either cause post-operative perivalvular regurgita-tion or annulus rupture. A short distance between aortic annulus and coronary ostia indicates elevated risk of coronary obstruction after valve deployment. Annulus plane angulation determines the position of an X-ray tube C-arm during operations to achieve an optimal view of valve delivery. Accurate segmentation of the aorta, aortic valve apparatus and detection of anatomic land-marks (coronary ostium, aortic commissures and aortic hinges) is the prerequisite for reliable meas-urement of the above parameters. Zheng et al. proposed a robust hierarchical approach by first segmenting the global aorta using marginal space learning from which the position of the anatomical landmarks can be roughly inferred, followed by us-ing specific landmark detectors to refine each land-mark.Elattar et al.used thresholding and connected component analysis to detect the region of interest, from which aortic root was extracted using 3D normalized cut.

Two coronary ostia and three valve hinge points were then detected on the surface of aortic root by intensity projection map and Gaussian curvature map. Lalys et al. used a hybrid approach which integrated thresholding, model-based method, statistical-based method and a 3D contour model in the procedure, however, a user-specific point is needed to define the vol-ume of interest. Recently, colonial walk algorithm, which is a machine learning method, was utilized by Al et al. to automatically localize the land-marks. Several commercial software including three mensio valves (3mensio Medical Imaging BV, the Netherlands) Syngo (Siemens Healthcare, Erlangen, Germany) , Intelli-Space Portal (Philips Medical Systems, Cleveland, OH) , have been available for routine clini-cal use.

Together with the aforementioned al-gorithms, these pioneering techniques showed reliable aortic annulus measurements A comparative study between 3 mensio, Intelli- Space Portal (version 7.0), IntelliSpace Portal (version 9.0) and manual measurement concerning annulus parameters, time-cost and reproducibility was performed . Results showed that Intelli-Space Portal (version 9.0) allowed the fastest and most reproducible measurements, parameters derived from either method can be used inter-changeably in prosthesis sizing. Moreover, Samim et al. performed a prospective cohort study to compare angiography and MSCT (using 3mensio) in predicting the annulus plane and choosing the C-arm position . The study included 35 patients in an angiography cohort and 36 patients in an MDCT cohort. The utilization of MDCT was as-sociated with a significant reduction of prosthesis implanting time, radiation exposure and contrast delivery. A reduction of postoperative complica-tions and 30-day mortality was observed in patients in the MDCT cohort.

AI-assisted interpretation of CMR

Cardiac magnetic resonance is the second-line technique in the assessment of VHDs. A standard CMR scan takes about an hour followed by tedi-ous image processing which is both time and labor consuming. However, it is the golden standard in the assessment of cardiac morphology, volume and function due to its high spatial resolution. MR cine imaging and phase-contrast velocity imaging are gaining increasing importance in studying val-vular function. Particularly, CMR have advantages over other imaging tools in the quantification of regurgitation when the regurgitant jet is highly eccentric. Automated cardiac chamber segmentation and cardiac volume measurement have been widely studied in MR images as reviewed by Bernard et al. and Petitjean etal.Several large CMR image datasets (Sunnybrook,STACOM, MICCAI RV and kaggle), which are free to access, have been released in the last decade in conjunction with international challenges to automatically segment left ventricle, right ventricle, end-diastolic volume and end-systolic volume Commercial software such as SuiteHEART® (Neosoft, Pewaukee, Wis-consin, USA) which allows automated quantifica-tion of biventricular volumes and function is now available .The regurgitant volume and fraction in isolated aortic or mitral regurgitation can be calculated from left ventricle and right ventricle stroke volume , however, to date, the afore-mentioned automated methods have not applied in quantification of valve regurgitation. AI-assisted CMR which allows automated diagnosis of VHDs is underexplored. However, several pioneering stud-ies have achieved many valuable results. Fries et al. developed a novel supervised deep learning model for aortic valve malformation classification using unlabeled MR images. 570 patients were classified as bicuspid aortic valve from a cohort of 9230 patients from the UK biobank. These indi-viduals showed a significant lower major adverse cardiac event-free survival rate compared to indi-viduals with a normal aortic valve.

Risk factor identification and in-hospital mortality prediction of cardiac surgery

Preoperative assessment of surgical risk is an important procedure in cardiac surgery which guides the selection of surgery, intervention or nonsurgical treatment. Great progress has been made in risk factor identification and mortality pre-diction. Risk score models including EuroSCORE, STS score and ACEF scores have been widely used . The linear regression model is the most widely used in analyzing a correlation between risk variables and cardiac adverse events. However, there is a growing trend of utilizing machine learn-ing methods in developing prediction models which outperform traditional scoring systems. Nilsson et al. were among the first to use an ANN model to identify risk factors and predict mortality in cardiac surgery. 72 risk factors were evaluated from 18,362 patients, 34 of the factors were identified as relevant to mortality. Receiver operating characteristic (ROC) area of the ANN model for mortality prediction was significantly larger than logistic EuroSCORE model (0.81 vs. 0.79). For isolated valve surgery (with or without coronary artery bypass grafting), the ROC area of the ANN model was 0.76 vs. 0.72 of the logistic models. Celi et al. achieved an even larger ROC area using ANN, Bayesian network and lo-gistic regression (0.941, 0.931, 0.854) compared to EuroSCORE (0.648). Allyn et al. utilized a novel ensemble machine learning method which integrates the results from four isolated machine learning algorithms to predict cardiac surgery mortality. 6250 patients were enrolled in the study,

Chi-square filtering was utilized to extract relevant variables. Results showed that the ensemble ma-chine learning model had a significantly stronger discriminatory power for operative mortality than EuroSCORE II (ROC area: 0.795 vs. 0.737). Recently, Hernandez-Suarez firstly applied four machine learning algorithms in mortality predic-tion after TAVI 10,883 patients were enrolled in the study. Logistic regression, ANN, Naïve bayes and random forest which are the four top supervised learning algorithms all showed good discriminative performance. The best prediction model obtained by logistic algorithm (ROC area: 0.92) have close discriminative power with state-of-the-art National Inpatient Sample TAVR score model.

Moreover, ANN and machine learning algo-rithm have been applied in other fields such as pre-diction of length of stay in intensive care unit after cardiac surgery , post-operative complications , both short-term and long-term mortality after heart transplantation . However, the downside of current studies is that few studies have been dedicated to isolated cardiac surgery procedures which is partially due to a lack of sufficient samples to feed machine training. The introduction of minimally invasive strate-gies and a surgical robot in cardiac surgery prom-ises quicker recovery and less postoperative complications and mortality. While having many superiorities over human hands such as tremor resistance and scalable motion, current robotic systems are merely teleoperated devices under human control which entirely possess no autonomy. Since automation has gained great success in other robotic fields which have increased safety, accuracy and efficiency, it is reasonable to assume that the same benefit will be gained by developing autonomous surgical robots. To achieve the level of fully "autonomous", the surgical robot should possess the ability to "see", "think" and "act". "see" refers to perception of the surgical field and itself through sensors. "think" is the process of receiving information and calculating the future status that it needs to achieve in the following "act" . Recently, European research council launch the Autonomous Robotic Surgery (ARS) project aiming to developing a unified framework for the autonomous execution of robotic tasks . Main research objectives include establish-ment of global action model by analyzing current robotic surgical data, patient specific intervention

Intelligent cardiac operating room: Towards autonomous robotic surgery

models, design of controllers, perception of overall surgical situations, and assessment of the surgical robot capability.Though at an experimental stage, the feasi-bility of autonomous robots performing simple surgical tasks like suture and knot typing have been demonstrated. Penesar et al. developed a novel Smart Tissue Autonomous Robot (STAR) which was able to perform linear continuous suture, it successfully completed in-vivo end-to-end anastomosis of porcine small intestine with few suturing mistakes, no complications were observed in 7 day follow-up. Although the STAR system realized autonomous suture, the step of knot typing remained manual. In the context of endoscopic surgery or robot-assisted surgery,the task of knot typing is cumbersome which re-quires manipulation of many subtle movements in a confined space. Through training a recurrent neural network on 3D loop trajectories generated by human surgeon, the Endoscopic Partial-Auton-omous Robot (EndoPAR) was able to accurately perform the winding portion of a knot-tying task [99]. To date however, robots are unable to fully perform autonomous knot tying.

Transcatheter therapy has been accepted as an alternative to traditional cardiac valvular surgery especially in patients with high surgical risk in recent years. Catheters are inserted either from peripheral vessel or the cardiac apex to deploy valve prothesis or occlusion device. In either case, the catheters need to be precisely navigated to the intervention site which is a very challenging task in a beating heart. Inspired by wall following, which is used by thigmotactic animals to locate and navi-gate themselves in low-visibility environments,

Fagogenis et al. developed an autonomous intracardiac catheter navigation system. With hybrid imaging and touch sensor installed on the catheter tip, which can provide clear images of what it has touched and identify it as blood, valve or myocardium. The catheter created continuous low-force contact with the surrounding tissue and followed the cardiac wall to achieve autonomous navigation. With the navigation system, authors designed a robotic catheter, inserted from the cardiac apex, which can autonomously navigate to the aortic valve and deploy an occlusion device into the leak site on a porcine model. The in-vivo animal experiments demonstrate that an autono-mous robot catheter was non-inferior to human experts

Conclusions

Artificial intelligence is changing the land-scape of healthcare. The inclusion of AI and automated algorithms in medical image analysis are very promising for they require less measure-ment time and meanwhile provide more accurate and reproducible results, which make them ideal helpers in a busy clinical flow. Machine learning methods can make full use of patient data and build more powerful prediction models of cardiac surgery compared to traditional statistical ap-proaches. Moreover, the autonomous surgical robot, although in its infancy, holds great promise for improved safety and efficiency in cardiac surgery and intervention.

Bibliography And Acknowledgement

- Al WA, Jung HoY, Yun IlD, et al. Automatic aortic valve land-mark localization in coronary CT angiography using colonial walk.PLoSOne.2018;13(7):
- Allyn J, Allou N, Augustin P, et al. A Comparison of a Machine Learning Model with EuroSCORE II in Predicting Mortality after Elective Cardiac Surgery: A Decision Curve Analysis. PLoS One. 2017; 12(1
- Backhaus SJ, Staab W, Steinmetz M, et al. Fully automated quan-tification of biventricular volumes and function in cardiovascular magnetic resonance: applicability to clinical routine settings. J Cardiovasc Magn Reson. 2019; 21(1): 24,
- Baeßler B, Mauri V, Bunck AC, et al. Software-automated multi-detector computed tomography-based prosthesis-sizing in tran-scatheter aortic valve replacement: Inter-vendor comparison and relation to patientoutcome.IntJCardiol.2018;272:267–272,
- Beam AL, Kohane IS. Big data and machine learning in health care.JAMA.2018;319(13):13171318,doi:10.1001jama.2017.18391,indexedinPubmed:29532063.
- Benjamin EJ, Muntner P, Alonso A, et al. Heart Disease and Stroke Statistics — 2019 Update: A Report From the American Heart Association.Vol.139,Circulation.2019.
- Bernard O, Cervenansky F, Lalande A, et al. Deep learning tech-niques for automatic MRI cardiac multi-structures segmentation and diagnosis: is the problem solved? IEEE Trans Med Imag-ing. 2018;37(11):2514–2525
- Calleja A, Thavendiranathan P, Ionasec RI, et al. Automated quantitative 3-dimensional modeling of the aortic valve and root by 3-dimensional transesophageal echocardiography in normals, aortic regurgitation, and aortic stenosis: comparison to computed tomography in normals and clinical implications. Circ Cardio-vasc Imaging.2013;6(1):99–108,
- Celi LA, Galvin S, Davidzon G, et al. A database-driven deci-sion support system: customized mortality prediction. J Pers Med. 2012; 2(4): 138–148, doi: 10.3390/jpm2040138, indexed in Pubmed: 23766893.
- Chen C. Computer vision in medical imaging. Vol. 2. World Scientific.2014.
- Chen TE, Yang SI, Ho LT, et al. S1 and S2 Heart Sound Rec-ognition Using Deep Neural Networks. IEEE Trans Biomed Eng. 2017;64(2):372–380,
- Choi J, Hong GR, Kim M, et al. Automatic quantification of aortic regurgitation using 3D full volume color doppler echocardiogra-phy: a validation study with cardiac magnetic resonance imaging. Int J CardiovascImaging.2015;31(7):1379–1389
- Cobey FC, McInnis JA, Gelfand BJ, et al. A method for automat-ing 3-dimensional proximal isovelocity surface area measure-ment. J Cardiothorac Vasc Anesth. 2012; 26(3): 507–511,
- de Agustin JA, Viliani D, Vieira C, et al. Proximal isovelocity sur-face area by single-beat three-dimensional color Doppler echo-cardiography applied for tricuspid regurgitation quantification. J Am SocEchocardiogr.2013;26(9):1063–1072
- Delgado V, Ng ACT, Schuijf JD, et al. Automated assessment of the aortic root dimensions with multidetector row com-puted tomography. AnnThoracSurg.2011;91(3):716–723,
- Dwivedi AK, Imtiaz SA, Rodriguez-Villegas E. Algorithms for au-tomatic analysis and classification of heart sounds-A systematic review. IEEE Access. 2019; 7(c): 8316–45.
- Elattar M, Wiegerinck E, van Kesteren F, et al. Automatic aortic root landmark detection in CTA images for preprocedural plan-ning of transcatheter aortic valve implantation. Int J Cardiovasc Imaging.2016;32(3):501–511,
- Elattar MA, Wiegerinck EM, Planken RN, et al. Automatic seg-mentation of the aortic root in CT angiography of candidate pa-tients for transcatheter aortic valve implantation. Med Biol Eng Comput.2014;52(7):611–618,
- Ernande L, Audureau E, Jellis CL, et al. Clinical implications of echocardiographic phenotypes of patients with diabetes mel-litus. J Am Coll Cardiol. 2017; 70(14): 1704–1716,
- Fagogenis G, Mencattelli M, Machaidze Z, et al. Autonomous Ro-botic Intracardiac Catheter Navigation Using Haptic Vision. SciRobot.2019;4(29),
- Fahad HM, Ghani Khan MU, Saba T, et al. Microscopic abnormal-ity classification of cardiac murmurs using ANFIS and HMM. Mi-crosc ResTech.2018;81(5):449–457,
- Falk V, Baumgartner H, Bax JJ, et al. ESC/EACTS Guidelines for the management of valvular heart disease. Eur J Cardio-thoracic Surg.2017;52:616–664.
- Fries JA, Varma P, Chen VS, et al. Weakly supervised classifica-tion of rare aortic valve malformations using unlabeled cardiac MRIsequences.bioRxiv.2018;2019:1–25,
- Garcia-RuizA,GagnerM,MillerJH, et al. Manual vs robotically assisted laparoscopic surgery in the performance of basic ma-nipulation and suturing tasks. Arch Surg. 1998; 133(9):957–961,
- Gill D, Gavrieli N, Intrator N. Detection and identification of heart sounds using homomorphic envelogram and self-organiz-ing probabilistic model. Comput Cardiol. 2005; 32: 957–60.
- Grady L, Datta S, Kutter O, et al. Regurgitation Quantification Using 3D PISA in Volume Echocardiograhy. In: Fichtinger G, editors. pMedical Image Comuting and Comuter-AssisteInter-vention MICCAI 2011. Berlin, Heidelberg: Sringer Berlin Heidelberg. 2011: 512–519.
- Grbic S, Ionasec R, Mansi T, et al. Advanced intervention plan-ning for Transcatheter Aortic Valve Implantations (TAVI) from CT using volumetric models. Proc Int Symp Biomed Imaging. 2013: 1424–1427.
- Grbic S, Ionasec R, Vitanovski D, et al. Complete valvular heart apparatus model from 4D cardiac CT. Med Image Anal. 2012; 16(5): 1003–1014.
- Grespan L, Fiorini P, Colucci G. Looking Ahead: The Future of Robotic Surgery. In: The Route to Patient Safety in Robotic Sur-gery [Internet]. Cham: Springer International Publishing. 2019: 157–162,
- Guez D, Boroumand G, Ruggiero NJ, et al. Automated and Manual Measurements of the Aortic Annulus with ECG-Gated Cardiac CT Angiography Prior to Transcatheter Aortic Valve Replacement: Comparison with 3D-Transesophageal Echocar-diography. Acad Radiol. 2017; 24(5): 587–593

- Hernandez-Suarez DF, Kim Y, Villablanca P, et al. Machine Learning Prediction Models for In-Hospital Mortality After Transcatheter Aortic Valve Replacement. JACC Cardiovasc In-terv. 2019; 12(14): 1328–1338,
- Hinton GE, Osindero S, Teh YW. A fast learning algorithm for deep belief nets. Neural Comput. 2006; 18(7): 1527–1554,
- Ionasec RI, Georgescu B, Gassner E, et al. Dynamic Model-Driven Quantitative and Visual Evaluation of the Aortic Valve from 4D CT. In: Metaxas D, editors. Medical Image Comuting and Comuter-Assisted Intervention. MICCAI 2008. Berlin, Hei-delberg: Sringer Berlin Heidelberg.2008:686–694.
- Ionasec RI, Voigt I, Georgescu B, et al. Patient-specific modeling and quantification of the aortic and mitral valves from 4-D cardiac CT and TEE. IEEE Trans Med Imaging. 2010; 29(9): 1636–1651,
- Iwata A, Ishii N, Suzumura N, et al. Algorithm for detecting the first and the second heart sounds by spectral tracking. Med Biol Eng Comput.1980;18(1):19–26,
- Jiang Z, Choi SA. cardiac sound characteristic waveform method for in-home heart disorder monitoring with electric stethoscope. Expert Syst Appl. 2006; 31(2): 286–98.
- Kagiyama N, Toki M, Hara M, et al. Efficacy and Accuracy of Novel Automated Mitral Valve Quantification: Three-Dimensional Transesophageal Echocardiographic Study. Echocardiography. 2016; 33(5):756–763,
- Khalid S, Khalil T, Nasreen SA. survey of feature selection and feature extraction techniques in machine learning. Proc 2014 Sci Inf ConfSAI.2014;2014:372–378.
- Koos R, Mahnken AH, Dohmen G, et al. Association of aortic valve calcification severity with the degree of aortic regurgitation after transcatheter aortic valve implantation. Int J Cardiol. 2011; 150(2): 142–145.
- Kumar D, Carvalho P, Antunes M, et al. Heart murmur clas-sification with feature selection. Conf Proc IEEE Eng Med Biol Soc. 2010;2010:4566–4569,
- Kwak C. Kwon O-W. Cardiac disorder classification by heart sound signals using murmur likelihood and hidden Markov model state likelihood.IETSignalProcess.2012;6(4):326.
- LaFaro RJ, Pothula S, Kubal KP, et al. Neural Network Predic-tion of ICU Length of Stay Following Cardiac Surgery Based on Pre-IncisionVariables.PLoSOne.2015;10(12):
- Lalys F, Esneault S, Castro M, et al. Automatic aortic root seg-mentation and anatomical landmarks detection for TAVI pro-edure planning. Minim Invasive Ther Allied Technol. 2019; 28(3): 157–164,
- Lehner RJ, Rangayyan RM. A three-channel microcomputer system for segmentation and characterization of the phonocar-diogram. IEEETransBiomedEng.1987;34(6):485–489,
- Liang H, Lukkarinen S, Hartimo I. Heart sound segmentation algorithm based on heart sound envelogram. 1997; 24: 105–108.
- Liu X, Cheung Y, Ming Y, et al. Automatic mitral valve leaflet tracking in Echocardiography via constrained outlier pursuit and region-scalable active contours. Neurocomputing. 2014; 144: 47–57
- Mayer H, Gomez F, Wierstra D, et al. system for robotic heart surgery that learns to tie knots using recurrent neural networks. Adv Robot. 2008; 13(14): 1521–1537.
- Mediratta A, Addetia K, Medvedofsky D, et al. 3D echocardio-graphic analysis of aortic annulus for transcatheter aortic valve replacement using novel aortic valve quantification software: Comparison with computed tomography. Echocardiography. 2017; 34(5): 690–699
- Moustris GP, Hiridis SC, Deliparaschos KM, et al. Evolution of autonomous and semi-autonomous robotic surgical systems: a review of the literature. Int J Med Robot. 2011; 7(4): 375–392
- Nashef SAM, Roques F, Sharples LD, et al. EuroSCORE II. Eur J Cardiothorac Surg. 2012; 41(4): 734–44; discussion 744, doi: 10.1093/ejcts/ezs043, indexed in Pubmed: 22378855.
- Nilsson J, Ohlsson M, Höglund P, et al. The International Heart Transplant Survival Algorithm (IHTSA): a new model to improve organ sharing and survival. PLoS One. 2015; 10(3):
- Nilsson J, Ohlsson M, Thulin L, et al. Risk factor identification and mortality prediction in cardiac surgery using artificial neural networks. J Thorac Cardiovasc Surg. 2006; 132(1): 12–19, doi: 10.1016/j.jtcvs.2005.12.055, indexed in Pubmed: 16798296.
- Noble JA, Boukerroui D. Ultrasound image segmentation: a survey. IEEE Trans Med Imaging. 2006; 25(8): 987–1010 Olmez T, Zumray D. Classification of heart sounds using an arti-ficial neural network. Pattern Recognit Lett. 2003; 24: 617–629.
- Panesar S, Cagle Y, Chander D, et al. Artificial Intelligence and the Future of Surgical Robotics. Ann Surg. 2019; 270(2): 223– 226 Pennell DJ Cardiovascular magnetic resonance Circulation. 2010;121(5):692–705.
- Petitjean C, Dacher JN. A review of segmentation methods in short axis cardiac MR images. Med Image Anal. 2011; 15(2): 169–184, doi: 10.1016/j.media.2010.12.004, indexed in Pubmed: 21216179.
- Potes C, Parvaneh S, Rahman A, et al. Ensemble of feature-based and deep learning-based classifiers for detection of abnormal heart sounds. Comput Cardiol. 2016; 43: 621–624.
- Pouch AM, Wang H, Takabe M, et al. Fully automatic segmenta-tion of the mitral leaflets in 3D transesophageal echocardio-graphic images using multi-atlas joint label fusion and deform-able medial modeling. Med Image Anal. 2014; 18(1): 118–129,
- Puppe F. Systematic introduction to expert systems: Knowledge representations and problem-solving methods. Springer Science &BusinessMedia.2012.
- Safara F, Doraisamy S, Azman A, et al. Multi-level basis selection of wavelet packet decomposition tree for heart sound classifica-tion. Comput Biol Med. 2013; 43(10): 1407–1414,
- Samim M, Stella PR, Agostoni P, et al. Automated 3D analysis of pre-procedural MDCT to predict annulus plane angulation and C-arm positioning: benefit on procedural outcome in patients re-ferred for TAVR. JACC Cardiovasc Imaging. 2013; 6(2): 238–248
- Schmidt SE, Holst-Hansen C, Graff C, et al. Segmentation of heart sound recordings by a duration-dependent hidden Markov model.PhysiolMeas.2010;31(4):513–529,doi: 10.1088/0967-3334/31/4/004,indexedinPubmed:20208091.
- Schneider RJ, Perrin DP, Vasilyev NV, et al. Mitral annulus segmentation from 3D ultrasound using graph cuts. IEEE Trans MedImaging.2010;29(9):1676–1687,
- Schwartz WB, Patil RS, Szolovits P. Artificial intelligence in medicine. Where do we stand? N Engl J Med. 1987; 316(11): 685–688
- Shortliffe EHA. rule-based comuter rogram for advising hysi-cians regarding antimicrobial theray selection. In: Proceedings of the AnnualACMConference.ACM.1974;739.
- Siefert AW, Icenogle DA, Rabbah JPM, et al. Accuracy of a mitral valve segmentation method using J-splines for real-time 3D echocardiography data. Ann Biomed Eng. 2013; 41(6): 1258–1268

- Springer DB, Tarassenko L, Clifford GD. Logistic Regression-HSMM-Based Heart Sound Segmentation. IEEE Trans Biomed Eng.2016;63(4):822–832,
- Sultan MS, Martins N, Costa E, et al. Virtual M-Mode for Echocardiography: A New Approach for the Segmentation of the Anterior Mitral Leaflet. IEEE J Biomed Health Inform. 2019; 23(1): 305–313
- Sun S, Jiang Z, Wang H, et al. Automatic moment segmentation and peak detection analysis of heart sound pattern via short-time modified Hilbert transform. Comput Methods Programs Biomed. 2014;114(3):219–230,
- Sun S. An innovative intelligent system based on automatic diagnostic feature extraction for diagnosing heart diseases. Knowledge-Based Syst. 2015; 75: 224–238, doi: 10.1016/j.knosys.2014.12.001.
- Swee JKY, Grbić S. Advanced transcatheter aortic valve implantation (TAVI) planning from CT with ShapeForest. Lect Notes Comput Sci. (including Subser Lect Notes Artif Intell Lect Notes Bioinformatics).2014;8674LNCS(Part2):17–24.
  Szolovits P, Pauker SG. Categorical and probabilistic reason-ing in medical diagnosis. Artif Intell [Internet]. 1978 Aug 1; 11(1–2):115–44.
- Tavel ME. Cardiac auscultation. A glorious past -- but does it have a future? Circulation. 1996; 93(6): 1250–1253,
- Thavendiranathan P, Liu S, Datta S, et al. Quantification of chronic functional mitral regurgitation by automated 3-dimensional peak and integrated proximal isovelocity surface area and stroke volume techniques using real-time 3-dimensional volume color doppler echocardiography: In vitro and clini. Circ Cardiovasc Imaging. 2013; 6(1): 125–133.
- Thavendiranathan P, Phelan D, Thomas JD, et al. Quantitative assessment of mitral regurgitation: validation of new methods. J Am Coll Cardiol. 2012; 60(16): 1470–1483,
- Thompson WR, Reinisch AJ, Unterberger MJ, et al. Artificial intelligence-assisted auscultation of heart murmurs: validation by virtual clinical trial. Pediatr Cardiol. 2019; 40(3):623–629,
- Thottakkara P, Ozrazgat-Baslanti T, Hupf BB, et al. Application of Machine Learning Techniques to High-Dimensional Clinical Data to Forecast Postoperative Complications. PLoS One. 2016; 11(5
- Topol EJ. High-performance medicine: the convergence of human and artificial intelligence. Nat Med. 2019; 25(1): 44–56, doi: 10.1038/s41591-018-0300-7, indexed in Pubmed: 30617339.
- Ton J. Cleophas AHZ. Machine Learning in Medicine. 2013;1920–30. LeCun Y, Bengio Y, Hinton G. Deep learning. Nature. 2015; 521(7553):436–444
- Uğuz H. A biomedical system based on artificial neural network and principal component analysis for diagnosis of the heart valve diseases. J Med Syst. 2012; 36(1): 61–72
- Waechter I, Kneser R, Korosoglou G, et al. Patient Secific Mod-els for Planning and Guidance of Minimally Invasive Aortic Valve Imlantation. In: Jiang T, Navab N, Pluim JPW, Viergever MA, editors. Medical Image Comuting and Comuter-Assisted Intervention -- MICCAI 2010. Sringer Berlin Heidelberg. 2010: 526–533.
- Wang Y, Georgescu B, Datta S, et al. Automatic cardiac flow quantification on 3D volume color Doppler data. Proc - Int Symp Biomed Imaging. 2011; C(Lv): 1688–1691.
- Watanabe Y, Morice MC, Bouvier E, et al. Automated 3-dimensional aortic annular assessment by multidetector computed tomography in transcatheter aortic valve implantation. JACC Cardiovasc Interv. 2013; 6(9): 955–964,
- Zhang J, Gajjala S, Agrawal P, et al. Fully automated echocardiogram interpretation in clinical practice. Circulation. 2018; 138(16):1623–1635,
- Zhang W, Guo X, Yuan Z, et al. Heart sound classification and recognition based on eemd and correlation dimension. J Mech Med Biol.2014;14(04):1450046.
- Zhang W, Han J, Deng S. Heart sound classification based on scaled spectrogram and tensor decomposition. Expert Syst Appl. 2017; 84: 220–231.
- Zhao Y, Zeng D, Socinski MA, et al. Reinforcement learning strategies for clinical trials in nonsmall cell lung cancer. Biometrics. 2011;67(4):1422–1433,
- Zheng Y, John M, Liao R, et al. Automatic aorta segmentation and valve landmark detection in C-arm CT for transcatheter aortic valve implantation. IEEE Trans Med Imaging. 2012; 31(12): 2307–2321.
- Zhou X, Yang C, Yu W. Automatic mitral leaflet tracking in echocardiography by outlier detection in the low-rank representation. Proc IEEE Comput Soc Conf Comput Vis Pattern Recognit. 2012: 972–979.

CHAPTER

10

Artificial Intelligence In The Diagnosis And Management Of Cardiac Arrhythmias

As artificial intelligence (AI) has entered the medical field in recent years, machine learning (ML) approaches have made progress in assisting healthcare professionals in optimizing personalized treat-ment in a given situation, in particular in electrocardiography and image interpretation. Artificial intelligence methodologies are increas-ingly being adopted into all aspects of patient care and are paving the way to minimally invasive or non-invasive treatment modalities. This article offers a state-of-the-art overview on milestones achieved, but also on future integration of this information into diagnostic and therapeutic measures, and its likely impact on all aspects of arrhyth-mia care. Integration of all individual information in combination with AI solutions is likely to revolutionize electrophysiology (EP) interven-tions in the near future

Cardiac electrical signal analysis using artificial intelligence methodologies

Human intelligence is characterized by the capability of learning, reasoning, analysing, and decision-making. When machines mimic the use of these capabilities, it can be termed AI. Although the concept and the term AI have been used for over six decades.its usage has skyrocketed over the last decade. Whilst ML is the most commonly used term for AI, it only denotes one of the methodologies of AI Most of the AI applications in EP are based on the analysis of signals that represent cardiac electrical activity, with the signal varying with the type of sensor and underlying technology. Two of the most com-monly used signals are electrocardiogram (ECG) and photo plethys-mography (PPG). Photo plethysmography is more contemporary and has been used in some of the wearable devices including watches, wrist bands, and smartphones. Fundamental AI processes employed in analysing data obtained from these devices are essentially similar Following data collection, data are pre-processed, feature engin-eering carried out, and followed by classification by one of the ML methodologies.The ML methodology is first trained using the 'training data' with appropriate labels. The second stage involves ML methodology assessment using a 'validation data set' and fine tuning the algorithm. Following these two steps, the ML algo-rithm would then be ready to be used with a third 'test set'. Performance of the algorithm is expressed using values such as sensi-tivity, specificity, accuracy, receiver operating curve (ROC), and area under ROC (AUC).

Arrhythmia detection using artificial intelligence

Since digitalization of ECG, AI methods have been employed in com-puterized interpretation of ECGs. Whilst ML methods revealed high sensitivity and specificity for detecting normal sinus rhythm, their abilities were lower than expert cardiologists for the identification of cardiac arrhythmias. One of the main deterrents have been the pres-ence of noise, small or varying P waves resulting in over diagnosis of atrial fibrillation (AF), paced rhythms, poor-quality ECGs, tremor, and previously untrained rhythms. With better ML algorithms, noise reduction techniques and advanced feature extraction, selection and reduction methods [including use of the unsupervised deep neural network (DNN)], computerized interpretation of ECGs has clearly improved arrhythmia detection achieving an accuracy close to 95% Hannun et al.8 developed an end to end deep learning (DL) ap-proach for ECG analysis by using a DNN for identifying 12 rhythm abnormalities by using 91 232 single-lead ECGs. When validated against independent data reported by a committee of certified cardiologists, their algorithm was shown to be superior to an average car-diologist in identifying these rhythm abnormalities (ROC 0.97 vs. 0.78). With the development of unsupervised DNN algorithms, more interest has been generated amongst researchers for identifying hid-den diseased state signatures in a 12-lead ECG. So far, it has been shown to be feasible to detect hyperkalaemia, heart failure,hypoglycaemia, and even changes in emotional states using 12-lead ECG. Attia et al. at Mayo Clinic Rochester assessed the feasibility of identifying previous episodes of or impending AF using an AI-enabled 12-lead ECG in normal sinus rhythm. They used 0.65 million ECGs to train, validate, and test the AI algorithm in a 7:1:2 ratio and found that AI-enabled ECG recorded during normal sinus rhythm performed well as a screening test to identify AF with an accuracy of 79.4% and this improved to 83.4% when it was a first ECG following an episode of AF. Additional multiple ECGs improved the model accuracy lead-ing to the hypothesis that structural changes that may precede AF including myocyte hypertrophy, fibrosis, or chamber dilatation may result in subtle multifaceted changes in ECG that may otherwise be unrecognized by the human eye but are detectable by a DNN. This observation has important clinical implications with potential point-of-care identification of individuals at the risk of AF and for the em-bolic stroke of undetermined source.Deep neural network has also been used to predict hypertrophic cardiomyopathy (HCM), age and sex, and plasma dofetilide concentration from ECG. Advancements in sensor technology, telecommunications (increased availability of wireless, Wi-Fi, Bluetooth and smartphone technologies), availability of web-based data storage, and AI-aided analysis have seen rapid growth of handheld and wearable cardiac monitoring systems. Whilst several handheld devices are available, the AliveCor Heart Monitor, an ECG-based system, has been studied extensively for AF detection in symptomatic patients. In most of these studies, AliveCor Heart Monitor achieved well over 90% sensitivity and speci-ficity for AF detection both in outpatient and hospital settings. In a comparison with traditional transtelephonic monitor, AliveCor Heart Monitor achieved 100% sensitivity and 97% specificity for AF and atrial flutter detection. Similar results were seen with the use of PPG-based systems coupled with AI-aided analysis. In the WATCH AF trial, Do¨rr et al. studied the efficacy of a smartphone PPG-based algorithm in AF detection. The PPG algorithm achieved a sensitivity of 93.7%, a specificity of 98.2%, and an accuracy of 96.1%to detect AF. In a recent community-based trial on the utility of a smartwatch in AF detection (Apple Heart Study), smartwatch in conjunction with a pulse notification algorithm showed promising results in 0.41 million participants with no prior history of AF. The smartwatch application collected single 1-min tachograms every 2 h. If a smartwatch-based irregular pulse notification algorithm identified possible AF, the partici-pant was notified to have further simultaneous 7-day monitoring using an ECG patch. The smartwatch-based algorithm had a positive predictive value of 0.84 (95% confidence interval 0.76–0.92) for iden-tifying AF during the simultaneous monitoring period. Similar results were shown in yet another population-based AF screening study using a PPG algorithm in conjunction with smart devices.Chen et al.studied AF detection using a smart wristband equipped with both ECG and PPG sensors, comparing ECG and PPG individually as well as in combination. They demonstrated higher ac-curacy of 97.5% for AF detection with the combination against 94.7%and 93.2% with ECG and PPG, respectively. Wasserlauf et al. compared smartwatch detection of AF using a DL algorithm (episodes lasting >_1 h) with an insertable loop record-er. They analysed 348 h of simultaneously recorded data. The smartwatch algorithm achieved 97.5% and 97.7% for episode sensitivity and duration sensitivity, respectively. Artificial intelligence-enabled monitoring systems are affordable and reliable, can be used for continuous ambulatory monitoring, and will facilitate the detection of vulnerable groups. A step closer to the holy grail of early AF detection within the community in otherwise symptomatic patients may in fact initiate a paradigm shift in arrhythmia detection.

Artificial intelligence and cardiac devices

Most of the pacemaker and defibrillator functions use rule-based algorithms. Rate response feature in a pacemaker, which incorpo-rates the ability of the device to vary the pacing rate based on an input from a biosensor; tachycardia detection and deliverance of an appro-priate therapy by an implantable defibrillator, are some of the illustra-tions of the rule-based decision-making. A rule-based algorithm is referred to as a simplest form of AI but it differs from ML in its inabil-ity to learn.

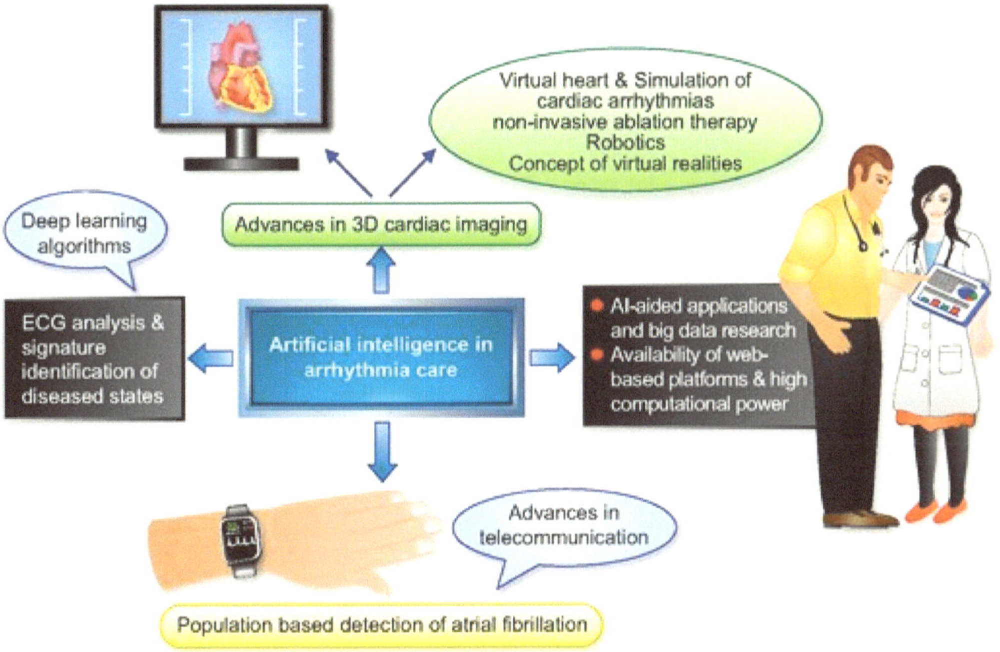

Fig. 10.1 Graphical Abstract Artificial intelligence-enhanced arrhythmia care.

In rule-based algorithms, rules are laid down by humans based on the domain expertise, whereas ML methodologies learn ac-tively from the training data and create their own rules for decision-making, which may not be transparent in some instances.Machine learning algorithms are finding their use with cardiac devices both in arrhythmia detection and prediction of future events. Machine learning methods have been employed in automatedexternal defibrillators in thedevelopment of shock advice algorithms.

Recently, Nguyen et al. developed an algorithm for the detection of shockable and non-shockable rhythms using ML. They used both boosting classifier and convolutional neural network as a feature extractor with a sensitivity and specificity of 95.21% and 99.31%, respectively. This shock advice algorithm was a considerable improvement over existing algorithms and in keeping with the stand-ards set by the American Heart Association guidelines. More re-cently, a DL technique was introduced to identify any cardiac device model from a chest radiograph.Machine learning methods have been used to improve cardiac resynchronization therapy (CRT) outcomes prediction, paving the way for better patient selection. In a proof of concept, single centre study, ML algorithm in conjunction with natural language proc-essing was applied to electronic health records.

This model suc-cessfully identified subgroups of patients who were unlikely to benefit from CRT. An ML algorithm using naive Bayes classifier using patient variables including age, sex, QRS duration and morphology, left ventricular ejection fraction and end-diastolic diameter, New York Heart Association functional class, presence of AF, and epicar-dial left ventricular lead was superior to existing guidelines in predict-ing event-free survival post-CRT.

Machine learning algorithms including random forests and convo-luted neural networks, when applied to the AF signature burden obtained using continuous remote monitoring data in patients with cardiac implantable electronic devices, were superior in predicting stroke compared to the widely used CHA2DS2-VASc score. An en-semble method using ML model in conjunction with CHA2DS2-VASc score had better sensitivity and specificity when compared to using CHA2DS2-VASc score alone and improved AUC from 0.52 to 0.63.

Multimodal integrative approach to predict sites of arrhythmia origins and role of machine learning

Non-invasive characterization of arrhythmia prior to attempting abla-tive therapy is gaining favour amongst electrophysiologists. This ap-proach aids in focused targeting of the cardiac region of

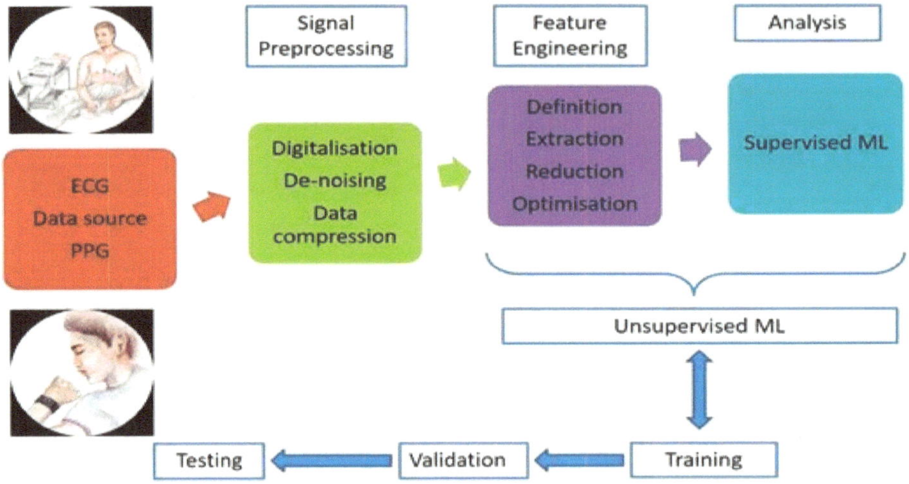

Fig 10.2 Schematic representation of steps involved in cardiac impulse analysis from the data acquisition to analysis by machine learning algorithm. ECG, electrocardiogram; ML, machine learning; PPG, photo plethysmography.

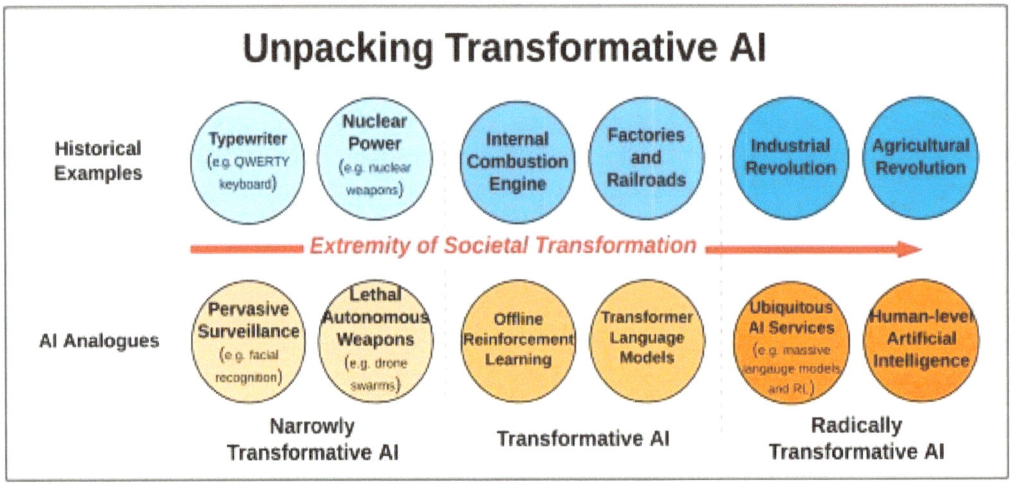

Fig.10.3 Our proposed levels of transformative AI and analogous AI technologies compared with historical examples of transformative GPTs

interest. One of the important contributors to this being ML aided advances in car-diac 3D imaging. Application of DL methods including convolutional neural net-work has improved the speed of acquisition, time efficiency, reconstruction quality of images,and accuracy of cardiac magnetic resonance (CMR) segmentation. Machine learning techniques have been applied to improve myocardial tissue characterization and texture analysis and define the heterogeneous nature of the scarred myocardium in late gadolinium enhancement (LGE) CMR images in patients post-myocardial infarction. Automated CMR analysis using a convolutional neural network al-gorithm was shown to be similar in precision to human analysis for measuring left ventricular ejection fraction and left ventricular mass but was 186 times faster. In a proof of concept study, Fahmy et al. used U-Net deep convo-luted networks with 150 operational layers to quantify scar volumes in patients with HCM. A strong correlation was observed between the manually and automatically segmented scar volumes. Cardiac magnetic resonance-defined scar regions have gained con-siderable importance and form the basis of some of the ablation strat-egies including scar homogenization and scar dechannelling in ventricular tachycardia (VT) ablation.

These advancements have also paved the way for the concept of targeting fibrotic substrate that can perpetuate rotors, in addition to pulmonary vein isolation in patients with persistent AF.

Advances of ML-aided imaging have set the stage for the devel-opment of several novel concepts in EP including non-invasive local-ization of arrhythmia foci with high precision, personalized virtual heart modelling including simulation of cardiac arrhythmias and con-cept of non-invasive ablation. In parallel with developments in cardiac imaging, further advance-ments have been made in ECG acquisition with the development of body surface mapping (using up to 252 electrodes instead of standard 12 leads). Electrocardiography imaging systems that integrate body surface mapping with non-contrast computed tomography (CT) that simultaneously records electrode location and geometry of cardiac surface can localize focal activation of atrial or ventricular ectopy on the 3D reconstruction of the patient's heart using an inverse solution approach.The Amycard 01C (EP Solutions SA, Yverdonles-Bains,Switzerland)and ECVUE (CardioInsight Technologies Inc., Cleveland, OH, USA) systems are now commercially available and are able to locate atrial and ventricular arrhythmias. As they provide a simultaneous, quasi global view of the entire atrial or ventricular ac-tivation, these systems allow to visualize even AF. Using this technique, focal trigger and rotor sites are identified, which is impossible using the conventional sequential mapping techniques . View into ventricular onset (VIVO, Catheter Precision) is a next-generation non-invasive mapping system that combines knowledge of the exact location of the surface 12-lead ECG stickers with carefully reconstructed cardiac anatomy from either CMR or CT imaging . With the VIVO platform, prediction of the focus of premature ventricular electrical activity and VT focus is correct in 85% and 88% of patients, respectively.

Using a multimodal integrative approach, feasibility of combining body surface mapping, cardiac gated multidetector CT, and/or delayed contrast-enhanced magnetic resonance (MR) imaging on a common platform This approach was useful in understanding complex accessory pathway previously resistant to ablation and to identify rotor trajectories in patients with AF Software (Automatic Detection of Arrhythmic Substrate, ADAS-VT, Galgo Medical SL, Barcelona, Spain), which processes LGE CMR images offline to characterize 3D scar architecture to be merged with electro anatomical mapping (EAM) during the ablation procedure, has been shown to facilitate the ablation procedure.

With the development of methods for non-invasive localization of arrhythmia focus, several groups have reported on their experience of using radiation therapy in patients with mostly ischaemic ventricular arrhythmia. Robinson et al. reported successful utilization of radiotherapy in a cohort of patients with treatment-refractory episodes of VT or cardiomyopathy related to premature ventricular contractions. They identified scar regions using ECG imaging, cardiac anatomical imaging and delivered Focused stereotactic body radiation therapy (SBRT) with marked reduction in arrhythmia burden, reduced use of anti-arrhythmic medication and improved quality of life following therapy. Overall survival was 89% and 72% at the end of 6 and 12months,respectively.

In addition,first-in-man treatment of paroxysmal AF using SBRT in two patients has been reported with the demonstration of safety and efficacy of delivering SBRT lesion set in the left atrium confirmed by presence of fibrosis. Results from these initial pilot studies and case reports are encouraging. However, more robust data are required from larger clinical trials with longer follow-up to show long-term safety of these techniques, which are of great interest but still under evaluation.

Personalized virtual heart modelling—a new paradigm

Considerable advances in cellular modelling technology have paved the way for the development of a computerized human cardiac myo-cyte.68 Virtual ventricular myocytes, with predefined electrophysio-logical properties, and predictable functional changes in response to surroundings including ion channel changes and myocardial ischaemia have been developed. Trayanova et al. envisaged the creation of a computerized but per-sonalized virtual heart mode.

Contrast-enhanced MR images of the patient's heart were used to create near identical geometrical models of the cardiac chambers and were populated with virtual car-diac myocytes with physiological properties pertaining to the cells from a designated location. Previously validated rule-based algo-rithms were applied for fibre orientation to compute heart models. These computed virtual hearts were electrophysiological twins to the patient's heart on which various stimulation protocols could be applied to induce ventricular arrhythmias of different morphologies and identify critical isthmus zones for these arrhythmias.

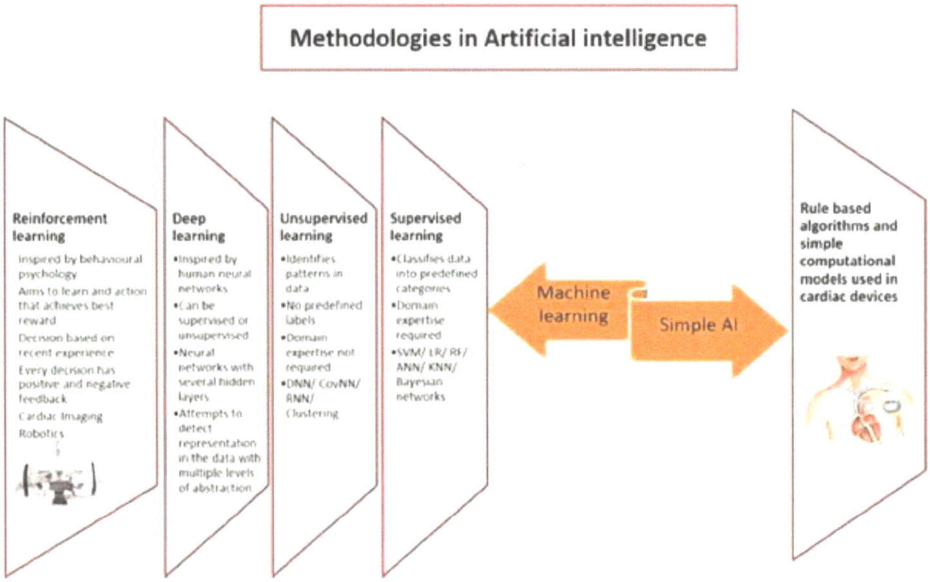

Fig. 10.4 Artificial intelligence methodologies with their individual characteristics. AI, artificial intelligence; ANN, artificial neural network; CovNN, convolutional neural network; DNN, deep neural network; KNN, K-nearest neighbours; LR, logistic regression; RF, random forest; RNN, recurrent neural network; SVM, support vector machine.

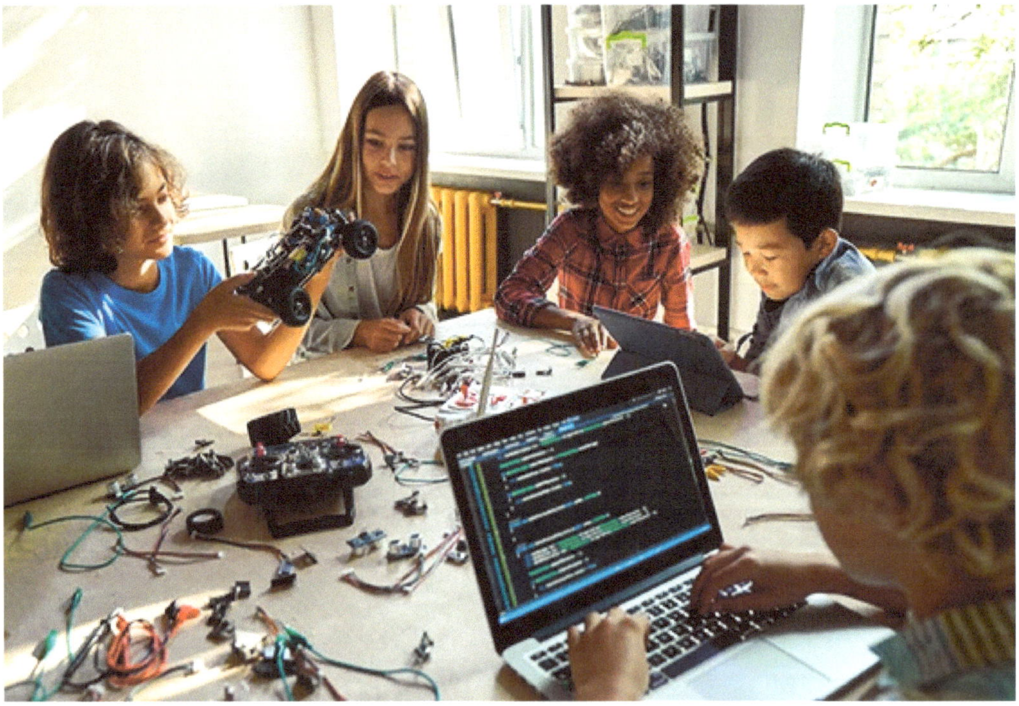

Fig. 10.5 Generative AI opens new horizons and challenges for education. But we urgently need to take action to ensure that new AI technologies are integrated into education on our terms. It is our duty to prioritize safety, inclusion, diversity, transparency and quality — as stated in the UNESCO Recommendation on the Ethics of Artificial Intelligence adopted unanimously by our Member States.Stefania Giannini UNESCO Assistant Director-General for Education

As a proof of concept, this study of virtual heart modelling was used for non-invasive risk assessment of sudden cardiac death in a high-risk population undergoing cardioverter defibrillator implant-ation. The virtual heart arrhythmia risk predictor approach (VARP) was evaluated retrospectively in a cohort of 41 patients executing simulations to evaluate patient specific VT inducibility and found to be superior to other predictors including left ventricular ejection fraction. Predictive capability of this novel targeted approach needs further evaluation in larger studies. Yet another proof of concept study evaluated the use of virtual heart modelling in patients undergoing VT ablation. Virtual hearts were modelled from patients' contrast-enhanced MR images and VT induction carried out as in the VARP study.

Once VT induction was carried out, the optimal ablation strategy was performed virtually. This technique was termed virtual heart arrhythmia ablation targeting (VAAT). When compared retrospectively in 21 patients undergoing VT ablation, it was found to correspond well with real ablation lesions. The VAAT strategy was further tested prospectively in 5 patients undergoing VT ablation in two different centres. VAAT lesions were merged with an EAM system and an ablation was carried out at these sites without further prior mapping. The clinical outcomes for these patients were encouraging with no further VT episodes post-ablation.

Virtual hearts and machine learning in atrial fibrillation

Machine learning methodologies in conjunction with atrial computa-tional models were used to define re-entrant driver locations in AF.80 Segmented LGE CMR scans were used to identify atrial fibrosis in 21 patients with persistent AF. Fibrotic and non-fibrotic regions were identified and were assigned with region-specific tissue properties. Atrial fibrillation was induced using multisite atrial pacing in these vir-tual atrial models. Phase mapping with an unsupervised density-based spatial cluster algorithm was used to define re-entrant driver locations.Over 80% of re-entrant driver locations matched to the fibrosis border zones. The first-in-human clinical study of virtual heart models to guide ablation in patients with persistent AF used personalized atrial geo-metric models created using segmented LGE MR scans done prior to the procedure. Rapid pacing was carried out from 40 uniformly distributed bi-atrial sites. The model response was analysed to determine the optimal ablation lesion set to eliminate all possible persistent re-entrant drivers identified using above mentioned MLmethodologies sustaining AF and other atrial arrhythmias; the opti-mal ablation lesion set created using this approach was called OPTIMA: OPtimal Target Identification via Modelling of Arrhythmogenesis was then loaded onto the EAM mapping system and the ablation was carried out without prior mapping. This was a proof of concept feasibility study and was not designed to evaluate procedure outcomes. In fact, outcomes reported from 10 patients were encouraging with no further recurrence of persistent AF.

In a study combining ML and personalized computational modelling, an ML algorithm was shown to predict AF recurrence post-pulmonary vein isolation in patients with paroxysmal AF. In this proof of concept study, features were derived from patient's pre-pulmonary vein isolation LGE MR images and also from the results of AF simulations carried out on their personalized computational model. Random forests were used for unbiased feature selection, and ten-fold nested cross-validation was used to train, validate, and test quadratic discriminant analysis ML classifier. Most predictive features were used as input to this classifier. This ML algorithm predicted post-pulmonary vein isolation AF recurrence with an average valid-ation sensitivity and specificity of 82% and 89%, respectively,

Intracardiac data and machine learning applications in atrial fibrillation

and a validation AUC of 0.82.Large quantities of intracardiac data are recorded during EP procedures. Recent advances in ML methodologies have encouraged researchers to apply these techniques to the intracardiac electro-grams and EAM data with a view to define extra pulmonary ablation sites in AF. Schilling et al. showed the feasibility of classifying complex frac-tionated atrial electrograms in an objective way using fuzzy decision tree algorithm retrospectively on intracardiac electrograms. Atrial electrograms were classified into four subgroups ranging from non-fractionated with high frequency to continuous activity achieving a correct rate of 81 ± 3%. Electrograms with

Table 10.1 Overview of feature engineering processes employed during development of machine learning methods

Feature engineering	Extraction	Optimization
Definition • Most informative and non-redundant characteristics of data signals • Represented in a numerical form and together form a feature vector • Data represented as features is computationally processed by ML algorithms	• In supervised ML methods feature extraction is done by experts in the domain • In unsupervised and DL methodologies feature engineering is done by the algorithm itself • Features used for cardiac signal analysis—time intervals, morphological amplitudes, areas or distances	• Selection of appropriate features is crucial for the success of ML methodology • Algorithms used for relevant feature identi-fication—particle swarm optimization, etc. • Algorithms used for dimensionality reduction—principal component analysis and linear discriminant analysis

DL, deep learning; ML, machine learning.

Table 10..2 Commonly used machine learning classification algorithms

Algorithm	Learning method	Description	Utility in EP ML
Support vector machine	• Most commonly used supervised learning method	• Used to classify complex non-linear data • Creates 'hyperplane' that non-linearly separates the two classes in a feature space • Good classification and generalization properties	• Arrhythmia classification using heart rate variability • VF detection algorithm in automated external defibrillators
Random Forest	• Supervised learning method	• Ensemble learning methods that combine multiple decision trees (algorithms) • Decision trees arranged in a hierarchical manner • Final prediction derived by calculating the mean or mode of the individual DT's decision	• Classification of ECG beats • CRT outcomes prediction
Bayesian networks	• Supervised learning method	• Graphical structures to represent know-ledge about an uncertain domain • Represent variables and their probabilistic relationships • HMM—one of the frequently used exam-ples of BNs	• Classification of ECG beats • CRT outcomes prediction
Neural networks	• Can be supervised or unsupervised learning method	• Computational model mimicking biologic-al neural networks • Data is propagated in a hierarchical man-ner via nodes in each layer • Input/target pairs are used during model training	• Classifying large amounts of data • Classification of ECG beats
Convolutional neuranetworksl	• Can be supervised or unsupervised learning method	• Evolved form of deep neural networks (multiple hidden layers between input and output) • Convolution layers produce a spatially de-pendent feature for the subsequent layer • Most widely used DL	• For deciphering diseased state footprints in 12-lead ECG • Cardiac imaging

BN, bayesian networks; CRT, cardiac resynchronization therapy; DL, deep learning; ECG, electrocardiogram; EP, electrophysiology; HMM, Hidden Markov Models; ML, machine learning; VF, ventricular fibrillation.

Table 11.3 Diagnostic accuracy of artificial intelligence-aided devices in identifying atrial fibrillation

Study	Device and AI algorithm	Signal analysed	AF detection
The iREAD Study William et al.17	Algorithm using smartphone (Kardia Mobile Cardiac Monitor) and handheld cardiac rhythm recorder vs. physician-interpreted ECG	ECG	96.6% sensitivity and 94.1% specificity for AF detection
HUAWEI Heart Study Guo et al.18 Apple Heart Study Do¨rr et al.19	Wristband/wristwatch-based irregular pulse notification algorithm Smartwatch-based irregular pulsenotifi-cation algorithm vs. subsequent moni-toring with ECG patch	PPG Initial PPG followed by simultaneous PPG and ECG	Positive predictive value of PPG signals being 91.6%(95%CI91.5–91.8%)Smartwatch-based algorithm had a positive pre-dictive value of 0.84 (95% CI 0.76–0.92) for observing AF during the simultaneous moni-toring period
Chen et al.[20]	Smart wristband device enabled by AF-identifying AI algorithm vs. wristband ECG reviewed by physicians	PPG and ECG	Sensitivity, specificity, and accuracy were 88.00%, 96.41%, and 93.27%, respectively, for PPG and 87.33%, 99.20%, and 94.76% for ECG
Wasserlauf et al.[21]	Apple Watch with KardiaBand (enabled by convoluted neural network algorithm) vs. insertable cardiac monitor	ECG	97.5% and 97.7% for episode sensitivity and duration sensitivity, respectively
WATCH AF trial Do¨rr et al.[22]	Smartwatc based algorithm vs. cardiolo-gists' diagnosis by electrocardiography	PPG	Sensitivity of 93.7% (95% CI 89.8–96.4%), specificity of 98.2% (95% CI 95.8–99.4%), and 96.1% accuracy (95% CI 94.0–97.5%)-

AF, atrial fibrillation; AI, artificial intelligence; CI, confidence interval; ECG, electrocardiogram; PPG, photo plethysmography.

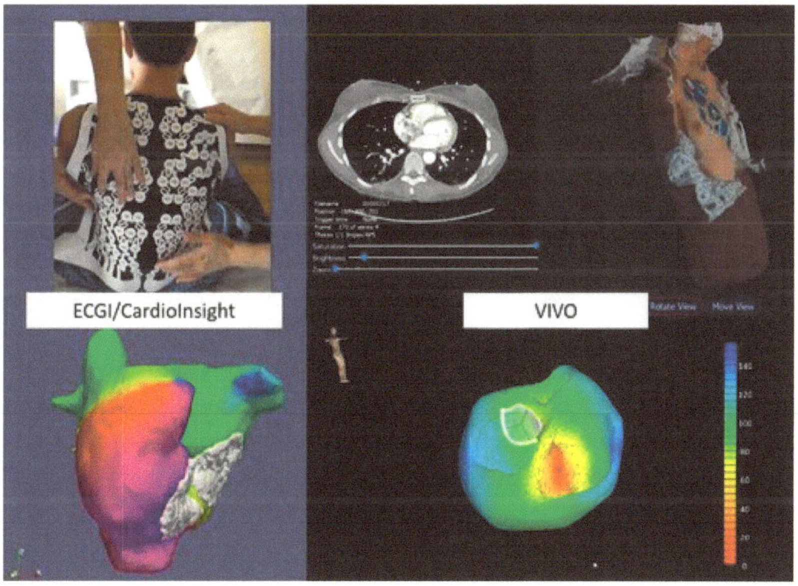

Fig.10.6 Left panel: Example of non-invasive simultaneous mapping of atrial fibrillation of both the right and left atrium using the electrocardiogram imaging technology. Several mechanisms occur in various areas of the atria simultaneously and thereby maintain atrial fibrillation. Right panel: Example of non-invasive simultaneous mapping of ventricular ectopy using the view into ventricular onset technology.

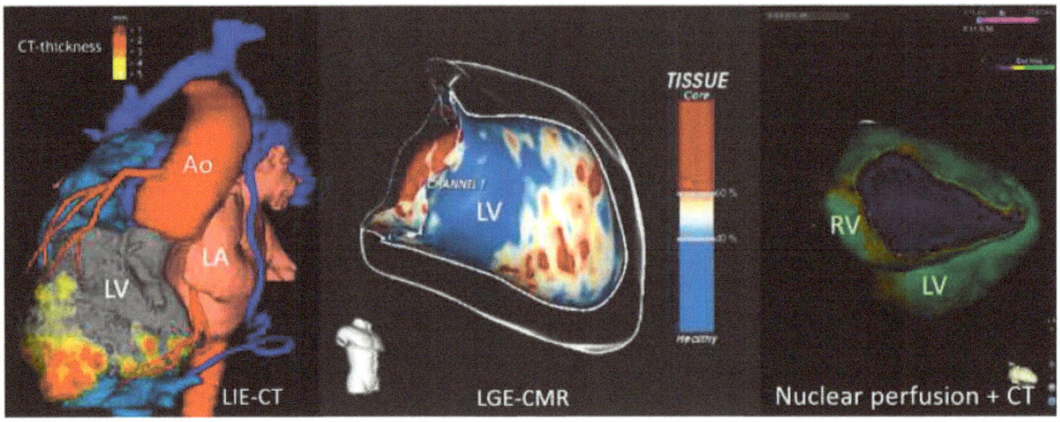

Fig.10.7 Left panel: 3D image information from computed tomography and myocardial thickness in a patient with coronary artery disease and ap-ical scar after myocardial infarction. Middle panel: Image information of late gadolinium enhancement from cardiac magnetic resonance imaging of the left ventricle with identification of the potentially arrhythmogenic channels within the scar responsible for ventricular re-entrant tachycardia. Right panel: Example of perfusion information from functional nuclear imaging superimposed on a contrast computed tomography scan in a patient with arrhythmogenic right ventricular disease. Ao, aorta; CMR, cardiac magnetic resonance; LA, left atrium; LGE, late gadolinium enhancement; LV, left ventricle; RV, right ventricle.

continuous activity were detected correctly 100% of the time.In a proof of concept study, McGillivray et al. developed random forest supervised ML algorithm to locate re-entrant circuits driving AF using indirect feature measurements, derived from electrograms in a simulated model. The model correctly identified 95.4% of drivers in the simulation model.In a recent study, Alhusseini et al.85 developed an ML algorithm to classify intracardiac electrical patterns during AF. They used a convo-luted neural network DL approach to analyse EAM data obtained from bi-atrial sites using basket catheters. Spatial maps of activation were created to identify the presence of rotational activation fea-tures. Algorithm compared well with a team of experts with an ac-curacy of 97.3% when the experts were in unanimous agreement and 85.1% in more difficult instances. Convoluted neural network accur-acy in the test set was similar for locations containing termination sites (95.6%) or otherwise (94.2%). With ML-guided ablation strategies becoming a possibility for the near future, electrophysiologists would need real-time access to inte-grated data from different sources including EAM and 3D cardiac imaging.

Availability of this information with the ability to manipulate the data for better visualization whilst still operating in a sterile field would enhance operator dexterity and procedural efficacy during complex ablations. Holographic visualization of real-time catheter position, cardiac geometry, EAM, and ablation data in an EP lab has been shown to be feasible. Systems to provide augmented reality solutions in EP labs are currently being developed for future use87 and would certainly aid in better and efficient work flow.

Robotics in electrophysiology and potential role of machine learning

To deliver catheter ablation safely to a high degree of precision reducing the impact of operator variability in level of training and technical skill, robotic ablation can be seen as a valuable tool to help improve access to the same level of accuracy in a reproducible fashion.In the field of EP, robotic navigation was introduced 20 years ago. The two concepts proposed were either a mechanical sheath system guiding a conventional ablation catheter via computer-enhanced technique (Hansen & Amigo) or a magnetic platform (Stereotaxis). A more recent contender is another mechanical system, which uses acoustic energy for both imaging and lesion deployment (Vytronus).3Dreconstruction using ultrasound imaging is performed automatically and the robotic system months deploys acoustic energy completely automatically along an operator designed ablation line.First-in-human experience was reported in a cohort of 52 patients with paroxysmal AF undergoing pulmonary vein isolation using low intensity collimated ultrasound (LICU). Acute pulmonary vein isolation was achieved in 77.3% and 94.2% of patients using LICU only and LICU with enhanced software, respectively, with continued freedom from atrial arrhythmia recurrence at 12 months A vast body of evidence has been published for the magnetic navi-gation system (Niobe, Stereotaxis), which in combination with 3D EAM systems (CARTO or ACUTUS) plus 3D image integration, can be applied to all arrhythmias. Feasibility of using an ML algorithm to guide automated electro-anatomical voltage mapping was previously demonstrated using re-mote magnetic navigation system. The ML algorithm used learning from demonstration framework utilizing prior knowledge from ex-pert mapping procedures and Gaussian process model-based active learning.

Non-invasive ML-aided identification of the ablation targets using 3D imaging and personalized heart modelling followed by robotic ab-lation of these pre-defined locations appears to be an exciting pro-spect for the future. This approach, if successful, could limit the number of catheters to a minimum and could be both more time and cost-efficient.

Is artificial intelligence bridging the gaps in arrhythmia care?

Recent research into AI-enabled ECG has rekindled interest into ob-servational-based research. Artificial intelligence-enabled ECG has been shown to identify patients with persistent AF, left ventricular systolic dysfunction, and HCM and the list is likely to grow in time with emerging evidence from ongoing research. This ubiquitous car-diac investigation has a potential to be a powerful screening tool at point of care, an innovation that may have a significant impact on community-based diagnosis of latent cardiac conditions, even more so in the under privileged parts of the world. In an acute setting, AI-enabled ECG may aid in the rapid identification of life threatening electrolyte imbalance and patients at imminent risk of cardiac arrest who may need more intensive moni-toring. Severe restrictions imposed by the recent COVID-19 pan-demic resulted in some of the AI-enabled technologies such as QT interval monitoring using AI-enabled mobile devices, approved by regulatory authorities to see the light of the day in clinical practice.Advancements in sensor technology and wireless communications with ability to link devices overinternet of things have made continuous heart rhythm monitoring feasible, albeit resulting in an exponen-tial increase in data to be analysed. Review of such data by a skilled personnel is nearly impossible due to time and resource constraints. Artificial intelligence solutions can effectively analyse these data in a time and a resource efficient manner. Artificial intelligence-assisted near real-time analysis of data from wearable devices has prompted the contemplation of newer research into novel treatment strategies such as pill in the pocket anticoagulation following an epi-sode of AF.Machine learning algorithms have shown their utility to further personalized patient care by improving existing guidelines, which aid in clinical decision-making regarding anticoagulation in the at-risk population and patient selection for cardiac device therapy.

Superiority of ML methodologies over traditional rule-based algo-rithms in handling big data may facilitate data analysis from multiple data sources to identify the impending risk of life threatening arrhyth-mia or heart failure episodes in a timely manner. Artificial intelligence-enabled technological advancements are aid-ing in arrhythmia focus identification prior to EP procedures. In time, AI-enabled ECG may better contribute to accurate localization of ac-cessory pathway or arrhythmia focus. There is a vast potential for the application of ML methodologies to intracardiac data including EAM, for better characterization of an arrhythmia to aid in selection of the ideal ablation strategy.

Limitations and challenges

Machine learning methodologies are not error free, best example being overfitting,a phenomenon resulting from a disproportionate number of features in comparison to the amount of data in the training set.As a result of overfitting, the ML algorithm performs very well on the training set whilst performing poorly on the test set with poor generalizability.

It has to be appreciated that traditional statistical methods may be superior in analysing lesser amount of data whilst ML offers the ability to handle high computational power to classify large amounts of data efficiently.

Some of the ML methodologies are opaque, and as a consequence, it may not possible to verify how an algorithm arrives at its conclu-sions. This current lack of transparency in methodology, often referred to as black box nature of ML can affect clinicians' confidence when applying ML-based technologies in active clinical decision-making. Defining regulatory guidelines forhese self-learning, non-transparent yet accurate ML methods can be challenging Artificial intelligence is a data science, and hence, the importance of the quality of the data used to train and validate ML algorithms can-not be overstated.

There is a greater need for collaboration and data sharing between research centres to collate large quantities of robust healthy data to improve the generalizability of ML methodolo-gies. This highlights yet another challenge relating to data security and privacy. More transparency about how data are shared and stricteradherence to data management laws is essential in research involving ML methodologies. Increasing use of ML algorithms in clinical decision-making101 is likely to challenge the concept of personal responsibility and a physi-cians fiduciary relationship towards patients, necessitating regula-tory guidelines to clarify the distribution of liability in the event of mishaps involving AI-aided technologies. Cardiologists in the near term are likely to be keen on AI-aided rather than AI-dictated clinical decision-making for patient management.

Abstract

The field of cardiac electrophysiology (EP) had adopted simple artificial intelligence (AI) methodologies for decades. Recent renewed interest in deep learning techniques has opened new frontiers in electrocardiography analysis including signature identification of diseased states. Artificial intelligence advances coupled with simultaneous rapid growth in computational power, sensor technology, and availability of web-based platforms have seen the rapid growth of AI-aided applications and big data research. Changing lifestyles with an expansion of the concept of internet of things and advancements in telecommunication technology have opened doors to population-based detec-tion of atrial fibrillation in ways, which were previously unimaginable. Artificial intelligence-aided advances in 3D cardiac imaging heralded the concept of virtual hearts and the simulation of cardiac arrhythmias. Robotics, completely non-invasive ablation therapy, and the con-cept of extended realities show promise to revolutionize the future of EP.

In this chapter , we discussed the impact of AI and recent technological advances in all aspects of arrhythmia care.

Conclusion

Artificial intelligence has considerable impact on all aspects of patient management in the field of cardiac EP from the identification of ar-rhythmia to therapy (invasively and non-invasively). Simple AI techni-ques have been established in the form of computerized interpretation of electrocardiography and rule-based algorithms for cardiac devices. Recent advances with the use of DL techniques are paving the way for newer research in arrhythmia detection and arrhythmogenic focus identification. The most recent AI-aided advancements in cardiac imaging invigorated the attempts to develop better non-invasive mapping techniques to guide targeted ablation therapies (invasive and non-invasive). This is a new paradigm shift and promises personalized 'state of the art' precision care for patients with complex cardiac arrhythmias. The combination of advanced communication and imaging technologies have helped the rapid adoption of AI techniques and big data research as evidenced by the exponential growth of literature on AI-aided research. It may well be that we are in the midst of an AI-led profound change in patient care.

Bibliography And Acknowledgement

- Acharya UR, Oh SL, Hagiwara Y, Tan JH, Adam M, Gertych A, Tan R. A deep convolutional neural network model to classify heartbeats.ComputBiolMed2017;89:389–396.
- Al'Aref SJ, Anchouche K, Singh G, Slomka PJ, Kolli KK, Kumar A, Pandey M, Maliakal G, van Rosendael AR, Beecy AN, Berman DS, Leipsic J, Nieman K, Andreini D, Pontone G, Schoepf UJ, Shaw LJ, Chang HJ, Narula J, Bax JJ, Guan Y, Min JK. Clinical applications of machine learning in cardiovascular disease and its relevance to cardiacimaging.EurHeartJ2019;40:1975–1986.
- Al-Ahmad A, Grossman JD, Wang PJ. Early experience with a computerized ro-botically controlled catheter system. J Interv Card Electrophysiol 2005;12:199–202. Alhusseini MI, Abuzaid F, Rogers AJ, Zaman JAB, Baykaner T, Clopton P, Bailis P, Zaharia M, Wang PJ, Rappel WJ, Narayan S. Machine learning to classify intra-cardiac electrical patterns during atrial fibrillation: machine learning of atrial fib-rillation. Circ Arrhythm Electrophysiol2020;13:e008160.
- Al-Khatib SM, Stevenson WG, Ackerman MJ, Bryant WJ, Callans DJ, Curtis AB, Deal BJ, Dickfeld T, Field ME, Fonarow GC, Gillis AM, Granger CB, Hammill SC, Hlatky MA, Joglar JA, Kay GN, Matlock DD, Myerburg RJ, Page R. 2017 AHA/ACC/HRS
- Guideline for management of patients with ventricular arrhythmias and the prevention of sudden cardiac death: a report of the American College of Cardiology/American Heart Association Task Force on Clinical Practice Guidelines and the Heart Rhythm Society. JAmCollCardiol2018;72

- Alonso-Atienza F, Morgado E, Ferna´ndez-Martı´nez L, Garcı´a-Alberola A, Rojo-lvarez JL. Detection of life-threatening arrhythmias using feature selection and support vector machines. IEEE Trans Biomed Eng 2014;61:832–840.
- Aronis KN, Ali RL, Liang JA, Zhou S, Trayanova N. Understanding AF mecha-nisms through computational modelling and simulations. ArrhythmElectrophysiolRev2019;8:210–219.
- Attia ZI, Friedman PA, Noseworthy PA, Lopez-Jimenez F, Ladewig DJ, Satam G, Pellikka PA, Munger TM, Asirvatham SJ, Scott CG, Carter RE, Kapa S. Age and sex estimation using artificial intelligence from standard 12-lead ECGs. Circ Arrhythmia Electrophysiol 2019;12:
- Attia ZI, Kapa S, Lopez-Jimenez F, McKie PM, Ladewig DJ, Satam G, Pellikka PA, Enriquez-Sarano M, Noseworthy PA, Munger TM, Asirvatham SJ, Scott CG, Carter RE, Friedman PA. Screening for cardiac contractile dysfunction using an artificial intelligence-enabled electrocardiogram.NatMed2019;25:70–74.
- Attia ZI, Noseworthy PA, Lopez-Jimenez F, Asirvatham SJ, Deshmukh AJ, Gersh BJ, Carter RE, Yao X, Rabinstein AA, Erickson BJ, Kapa S, Friedman P. An artifi-cial intelligence-enabled ECG algorithm for the identification of patients with atrial fibrillation during sinus rhythm: a retrospective analysis of outcome pre-diction. Lancet2019;394:861–867.
- Attia ZI, Sugrue A, Asirvatham SJ, Ackerman MJ, Kapa S, Friedman PA, Noseworthy P. Noninvasive assessment of dofetilide plasma concentration using a deep learning (neural network) analysis of the surfaceelectrocardio-gramproof ofconceptstudy.PLoSOne2018;13:e0201059.
- Avendi MR, Kheradvar A, Jafarkhani H. A combined deep-learning and deformable-model approach to fully automatic segmentation of the left ven-tricle in cardiac MRI. Med Image Anal2016;30:108–119.
- Bertagnolli L, Torri F, Paetsch I, Jahnke C, Hindricks G, Arya A, Dinov B. Cardiac magnetic resonance imaging for coregistration during ablation of ische-mic ventricular tachycardia for identification of the critical isthmus.Heart Rhythm Case Rep2018;4:70–72.
- Bhaskaran A, Downar E, Chauhan VS, Lindsay P, Nair K, Ha A, Hope A, Nanthakumar K. Electroanatomical mapping–guided stereotactic radiotherapy for right ventricular tachycardia storm. HeartRhythm Case Rep 2019;5:590–592.
- Bhuva AN, Bai W, Lau C, Davies RH, Ye Y, Bulluck H, McAlindon E, Culotta V, Swoboda PP, Captur G, Treibel TA, Augusto JB, Knott KD, Seraphim A, Cole GD, Petersen SE, Edwards NC, Greenwood JP, Bucciarelli-Ducci C, Hughes AD, Rueckert D, Moon JC, Manisty C. A multicenter, scan-rescan, human and machine learning CMR study to test generalizability and precision in imaging biomarker analysis. CircCardiovascImaging2019;12:
- Boyle PM, Zghaib T, Zahid S, Ali RL, Deng D, Franceschi WH, Hakim JB, Murphy MJ, Prakosa A, Zimmerman SL, Ashikaga H, Marine JE, Kolandaivelu A, Nazarian S, Spragg DD, Calkins H, Trayanova N. Computationally guided personalized tar-geted ablation of persistent atrial fibrillation.Nat Biomed Eng2 019;3:870–879.
- Chen E, Jiang J, Su R, Gao M, Zhu S, Zhou J, Huo Y. A new smart wristband equipped with an artificial intelligence algorithm to detect atrial fibrillation. Heart Rhythm 2020;17:847–853.
- Cheniti G, Puyo S, Martin CA, Frontera A, Vlachos K, Takigawa M, Bourier F, Kitamura T, Lam A, Dumas-Pommier C, Pillois X, Pambrun T, Duchateau J, Klotz N, Denis A, Derval N, Cochet H, Sacher F, Dubois R, Jais P, Hocini M, Haissaguerre M. Noninvasive mapping and electrocardiographic imaging in atrial and ventricular arrhythmias (CardioInsight). Card Electrophysiol Clin 2019;11: .459–471.
- Cuculich PS, Schill MR, Kashani R, Mutic S, Lang A, Cooper D, Faddis M, Gleva M, Noheria A, Smith TW, Hallahan D, Rudy Y, Robinson CG. Noninvasive car-diac radiation for ablation of ventricular tachycardia. N Engl J Med 2017;377: 2325–2336.
- Desteghe L, Raymaekers Z, Lutin M, Vijgen J, Dilling-Boer D, Koopman P, Schurmans J, Vanduynhoven P, Dendale P, Heidbuchel H. Performance of hand-held electrocardiogram devices to detect atrial fibrillation in a cardiology and geriatric wardsetting.Europace2017;19:29–39.
- Dissanayake T, Rajapaksha Y, Ragel R, Nawinne I. An ensemble learning ap-proach for electrocardiogram sensor based human emotion recognition.Sensors2019;19:4995.
- Do¨rr M, Nohturfft V, Brasier N, Bosshard E, Djurdjevic A, Gross S, Raichle CJ, Rhinisperger M, Sto¨ckli R, Eckstein J. The WATCH AF trial: SmartWATCHes for detection of atrial fibrillation. JACC Clin Electrophysiol2019;5:199–208.
- Ernst S, Babu-Narayan SV, Keegan J, Horduna I, Lyne J, Till J, Kilner PJ, Pennell D, Rigby ML, Gatzoulis MA. Remote-controlled magnetic navigation and abla-tion with 3D image integration as an alternative approach in patients with intra-atrial baffle anatomy. Circ Arrhythmia Electrophysiol 2012;5:131–139.
- Ernst S, Ouyang F, Linder C, Hertting K, Stahl F, Chun J, Hachiya H, Ba¨nsch D, Antz M, Kuck KH. Initial experience with remote catheter ablation using a novel magnetic navigation system: magnetic remote catheter ablation. Circulation 2004; 109:1472–1475.
- Faddis MN, Blume W, Finney J, Hall A, Rauch J, Sell J, Bae KT, Talcott M, Lindsay B. Novel, magnetically guided catheter for endocardial mapping and radiofrequency catheter ablation. Circulation2002;106:2980–2985.
- Fahmy AS, El-Rewaidy H, Nezafat M, Nakamori S, Nezafat R. Automated ana-lysis of cardiovascular magnetic resonance myocardial native T1 mapping images using fully convolutional neural networks. J Cardiovasc Magn Reson 2019;21:7.
- Fahmy AS, Neisius U, Chan RH, Rowin EJ, Manning WJ, Maron MS, Nezafat R. Three-dimensional deep convolutional neural networks for automated myocardial scar quantification in hypertrophic cardiomyopathy: amulticenter multivendor study. Radiology2020;294:52–60.
- Fahmy AS, Rausch J, Neisius U, Chan RH, Maron MS, Appelbaum E, Menze B, Nezafat R. Automated cardiac MR scar quantification in hypertrophic cardiomy-opathy using deep convolutional neural networks. JACC Cardiovasc Imaging 2018;11:1917–1918.
- Fan YY, Li YG, Li J, Cheng WK, Shan ZL, Wang YT, Guo Y. Diagnostic performance of a smart device with photoplethysmography technology for atrial fibrillation detec-tion: pilot study (Pre-mAFA II Registry). JMIR Mhealth Uhealth 2019;7:e11437.
- Feeny AK, Rickard J, Patel D, Toro S, Trulock KM, Park CJ, LaBarbera MA, Varma N, Niebauer MJ, Sinha S, Gorodeski EZ, Grimm RA, Ji X, Barnard J, Madabhushi A, Spragg DD, Chung M. Machine learning prediction of response to cardiac resynchronization therapy: improvement versus current guidelines. Circ Arrhythm Electrophysiol2019;12:e00731625.
- Feng Y, Guo Z, Dong Z, Zhou XY, Kwok KW, Ernst S, Lee SL. An efficient car-diac mapping strategy for radiofrequency catheter ablation with active learning. Int J Comput Assist Radiol Surg 2017;12:1199–1207.
- Figuera C, Irusta U, Morgado E, Aramendi E, Ayala U, Wik L, Kramer-Johansen J, Eftestøl T, Alonso-Atienza F. Machine learning techniques for the detection of shockable rhythms in automated external defibrillators. PLoS One 2016;11:e0159654.

- Galloway CD, Valys AV, Shreibati JB, Treiman DL, Petterson FL, Gundotra VP, Albert DE, Attia ZI, Carter RE, Asirvatham SJ, Ackerman MJ, Noseworthy PA, Dillon JJ, Friedman P. Development and validation of a deep-learning model to screen for hyperkalemia from the electrocardiogram. JAMA Cardiol 2019;4: 428–436.
- Goldenthal IL, Sciacca RR, Riga T, Bakken S, Baumeister M, Biviano AB, Dizon JM, Wang D, Wang KC, Whang W, Hickey KT, Garan H. Recurrent atrial fibril-lation/flutter detection after ablation or cardioversion using the AliveCor KardiaMobile device: iHEART results. Cardiovasc Electrophysiol 2019;30: 2220–2228.
- Goldstein BA, Navar AM, Carter RE. Moving beyond regression techniques in cardiovascular risk prediction: applying machine learning to address analytic challenges. Eur Heart J 2017;38:1805–1814. Grosan C, Abraham A. Intelligent systems. In: Rule-Based Expert Systems. ISRL. Vol. 17. Berlin, Heidelberg: Springer-Verlag;2011.p.149–187.
- Guo Y, Wang H, Zhang H, Liu T, Liang Z, Xia Y, Yan L, Xing Y, Shi H, Li S, Liu Y, Liu F, Feng M, Chen Y, Lip GYH; MAFA II Investigators. Mobile photoplethys-mographic technology to detect atrial fibrillation. J Am Coll Cardiol 2019;74: 2365–2375.
- Han L, Askari M, Altman RB, Schmitt SK, Fan J, Bentley JP, Narayan SM, Turakhia MP. Atrial fibrillation burden signature and near-term prediction of stroke: a machine learning analysis. Circ Cardiovasc Qual Outcomes 2019;12: e005595.
- Hannun AY, Rajpurkar P, Haghpanahi M, Tison GH, Bourn C,TurakhiaMP, Ng AY. Cardiologist-level arrhythmia detection and classification in ambulatory electrocardiograms using adeepneuralnetwork.NatMed2019;25:65–69.
- Himmelreich JCL, Karregat EPM, Lucassen WAM, van Weert HCPM, de Groot JR, Handoko ML, Nijveldt R, Harskamp R. Diagnostic accuracy of a smartphone-operated, single-lead electrocardiography device for detection of rhythm and conduction abnormalities in primary care. Ann Fam Med 2019;17: 403–411
- Howard JP, Fisher L, Shun-Shin MJ, Keene D, Arnold AD, Ahmad Y, Cook CM, Moon JC, Manisty CH, Whinnett ZI, Cole GD, Rueckert D, Francis DP. Cardiac rhythm device identification using neural networks. JACC Clin Electrophysiol 2019; 5:576–586.
- Hu SY, Santus E, Forsyth AW, Malhotra D, Haimson J, Chatterjee NA, Kramer DB, Barzilay R, Tulsky JA, Lindvall C. Can machine learning improve patient se-lection for cardiac resynchronization therapy? PLoSOne2019;14:
- Kalscheur MM, Kipp RT, Tattersall MC, Mei C, Buhr KA, DeMets DL, Field ME, Eckhardt LL, Page C. Machine learning algorithm predicts cardiac resynchroniza-tion therapy outcomes: lessons from the COMPANION trial. Circ Arrhythm Electrophysiol 2018;11
- Kim EJ, Davogustto G, Stevenson WG, John RM. Non-invasive cardiac radiation for ablation of ventricular tachycardia: A new therapeutic paradigm in electro-physiology. Arrhythmia Electrophysiol Rev 2018;7:8–10.
- Ko W-Y, Siontis KC, Attia ZI, Carter RE, Kapa S, Ommen SR, Demuth SJ, Ackerman MJ, Gersh BJ, Arruda-Olson AM, Friedman PA, Noseworthy P. Detection of hyper-trophic cardiomyopathy using a convolutional neural network-enabled electro-cardiogram. J Am Coll Cardiol 2020;75:722–733.
- Koivuma¨ki JT, Korhonen T, Tavi P. Impact of sarcoplasmic reticulum calcium re-lease on calcium dynamics and action potential morphology in human atrial myocytes: a computational study. PLoS Comput Biol 2011;7:e1001067.
- Kotu LP, Engan K, Skretting K, Ma°løy F, Ørn S, Woie L, Eftestøl T. Probability mapping of scarred myocardium using texture and intensity features in CMR images. Biomed Eng Online 2013;12:91.
- Krittanawong C, Johnson KW, Rosenson RS, Wang Z, Aydar M, Baber U, Min JK, Tang WHW, Halperin JL, Narayan SM. Deep learning for cardiovascular medicine: a practical primer. Eur Heart J 2019;40:2058–2073.
- Krittanawong C, Rogers AJ, Johnson KW, Wang Z, Turakhia MP, Halperin JL, Narayan SM. Integration of novel monitoring devices with machine learning tech-nology for scalable cardiovascular management. Nat Rev Cardiol 2021;18:75–91.
- Lascano EC, Said M, Vittone L, Mattiazzi A, Mundi~na-Weilenmann C, Negroni J. Role of CaMKII in post acidosis arrhythmias: a simulation study using a human myocyte model. J Mol Cell Cardiol 2013;60:172–183.
- Lau JK, Lowres N, Neubeck L, Brieger DB, Sy RW, Galloway CD, Albert DE, Freedman S. iPhone ECG application for community screening to detect silent atrial fibrillation: a novel technology to prevent stroke. Int J Cardiol 2013;165:193–194.
- Leiner T, Rueckert D, Suinesiaputra A, Baeßler B, Nezafat R, I sgum I, Young AA. Machine learning in cardiovascular magnetic resonance: basic concepts and applications. J Cardiovasc Magn Reson 2019;21:61.
- Li Q, Rajagopalan C, Clifford G. Ventricular fibrillation and tachycardia classifica-tion using a machine learning approach. IEEE Trans Biomed Eng 2014;61: 1607–1613.
- Li Y, Bisera J, Weil MH, Member S, Tang W. An algorithm used for ventricular fibrillation detection without interrupting chest compression. IEEE Trans Biomed Eng 2012;59:78–86.
- Loo BW, Soltys SG, Wang L, Lo A, Fahimian BP, Iagaru A, Norton L, Shan X, Gardner E, Fogarty T, Maguire P, Al-Ahmad A, Zei P. Stereotactic ablative radiotherapy for the treatment of refractory cardiac ventricular arrhythmia. Circ Arrhythmia Electrophysiol 2015;8:748–750.
- Lowres N, Neubeck L, Salkeld G, Krass I, McLachlan AJ, Redfern J, Bennett AA, Briffa T, Bauman A, Martinez C, Wallenhorst C, Lau JK, Brieger DB, Sy RW, Freedman S. Feasibility and cost-effectiveness of stroke prevention through community screening for atrial fibrillation using iPhone ECG in pharmacies. The SEARCH-AF study. Thromb Haemost2014;111:1167–1176.
- Marques E, Filho DS, Fernandes FDA, Lacerda C, Soares DA, Seixas L, Augusto A, Sarmet MD, Gismondi RA, Mesquita ET, Mesquita CT. Artificial intelligence in cardiology: concepts, tools and challenges —"the horse is the one who runs, you must be the jockey". Arq Bras Cardiol020;114:718–725.
- Martin-Isla C, Campello VM, Izquierdo C, Raisi-Estabragh Z, Baeßler B, Petersen SE, Lekadir K. Image-based cardiac diagnosis with machine learning: a review. Front Cardiovasc Med 2020;7:1.
- McGillivray MF, Cheng W, Peters NS, Christensen K. Machine learning methods for locating re-entrant drivers from electrograms in a model of atrial fibrillation. R Soc Open Sci 2018;5:172434.
- Misra S, van Dam P, Chrispin J, Assis F, Keramati A, Kolandaivelu A, Berger R, Tandri H. Initial validation of a novel ECGI system for localization of premature ventricular contractions and ventricular tachycardia in structurally normal and abnormal hearts. J Electrocardiol 2018;51:801–808.
- Moore J. The Dartmouth College Artificial Intelligence Conference: the nextfiftyyears.AIMag2006;27:87–91.
- Nguyen MT, Nguyen BV, Kim K. Deep feature learning for sudden cardiac ar-rest detection in automated external defibrillators. Sci Rep 2018;8:17196.

- Nygren A, Fiset C, Firek L, Clark JW, Lindblad DS, Clark RB, Giles WR. Mathematical model of an adult human atrial cell: the role of Kþ currents in repolarization. Circ Res 1998;82:63–81.
- O'Hara T, Vira´g L, Varro´ A, Rudy Y. Simulation of the undiseased human car-diac ventricular action potential: model formulation and experimental valid-ation. PLoS Comput Biol 2011;7:e1002061.
- Petersen SE, Abdulkareem M, Leiner T. Artificial intelligence will transform car-diac imaging—opportunities and challenges. Front Cardiovasc Med 2019;6:133.
- Porumb M, Stranges S, Pescape` A, Pecchia L. Precision medicine and artificial in-telligence: a pilot study on deep learning for hypoglycemic events detection based on ECG. Sci Rep 2020;10:170.
- Prakosa A, Arevalo HJ, Deng D, Boyle PM, Nikolov PP, Ashikaga H, Blauer JJE, Ghafoori E, Park CJ, Blake RC 3rd, Han FT, MacLeod RS, Halperin HR, Callans DJ, Ranjan R, Chrispin J, Nazarian S, Trayanova N. Personalized virtual-heart technology for guiding the ablation of infarct-related ventricular tachycardia. Nat BiomedEng2018;2:732–740.
- Qian PC, Azpiri JR, Assad J, Gonzales Aceves EN, Cardona Ibarra CE, de la Pena C, Hinojosa M, Wong D, Fogarty T, Maguire P, Jack A, Gardner EA, Zei PC. Noninvasive stereotactic radioablation for the treatment of atrial fibrilla-tion: first-in-man experience. J Arrhythmia2020;36:67–74.
- Qin C, Schlemper J, Caballero J, Price AN, Hajnal JV, Rueckert D. Convolutional recurrent neural networks for dynamic MR image reconstruc-tion. IEEE Trans Med Imaging 2019;38:280–290.
- Reddy VY, Neuzil P, Malchano ZJ, Vijaykumar R, Cury R, Abbara S, Weichet J, McPherson CD, Ruskin JN. View-synchronized robotic image-guided therapy for atrial fibrillation ablation: experimental validation and clinical feasibility. Circulation 2007;115:2705–2714.
- Reed MJ, Grubb NR, Lang CC, O'Brien R, Simpson K, Padarenga M, Grant A, Tuck S, Keating L, Coffey F, Jones L, Harris T, Lloyd G, Gagg J, Smith JE, Coats T.Multi-centre randomised controlled trial of a smartphone-based event re-corder alongside standard care versus standard care for patients presenting to the emergency department with palpitations and pre-syncope: the IPED (Investigation of Palpitations in the ED) study. EClinicalMedicine 2019;8:37–46.
- Robinson CG, Samson PP, Moore KMS, Hugo GD, Knutson N, Mutic S, Goddu SM, Lang A, Cooper DH, Faddis M, Noheria A, Smith TW, Woodard PK, Gropler RJ, Hallahan DE, Rudy Y, Cuculich PS. Phase I/II trial of electrophysiology-guided noninvasive cardiac radioablation for ventricular tachycardia. Circulation2019;139:313–321.
- Sana F, Isselbacher EM, Singh JP, Heist EK, Pathik B, Armoundas A. Wearable devices for ambulatory cardiac monitoring: JACC state-of-the-art review. JAm Coll Cardiol 2020;75:1582–1592.
- Saucerman JJ, Healy SN, Belik ME, Puglisi JL, McCulloch A. Proarrhythmic con-sequences of a KCNQ1 AKAP-binding domain mutation: computational models of whole cells and heterogeneous tissue.CircRes2004;95:1216–1224.
- Scara` A, Sciarra L, De Ruvo E, Borrelli A, Grieco D, Palama` Z, Golia P, De Luca L, Rebecchi M, Calo` L. Safety and feasibility of atrial fibrillation ablation using AmigoRV system versus manual approach: a pilot study. Indian Pacing Electrophysiol J 2018;18:61–67.
- Schilling C, Keller M, Scherr D, Oesterlein T, Haı¨ssaguerre M, Schmitt C, Do¨ssel O, Luik A. Fuzzy decision tree to classify complex fractionated atrial electrograms. Biomed Tech Schla¨pfer J, Wellens HJ. Computer-interpreted electrocardiograms benefits and limitations. J Am Coll Cardiol 2017;70:1183–1192.
- Schlemper J, Caballero J, Hajnal JV, Price AN, Rueckert D. A deep cascade of convolutional neural networks for dynamic MR image reconstruction. IEEE Trans Med Imaging 2018;37:491–503.
- Scholz EP, Seidensaal K, Naumann P, Andre´ F, Katus HA, Debus J. Risen from the dead: cardiac stereotactic ablative radiotherapy as last rescue in a patient with refractory ventricular fibrillation storm. HeartRhythm Case Rep 2019;5: 329–332.
- Shade JK, Ali RL, Basile D, Popescu D, Akhtar T, Marine JE, Spragg DD, Calkins H, Trayanova N. Pre-procedure application of machine learning and mechanistic simulations predicts likelihood of paroxysmal atrial fibrillation recurrence fol-lowing pulmonary vein isolation. Circ Arrhythm Electrophysiol 2020;13:e008213.
- Silva JNA, Southworth M, Raptis C, Silva J. Emerging applications of virtual real-ity in cardiovascular medicine. JACC Basic Transl Sci2018;3:420–430.
- Southworth MK, Silva JR, Silva JNA. Use of extended realities in cardiology. Trends Cardiovasc Med 2020;30:143–148.
- Stavrakis S, Stoner JA, Kardokus J, Garabelli PJ, Po SS, Lazzara R. Intermittent vs. Continuous Anticoagulation theRapy in patiEnts with Atrial Fibrillation (iCARE-AF): a randomized pilot study. J Interv Card Electrophysiol 2017;48:51–60.
- Tarakji KG, Wazni OM, Callahan T, Kanj M, Hakim AH, Wolski K, Wilkoff BL, Saliba W, Lindsay B. Using a novel wireless system for monitoring patients after the atrial fibrillation ablation procedure: the iTransmit study. Heart Rhythm 2015;12:554–559.
- Tison GH, Sanchez JM, Ballinger B, Singh A, Olgin JE, Pletcher MJ, Vittinghoff E, Lee ES, Fan SM, Gladstone RA, Mikell C, Sohoni N, Hsieh J, Marcus G. Passive detection of atrial fibrillation using a commerciallyavailable smart watch.JAMA Cardiol 2018;3:409–416.
- Trayanova NA. How personalized heart modeling can help treatment of lethal arrhythmias: a focus on ventricular tachycardia ablation strategies in post-infarction patients. Wiley Interdiscip Rev Syst Biol Med 2020;12:e147
- Tsyganov A, Wissner E, Metzner A, Mironovich S, Chaykovskaya M, Kalinin V, Chmelevsky M, Lemes C, Kuck K. Mapping of ventricular arrhythmias using a novel noninvasive epicardial and endocardial electrophysiology system. J Electrocardiol 2018;51:92–98.
- Turagam MK, Petru J, Neuzil P, Kakita K, Kralovec S, Harari D, Phillips P, Piazza D, Whang W, Dukkipati SR, Reddy V. Automated noncontact ultrasound imag-ing and ablation system for the treatment of atrial fibrillation: outcomes of the first-in-human VALUE trial. Circ Arrhythm Electrophysiol 2020;13:e007917
- Turing A. Computing machinery and intelligence. Mind 1950;LIX:433–460.
- Wasserlauf J, You C, Patel R, Valys A, Albert D, Passman R. Smartwatch per-formance for the detection and quantification of atrial fibrillation. Circ Arrhythmia Electrophysiol 2019;12:e006834.
- William AD, Kanbour M, Callahan T, Bhargava M, Varma N, Rickard J, Saliba W, Wolski K, Hussein A, Lindsay BD, Wazni OM, Tarakji KG. Assessing the accur-acy of an automated atrial fibrillation detection algorithm using smartphone technology: the iREAD study. Heart Rhythm 2018;15:1561–1565.
- Zahid S, Cochet H, Boyle PM, Schwarz EL, Whyte KN, Vigmond EJ, Dubois R, Hocini M, Haı¨ssaguerre M, Jaı¨s P, Trayanova N. Patient-derived models link re-entrant driver localization in atrial fibrillation to fibrosis spatial pattern. Cardiovasc Res 2016;110:443–454.

CHAPTER 11

Ocular images-based Artificial Intelligence In Diagnosis of Systemic Diseases Including Cardiovascular Ailments

Artificial intelligence (AI) is intelligence—perceiving, synthesizing, and inferring information—demonstrated by computers, as opposed to intelligence displayed by humans or by other animals. "Intelligence" encompasses the ability to learn and to reason, to generalize, and to infer meaning.Example tasks in which this is done include speech recognition, computer vision, translation between (natural) languages, as well as other mappings of inputs. AI applications include advanced web search engines (e.g., Google Search), recommendation systems (used by YouTube, Amazon, and Netflix), understanding human speech (such as Siri and Alexa), self-driving cars (e.g., Waymo), generative or creative tools (ChatGPT and AI art), automated decision-making, and competing at the highest level in strategic game systems (such as chess and Go). This has changed the purchasing process, being the AI application functions a mediator between the consumer, product, and brand by providing personalized recommendations based on previous consumer purchasing decisions. As machines become increasingly capable, tasks considered to require "intelligence" are often removed from the definition of AI, a phenomenon known as the AI effect. For instance, optical character recognition is frequently excluded from things considered to be AI, having become a routine technology Artificial intelligence was founded as an academic discipline in 1956, and in the years since it has experienced several waves of optimism, followed by disappointment and the loss of funding (known as an "AI winter"), followed by new approaches, success, and renewed funding. AI research has tried and discarded many different approaches, including simulating the brain, modeling human problem solving, formal logic, large databases of knowledge and imitating animal behavior.

In the first decades of the 21st century, highly mathematical and statistical machine learning has dominated the field, and this technique has proved highly successful, helping to solve many challenging problems throughout industry and academia. The various sub-fields of AI research are centered around particular goals and the use of particular tools. The traditional goals of AI research include reasoning, knowledge representation, planning, learning, natural language processing, perception, and the ability to move and manipulate objects.[a] General intelligence (the ability to solve an arbitrary problem) is among the field's long-term goals. To solve these problems, AI researchers have adapted and integrated a wide range of problem-solving techniques, including search and mathematical optimization, formal logic, artificial neural networks, and methods based on statistics, probability, and economics. AI also draws upon computer science, psychology, linguistics, philosophy, and many other fields.The field was founded on the assumption that human intelligence "can be so precisely described that a machine can be made to simulate it".[b] This raised philosophical arguments about the mind and the ethical consequences of creating artificial beings endowed with human-like intelligence; these issues have previously been explored by myth, fiction (science fiction), and philosophy since antiquity.Computer scientists and philosophers have since suggested that AI may become an existential risk to humanity if its rational capacities are not steered towards goals beneficial to humankind. [c] Economists have frequently highlighted the risks of redundancies from AI, and speculated about unemployment if there is no adequate social policy for full employment. The term artificial intelligence has also been criticized for overhyping AI's true technological capabilities

In Ayurvedic and TCM ,much stress had been layed in the examination of eyes for not only diagnosis of eye diseases but also many systemic ailments.

Chakshu- Eyes: (Changes in the eye condition are indicative of many health conditions. A big whitish slow moving eye is indicative of kapha, a sharp bright, moist pinkish eye indicative of pitta, and a small flickering, dry, dusky and pigmented eye is indicative of vata. The shape of the eyes reveal the nature of the person's original constitution. Also on examination, the eyes reveal what is the nature of the ailment and the doshas responsible for it.

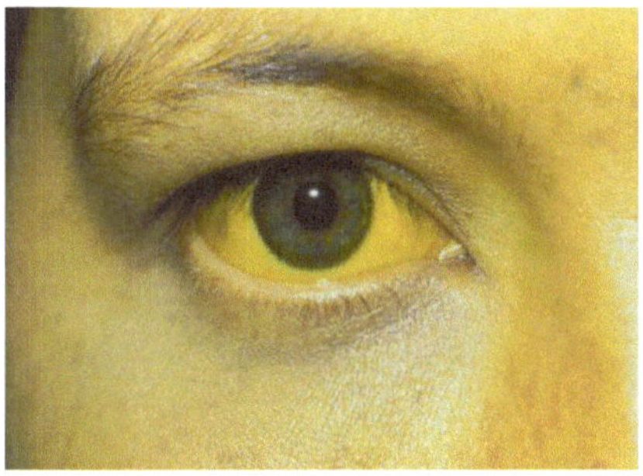

Fig 11.1 Showing face and eyes examination of a patient with jaundice in TCM in a patient with liver disease.

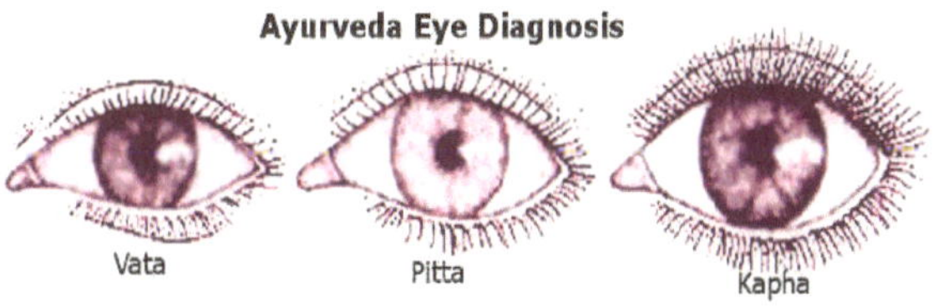

Fig 11.2 Changes in eyes in tridosha imbalance

Iriscopic Examination with TCM

- Iriscope is a diagnostic tool used to detect underlying signs of developing disease to recognize health problems at their earliest stages and to suggest ways to keep disease from developing.
- Safe, non-invasive and painless
- Analysis body constitutional strengths and weaknesses and nutritional deficiencies.
- Detect areas of injury, inflammation or degeneration and accumulation of toxins.
- Find emotional issues.
- Detect precancerous cell which may not be detected from western examination
- High percentage of accuracy in terms of diagnosis
- Right side reflects organs at right side such as Liver, Kidney etc and left side reflects organs at left side such as Heart, Spleen, Kidney etc.

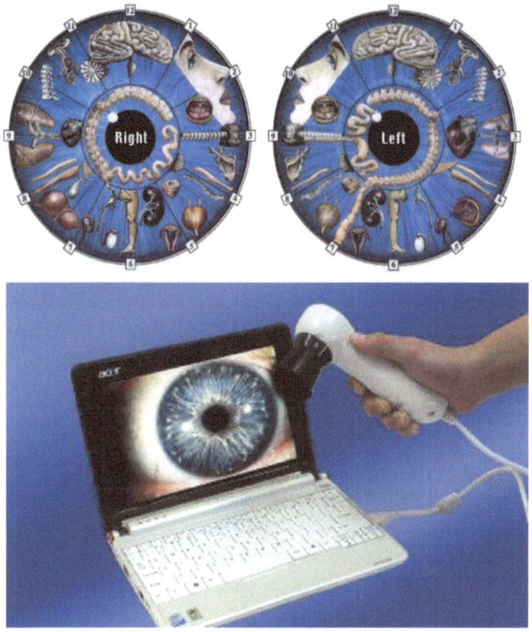

Fig.11.3 (Upper panel) shows diagnostic tool used for iris and (lower) localization of different bodly organs for detection of any developing disease .

artificial intelligence (AI), Ability of a machine to perform tasks thought to require human intelligence. Typical applications include game playing, language translation, expert systems, and robotics. Although pseudo-intelligent machinery dates back to antiquity, the first glimmerings of true intelligence awaited the development of digital computers in the 1940s. AI, or at least the semblance of intelligence, has developed in parallel with computer processing power, which appears to be the main limiting factor. Early AI projects, such as playing chess and solving mathematical problems, are now seen as trivial compared to visual pattern recognition, complex decision making, and the use of natural language

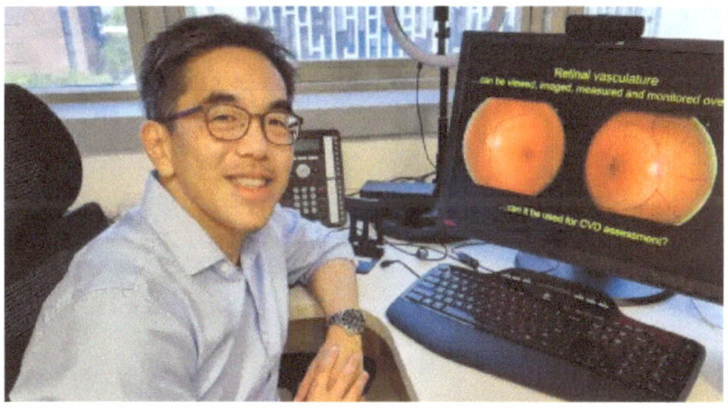

Fig.11.4 The application of AI to retinal image analysis may allow physicians, in milliseconds, to predict the risk for specific systemic diseases, according to Tien Yin Wong, MD, PhD

Artificial Intelligence (AI), which sprung from Alan Turing's paper in 1950, has revolutionized numerous real-world industries, such as translation, natural language processing, and image recognition after decades of development; and medicine is no exception. Machine learning (ML) and its important subset deep learning (DL) achieved prominent performance in multiple tasks of medical image processing: classification, object detection, tracking, and semantic segmentation. Powered by DL, AI is now used as a classifier and screening tool in some real-time in-vivo imaging processes, and also provides referral advice and reference diagnostics in image-centric specialties, such as ophthalmology,radiology, dermatology and cardiology. In ophthalmology, several AI-based diagnostic platforms based on retinal imaging such as IDx-DR and EyeArt AI Screening System for diabetic retinopathy (DR) have shown great application advantages in clinical practice.

To date, the US Foodand Drug Administration (FDA) has approved more than 300 AI medical products, and ophthalmic disease screening applications are among the first to be approved. Given the rich information on pathological changes and accessibility of retinal images in primary care settings, retinal imaging-based AI models are widely used for detecting and predicting diseases such as type 2 diabetes mellitus (T2DM),4 cardiovascular diseases (CVD), hepatobiliary diseases,and chronic kidney disease (CKD)

Detection of Cardiocerebral Vascular Diseases and Risk Stratification

Detection of Retinal Microvascular Morphological Parameters for Stratification Certain visible changes in the retinal arterioles, such as vessel caliber , bi-furcation, or tortuosity , have been highly valuable for suggesting that altered arteriolar function may exist throughout the body

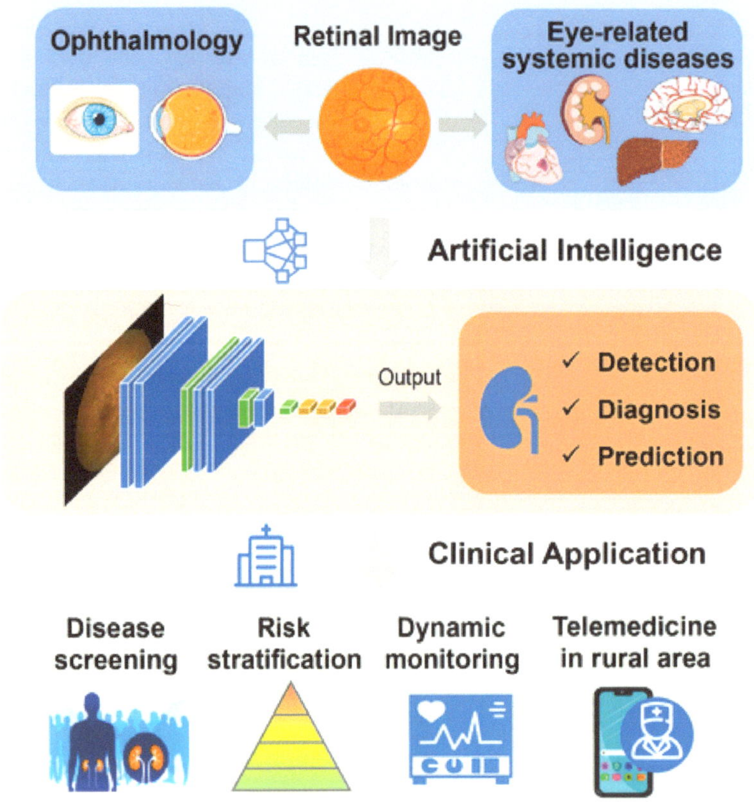

Fig.11.5 Graphical schematic illustration of retinal image-based artificial intelligence for the detection, diagnosis, and prediction of kidney diseases.

Deep learning models designed by Cheung et al. for the automatic measurement of retinal-vessel caliber in fundus photographs performed well. Their performance was comparable to expert graders in associations between measurements of retinal-vessel caliber, and cardiovascular disease (CVD) risk factors, including blood pressure, body-mass index, total cholesterol, and glycated-hemoglobin levels. This demonstrated that reduced retinal arteriolar caliber and increased retinal venular caliber were both independently associated with an increased risk of incident CVD events. Zekavat et al. leveraged deep learning to quantify geometric microvasculature indices, and thereby characterized phenome-wide clinical associations and genomic risk factors. They reported that low retinal vascular fractal dimension and density were significantly associated with a higher risk of incident mortality, hypertension, and congestive heart failure. This novel framework emphasized how deep learning of images can quantify an interpretable phenotype that can then be integrated into clinical metadata, genetic data, and biomarker datasets to predict risk.

In another study, Duan et al. applied AI to assess morphological changes in retinal microvasculature and foveal avascular zone (FAZ) using optical coherence tomography angiography (OCTA), including three vascular parameters and four FAZ-related parameters. This investigation demonstrated that retinal microvascular and macular morphology exhibited damage patterns specific to different subtypes of ischemic stroke.

Prediction of Additional Risk Factors for Stratification

Given the anatomical and physiological similarity between cerebral and coronary circulation , non-invasive and accessible retinal abnormalities can directly reflect systemic vascular properties. Thus, in addition to demographic data including age and gender, coronary artery calcium (CAC) and carotid artery atherosclerosis are also frequently used to evaluate CVD risk index.

Poplin et al. proposed a deep-learning model to extract and quantify multiple cardiovascular risk factors from retinal images. The factors used by this model included age, gender, smoking status, HbA1c, and systolic blood pressure, all of which were considered essential for predicting incident CVD. Retinal age has also been used as a proxy for predisposition to CVD. For example, Nusinovici et al. evaluated the retina-based biological age (RetiAGE) based on a deep learning approach. They reported that RetiAGE, independently of phenotypic biomarkers (e.g., creatinine, glucose, C-reactiveprotein, etc.) and chronological age, indicated the potential presence of CVD. Moreover, retinal age prediction based on fundus images was also investigated by Zhu et al., who found that the retinal age gap (i.e., predicted retinal age minus chronological age) was significantly associated with arterial stiffness index, incident CVD events and stroke .

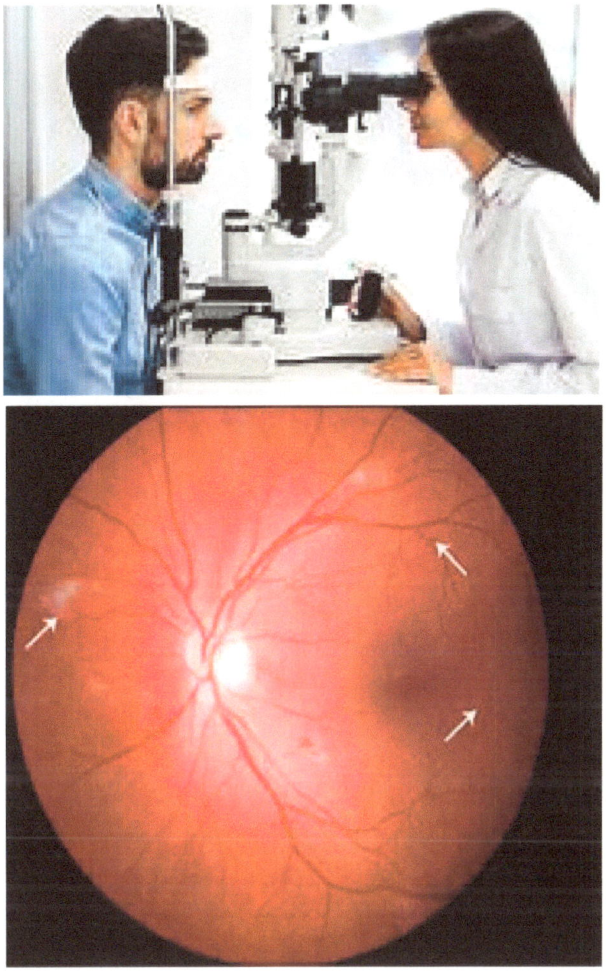

Fig.11.6 **Retinopathy Can Signal Coronary Heart Disease** Retinal abnormalities usually have no symptoms in the early stages.It may not just be diabetics who have a higher risk of coronary heart disease (CHD) if they develop the eye condition retinopathy. Its reputation as a sign of systemic disease could extend to non-diabetics. "New studies have proven that retinopathy may occur parallel to small vessel disease in other organs such as the heart," says Jonathan Sears, MD, associate professor of ophthalmology at Cleveland Clinics Cole Eye Institute. "This means that a simple eye exam could potentially help assess a patients risk of CHD. Diabetes is a known risk factor, because this disease affects small vessels-but new clinical research has revealed a similar association in non-diabetics."

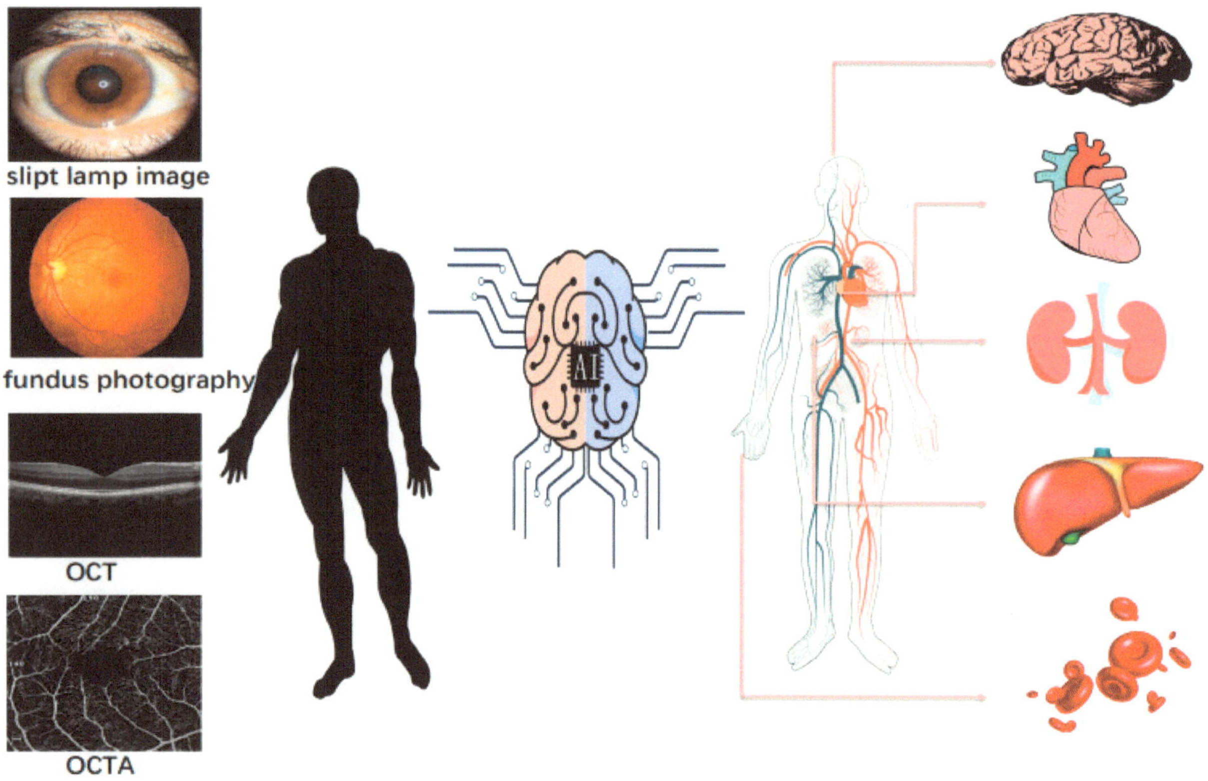

Fig.11.7 Overview of predictable systemic diseases capable of being assessed using primary ophthalmic imaging modalities and AI technology. These ocular images were derived from the authors' research database.

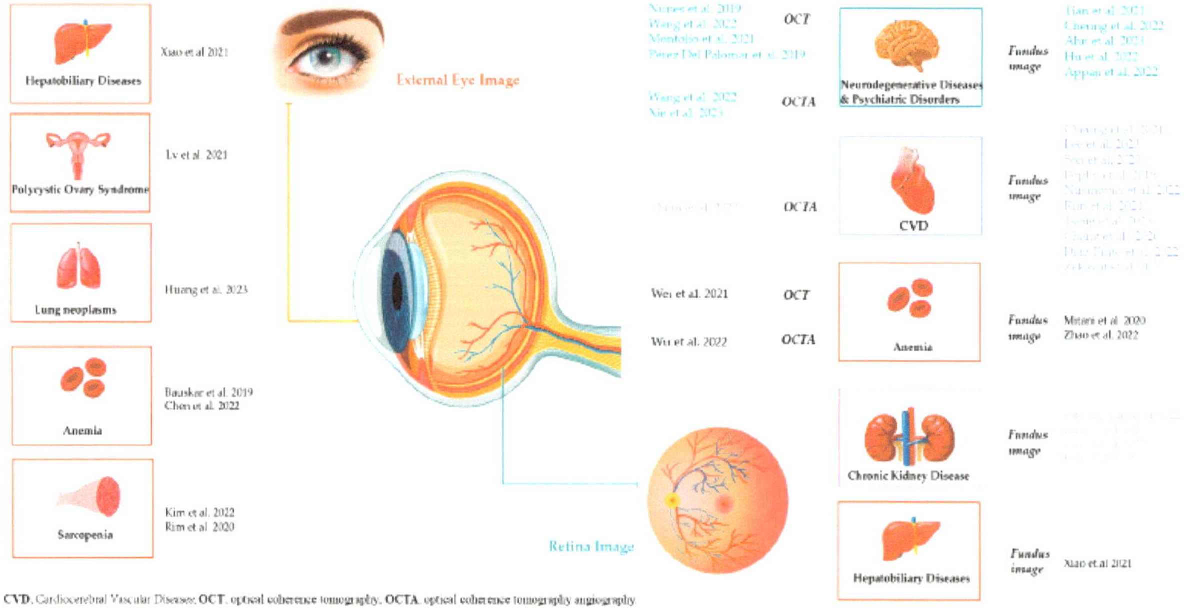

Fig.11.8 Classification of the included articles according to the image modalities used and the target systemic diseases

Many investigations have suggested that retinal image-based deep learning may be a beneficial alternative measure of CAC. For instance, a study conducted by Son et al. demonstrated a high accumulation of CAC. This accumulation was highly correlated with CVD and could be recognized by deep learning algorithms. In another study, Rim et al. developed a three-tier CVD risk stratification system based on Reti-CVD, which showed comparable effectiveness to traditional CT scan measurement in predicting future CVD risk. Furthermore, the authors validated the decent capabilities of Reti-CVD to serve as a risk enhancer tool to predict CVD events using UK biobank data.

Using retinal fundus images, Chang et al. predicted atherosclerosis using a similar image analysis strategy. However, the low specificity (i.e., 0.404) suggested that the current algorithm was not suitable for the specific detection of atherosclerosis. Furthermore, they conducted a retrospective cohort analysis to prove that the deep-learning funduscopic atherosclerosis score (DL-FAS), as an independent predictor of CVD mortality, added predictive value over the standard Framingham risk score.

Prediction of Major Cardiocerebral Vascular Events Previous studies have consistently suggested that major CVD events are predictable using AI algorithms. The aforementioned model by Poplin et al.] simultaneously predicted major adverse cardiac events (MACE) based on specific risk factors and obtained an area under the curve (AUC) value of 0.70 (0.65–0.74). Nevertheless, the retinal fundus algorithm did not have an additive effect on the predictive performance of SCORE risk calculation for MACE. In the hybrid system proposed by Diaz-Pinto et al. , retinal images and relevant clinical metadata were analyzed together to estimate cardiac indices—including left ventricular mass and left ventricular end-diastolic volume—and to predict incident myocardial infarction; this model showed an AUC of 0.80. In another study, a multimodal deep learning system was proposed by Lee et al. to predict current CVD and assess its performance against a clinical risk factors data-input model simultaneously. The authors found that the integrated network, which combined two networks using two different modalities and made full use of clinical metadata and fundus images, achieved the best performance, with an AUC of 0.872 in the external validation set. Given these results, many patients at high risk of future CVD events may benefit from available retinal image-based AI technology soon.

Detection of Chronic Kidney Disease and Renal Function

Homology in microvascular structure between the eye and the kidney suggests that incipient kidney diseases and renal function may be diagnosed using noninvasive ocular images

Sabanayagam et al. developed a deep learning algorithm to detect chronic kidney disease (CKD) from retinal images, and assessment of this model showed that it achieved both good performance and favorable generalization. Although slightly inferior to the combination model that incorporates clinical metadata of risk factors, it implied that accessible retinal photography can be used independently for CKD screening even without detailed medical history acquisition. In one interesting study, Zhang et al. further validated the potential value of an AI-derived image analysis system designed to predict the development of CKD in longitudinal cohorts. Risk stratification performance and the prognostic accuracy of the AI system were both positively assessed, and this model showed an AUC of 0.771 (0.677–0.840) for predicting the onset of CKD in four-year longitudinal data. To explore more predictive biomarkers, Zhang et al. conducted a prospective cohort study to assess the association between the retinal age gap (defined above) and incident kidney failure. Although a significant relationship was revealed, various confounding factors and selection bias were imputed for the limited generalizability of this model

Additionally, deterioration of renal function reflects a propensity to advance to chronic kidney disease. Rim et al. attempted to use retinal photographs to predict the relative abundances of a series of systemic biomarkers, including creatinine, whose dynamic fluctuations are directly related to renal function. However, this analysis showed relatively poor predictive performance in the European external test. As a result, more comprehensive work is required to explore more precise predictive factors for incident CKD.

Application of retinal image-based AI models in diabetes

Currently, 425 million people are affected by diabetes mellitus worldwide.44 And at least one-third of patients with diabetes suffer from DR, leading to different stages of microaneurysms, exudates, hemorrhages, and eventually irreversible blindness. A DL algorithm developed by Gulshan et al.4 can check for signs of retinal photographs to help physicians screen more patients. A dataset of more than 128,000 images was created to train a deep neural network to detect DR, achieving 90.3% and 87.0% sensitivity

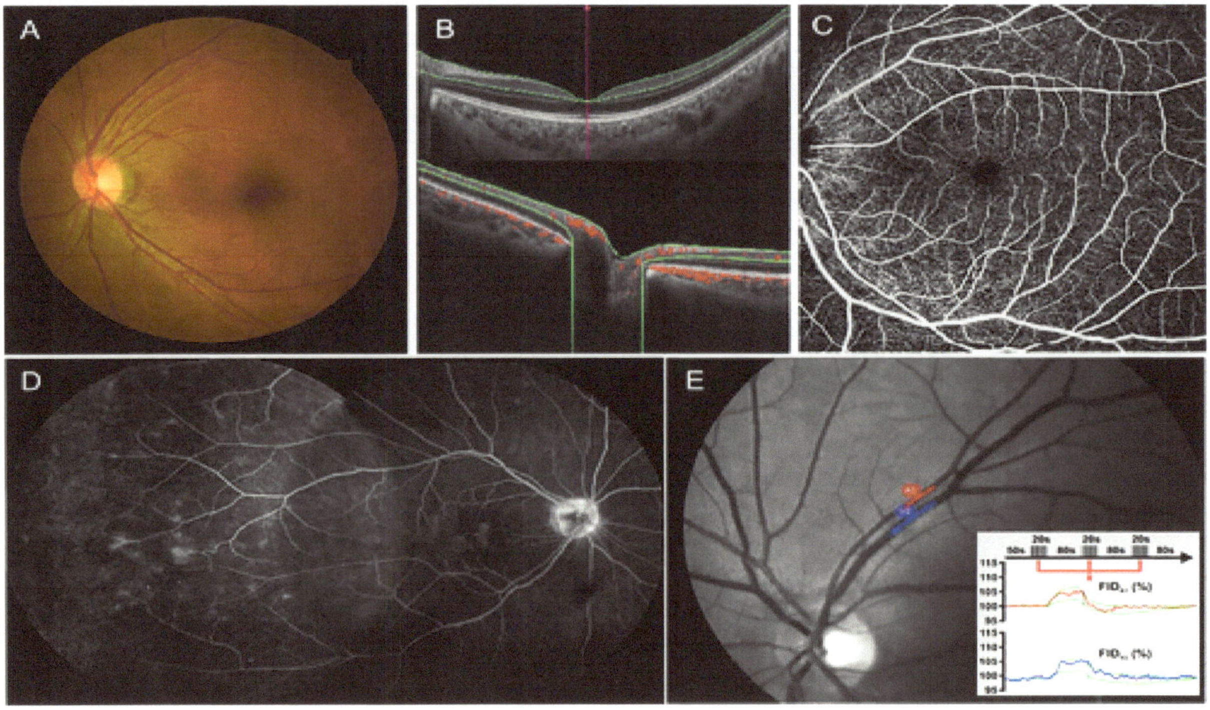

Fig.11.9 Retinal imaging modalities. (A) Color fundus photography; (B) Optical coherence tomography (OCT); (C) optical coherence tomography angiography (OCT-A); (D) Fluorescein angiography (FA); (E) dynamic retinal vessel analysis (DVA). Source: (D) Copyright 2021, Association for Research in Vision and Ophthalmology; (E) Copyright 2020, MDPI

and 98.1% and 98.5% specificity in 2 validation sets, performed with comparable accuracy as the ophthalmologists. Later numerous AI models detecting DR were developed and validated in multiethnic populations, multi-continent levels, and also in different levels of care.47 The system was put in a primary setting to help predict the DR development with an area under the curve (AUC) of 0.79 (95% confidence interval [CI]: 0.77–0.81) in the internal validation set and 0.70 in the external validation set. And the economic analysis has proved that the AI screening of DR combined with specialists can reach the lowest cost, which is US$62 per patient per year, compared to $66 for a fully automated model and $77 for the human assessment model However, real-world studies have somehow shown that AI screening fell short in clinical practice, especially in remote rural areas with few medical resources. The project is being carried out in Thailand, where the same DL system has been installed in 11 clinics in the provinces of Pathum Thani and Chiang Mai. With inexperienced operators and unmet conditions, acquired images were somewhat different from the images required by the algorithm, and connect speed impeded the future applications of algorithms

TheEye/Kidney Connection: From Molecular To Clinical

The eye is a window for direct observation of many diseases, and the eye and kidney share similar development, structure, and pathogenic mechanisms. The alteration of ocular vascular structure and function is closely related to different kinds of kidney diseases, including diabetic nephropathy and hypertension nephropathy. Herein kidney diseases can be studied non-invasively by the in vivo visualization of the retinal microvasculature

Shared physiological and molecular pathways of eye and kidney diseases

The link between kidney diseases and blindness was first reported by Richard Bright in 1836.60 Nowadays, scientists identify that both choroids of the eye and kidney develop from mesoderm around the fourth week, and they can be both affected by the same factors during this period. Basically, nephrons and choroids share some similar structures consisting ofnerve fibers, stroma, and fenestrated microvessels, which are highly permeable to proteins and result in stroma edema.They both expressedrenin-angiotensin-aldosterone receptors, innervated by the autonomic nervous system, and regulated by systemic perfusion pressure

Epidemiologic and clinical association of eye and kidney diseases

Common risk factors of old age, smoking, diabetes mellitus, hyperlipidemia, and hypertension were reported shared

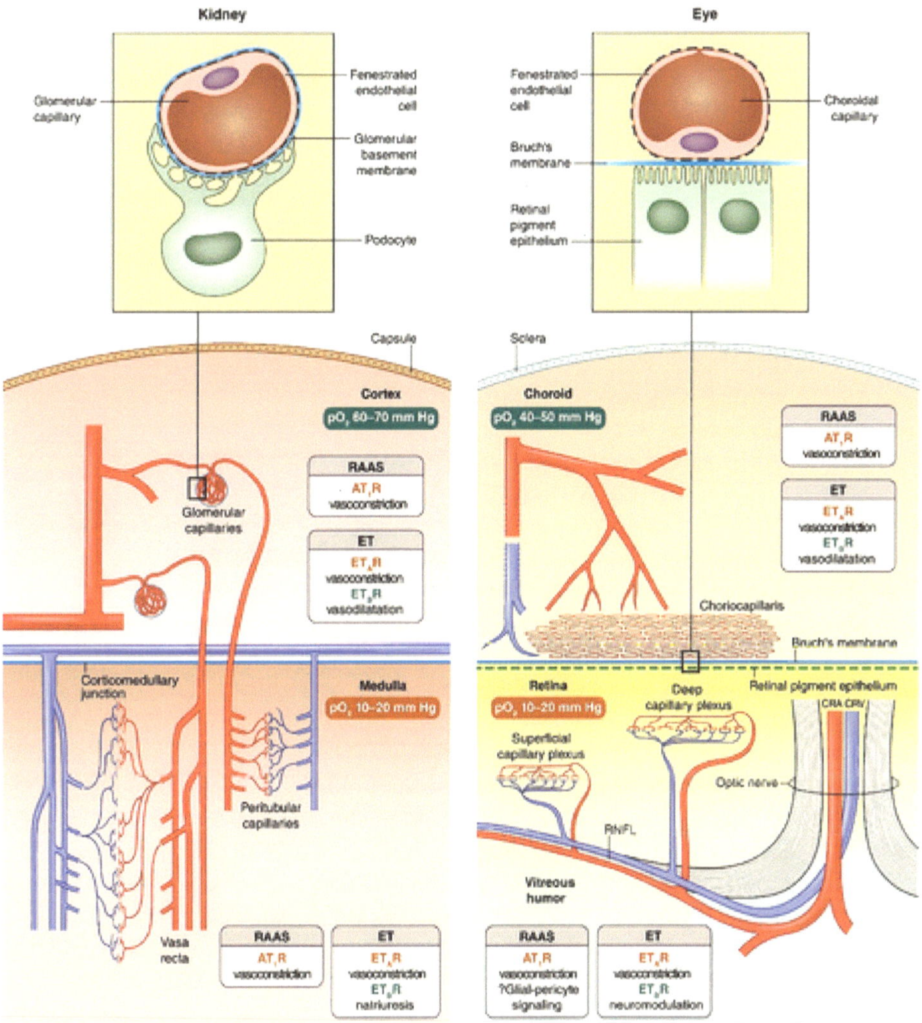

Fig. 11.10 The eye as a window to the kidney: common microcirculation organization and physiological regulation in kidney and eye. AT1R, angiotensin II type 1 receptor; CRA, central retinal artery; CRV, central retinal vein; ET, endothelin; ETAR, endothelin type A receptor; ETBR, endothelin type B receptor; pO2, partial pressure of oxygen; RAAS, renin-angiotensin-aldosterone system; RNFL, retinal nerve fiber layer. Source: Copyright 2020, Elsevier. Eye and kidney diseases have common embryonic, structural, pathogenic, and underlying molecular pathways. A variety of human congenital oculorenal syndromes have been described.63 Pax genes consist of a group of gene families that control development in encoding nuclear transcription factors, such as Waardenburg syndrome (Pax3), Aniridia (Pax6), Peter's anomaly (Pax6), and renal coloboma syndrome (Pax2).64 Bone morphogenetic protein-7 (BMP-7)41 is from another important growth factor-secreting family, the transforming growth factor-beta (TGF-beta) family. During embryogenesis of the mammalian kidney and eye, they would be both affected by the lack of BMP-7, exhibiting renal dysplasia and anophthalmia. Wilms' tumor suppressor (WT1)65 could also cause aniridia, cataract, corneal clouding, and nephroblastoma (Wilms' tumor) in children.

between CKD and ocular problems, either alone or in combination.66 Clinically, the comorbid eye diseases in patients with CKD and ESRD have some common manifestations. Retinopathies and certain ocular fundus signs of cotton-wool spots and hemorrhages in superficial or deep capillaries of the retina were often found in CKD patients. Systemic or retinal edema is caused by hypoalbuminemia and retention of excess fluid accumulation in interstitial spaces or subretinal spaces. Renal anemia may cause retinal hypoxia, which leads to infarction of the nerve fiber layer and results in cotton wool spots. And the elevated blood cholesterol is associated with increased severity and extent of hard exudates Epidemiologic studies reveal a high prevalence of retinopathies in patients with CKD, independent of diabetes, hypertension, and other risk factors. A population-based cross-sectional study of 9670 Chinese participants in Beijing by Gao et al., found that retinopathy is more prevalent in patients with CKD (28.5% vs. 16.3%, $p < 0.001$). Also, the severity of retinopathy is associated with the level of kidney function loss (estimated glomerular filtration rate, eGFR) and predicts the future progression of CKD. In the Chronic Renal Insufficiency Cohort (CRIC) study of 1904 CKD patients in the United States found CKD patients with eGFR <30 ml/min/1.73m2 are associated with three times higher risk of retinopathies. A later serial study of 1583 CRIC participants showed that with the progression of retinopathy, the odds ratio (OR) for CKD progression was 2.24 (95% CI: 1.28–3.91) compared with participants with stable retinopathy, indicating a bidirectional link between the severity of kidney and eye diseases.Most kidney diseases and retinopathies start or worsen from vascular dysfunction and systemic diseases like diabetes mellitus and hypertension.The narrowing diameters of arterioles and widening of venules are thought to reflect the severity of both diseases. In the past two decades, studies have been focused on the qualitative measurement of retinal vessel calibers, including central retinal arteriolar equivalent (CRAE), central retinal venular equivalent (CRVE), arteriole-to-venule ratio (AVR), and the analysis of vessel network geometry, fractal dimension. Bao et al. aimed to examine the association between CRAE, CRVE, and AVR with CKD in rural China to provide the scientific basis for the early detection and diagnosis of CKD. After controllingforpotentialconfoundingfactors, participants with the first quartile of AVR were shown to have a greater risk of were shown to have a greater risk of albuminuria (OR = 1.261, 95% CI: 1.02–1.57) and CKD (OR = 1.240, 95% CI: 1.00–1.54) than the fourth quartile. It was investigated by Sabanayagam et al.75 if baseline retinal vessel diameters were related to future risk of impaired kidney function or vice versa, in prospective research involving numerous assessments of serum creatinine and retinal artery diameters (CRAE and CRVE). Retinopathy was also assessed whether it could predict future CVD events in participants of the CRIC study. Worsening early treatment DR study retinopathy scores were reported in 9.8% of individuals and were related to an elevated risk of incidence of any CVD (OR = 2.56, 95% CI: 1.25–5.22).A large scale of studies show that these retinal vascular indices are associated with

CKD prevalence, but their abilities to predict CKD incidence or progression are equivocal.The measurement of consistent retinal vascular metrics may overlook the heterogeneity of different study populations and other information on fundus signs (e.g., microaneurysms, exudates, hemorrhages, and papilledema),And it also suggests that the sensitivity of conventional analysis of fundus photography cannot meet the need for precise identification of patients at risk

Detecting And Diagnosing Kidney Diseases From Retinal Imaging

Kidney diseases, like glomerulonephritis and acute kidney injury, usually entail some decline in renal function, eventually developing CKD or kidney failure over time. CKD is the most common type of kidney disease. The high prevalence of CKD has become a major public health problem worldwide, affecting almost 10%–16% of the population in Asia, Europe, Australia, and the United States.With an increasing incidence of obesity and T2DM, combined with an aging population worldwide, a heavier burden is expected in the future decades, especially in low- and middle-income countries. Despite its severity, CKD is usually asymptomatic and progresses insidiously until the very late stage or ESRD, leading to complications like CVD and higher mortality. The idea of early detection is appealing because the inexpensive intervention can ameliorate renal function at an early stage and prevent continuous deterioration. The shortcomings of traditional analysis methods make a new comprehensive assessment approach urgently needed in kidney disease patients and a larger scale of population. The use of ML and DL combined withretinal imaging is a relatively prominent frontier in this research area

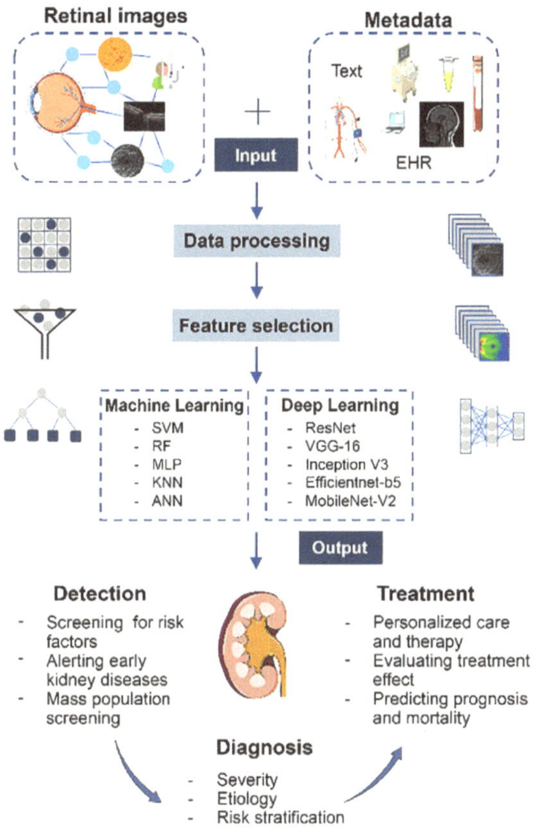

Fig.11.11 An illustration of the general workflow of retinal detection and prediction of kidney diseases. First, input data includes retinal information and metadata (text, electrical health record (EHR) and results from ultrasound or magnetic resonance imaging (MRI)), second: data processing (e.g., missing data imputation, image enhancement, etc.), third: feature selection, forth: model building with different machine learning (ML)/deep learning (DL) approaches, fifth: output classified into detection, diagnosis, and treatment of kidney diseases, and their applications in clinical practice and research. EHR, electrical health record; SVM, support vector machines; RF, random forest; MLP, multilayer perceptron; KNN, k-nearest neighbors; ANN, artificial neural network; RRT, renal replacement therapy.

Screening for risk factors of CKD

The increasing prevalence of kidney diseases worldwide is closely associated with risk factors, including smoking, obesity, hypertension, and metabolic syndromes like hyperlipidemia and diabetes. Retinal images were used to predict these important risk factors (age, gender, smoking, body mass index [BMI], etc.) in different studies. Kim et al. built a CNN model based on retinal fundus images to accurately predict age and sex. The R2 and MAE were 0.92 and 3.06 years for age prediction and sex was predicted with AUC>0.96 in test sets of normal, diabetes, and hypertensive participants, independent from the pathologic changes caused by systemic vascular diseases. Smokers and non-smokers were identified by aCNN model built by Vaghefi et al. using 165,104 retinal photographs, achieving 88.8% accuracy and 93.87% specificity in the contrast-enhanced model, while the skeletonized model was only 63.63% accuracy and 65.60% specificity. BMI, as well as other body composition factors like body muscle mass, weight, height, and percentage of body fat, were also predicted from retinal photographs, but the performance of current algorithms was generally poor with low R2 values (R2 = 0.13–0.17). Other models were also developed to detect different factors related to kidney diseases, like dyslipidemia with elevated triglyceride (MAE = 0.49, R2 = 0.03), total cholesterol (MAE = 0.75, R2 = 0.03) and low-density lipoprotein cholesterol (LDL-c, MAE = 0.72, R2 = -0.03).80 The performance of the models was relatively poor in test sets and needed to be improved. Classification models of dyslipidemia81 identification show a better ability with an accuracy of 66.7% and an AUC of 0.703. Diabetes and hypertension are common underlying conditions associated with CKD. In patients with diabetes, the prevalence of CKD is approximately 30% to 40%, and the numbers are rising with socioeconomic change and population aging. And hypertension accounts for 30% of all kidney diseases, only secondary to diabetes, leading to hypertensive nephropathy. The renal injury can be insidious and progressive, but the retinal signs can be the earliest findings to identify target organ damages, even before the presence of proteinuria and decrease of eGFR.

Alerting signs of early kidney diseases

CKD is often insidious, with patients remaining asymptomatic (stages G1 and G2) for long periods and consequential low awareness. When progressing to stage G3, a symptomatic stage with polyuria or fatigue caused by anemia, patients are at a significantly higher risk of complications and progression to ESRD. The assessment of kidney function chiefly depends on the level of GFR, and serum creatinine concentration is generally measured to calculate the value of eGFR by specific formula (for example, the CKD-EPI formula). CKD could also be alerted by abnormal laboratory blood tests of urea nitrogen, cystatin C, and proteinuria/microalbuminuria from urine tests in routine health checks or population screening.Patients with increased blood urea nitrogen and creatinine were associated with the incidence of posterior subcapsular cataract84 (OR = 1.22, 95% CI: 1.03–1.54), late AMD85 (OR = 3.05, 95% CI: 1.51–1.61) and DR78 (OR = 3.20, 95% CI: 1.58–6.40). Vice versa, the change in retinal signs can indicate changes in kidney functions. The level of creatinine was predicted by Rim et al.86 with moderate performance (MAE = 0.11, R2 = 0.12) in the Korean dataset, however, it falls far short of robustness in multi-ethnic datasets (R2 = 0.06, 0.01 for Singapore Epidemiology of Eye Diseases and UK Biobank, respectively). Serum creatinine level may be affected by age, food intake, inflammation status, and drugs, the calculated eGFR was adopted as a more reliable indicator, whose decline could be observed at the early stage of kidney injury. Kang et al.87 attempted to predict early renal impairment, defined as eGFR < 90 ml/min/1.73m2, trained and tested with 25,706 fundus images from 6212 patients (Figure 4A). The AUC was 0.81 in the overall population, higher in subgroups of elevated serum hemoglobin A1c (HbA1c) level (0.81, 0.84, 0.85, and 0.87 for HbA1c level of ≤6.5%, >6.5%, >7.5%, and>10%, respectively), but observed poor specificity (60%) in diabetes patients. The performance of this model lacked external validation, and it should be noted that the concerned retinal-vessel features, and abnormal retina signs marked by saliency maps, like exudation and hemorrhage, may be due to pathological changes caused by other ophthalmic or systemic comorbidities. Proteinuria or microalbuminuria, which is defined as albumin/creatinine ratio (ACR)17.0 for males or ACR>25.0 for females, is recommended as the preferred screening strategy for all patients with diabetes and hypertension. Lim et al.88 quantitatively measured fundus photographs by a semiautomated program to predict the presence of albuminuria, and the retinal vascular parameters were considered associated with renal function from regression models, showing better discriminative ability than the traditional risk factors model (AUC 0.80 vs. 0.77).

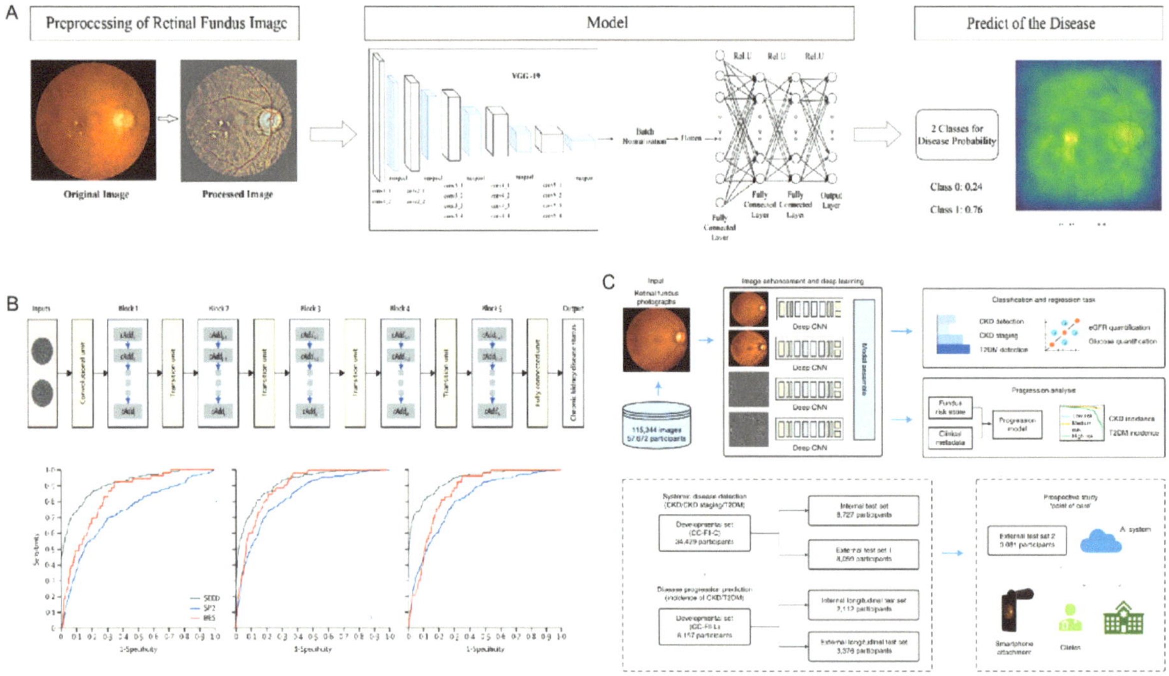

Fig.11.12 Retinal image-based AI models for screening and diagnosing kidney diseases: (A) schematic illustration of deep learning model detecting early renal function impairment; (B) Structure of deep learning models using retinal images to identify chronic kidney disease in community populations (upper panel) and the performance of image-only, risk factors and hybrid models (lower panel); (C) AI system for the diagnosis and incidence prediction of chronic kidney diseases using retinal fundus images. Source: (A) Copyright 2020, JMIR Publications; (B) Copyright 2020, Elsevier; (C) Copyright 2021, Springer Nature.

Diagnosing and Grading CKD

For the early diagnosis of CKD in community and primary care clinics, two important studies have pointed out a new direction for renal disease screening mode based on retinal fundus images. In 2020, Sabanayagam et al.89 developed and validated a DL algorithm to detect CKDs in three population-based, multi-ethnic datasets (12,970 participants in total). In this study, multi-modal data were added into three models: a model of only fundus images, a model of CKD risk factors (age, sex, ethnicity, diabetes, and hypertension), and a hybrid model combining images and risk factors.They all showed similar good performance in the internal validation set (AUC = 0.911, 0.916, and 0.914, respectively) and moderate performance in the external validation cohort (AUC0.733–0.858). In subgroups of diabetes and hypertension patients, AUC was estimated similar to the whole population. Given that both the image-only model and the risk-factor model could predict CKD with high AUCs, and their combination only slightly improved the performance, fundus images alone could be employed as an auxiliary or opportunistic screening tool for CKDs in community populations, even without the collection of patient information. While the positive predictive value was high (54%) in the internal validation set, it was only 14% and 9% in external validation sets due to the high prevalence of CKD in the internal validation set. To improve the positive predictive value, the image-only model is recommended only to be applied to high-risk groups, such as diabetes and hypertension patients, however, this would limit its clinical utility in a larger population.Following this study, Zhang et al.16 built a DL model using ResNet-50 to identify CKD and early CKD patients only with fundus Images or combined with clinical metadata (age, sex, height, weight, BMI, and BP). The models were trained and validated with 115,344 images from 57,672 patients. In the diagnosis model of CKD, the AUCs were 0.861 for the metadata model, and 0.918 for the model with only retinal images (Figure 4C). If the two models are combined, the accuracy rate will further increase (AUC = 0.930), providing better solutions for capturing features of CKDs. Then patient's eGFR, the key index of renal function and grading of CKD, was predicted using retinal fundus images with R2 of 0.327–0.507, and MAE of 11.1–13.4 ml/min/1.73m2, showing consistency with the measured eGFR (intraclass correlation coefficient [ICC] = 0.65, 95% CI: 0.63–0.66). For the grading of CKD, the thresholds of predicted eGFR were used to train regression models of differentiating advanced (stage G3) or severe+ CKD (stages G4 and G5) from early CKD (stages G1 and G2), which achieved good performance with AUCs of 0.853 and 0.825.Images captured by smartphone-based devices were introduced as an external test set to further evaluate the generalizability of the AI model and assess the feasibility of a massive population in a longitudinal cohort, achieving comparably good CKD detection performance (AUC = 0.897, 95% CI: 0.85–0.89, for image-only model) and non-inferior performance of eGFR prediction (ICC = 0.53, 95% CI: 0.50–0.55). The deployment of smartphone- and cloud-based AI diagnosis systems could build a bidirectional relationship between patients and clinics to improve the feasibility and broaden healthcare access by encouraging patients to self-monitor and allowing doctors to diagnose and follow up with patients remotely. However, current studies remain at the first stage of CKD diagnosis, only concerned about the qualitative value of eGFR, and did not include other important biomarkers for kidney function, like microalbuminuria or electrolytes. For CKD patients with different causes, such as glomerulonephritis or diabetic nephropathy, their treatment, and prognosis may vary. That's why the etiologic diagnosis (the so-called etiologic/ GFR/albuminuria classification system) is emphasized. This helps to prioritize the diagnosis and treatment of the underlying disease to slow down the progression of CKD.

Individual management for common complications of CKD

The kidney is critical in maintaining volume, bone health, acid-base balance, electrolyte stability, and blood pressure. Decreased kidney function can lead to several serious complications such as anemia, hyperkalemia, mineral bone disease, hyperphosphatemia, hypertension, and CVDs. Renal anemia plays an important factor in affecting the quality of life and prognosis of the patients. Chen et al. applied retinal vessel images from OCT to directly and non-evasively observe the hemoglobin concentration in the retina for the first time. Later, Mitani et al.91 and Zhao et al. leverage retinal fundus images to predict hemoglobin concentration and detect the status of anemia accurately (MAE: 0.67, AUC: 0.87; MAE: 0.83, AUC: 0.93, respectively). For the predictions of electrolyte disorders, sodium was predicted with an R2 of 0.12 (95% CI: 0.10–0.13), while the performance was poor for potassium, calcium, and phosphorus (R2 = 0.07, 0.07, and 0.02, respectively).86 These studies indicate that retinal imaging has clinical potential to screen for and monitor renal anemia in patients with CKD, which could aid in deciding on treatment plans and improving patient outcomes.

Evaluating the treatment effect and predicting the complications of dialysis

When CKD patients progress to the end stage, their renal function fails to meet the basic need for body operation, and RRT is essentially needed, which consists of hemodialysis, peritoneal dialysis, and kidney transplant. The most common treatment for ESRD patients is hemodialysis, however, the occurrence of complications (intradialytic hypotension [IDH], adverse cardiovascular events, renal anemia, etc.) leads to dialysis failure and poor patient survival. To evaluate the treatment effect and prevent complications, many indicators were used to monitor and evaluate patients' fluid and metabolic status, which includes laboratory blood tests of creatine and bioimpedance for volume assessment. Retinal images and vessel measurements also represent novel and non-invasive methods to facilitate easy assessments of dialysis patients. It has been proved that the blood flow in the retina and choroid was significantly changed after a single session of hemodialysis and the decrease in SBP was associated with the subfoveal choroidal thickness. Thus, Coppolino et al. performed OCT-A before the dialysis session and predict the risk of IDH within 30 days of follow-up. IDH was shown to be associated with baseline foveal vessel density of superficial and deep capillary plexus in logistic regression analysis but inversely associated with the choroid. These metrics predict the occurrence of IDH with AUCs of 0.674-0.783, with limited small and single-center data without external validation and robustness tests. But a significantly high proportion of patients reported experiencing IDH emphasizes the importance of prediction and prevention of complications with rapid and non-invasive retinal examinations.

In another cohort of hemodialysis patients, Werfel et al. adopted flicker-induced dynamic retinal vessel signals to assess the microvascular function and improve the predictions of individual cardiovascular risk. For patients with ESRD and other chronic diseases, these algorithms provide a new potential for future applications of these clinically relevant outcome-specific impairments of microvascular function and will fill the gap in predictive tools for CKDs.

Predicting the prognosis and mortality of CKD

Prediction of CKD prognosis or mortality at the onset and primary assessment could help physicians identify patients at risk of ESRD progression and deliver intensive care and timely interventions. Retinal arteriolar narrowing reflects CKD and other vascular processes and predicts renal disease progression or renal endpoints (50% renal function loss or start of RRT). The relativerisk for renal endpoints of narrow arterioles was 3.7 (95% CI: 1.7-8.4) and the tertile of the narrowest arterioles was associated with more renal endpoints (log-rank p < 0.001).79 The incidence and severity of DR98, 99 also reveal that retinal vessel changes were associated with poor renal outcomes (hazard ratio (HR) = 1.69, 95% CI: 1.16–2.45).Zhang et al.16 implemented a DL-based AI model to predict the risk of progression to advanced (stage 3) and severe CKD (stages 4 and 5) based on a 6-year longitudinal cohort. Combined with clinical data, the model performed well with a C-index of 0.845 (95% CI: 0.789–0.910) on the internal test set and 0.719 (95% CI: 0.627–0.807) on the external test set. Applications also extend to healthy individuals, the Kaplan-Meier method was used to stratify participants into low, medium, and high-risk groups with high degrees of separation (p < 0.001). And the incidence of CKD or advanced CKD in high-risk groups was significantly different from medium-risk groups, while no differences were observed in low-risk groups of CKD (p = 0.212 and 0.689 in the internal and external longitudinal test sets, respectively). A DL model was developed by Zhang et al.100 to characterize retinal age from retinal images and the retinal age gap (difference between model-based retinal age and chronological age) was used to predict the risk of ESRD. Cox proportional hazards regression models showed a 10% increase in the risk of incident ESRD with each one-year increase in retinal age gap (HR = 1.10, 95% CI: 1.03–1.17). As the retinal images are highly amendable for early prediction and longitudinal evaluations, they could not only help estimate the progression of ESRD but also assist doctors to be a predictor of mortality,101 After multivariable adjustments, the retinal age gap was associated with a 2% increase in the risk of all-cause mortality (HR = 1.02, 95% CI: 1.00–1.03, p = 0.020) and a 3% increase in the risk of cause-specific mortality attributable to non-cardiovascular and non-cancer disease (HR = 1.03, 95% CI: 1.00–1.05, p = 0.041). This research suggests that retinal images have the potential to be used as a screening tool for risk assessment and the delivery of personalized treatment

Conclusion

As AI is transforming almost every aspect of our lives, researchers felt an urgent need to incorporate AI in medicine, including ophthalmology and other diseases. Many studies proved the capability of retinal image-based AI models for predicting systemic diseases, such as diabetes, CVDs, and CKDs

Neurological diseases

The eye is referred to as the "window to the soul" in literature, and the retina is an anatomical extension of the central nervous system. In reaction to internal and external environmental stimuli, the eye has a physiological and pathological state that is similar to that of the brain and spinal cord. As a result, research into the link between the eye and the neurological system is becoming increasingly common. For example, patients with Parkinson's disease can also exhibit visual impairment. Their retinal ganglion cells (RGCs) are injured, and the retinal nerve fibers layer (RNFL) in the retina is thinning Similarly, alterations in the structure and function of the retina have been seen in people with Alzheimer's disease (AD). Aβ and pTau proteins were found in the retina of Alzheimer's disease patients, which were representative molecules of Alzheimer's disease pathogenesis. OCT has produced evidence for considerable thinning of the peripapillary NFL, macular volume loss, and nerve fiber density reduction in individuals with moderate to severe AD, indicating that thinning could develop early in disease progression Besides, among older adults, thinner RNFL thickness at baseline was associated with a greater decline in cognitive function scores at follow-up . Given the retina's tight association with neurological illnesses, it's unsurprising that researchers have employed AI to investigate the eye's relationship with the neurological system.

Alzheimer's disease (AD)

The diagnosis of AD relies on clinical manifestations, imaging, and cognitive-psychological examinations, which may occur in the late stages of AD. As the aging process accelerates, early screening for AD is necessary. Cheung et al. retrospectively collected fundus images from AD patients and healthy individuals in 11 studies and different countries, to construct and validate a model for the diagnosis of AD . The AUCs of the external validation sets were from 0.73 to 0.91. They also found that the AI model was able to distinguish between beta amyloid-negative and positive patients, and had better performance in patients with ocular disease.Since retinal thickness correlates with AD , OCT images that present retinal thickness are a good source for constructing AI. The AI algorithm for texture acquisition from OCT images is well implemented for AD detection, with an AUC of 0.795 . In addition, the combination of multimodal imaging and clinical data may improve the efficacy of AI systems. Based on this, multimodal retinal images including OCT, OCT-A, Ultra-widefield scanning laser ophthalmoscopy, and the patients' data were combined to develop AI modelsto detect AD . Ganglion cell-inner plexiform layer thickness map in OCT and combined model made good results of AUC over 0.8.

Others Dysfunctions

For a subset of neurological diseases that are difficult and costly to diagnose, AI based on retinal images has provided a convenient tool of screening. An AI system to diagnose diabetic peripheral neuropathy based on retinal color images was developed , which could provide a chance to screen their peripheral neuropathy status when people with diabetes screened their eyes. In patients with diabetic retinopathy, the AUC reached over 0.85. Also, the retinal vascular trajectory was acquired with the help of an AI algorithm, which connected the retina with schizophrenia and bipolar disorder, and performed the accuracy of 0.86 and 0.73, respectively . Moreover, Lau et al. connected retinal images with MRI, and they detected white matter hyperintensities in healthy people, which was vital for the development of cerebral small vessel disease, and both of the sensitivity and specificity were over 0.9

Autoimmune Diseases

Multiple sclerosis

The relationship between the eyes and the immune system is so close that there are many autoimmune diseases with ocular characteristics, such as Sjögren syndrome, inflammatory bowel disease, multiple sclerosis, and many others. The patients can present as dry eyes, uveitis, optic neuritis, etc. The studies of eyes and multiple sclerosis suggested that the thickness of the retina was thing with the development of multiple sclerosis, and measurement of retinal thickness with OCT could be a biomarker of multiple sclerosis. Based on this, among the ocular images, OCT images are currently the main image source for AI diagnosis of multiple sclerosis. Cavaliere et al. collected OCT images from multiple sclerosis and controls. They got different regions of the retina and choroid with OCT ETDRS scan and TNSIT scan modes and calculated the variables with the highest AUC (0.97) to create a diagnosis model using a support vector machine algorithm.Similarly, Martin et al. got OCT images from 48 early-stage multiple sclerosis patients and 48 healthy people They measured the thickness of each layer of retina and choroid, and tried to find regions with the greatest discriminant capacity that could be used as a classifier. The best classifier showed a great performance (sensitivity = specificity = 0.98). Their work showed that the papillomacular bundle may be the first layer affected in the early stage of multiple sclerosis, and the OCT images-based AI system could be a new direction for the early diagnosis of multiple sclerosis.

Hematological Diseases

Anemia

Anemia is commonly defined as a low concentration of hemoglobin (Hb). Most of the anemia is easily corrected, while the key is to be detected. The "gold standard" of anemia is Hb concentration measured by venous blood samples. However, the invasive procedure is a risk of pollution for medical workers and painful for patients. Therefore, some non-invasive and painless methods of measuring Hb have been developed such as pulse oximetry, occlusion spectroscopy, photoplethysmography and reflectance spectroscopy Compared to the "gold standard", the stability and accuracy of these methods have yet to be proven.

During the physical examination, pallor of the skin mucosa such as lips and palpebral conjunctiva is often considered as an indication of anemia. Therefore, some researchers have attempted to estimate anemia status by AI through palpebral conjunctiva images. With the help of image processing programs, scientists extracted color information from segmented palpebral conjunctiva images. Early in 2007, Suner et al. took pictures of palpebral conjunctiva and got RGB values from them .

They developed an algorithm according to the manually delineated regions of the digital photos. This algorithm allowed for a crude calculation of the subjects' hemoglobin concentrations. However, the quality of the images was easily influenced by the environment. Algorithms and wearable devices were developed to overcome this challenge. However, despite the variety of methods, detecting Hb values seemed to be difficult for AI that relied on eye images. It might be easier to diagnose anemia rather than to detect Hb values for AI. On the other hand, the association between retina and anemia was discovered, and researchers tried to use AI based on retinal images to diagnose anemia.

Mitani et al. proposed a hypothesis that anemia could be detected from retinal images using deep learning They collected data from UK Biobank, and developed deep learning systems based on fundus images and metadata to determine Hb and anemia status. Also, the combined AI system made a good performance on diabetes patients (AUC = 0.89).

Along with the wide application of OCT . technology in the field of ophthalmology, Wei et al. used retinal OCT images and deep learning to predict anemia for the first time . Their work has led to a new level of efficacy in assessing anemia status, with a high accuracy of 98.65%.

Sleep disorders

Obstructive sleep apnea (OSA) and narcolepsy

These are two main types of sleep disorders. The former is characterized by recurrent apnea during sleep, and the latter is characterized by drowsiness when awake and disturbed sleep. The diagnosis of OSA depends on a sleep breathing test, while the "gold standard" for the diagnosis of narcolepsy is the multiple sleep latency test. Relatively difficult diagnostic criteria limit the diagnosis of sleep disorders. With the deeper research of sleep disorders, the sleep status of patients with sleep disorders was gradually being understood and it had been found that electroencephalogram (EEG) and pupil size can represent such alterations . Based on this, Liu et al. developed a neural network method to detect OSA and narcolepsy according to EEG and pupil size The accuracy of the algorithm was above 90%

Hepatobiliary Diseases

Previously, it appeared that ocular symptoms such as scleral yellowing due to jaundice and K-F rings due to hepatomegaly could only offer suggestive information for particular disorders. However, Xiao et al. innovated the use of ocular images in the detection of hepatobiliary diseases with AI . They collected clinical data and ocular images (fundus images and slit-lamp images) of patients with seven hepatobiliary diseases from multiple centers and built an AI detection system based on the ocular images. Their algorithm has achieved good results in diseases such as cirrhosis and liver cancer (both of AUCs were over 0.83). In comparison to the AI, it was difficult for the six ophthalmologists to determine whether the subjects had hepatobiliary disease based on the ocular images, let alone diagnose the specific type of diseases. When using the heat map to interpret AI concerns, the highlighted areas are the optic disc and blood vessels of the fundus images and the conjunctiva, sclera, and iris of the slit-lamp images. This may help to discover new mechanisms of hepatobiliary diseases

Systemic parameters

The previous studies demonstrated that we could observe the whole body non-invasively through the eye. The above discussion shows that ocular images can be used for diabetes, cardiovascular disease, anemia, and many other systemic diseases. In 2019, Banowati et al. detected cholesterol levels by iris images with the help of AI, whose accuracy was 97.45% . And in the same year, Vaghefi et al. were able to determine the smoking status of the subjects based on retinal images.However, as AI is still in the developmental stage, reflecting the the whole-body state through ocular images still requires careful and comprehensive research. Thus, Rim et al. did the largest study to date in a related field. Collecting more than 230,000 fundus photographs, as well as setting 47 systemic parameters (age, sex, body-mass index, blood pressure, and some laboratory measurements, such as creatinine) as outputs, they evaluated the diagnostic efficacy of the AI more comprehensively. And the impact of different races on AI was also compared. Despite the poor detection efficacy of AI systems in some biomarkers, especially in external validation sets, it demonstrated the relevance of the eye to the whole body from another perspective. In addition, considering parameters with poor predictive performance, Rim et al. suggested that retinal changes may better reflect chronic diseases such as cardiovascular disease and chronic kidney disease

Heighlights of ocular based Artificial studies in systemic studies

1.Current studies are mainly focused on diseases that are very closely associated with the eye, such as diabetes, cardiovascular disease, CKD and AD. Researchers haven't often used AI to examine the connection between other diseases and the eye because there hasn't been much study on intrinsic connections. And this relies on researchers to further explore the ocular features associated with systemic diseases. Most current studies have focused on the use of ocular images to diagnose systemic diseases, with a small number being predictions of future incidence or progression, while clustering tasks are rare. This is mainly due to the level of difficulty in obtaining data. Future researchers may focus more on the task of predicting disease progression and assisting physicians in developing treatment plans.

2.Ocular images-based AI has benefits in several aspects, including reducing screening costs, improving efficiency and coverage, and reducing the burden on physicians. In the future, ocular images-based AI may be more widely used in screening, as it is presently used clinically to detect retinal diseases . In places with limited medical resources, AI can perform routine screening by integrating software into fundus cameras. Fundus images can simultaneously detect retinal diseases, systemic diseases, and risk factors with the help of AI, which may help us to identify problems at an early or even pre-clinical stage of the disease.

3.In the future, many areas still require research. Firstly, apartfrom diagnosis, researchers can explore predicting the prognosis of diseases through eye imaging. This can help doctors in planning medical treatments. Secondly, most current researches use two-dimensional ocular images, and the acquisition of three-dimensional images from OCTA or other devices may be a new direction. Treating the entire eye as a single entity may help us uncover more differences in diseases. Thirdly, more innovative algorithms must be developed and incorporated to enhance disease detection performance.

4.Currently, the application of ocular images to detect systemic diseases confronts many challenges. First, a large number of images are needed in AI systems. Not only the construction of the model, but also testing the performance of the model requires an external validation set. In addition, the number of ocular images needed for each type of disease is currently unknown. However, for most departments, eye examinations are not routine. Therefore, to study the relationship between systemic diseases and the eyes, the acquirement of high-quality ocular images and a complete database of clinical information needs to be fully supported. This requires close collaboration between doctors in ophthalmology and other departments, as well as the assistance of AI engineers. To eliminate the interference of the number of images, the researchers must make images "better and more".

5.There are a lot of "black boxes" in the field of AI. There is still a great deal unknown about the mechanisms of image recognition by artificial intelligence, especially by deep learning systems. Some scientists have attempted to debunk AI systems, but no better explanatory views have emerged yet. Therefore, although some studies have attempted to represent the regions of interest of AI in the form of heat maps, we cannot understand the principles by which the system establishes the association of ocular and systemic diseases. Machine learning algorithms apart from deep learning may have better interpretations and should be applied more often to obtain more highly interpretable eye features.

6.Some rare diseases are difficult to study with AI. Based on the need for AI systems to extract features, a large number of high-quality images are indispensable to build a diagnostic system. However, this is difficult to do for some rare diseases. In these areas, it is likely that manual diagnosis will still dominate in the future. Although there are algorithms to increase the number of images by image enhancement, this is still of limited help for diversity. Multicenter studies and interpretable machine learning algorithms may be the solutions.

7.Ophthalmic imaging devices vary widely and produce different types of images. For example, fundus images from different devices may differ in size, resolution, image format, and color. Using images from different devices to build AI models may reduce model performance. Conversely, if a model can perform well in different styles of image datasets, it indicates that the model has good robustness. Therefore, we need an algorithm or image standard to make different images easy for AI recognition.

8.There are many ethical and legal issues before AI can be used in the clinical setting. There is a risk of information leaking when using AI systems because they need a lot of patient data to build them. To make sure that patient information is not utilized in other ways, strict legal restrictions and information protection measures are required. Blockchain technology has been used in data transfer to ensure that patients' personal information was not misused.

Predicting Body Composition Factors From RFPBody composition factors predicted from RFP include body massindex (BMI), body muscle mass, height, weight, relative fat mass,and waist-hip ratio (WHR) . Performance of current algorithms in BMI prediction is generally poor withlow R2-values (R2: 0.13–0.17). Model generalizability across ethnically distinct datasets was poor as well. Rim et al. found that DL algorithms for prediction of height, body weight,BMI (and other non-body composition factors), trained on aSouth Korean dataset, showed limited generalizability in the UK Biobank dataset (majority White ethnicity) (R^2 ≤0.08).Proportional bias was observed, where predicted values in thelower range were overestimated and those in the higher rangewere underestimated. While BMI is a parameter of interest dueto its well-established associations withall-causeandcause-specificmortality,prediction of other plausible parametersof body composition have been described. The prediction of bodymuscle mass is noteworthy, as it is a potentially more reliablebiomarker than BMI for cardiometabolic risk and nutritionalstatus Rim et al. reported that body muscle masscould be predicted with an R^2 of 0.52 (95% CI: 0.51–0.53) i

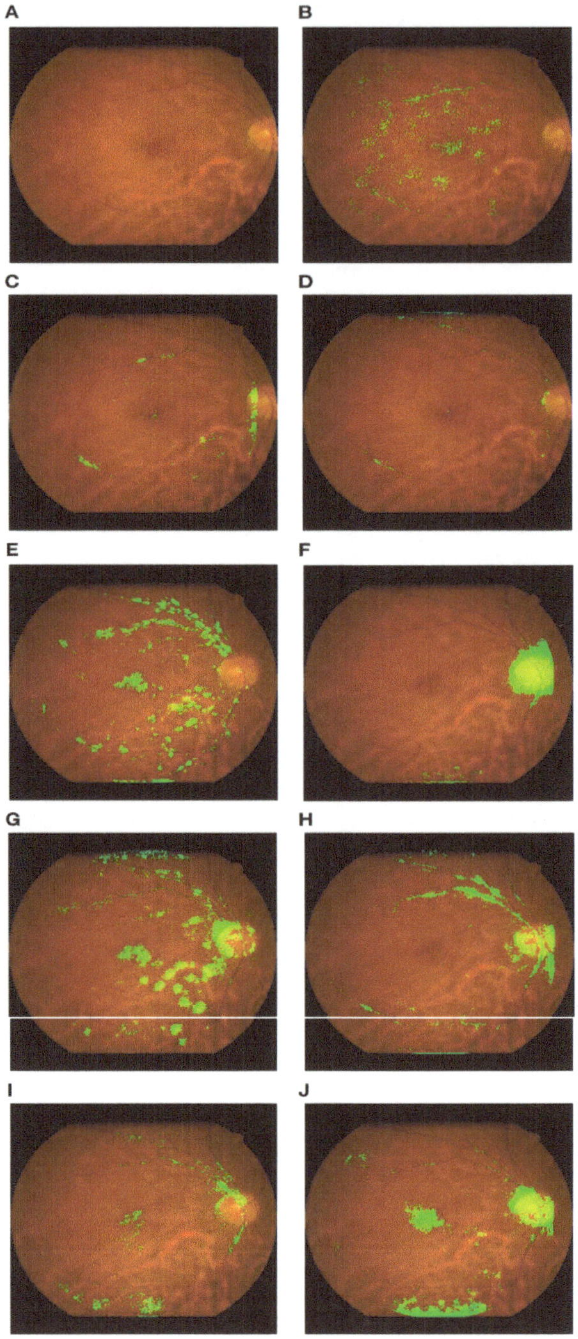

Fig 11.13 Example heatmaps overlaid on retinal fundus photographs highlighting areas of interest. These examples were derived from the authors' research database. (A) Original photograph with no overlay; (B) red blood cell count; (C) systolic blood pressure; (D) Weight; (E) age; (F) body mass index; (G) creatinine; (H) diastolic blood pressure; (I) hemoglobin; (J) height.

Bibliography and Acknowledgement

- Aldrich TK, Moosikasuwan M, Shah SD, Deshpande KS. Length-normalized pulse photoplethysmography: a noninvasive method to measure blood hemoglobin, Bronx, NY. Ann Biomed Eng. 2002;30(10):1291–1298.
- Appaji A, Nagendra B, Chako DM, Padmanabha A, Jacob A, Hiremath CV, et al. Examination of retinal vascular trajectory in schizophrenia and bipolar disorder. Psychiatry Clin Neurosci. 2019;73(12):738–744
- Banowati C, Novianty A, Setianingsih C. Cholesterol level detection based on iris recognition using convolutional neural network method. In: 2019 IEEE Conference on Sustainable Utilization and Development in Engineering and Technologies (CSUDET). Penang, Malaysia: IEEE; 2019. p. 116–21
- Barker SJ, Badal JJ. The measurement of dyshemoglobins and total hemoglobin by pulse oximetry. Curr Opin Anaesthesiol. 2008;21(6):805–810.
- Campbell JP, Kim SJ, Brown JM, Ostmo S, Chan RVP, Kalpathy-Cramer J, et al. Evaluation of a deep learning-derived quantitative retinopathy of prematurity severity scale. Ophthalmology. 2021;128(7):1070–1076. doi: 10.1016/j.ophtha.2020.10.025
- Cavaliere C, Vilades E, Alonso-Rodríguez M, Rodrigo M, Pablo L, Miguel J, et al. Computer-aided diagnosis of multiple sclerosis using a support vector machine and optical coherence tomography features. Sens. 2019;19(23):5323.
- Cervera DR, Smith L, Diaz-Santana L, Kumar M, Raman R, Sivaprasad S. Identifying peripheral neuropathy in colour fundus photographs based on deep learning. Diagnostics. 2021;11(11):1943.
- Chang J, Ko A, Park SM, Choi S, Kim K, Kim SM, et al. Association of cardiovascular mortality and deep learning-funduscopic atherosclerosis score derived from retinal fundus images. Am J Ophthalmol. 2020;217:121–130.
- Chen YM, Miaou SG. A Kalman filtering and nonlinear penalty regression approach for noninvasive anemia detection with palpebral conjunctiva images. J Healthc Eng. 2017;2017:9580385.
- Cheung CY, Ran AR, Wang S, Chan VTT, Sham K, Hilal S, et al. A deep learning model for detection of Alzheimer's disease based on retinal photographs: a retrospective, multicentre case-control study. Lancet Digit Health. 2022
- Cheung CY, Xu D, Cheng CY, Sabanayagam C, Tham YC, Yu M, et al. A deep-learning system for the assessment of cardiovascular disease risk via the measurement of retinal-vessel calibre. Nat Biomed Eng. 2021;5(6):498–508. doi: 10.1038/s41551-020-00626-4
- Dimauro G, Caivano D, Girardi F. A new method and a non-invasive device to estimate anemia based on digital images of the conjunctiva. Ieee Access. 2018;6:46968–46975.
- Frank Z, Timothy R, Robert W, James L, Jeanne S, Thomas R. Sleep-wake abnormalities in narcolepsy. Sleep. 1986;1:189–193
- Garcia-Martin E, Ortiz M, Boquete L, Sánchez-Morla EM, Barea R, Cavaliere C, et al. Early diagnosis of multiple sclerosis by OCT analysis using Cohen's d method and a neural network as classifier. Comput Biol Med. 2021;129:104165.
- Grzybowski A, editor. Artificial intelligence in ophthalmology. Cham: Springer; 2021
- Gu C, Wang Y, Jiang Y, Xu F, Wang S, Liu R, et al. Application of artificial intelligence system for screening multiple fundus diseases in Chinese primary healthcare settings: A real-world, multicentre and cross-sectional study of 4795 cases. Br J Ophthalmol. 2023 Mar 6
- Hannappe MA, Arnould L, Méloux A, Mouhat B, Bichat F, Zeller M, et al. Vascular density with optical coherence tomography angiography and systemic biomarkers in low and high cardiovascular risk patients. Sci Rep. 2020;10(1):16718. doi: 10.1038/s41598-020-73861-z.
- Hart NJ, Koronyo Y, Black KL, Koronyo-Hamaoui M. Ocular indicators of Alzheimer's: exploring disease in the retina. Acta Neuropathol. 2016;132(6):767–787
- He J, Baxter SL, Xu J, Xu J, Zhou X, Zhang K. The practical implementation of artificial intelligence technologies in medicine. Nat Med. 2019;25(1):30–36. doi: 10.1038/s41591-018-0307-0.
- Huang L, Zhang D, Ji J, Wang Y, Zhang R. Central retina changes in Parkinson's disease: a systematic review and meta-analysis. J Neurol. 2021;268(12):4646–4654.
- Kang EY, Hsieh YT, Li CH, Huang YJ, Kuo CF, Kang JH, et al. Deep learning-based detection of early renal function impairment using retinal fundus images: model development and validation. JMIR Med Inform. 2020;8(11):e23472
- Kim HM, Han JW, Park YJ, Bae JB, Woo SJ, Kim KW. Association between retinal layer thickness and cognitive decline in older adults. JAMA Ophthalmol. 2022
- Kim O, McMurdy J, Jay G, Lines C, Crawford G, Alber M. Combined reflectance spectroscopy and stochastic modeling approach for noninvasive hemoglobin determination via palpebral conjunctiva. Physiol Rep. 2014;2(1):e00192.
- Lau AY, Mok V, Lee J, Fan Y, Zeng J, Lam B, et al. Retinal image analytics detects white matter hyperintensities in healthy adults. Ann Clin Transl Neurol. 2019;6(1):98–105.
- Li F, Su Y, Lin F, Li Z, Song Y, Nie S, et al. A deep-learning system predicts glaucoma incidence and progression using retinal photographs. J Clin Invest. 2022;132(11):e157968.
- Liew G, Mitchell P, Wong TY, Iyengar SK, Wang JJ. CKD increases the risk of age-related macular degeneration. J Am Soc Nephrol. 2008;19(4):806–811
- Liu D, Pang Z, Lloyd SR. A neural network method for detection of obstructive sleep apnea and narcolepsy based on pupil size and EEG. IEEE Trans Neural Netw. 2008;19(2):308–318.
- Liu N, Liang G, Li L, Zhou H, Zhang L, Song X. An eyelid parameters auto-measuring method based on 3D scanning. Displays. 2021;1(69):102063.
- Margulies LJ. Ocular manifestations of cardiovascular and hematologic disorders. Curr Opin Ophthalmol. 1994;5(6):99–104
Mitani A, Huang A, Venugopalan S, Corrado GS, Peng L, Webster DR, et al. Detection of anaemia from retinal fundus images via deeplearning. Nat Biomed Eng. 2020;4(1):18–27.
- Moraes G, Fu DJ, Wilson M, Khalid H, Wagner SK, Korot E, et al. Quantitative analysis of OCT for neovascular age-related macular degeneration using deep learning. Ophthalmology. 2021;128(5):693–705. doi: 10.1016/j.ophtha.2020.09.025
- Nunes A, Silva G, Duque C, Januario C, Santana I, Ambrosio AF, et al. Retinal texture biomarkers may help to discriminate between Alzheimer's, Parkinson's, and healthy controls. PLoS ONE. 2019;14(6):e0218826.
- O'Bryhim BE, Lin JB, Stavern GPV, Apte RS. OCT angiography findings in preclinical Alzheimer's disease: 3-year follow-up. Ophthalmology. 2021;128(10):1489–1491.
- Owen CG, Rudnicka AR, Welikala RA, Fraz MM, Barman SA, Luben R, et al. Retinal vasculometry associations with cardiometabolic risk factors in the european prospective investigation of cancer—norfolk study. Ophthalmology. 2019;126(1):96–106. doi: 10.1016/j.ophtha.2018.07.022.
- Pakzad-Vaezi K, Pepple KL. Tubulointerstitial nephritis and uveitis. Curr Opin Ophthalmol. 2017;28(6):629–635
Pinto M, Barjas-Castro ML, Nascimento S, Falconi MNA, Zulli R, Castro V. The new noninvasive occlusion spectroscopy hemoglobin measurement method: a reliable and easy anemia screening test for blood donors. Transfusion. 2012;53:766.
- Poplin R, Varadarajan AV, Blumer K, Liu Y, McConnell MV,

Corrado GS, et al. Prediction of cardiovascular risk factors from retinal fundus photographs via deep learning. Nat Biomed Eng. 2018;2(3):158–164

- Rim TH, Lee CJ, Tham YC, Cheung N, Yu M, Lee G, et al. Deep-learning-based cardiovascular risk stratification using coronary artery calcium scores predicted from retinal photographs. Lancet Digital Health. 2021;3(5):e306–e316.
- Rim TH, Lee G, Kim Y, Tham YC, Lee CJ, Baik SJ, et al. Prediction of systemic biomarkers from retinal photographs: development and validation of deep-learning algorithms. Lancet Digit Health. 2020;2(10):e526–e536.
- Ruamviboonsuk P, Tiwari R, Sayres R, Nganthavee V, Hemarat K, Kongprayoon A, et al. Real-time diabetic retinopathy screening by deep learning in a multisite national screening programme: a prospective interventional cohort study. Lancet Digit Health Saarela V, Nuutinen M, Ala-Houhala M, Arikoski P, Ronnholm K, Jahnukainen T. Tubulointerstitial nephritis and uveitissyndrome in children: a prospective multicenter study. Ophthalmology. 2013;120(7):1476–1481.
- Sabanayagam C, Xu D, Ting DSW, Nusinovici S, Banu R, Hamzah H, et al. A deep learning algorithm to detect chronic kidney disease from retinal photographs in community-based populations. Lancet Digit Health. 2020;2(6):e295–302.
- Sarabi MS, Khansari MM, Zhang J, Kushner-Lenhoff S, Gahm JK, Qiao Y, et al. 3D retinal vessel density mapping with OCT-angiography. IEEE J Biomed Health Inform. 2020;24(12):3466–3479.
- Sayin N. Ocular complications of diabetes mellitus. World J Diabetes. 2015;6(1):92.
- Smoking on age and sex prediction from retinal fundus images. Sci Rep. 2020;10(1):4623.
- Son J, Shin JY, Chun EJ, Jung KH, Park KH, Park SJ. Predicting high coronary artery calcium score from retinal fundus images with deep learning algorithms. Transl Vision Sci Technol. 2020;9(2):28. doi: 10.1167/tvst.9.2.28
- Suner S, Crawford G, McMurdy J, Jay G. Non-invasive determination of hemoglobin by digital photography of palpebral conjunctiva. J Emerg Med. 2007;33(2):105–111.
- Tan TE, Anees A, Chen C, Li S, Xu X, Li Z, et al. Retinal photograph-based deep learning algorithms for myopia and a blockchain platform to facilitate artificial intelligence medical research: a retrospective multicohort study. Lancet Digit Health. 2021;3(5):e317–e329.
- Vaghefi E, Yang S, Hill S, Humphrey G, Walker N, Squirrell D. Detection of smoking status from retinal images; a convolutional neural network study. Sci Rep. 2019;9(1):7180.
- Wang H, Abbas KM, Abbasifard M, Abbasi-Kangevari M, Abbastabar H, Abd-Allah F, et al. Global age-sex-specific fertility, mortality, healthy life expectancy (HALE), and population estimates in 204 countries and territories, 1950–2019: a comprehensive demographic analysis for the global burden of disease study 2019. Lancet. 2020;396(10258):1160–1203.
- Wei H, Shen H, Li J, Zhao R, Chen Z. AneNet: a lightweight network for the real-time anemia screening from retinal vessel optical coherence tomography images. Opt Laser Technol. 2021;136:106773.
- Wisely CE, Wang D, Henao R, Grewal DS, Thompson AC, Robbins CB, et al. Convolutional neural network to identify symptomatic Alzheimer's disease using multimodal retinal imaging. Br J Ophthalmol. 2022;106(3):388–395.
- Wong CW, Wong TY, Cheng CY, Sabanayagam C. Kidney and eye diseases: common risk factors, etiological mechanisms, and pathways. Kidney Int. 2014;85(6):1290–1302.
- Wong TY, Coresh J, Klein R, Muntner P, Couper DJ, Sharrett AR, et al. Retinal microvascular abnormalities and renal dysfunction: the atherosclerosis risk in communities study. J Am Soc Nephrol. 2004;15(9):2469–2476.
- Xiao W, Huang X, Wang JH, Lin DR, Zhu Y, Chen C, et al. Screening and identifying hepatobiliary diseases through deep learning using ocular images: a prospective, multicentre study. Lancet Digit Health. 2021;3(2):e88–97.
- Yoss RE, Moyer NJ, Hollenhorst RW. Pupil size and spontaneous pupillary waves associated with alertness, drowsiness, and sleep. Neurology. 1970;20(6):545–554.
- Zhang B, Chou Y, Zhao X, Yang J, Chen Y. Early detection of microvascular impairments with optical coherence tomography angiography in diabetic patients without clinical retinopathy: a meta-analysis. Am J Ophthalmol. 2021;222:226–237.
- Zhang K, Liu X, Xu J, Yuan J, Cai W, Chen T, et al. Deep-learning models for the detection and incidence prediction of chronic kidney disease and type 2 diabetes from retinal fundus images. Nat Biomed Eng. 2021;5(6):533–545
- Zhang L, Wu Y, Hu M, Guo W. Automatic image analysis of episcleral hemangioma applied to the prognosis prediction of trabeculotomy in Sturge-Weber syndrome. Displays. 2022;1(71):102118.
- Zhang L, Yuan M, An Z, Zhao X, Wu H, Li H, et al. Prediction of hypertension, hyperglycemia and dyslipidemia from retinal fundus photographs via deep learning: a cross-sectional study of chronic diseases in central China. PLoS ONE. 2020;15(5):e0233166.

Artificial Intelligence in Pediatric Cardiology: A Review

CHAPTER

12

The discipline of pediatric cardiology has evolved as a specialty over the past 60 years, deriving its roots from attempts to treat congenital heart diseases .Congenital heart diseases (CHD), in the wake of the burden of mortality and morbidity they bring in, have always been an issue of concern. A total of 3.12 million babies in the United States were born with congenital heart disease, and around 13.3 million individuals are living with congenital heart anomalies . CHD has a multifactorial etiology that consists of environmental stressors and genetic factors and accounts for 80% of all forms of CHD . Pediatric heart diseases remain a global burden on health services and are associated with lifelong comorbidities that carry into adulthood, ultimately decreasing the quality of life for children . The last decade has seen the increasing prevalence of hypertension and other 'adult' heart diseases among the pediatric population, especially adolescents, which has counterpoised the falling burden of rheumatic heart disease in the same age group. Advancements in pediatric cardiology care and surgical technology have helped with significant reductions in mortality . However, while high-income countries saw the mortality rates of CHD reduce by half, the needs for surgical care and advanced imaging for pediatric patients are unmet in middle- and lower-income countries .The absence of a timely diagnosis for suspected pediatric heart diseases significantly delays timely treatment and often presents a diagnostic dilemma. The clinically suspected diagnosis of CHD is confirmed by echocardiography, which can even be conducted during pre- and postnatal screening . The diagnosis thus requires adequate clinical suspicion, health infrastructure, and a skilled workforce .The growth of artificial intelligence (AI) in the context of medicine has contributed immensely to the streamlining of clinical processes and decision making in health care since 1960 . The concept of machine learning (ML) is integral to the evolution of AI. ML is defined as the ability of machines to learn tasks from a large amount of previous data and be able to predict the same for future instances . As a result, AI has multiple key applications in the diagnosis, surveillance, prevention, and intervention of congenital heart diseases and has created major advancements in pediatric cardiology as a specialty . Due to its widespread ability to improve the diagnostic value of cardiac magnetic resonance imaging (MRI), echocardiograms (ECHO), computer tomography (CT) scans, and electrocardiographs (ECG), AI can augment the diagnostic accuracy of pediatric heart diseases .

While AI has already found its applications in a multitude of specialties, the notion of its use in almost any medical specialty is conceivable. CHD is an interesting area where AI can be applied owing to the burden of CHDs in pediatric and adult populations. AI-based algorithms have expanded their application in various domains of pediatric cardiology including but not limited to screening, clinical examination, diagnosis, image processing, prognosis, risk stratification, and precision medicine . Surprisingly, the full extent of AI applications in all stages of care for patients with congenital heart diseases has not yet been discussed. Evolving literature has pinpointed the efficiency of machine-learning algorithms in the interpretation of heart murmurs, a common sign of congenital heart diseases .The recent utilization of deep-learning computer networks has demonstrated the ability to perform MRI segmentation, allowing clinicians to detect valvular defects simultaneously in all four of the heart's chambers .Based on our knowledge, there is only one systematic analysis of a case series of atrial septal defect repair with robotic assistance and AI; the full extent of AI applications in all stages of care for patients with CHD has not yet been discussed. The objective of this systematic review is to compile all existing literature on AI applications in the specialty of pediatric cardiology with a focus on CHD. The review will attempt to appraise the evolving literature and compile clinically relevant data that can serve as a source of health information for clinicians.

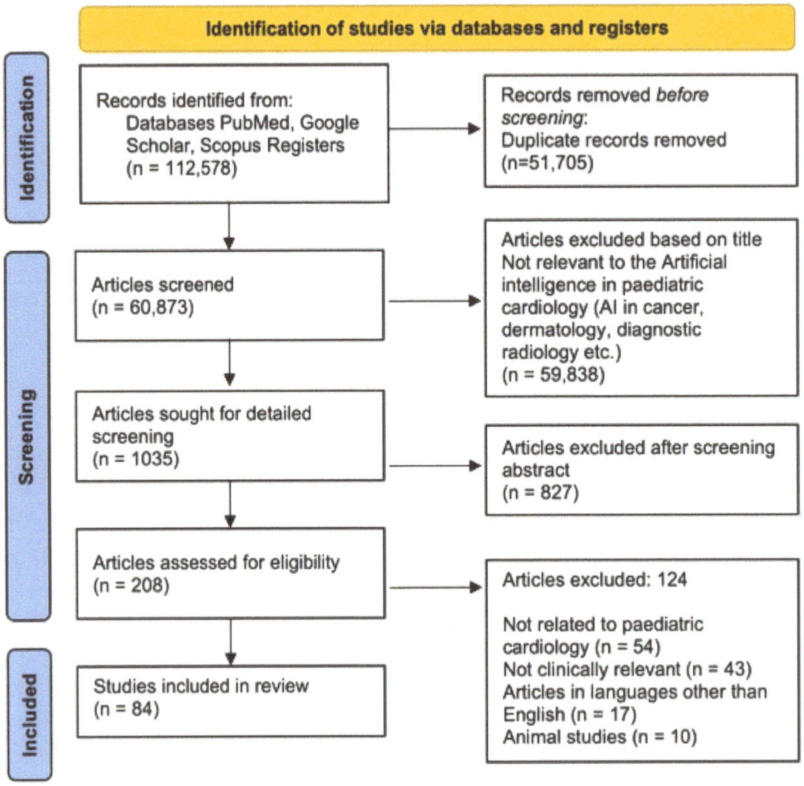

Fig. 12.1 Flow diagram showing selection process of studies included

AI and Murmurs

AI has the potential to improve the validity of auscultatory findings for diagnosing CHD .The limitations of objective performance data have restricted wide acceptability so far . The auscultatory findings of CHD are integral to the clinical diagnosis and have the benefit of being a low-cost tool, but are subject to clinical expertise, which becomes a limitation in resource-limited countries and creates a need for support to the clinician that is objective and reportable by even peripheral health workers. The lack of trained cardiologists at the peripheral level leads to an unavoidable miss of a timely clinical diagnosis of CHD, contributing to delayed intervention and thus a poor prognosis .The emergence of AI-based digital stethoscopes and cloud reporting for telemedicine has helped with the timely diagnosis and early intervention of CHD in reported samples . The AI-based technologies also seem affordable, helping the current interest. The use of an intelligent diagnostic system based on AI algorithms such as wavelet analysis and artificial neural networks has shown a specificity of 70.5% and a sensitivity of 64.7% . The developments in AI for detecting cardiac murmurs have shown promise in terms of sensitivity but still require clinical validation before wide clinical recommendation

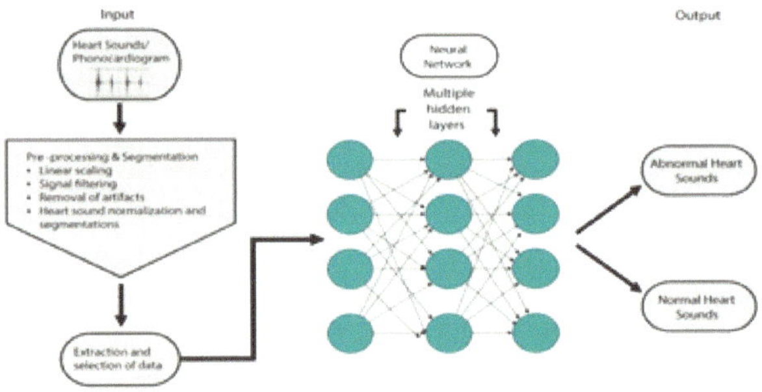

Fig.12.2 A model of application of neural networks in pediatric cardiology.

Image Processing with AI

Chest x-ray

CHDs present with some classical chest x-ray signs that can help with suspicion of the disease, including boot-shaped heart (Tetralogy of Fallot), egg-on-string (Transposition of Great Arteries), snowman sign (Total Anomalous Pulmonary Venous Return), scimitar sign (Partial Anomalous Pulmonary Venous Return), gooseneck sign (Endocardial cushion defects), a figure of three (Coarctation of Aorta) and box-shaped heart (Ebstein anomaly) .Chest radiography being easy, cost-effective, and readily available allows a direct or collaborative diagnostic approach to CHD. The evolution of deep learning models and machine learning models and the establishment of defined pediatric datasets have allowed the entry of AI for use in the pediatric population . AI can be immensely beneficial in various steps of imaging such as ordering tests, reporting communication, enhancing the quality of images, and aiding radiologists in interpreting images

MRI

Cardiac MRI has evolved as a precise method for structural and functional evaluations of the heart . The technology has evolved over the years from traditional techniques such as cardiac gating and the suspension of breathing to newer advanced techniques of high-field-strength magnets, high-performance gradient hardware and ultrafast pulse sequences. In the discipline of magnetic resonance imaging, the advancement of AI has allowed for shorter scan times, resulting in higher patient satisfaction; it also reduces errors by minimizing motion artefacts caused by patient movement. The segmentation of cardiac chambers helps visualize them better and aids in diagnosis. Currently, we do this manually, and a shift to AI will help with a faster diagnosis and reduce variation between different analysts .

Echocardiography

New AI-based technologies have revolutionized modern medicine in obtaining fetal echocardiograms with improved precision and accuracy. Combining it with machine learning has been quintessential in making predictions of future variables associated with disease progression using retrospective patient data. It has helped in eliminating limitations associated with a lack of expertise in fetal echocardiology, fetal movements, and fetal heart size . Machine learning-based systems have been useful in differentiating pathological versus physiological hypertrophic remodeling of the heart . Deep learning models have demonstrated superiority in terms of sensitivity and specificity up to 76% and 88%, respectively, in diagnosing atrial septal defect (ASD) compared with pediatric cardiologists who demonstrated sensitivity and specificity of 53% ± 0.04 and 67% ± 0.10 respectively .Automation, AI, and machine learning are game-changing as complementary tools to physicians and in areas with limited expert medical personnel or cardiologists.Fetal intelligent navigation echocardiography (FINE) has presented as a novel method for fetal echocardiographyusing "intelligent navigation" technology to obtain nine standard views—four-chamber, aortic arch, three vessels, and trachea—and display abnormalities with great sensitivity helping to detect CHD . New AI-based technologies have revolutionized modern medicine in obtaining fetal echocardiograms with improved precision and accuracy. Combining it with machine learning has been quintessential in making predictions of future variables associated with disease progression using retrospective patient data. It has helped in eliminating limitations associated with a lack of expertise in fetal echocardiology, fetal movements, and fetal heart size . Machine learning-based systems have been useful in differentiating pathological versus physiological hypertrophic remodeling of the heart . Deep learning models have demonstrated superiority in terms of sensitivity and specificity up to 76% and 88%, respectively, in diagnosing atrial septal defect (ASD) compared with pediatric cardiologists who demonstrated sensitivity and specificity of 53% ± 0.04 and 67% ± 0.10 respectively .Automation, AI, and machine learning are game-changing as complementary tools to physicians and in areas with limited expert medical personnel or cardiologists.Fetalintelligentnavigation echocardiography (FINE) has presented as a novel method for fetal echocardiography using "intelligent navigation" technology to obtain nine standard views—four-chamber, aortic arch, three vessels, and trachea—and display abnormalities with great sensitivity helping to detect CHD .

ECG

The use of deep learning (DL), an application of AI, in the field of adult cardiology has been well studied . Its application in pediatric cardiology has become especially relevant due to its potential for allowing early diagnosis, and thus better prognosis, in congenital heart diseases (CHDs). DL models such as convolutional neural network (CNN) and recurrent neural network (RNN) are used in conjunction with electrocardiograms, which remain the staple diagnostic tool for CHDs, to provide enhanced diagnostic information that is otherwise only deduced with input from specialists . Convolutional neural networks can perform image processing and classification, providing an advantage of extracting additional ECG information that would otherwise either be undetected . While the efficiency and utility of using AI models with ECGs for CHDs is evident, the enhancement of the interpretability and training of deep learning models is still needed for widespread implementation .

Prognosis and Risk Stratification

AI-based algorithms have proven to be of great help for pediatric cardiology in the clinical examination, diagnosis, procedural planning, and management of cardiac interventions AI models have also aided with the extraction of patient data for risk stratification and ambulatory health monitoring from wearables. Machine learning (ML)-based models such as optimal classification trees (OCTs) have accurately predicted mortality, postoperative mechanical ventilatory support time (MVST), and hospital length of stay (LOS) even with nonlinear data in patients with a history of congenital heart surgery . Similarly, ML algorithm-based models, extreme gradient boosting (XGBoost), and RCRnet have accurately predicted preoperative mortality odds in patients with CHDs and statistically significant prognostic indicators along with risk stratification markers in patients with Tetralogy of Fallot and left-to-right shunt CHDs, respectively . Importantly, the far-reaching utility of AI-based models in risk stratification and prognostic predictions is the trainability of models to work with various data cohorts .

Planning and Management of Cardiac Interventions

The current approach to planning and the execution of interventions in CHD relies primarily on generic treatment protocols derived from biological data and set guidelines. As such, there is a lack of tailor-made interventions based on each patient, which would drastically improve outcomes and post-intervention prognosis . Artificial intelligence (AI), with its applications in the form of machine learning (ML) and deep learning (DL) among many, has emerged as a tool aiding the creation of personalized intervention plans as well as an accurate data extractor to ascertain potential post-operative sequelae . The supervised machine learning models such as k-nearest neighbor classifier (KNN) and support vector machine classifier (SVM) have also aided in the intra-operative assessment of cardiac fluid kinematics, which are significant determinants of successful congenital heart surgeries . The subsequent post-operative management of CHDs is imperative for maintaining the structural fluid dynamics and thus the prognosis. This could be done seamlessly with the help of recurrent neural networks based on ML models and deep learning models, allowing for an integrated system that can enhance survival outcomes in pediatric patients .

AI in Cardiac Surgeries

AI can revolutionize pediatric surgery in all stages of surgery: preoperative, intraoperative and post-operative. Preoperative risk assessment and decision-making can be made easier by the tremendous processing and analyzing capacity of AI-enabled algorithms. Surgical decision support systems using ANN can predict post-op outcomes and can prevent morbidity and mortality arising from poor risk assessment pre-operatively.

Tech-enhanced (Hitech) operation theaters can enable intraoperative interventions and decision support and bring about a paradigm shift in telesurgery; it is especially useful in cardiac surgeries, where manual segmentation of retrieved images (CT/MRI) can take an unreasonable amount of time. Humans embarked on this path successfully when Xiaowei Xu et al. utilized AI to perform a cardiac surgery remotely in a patient having complications of long-standing ASD through the backbone of 5G technology. This was possible since AI replaced manual segmentation and provided accurate results in just two minutes compared to the traditional manual segmentation which takes 2–3 h even by experts . In this situation, the authors helped a patient who could not be transported to another hospital due to her frail condition; we can extend the same advantage to a remote inaccessible location especially in rural areas and developing countries . Postoperative AI can help in various aspects such as ambulatory patient monitoring post-discharge with AI wearables and automated risk stratification of patients to enable stricter follow-ups. Mahayni AA et al. described an ECG based AI algorithm that predicts ventricular dysfunction post-surgery, predicts long-term mortality in cardiac surgeries. Such algorithms can be developed and implemented for pediatric surgical procedures and drastically improve surgical outcomes.

AI in other Pediatric Heart Diseases

Kawasaki disease (KD) is an acquired pediatric vasculitis that can lead to coronary artery aneurysms and acute coronary syndrome . Very little is known about the pathogenesis of Kawasaki disease but a recent study using AI-guided signatures reveals a shared pathology with Multisystem inflammatory syndrome in children (MIS-C), COVID-19 associated vasculitis in children. Both these syndromes share systemic inflammatory storm with similar cytokines such as IL15/IL15RA. Such AI-based investigative approaches will further elucidate its complex pathogenesis and help decipher novel diagnostic and therapeutic targets

The appropriate and timely management of Kawasaki disease can significantly reduce the coronary complications associated with Kawasaki disease which contribute greatly to mortality in adulthood . AI-based approaches can prove to be extremely crucial in predicting the risk of developing a coronary aneurysm. It is widely known that Kawasaki patients with intravenous immunoglobulin resistance are at a higher risk of developing coronary artery aneurysms, but most scoring models present for predicting the resistance are impractical. Wang T et al. describe a machine learning-based model on patient data that can predict intravenous immunoglobulin resistance in Kawasaki disease patients successfully. The scope for several such prediction models is possible with the advent of AI and can support clinical decisions to improve patient outcomes . Distensibility changes in a coronary artery can be used to predict acute coronary disease in these patients. Benovoy M et al. calculated these changes in KD using an automated deep learning approach and correlated it with the severity of OCT (Optical coherence tomography) findings of KD-related CA damage . Despite, the limited studies using AI-based approaches, AI has the potential to revolutionize risk stratification and prognosis estimation of Kawasaki disease as well as paving way for newer drug targets by elucidating the pathogenesis.

RHD—The screening of RHD requires the clinician's expertise, and hence the grass-root level is limited by a lack of skilled human resources. Automatic diagnosis of echo-detected RHD is feasible and can form the core of the screening programs of the future covering the workload of experts . Recent data has also shown promise for a convolutional neural network-based deep learning algorithm to identify heart sounds as 'rheumatic' with an overall accuracy of 96.1% having 94.0% sensitivity and 98.1% specificity . Therefore, AI can form the backbone of future global screening programs for RHD.

AI Algorithms in Pediatric Cardiology

In many areas of pediatric cardiology, AI-based algorithms can be beneficial, including: (1) clinical examination and diagnosis, (2) image processing, (3) fetal cardiology, (4) prognosis and risk stratification, (5) precision cardiology, and (6) planning and management of cardiac interventions. Machine learning algorithms are a very promising tool for diagnosing and assessing critical and non-critical CHD; however, extensive research is still required to develop interpretable, robust, and generalizable models for clinical application, especially in light of the extreme heterogeneity of complex CHD. Various such AI algorithm models have gained interest over the past decade, and the present time has seen many motivating developments.

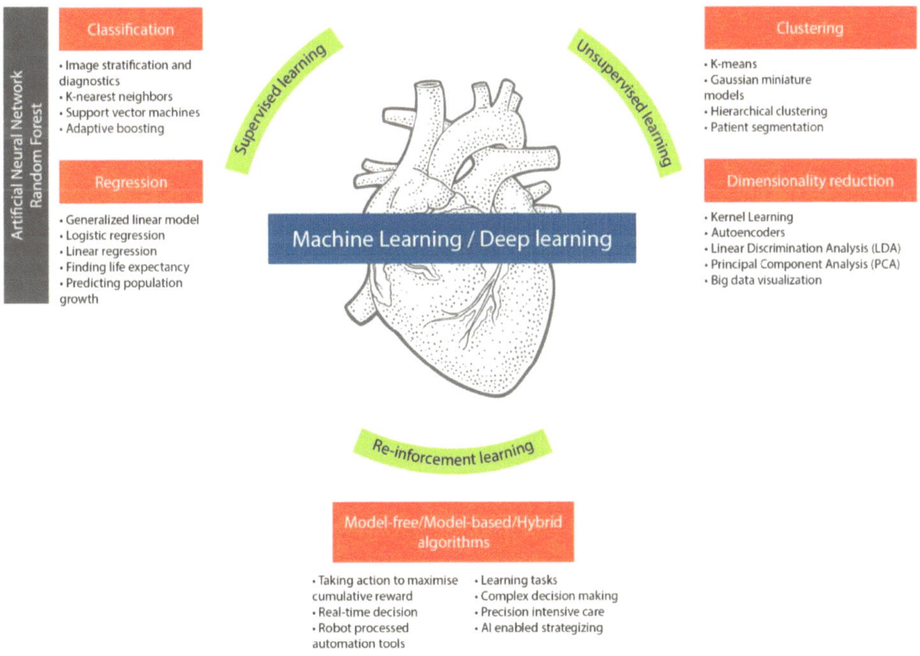

Fig. 12.3 AI-based algorithms and pediatric cardiology.

AI is rapidly growing, and its significance in clinical practice cannot be negated. It plays a crucial part in augmenting and standardizing care by adding to a physician's skills and expertise. The role of AI in pediatric cardiology has greatly evolved over the past two decades . It picks up subtle or unrecognizable features, preventing missed diagnoses and leading to a better prognosis. Physicians can combine their clinical expertise with AI to enhance their outputs in the domains of prevention, predictive intervention, and health maintenance. AI can make use of continuous data received from wearable devices to offer insight into patients' behaviors and health trends. These features of AI empower the professional to provide the best care to the patient earlier in the course of the disease, helping to improve prognosis and leading to better outcomes.

AI seems to be the tool of rich and economically advanced countries, but it can be the magic wand for risk stratification troubles in lower- and middle-income countries (LMICs). AI has the potential to reduce global health inequalities . It can help serve LMICs by bridging gaps in equity, availability, affordability, and accessibility . For instance, the major addition of AI is a reduction in the costs of dimensions requiring expensive equipment and specialized expertise, including tools of screening and planning that are unavailable in most hospitals, especially in LMICs. AI-based innovations can help overcome resource-constrained environments.The advent of AI has allowed smart tools to assist peripheral health workers in helping with a rough screening at the doorstep and in peripheral areas having poor doctor–patient ratios .

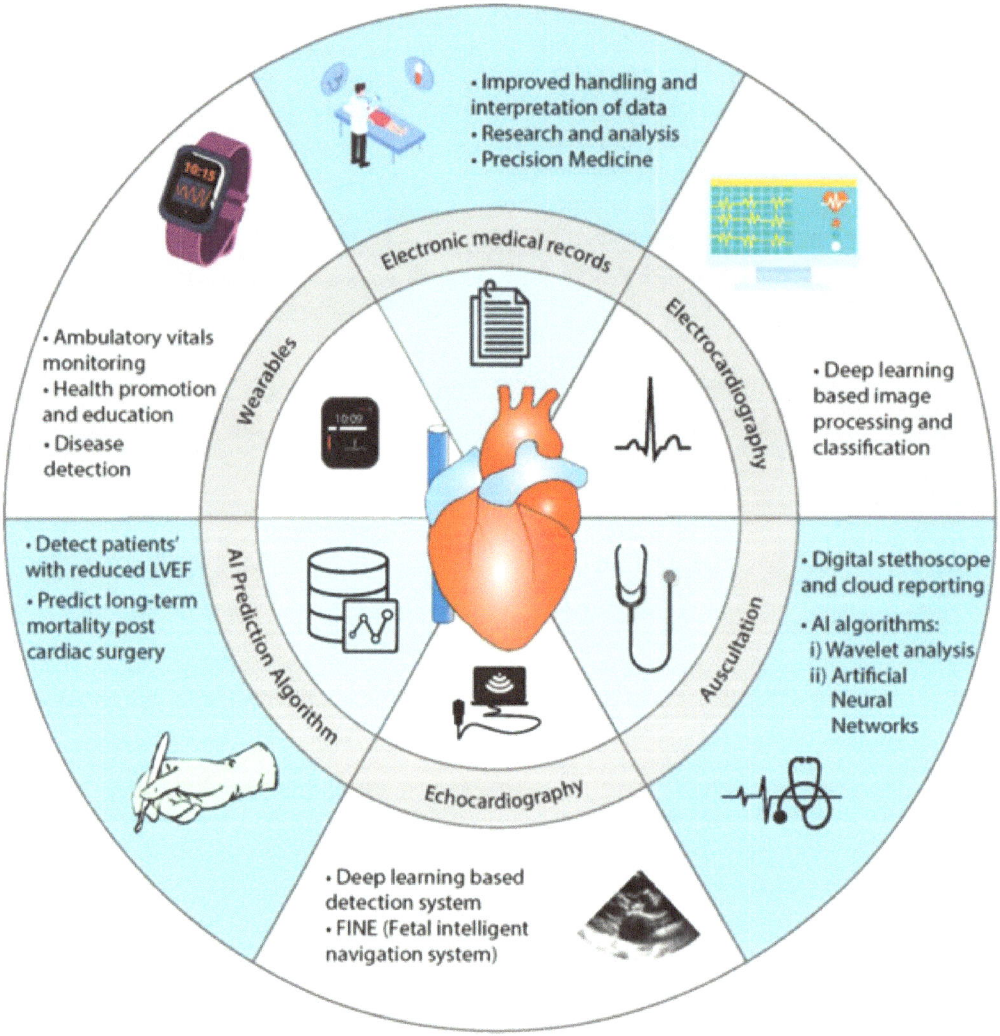

Fig. 12.4 Diagnostic and prognostic applications of AI in Pediatric Cardiology

The availability of skilled cardiologists to diagnose CHD in remote locations will require a giant leap in these countries. AI-based medical equipment can aid peripheral health care providers in helping with screening and referral. It can also help in terms of teleconsultation and remote radiology . Furthermore, with the availability of AI-based chatbots or virtual avatars and characters, we can offer greater help to populations suffering from stigmatizing pathologies (such as HIV/AIDS and psychiatric pathologies). This therefore can aid in improving access to health care and follow-up services. One of the biggest challenges to health care is language, with improving translation tools, AI can help cover this area well too .

AI: An Efficient Physician Assistant

The full-blown implementation of AI still is resisted by physicians and health care staff fearing inaccuracies, the exclusion of social variables, and possible unemployment. The mechanization of health care, loss of empathy, and human touch to this extent often invite skepticism from the traditional medical community. Despite the fear-mongering and skepticism of loss of human touch and jobs, we opine AI can be an efficient aid to physicians rather than a replacement . It can streamline insurance reviews, provide real-time data analysis, and assist in research. It can reduce the burden on physicians and burnout rates in the medical community. Thus, application in appropriate areas can contribute to the overall enhancement of health care delivery and experience .

Challenges to AI in Pediatric Cardiology

The incorporation of AI into pediatric cardiology has several challenges. The data available for pediatric cardiology is still very limited which is necessary to train AI algorithms to identify, assess and reduce inherent biases and overfitting. Furthermore, the heterogeneity in cardiac anatomy and the rarity of individual disease entities make data accessibility and AI incorporation into pediatric cardiology difficult. We can cater to this limitation by pooling data from all the different hospitals to get a large data set . Imaging in the pediatric population has another challenge owing to their smaller size and frequent movements during imaging, which lead to higher motion artifacts. This poses a technical challenge, for instance, requiring higher spatial resolution in the MRI . The doctor and patient may hesitate to use AI to replace the current protocols. The incorporation of AI will require health care providers to learn interpret data and accurately understand the many model parameters or model architectures. This challenge is being tackled in different ways. For example, some works have incorporated more intuitive interfaces in the models aiding easier interpretation .Additionally, AI is evolving and several ethical concerns are arising. These concerns include informed consent to data access, data security and privacy, algorithm fairness and biases, and transparency . Currently, there are no well-defined laws or regulations in place to address the legal and ethical issues that may arise with AI use in health care settings. However, as AI continues to grow and be used, laws and regulations can certainly be explored to ensure algorithmic transparency and protect data privacy.

Conclusions

AI can be touted as the next revolution in medicine. From making physicians' lives easier to enabling research with ease, it has variegated applications in the working environment as well as in the management of patients. Pediatric cardiology is a specialty requiring a great skill set in cognition and interpretation which makes it an ideal candidate for AI incorporation. AI has been successfully integrated into clinical examination, image interpretation, diagnoses, prognosis, risk stratification, precision medicine, and treatment in pediatric cardiology. The advent of AI has facilitated medicine to be more accurate and precise, but it is still a work in progress with challenges and limitations. Despite the roadblocks, we optimistically opine that AI with its current pace will streamline approaches in pediatric cardiology.

Bibliography and Acknowledgement

- Ahmad M.S., Mir J., Ullah M.O., Shahid M.L.U.R., Syed M.A. An Efficient Heart Murmur Recognition and Cardiovascular Disorders Classification System. Australas. Phys. Eng. Sci. Med. 2019;42:733–743.doi: 10.1007/s13246-019-00778-x. [PubMed] [CrossRef] [Google Scholar]
- Ali F., Hasan B., Ahmad H., Hoodbhoy Z., Bhuriwala Z., Hanif M., Ansari S.U., Chowdhury D. Detection of Subclinical Rheumatic Heart Disease in Children Using a Deep Learning Algorithm on Digital Stethoscope: A Study Protocol. BMJ Open. 2021;11:e044070. doi: 10.1136/bmjopen-2020-044070. [PMC free article] [PubMed] [CrossRef] [Google Scholar]
- Andrisevic N., Ejaz K., Rios-Gutierrez F., Alba-Flores R., Nordehn G., Burns S. Detection of Heart Murmurs Using Wavelet Analysis and Artificial Neural Networks. J. Biomech. Eng. 2005;127:899–904. doi: 10.1115/1.2049327. [PubMed] [CrossRef] [Google Scholar]
- Arafati A., Hu P., Finn J.P., Rickers C., Cheng A.L., Jafarkhani H., Kheradvar A. Artificial Intelligence in Pediatric and Adult Congenital Cardiac MRI: An Unmet Clinical Need. Cardiovasc. Diagn. Ther. 2019;9:S310–S325. doi: 10.21037/cdt.2019.06.09. [PMC free article] [PubMed] [CrossRef] [Google Scholar]
- Arnaout R., Curran L., Chinn E., Zhao Y., Moon-Grady A. Deep-Learning Models Improve on Community-Level Diagnosis for Common Congenital Heart Disease Lesions. arXiv. 2018 doi: 10.48550/arxiv.1809.06993.1809.06993 [CrossRef] [Google Scholar]

- Aufiero S., Bleijendaal H., Robyns T., Vandenberk B., Krijger C., Bezzina C., Zwinderman A.H., Wilde A.A.M., Pinto Y.M. A Deep Learning Approach Identifies New ECG Features in Congenital Long QT Syndrome. BMC Med. 2022;20:162. doi: 10.1186/s12916-022-02350-z. [PMC free article] [PubMed] [CrossRef] [Google Scholar]
- Basu K., Sinha R., Ong A., Basu T. Artificial Intelligence: How Is It Changing Medical Sciences and Its Future? Indian J. Dermatol. 2020;65:365. doi: 10.4103/ijd.IJD_421_20. [PMC free article] [PubMed] [CrossRef] [Google Scholar]
- Bayers S., Shulman S.T., Paller A.S. Kawasaki Disease. J. Am. Acad. Dermatol. 2013;69:513.e1–513.e8. doi: 10.1016/j.jaad.2013.06.040. [PubMed] [CrossRef] [Google Scholar]
- Begic E., Gurbeta Pokvic L., Begic Z., Begic N., Dedic M., Mrsic D., Jamakovic M., Vila N., Badnjevic A. From Heart Murmur to Echocardiography—Congenital Heart Defects Diagnostics Using Machine-Learning Algorithms. Psychiatr. Danub. 2021;33:236–246. [PubMed] [Google Scholar]
- Benke K., Benke G. Artificial Intelligence and Big Data in Public Health. Int. J. Environ. Res. Public Health. 2018;15:2796. doi: 10.3390/ijerph15122796. [PMC free article] [PubMed] [CrossRef] [Google Scholar]
- Benovoy M., Dionne A., McCrindle B.W., Manlhiot C., Ibrahim R., Dahdah N. Deep Learning-Based Approach to Automatically Assess Coronary Distensibility Following Kawasaki Disease. Pediatr. Cardiol. 2022;43:807–815. doi: 10.1007/s00246-021-02790-z. [PubMed] [CrossRef] [Google Scholar]
- Bertsimas D., Zhuo D., Dunn J., Levine J., Zuccarelli E., Smyrnakis N., Tobota Z., Maruszewski B., Fragata J., Sarris G.E. Adverse Outcomes Prediction for Congenital Heart Surgery: A Machine Learning Approach. World J. Pediatr. Congenit. Heart Surg. 2021;12:453–460. doi: 10.1177/21501351211007106. [PubMed] [CrossRef] [Google Scholar]
- Blue G.M., Kirk E.P., Sholler G.F., Harvey R.P., Winlaw D.S. Congenital Heart Disease: Current Knowledge about Causes and Inheritance. Med. J. Aust. 2012;197:155–159. doi: 10.5694/mja12.10811. [PubMed] [CrossRef] [Google Scholar]
- Bodenhofer U., Haslinger-Eisterer B., Minichmayer A., Hermanutz G., Meier J. Machine Learning-Based Risk Profile Classification of Patients Undergoing Elective Heart Valve Surgery. Eur. J. Cardiothorac. Surg. 2021;60:1378–1385. doi: 10.1093/ejcts/ezab219. [PubMed] [CrossRef] [Google Scholar]
- Bozkurt B., Germanakis I., Stylianou Y. A Study of Time-Frequency Features for CNN-Based Automatic Heart Sound Classification for Pathology Detection. Comput. Biol. Med. 2018;100:132–143. doi: 10.1016/j.compbiomed.2018.06.026. [PubMed] [CrossRef] [Google Scholar]
- Chang A. Artificial Intelligence in Pediatric Cardiology and Cardiac Surgery: Irrational Hype or Paradigm Shift? Ann. Pediatr. Cardiol. 2019;12:191. doi: 10.4103/apc.APC_55_19. [PMC free article] [PubMed] [CrossRef] [Google Scholar]
- Chang J.C., Binuesa F., Caneo L.F., Turquetto A.L.R., Arita E.C.T.C., Barbosa A.C., Fernandes A.M.D.S., Trindade E.M., Jatene F.B., Dossou P.-E., et al. Improving Preoperative Risk-of-Death Prediction in Surgery Congenital Heart Defects Using Artificial Intelligence Model: A Pilot Study. PLoS ONE. 2020;15:e0238199. doi: 10.1371/journal.pone.0238199. [PMC free article] [PubMed] [CrossRef] [Google Scholar]
- Chen C., Qin C., Qiu H., Tarroni G., Duan J., Bai W., Rueckert D. Deep Learning for Cardiac Image Segmentation: A Review. Front. Cardiovasc. Med. 2020;7:25. doi: 10.3389/fcvm.2020.00025. [PMC free article] [PubMed] [CrossRef] [Google Scholar]
- Chou F.-S., Ghimire L.V. Identification of Prognostic Factors for Pediatric Myocarditis with a Random Forests Algorithm-Assisted Approach. Pediatr. Res. 2021;90:427–430. doi: 10.1038/s41390-020-01268-7. [PubMed] [CrossRef] [Google Scholar]
- Davies R., Babu-Narayan S.V. Deep Learning in Congenital Heart Disease Imaging: Hope but Not Haste. Heart. 2020;106:960–961. doi: 10.1136/heartjnl-2019-316496. [PubMed] [CrossRef] [Google Scholar]
- Decourt C., Duong L. Semi-Supervised Generative Adversarial Networks for the Segmentation of the Left Ventricle in Pediatric MRI. Comput. Biol. Med. 2020;123:103884. doi: 10.1016/j.compbiomed.2020.103884. [PubMed] [CrossRef] [Google Scholar]
- DeGroff C.G., Bhatikar S., Hertzberg J., Shandas R., Valdes-Cruz L., Mahajan R.L. Artificial Neural Network–Based Method of Screening Heart Murmurs in Children. Circulation. 2001;103:2711–2716. doi: 10.1161/01.CIR.103.22.2711. [PubMed] [CrossRef] [Google Scholar]
- Dias R.D., Shah J.A., Zenati M.A. Artificial Intelligence in Cardiothoracic Surgery. Minerva Cardioangiol. 2020;68:532–538. doi: 10.23736/S0026-4725.20.05235-4. [PMC free article] [PubMed] [CrossRef] [Google Scholar]
- Diller G.-P., Babu-Narayan S., Li W., Radojevic J., Kempny A., Uebing A., Dimopoulos K., Baumgartner H., Gatzoulis M.A., Orwat S. Utility of Machine Learning Algorithms in Assessing Patients with a Systemic Right Ventricle. Eur. Heart J. Cardiovasc. Imaging. 2019;20:925–931. doi: 10.1093/ehjci/jey211. [PMC free article] [PubMed] [CrossRef] [Google Scholar]
- Diller G.-P., Kempny A., Babu-Narayan S.V., Henrichs M., Brida M., Uebing A., Lammers A.E., Baumgartner H., Li W., Wort S.J., et al. Machine Learning Algorithms Estimating Prognosis and Guiding Therapy in Adult Congenital Heart Disease: Data from a Single Tertiary Centre Including 10,019 Patients. Eur. Heart J. 2019;40:1069–1077. doi: 10.1093/eurheartj/ehy915. [PMC free article] [PubMed] [CrossRef] [Google Scholar]
- Diller G.-P., Lammers A.E., Babu-Narayan S., Li W., Radke R.M., Baumgartner H., Gatzoulis M.A., Orwat S. Denoising and Artefact Removal for Transthoracic Echocardiographic Imaging in Congenital Heart Disease: Utility of Diagnosis Specific Deep Learning Algorithms. Int. J. Cardiovasc. Imaging. 2019;35:2189–2196. doi: 10.1007/s10554-019-01671-0. [PubMed] [CrossRef] [Google Scholar]
- Diller G.P., Orwat S., Vahle J., Bauer U.M.M., Urban A., Sarikouch S., Berger F., Beerbaum P., Baumgartner H. Prediction of Prognosis in Patients with Tetralogy of Fallot Based on Deep Learning Imaging Analysis. Heart. 2020;106:1007–1014. doi: 10.1136/heartjnl-2019-315962. [PubMed] [CrossRef] [Google Scholar]
- Ding Y., Gudapati V., Lin R., Fei Y., Packard R.R.S., Song S., Chang C.-C., Baek K.I., Wang Z., Roustaei M., et al. Saak Transform-Based Machine Learning for Light-Sheet Imaging of Cardiac Trabeculation. IEEE Trans. Biomed. Eng. 2021;68:225–235. doi: 10.1109/TBME.2020.2991754. [PMC free article] [PubMed] [CrossRef] [Google Scholar]
- Dozen A., Komatsu M., Sakai A., Komatsu R., Shozu K., Machino H., Yasutomi S., Arakaki T., Asada K., Kaneko S., et al. Image Segmentation of the Ventricular Septum in Fetal Cardiac Ultrasound Videos Based on Deep Learning Using Time-Series Information. Biomolecules. 2020;10:1526. doi: 10.3390/biom10111526. [PMC free article] [PubMed] [CrossRef] [Google Scholar]

- El-Segaier M., Lilja O., Lukkarinen S., Sörnmo L., Sepponen R., Pesonen E. Computer-Based Detection and Analysis of Heart Sound and Murmur. Ann. Biomed. Eng. 2005;33:937–942. doi: 10.1007/s10439-005-4053-3. [PubMed] [CrossRef] [Google Scholar]
- Ernst S., Babu-Narayan S.V., Keegan J., Horduna I., Lyne J., Till J., Kilner P.J., Pennell D., Rigby M.L., Gatzoulis M.A. Remote-Controlled Magnetic Navigation and Ablation with 3D Image Integration as an Alternative Approach in Patients with Intra-Atrial Baffle Anatomy. Circ. Arrhythm. Electrophysiol. 2012;5:131–139. doi: 10.1161/CIRCEP.111.962993. [PubMed] [CrossRef]
- Ferguson E.C., Krishnamurthy R., Oldham S.A.A. Classic Imaging Signs of Congenital Cardiovascular Abnormalities. Radiographics. 2007;27:1323–1334. doi: 10.1148/rg.275065148. [PubMed] [CrossRef] [Google Scholar]
- Gaffar S., Gearhart A.S., Chang A.C. The Next Frontier in Pediatric Cardiology. Pediatr. Clin. N. Am. 2020;67:995–1009. doi: 10.1016/j.pcl.2020.06.010. [PubMed] [CrossRef] [Google Scholar]
- Gampala S., Vankeshwaram V., Gadula S.S.P. Is Artificial Intelligence the New Friend for Radiologists? A Review Article. Cureus. 2020;12:e11137. doi: 10.7759/cureus.11137. [PMC free article] [PubMed] [CrossRef] [Google Scholar]
- Gandhi S., Mosleh W., Shen J., Chow C.-M. Automation, Machine Learning, and Artificial Intelligence in Echocardiography: A Brave New World. Echocardiography. 2018;35:1402–1418. doi: 10.1111/echo.14086. [PubMed] [CrossRef] [Google Scholar]
- Garcia-Canadilla P., Isabel-Roquero A., Aurensanz-Clemente E., Valls-Esteve A., Miguel F.A., Ormazabal D., Llanos F., Sanchez-de-Toledo J. Machine Learning-Based Systems for the Anticipation of Adverse Events after Pediatric Cardiac Surgery. Front. Pediatr. 2022;10:930913. doi: 10.3389/fped.2022.930913. [PMC free article] [PubMed] [CrossRef] [Google Scholar]
- Garcia-Canadilla P., Sanchez-Martinez S., Crispi F., Bijnens B. Machine Learning in Fetal Cardiology: What to Expect. Fetal Diagn. Ther. 2020;47:363–372. doi: 10.1159/000505021. [PubMed] [CrossRef] [Google Scholar]
- Gerke S., Minssen T., Cohen G. Artificial Intelligence in Healthcare. Elsevier; Amsterdam, The Netherlands: 2020. Ethical and Legal Challenges of Artificial Intelligence-Driven Healthcare; pp. 295–336. [Google Scholar]
- Ghosh P., Katkar G.D., Shimizu C., Kim J., Khandelwal S., Tremoulet A.H., Kanegaye J.T., Abe N., Austin-Page L., Bryl A., et al. An Artificial Intelligence-Guided Signature Reveals the Shared Host Immune Response in MIS-C and Kawasaki Disease. Nat. Commun. 2022;13:2687. doi: 10.1038/s41467-022-30357-w. [PMC free article] [PubMed] [CrossRef] [Google Scholar]
- Gilboa S.M., Devine O.J., Kucik J.E., Oster M.E., Riehle-Colarusso T., Nembhard W.N., Xu P., Correa A., Jenkins K., Marelli A.J. Congenital Heart Defects in the United States. Circulation. 2016;134:101–109.doi: 10.1161/CIRCULATIONAHA.115.019307. [PMC free article] [PubMed] [CrossRef] [Google Scholar]
- Hauptmann A., Arridge S., Lucka F., Muthurangu V., Steeden J.A. Real-time Cardiovascular MR with Spatio-temporal Artifact Suppression Using Deep Learning–Proof of Concept in Congenital Heart Disease. Magn. Reason. Med. 2019;81:1143–1156. doi: 10.1002/mrm.27480. [PMC free article] [PubMed]
- Helman S.M., Herrup E.A., Christopher A.B., Al-Zaiti S.S. The Role of Machine Learning Applications in Diagnosing and Assessing Critical and Non-Critical CHD: A Scoping Review. Cardiol. Young. 2021;31:1770–1780.
- Higashi H., Barendregt J.J., Kassebaum N.J., Weiser T.G., Bickler S.W., Vos T. The Burden of Selected Congenital Anomalies Amenable to Surgery in Low and Middle-Income Regions: Cleft Lip and Palate, Congenital Heart Anomalies and Neural Tube Defects. Arch. Dis. Child. 2015;100:233–238. doi: 10.1136/archdischild-2014-306175. [PubMed] [CrossRef] [Google Scholar]
- Hong S., Zhou Y., Shang J., Xiao C., Sun J. Opportunities and Challenges of Deep Learning Methods for Electrocardiogram Data: A Systematic Review. Comput. Biol. Med. 2020;122:103801. doi: 10.1016/j.compbiomed.2020.103801. [PubMed] [CrossRef] [Google Scholar]
- Huang L., Li J., Huang M., Zhuang J., Yuan H., Jia Q., Zeng D., Que L., Xi Y., Lin J., et al. Prediction of Pulmonary Pressure after Glenn Shunts by Computed Tomography–Based Machine Learning Models. Eur. Radiol. 2020;30:1369–1377. doi: 10.1007/s00330-019-06502-3. [PubMed] [CrossRef] [Google Scholar]
- Johnson K.W., Torres Soto J., Glicksberg B.S., Shameer K., Miotto R., Ali M., Ashley E., Dudley J.T. Artificial Intelligence in Cardiology. J. Am. Coll. Cardiol. 2018;71:2668–2679. doi: 10.1016/j.jacc.2018.03.521. [PubMed] [CrossRef] [Google Scholar]
- Kang S., Doroshow R., McConnaughey J., Shekhar R. Automated Identification of Innocent Still's Murmur in Children. IEEE Trans. Biomed. Eng. 2017;64:1326–1334. doi: 10.1109/TBME.2016.2603787. [PubMed] [CrossRef] [Google Scholar]
- Karimi-Bidhendi S., Arafati A., Cheng A.L., Wu Y., Kheradvar A., Jafarkhani H. Fully-automated Deep-learning Segmentation of Pediatric Cardiovascular Magnetic Resonance of Patients with Complex Congenital Heart Diseases. J. Cardiovasc. Magn. Reson. 2020;22:80. doi: 10.1186/s12968-020-00678-0.
- Khurshid S., Friedman S., Pirruccello J.P., di Achille P., Diamant N., Anderson C.D., Ellinor P.T., Batra P., Ho J.E., Philippakis A.A., et al. Deep Learning to Predict Cardiac Magnetic Resonance–Derived Left Ventricular Mass and Hypertrophy from 12-Lead ECGs. Circ. Cardiovasc. Imaging. 2021;14:e012281.
- Ko W.-Y., Siontis K.C., Attia Z.I., Carter R.E., Kapa S., Ommen S.R., Demuth S.J., Ackerman M.J., Gersh B.J., Arruda-Olson A.M., et al. Detection of Hypertrophic Cardiomyopathy Using a Convolutional Neural Network-Enabled Electrocardiogram. J. Am. Coll. Cardiol. 2020;75:722–733.
- Kokol P., Završnik J., Blažun Vošner H. Artificial Intelligence and Pediatrics: A Synthetic Mini Review. Pediatr. Dimens. 2017;2 doi: 10.15761/PD.1000155. [CrossRef] [Google Scholar]
- Lakhe A., Sodhi I., Warrier J., Sinha V. Development of Digital Stethoscope for Telemedicine. J. Med. Eng. Technol. 2016;40:20–24.
- Lemaire J.B., Schaefer J.P., Martin L.A., Faris P., Ainslie M.D., Hull R.D. Effectiveness of the Quick Medical Reference as a Diagnostic Tool. CMAJ. 1999;161:725–728. [PMC free article] [PubMed] [Google Scholar]
- Leng S., Tan R.S., Chai K.T.C., Wang C., Ghista D., Zhong L. The Electronic Stethoscope. Biomed. Eng. Online. 2015;14:66. doi: 10.1186/s12938-015-0056-y. [PMC free article]
- Li H., Luo M., Zheng J., Luo J., Zeng R., Feng N., Du Q., Fang J. An Artificial Neural Network Prediction Model of Congenital Heart Disease Based on Risk Factors. Medicine. 2017;96:e6090.

- Liu J., Wang H., Yang Z., Quan J., Liu L., Tian J. Deep Learning-Based Computer-Aided Heart Sound Analysis in Children with Left-to-Right Shunt Congenital Heart Disease. Int. J. Cardiol. 2022;348:58–64. doi: 10.1016/j.ijcard.2021.12.012. [PubMed] [CrossRef] [Google Scholar]
- Lv J., Dong B., Lei H., Shi G., Wang H., Zhu F., Wen C., Zhang Q., Fu L., Gu X., et al. Artificial Intelligence-Assisted Auscultation in Detecting Congenital Heart Disease. Eur. Heart J. Digit. Health. 2021;2:119–124. doi: 10.1093/ehjdh/ztaa017.
- Lytzen R., Vejlstrup N., Bjerre J., Petersen O.B., Leenskjold S., Dodd J.K., Jørgensen F.S., Søndergaard L. Live-Born Major Congenital Heart Disease in Denmark. JAMA Cardiol. 2018;3:829. doi: 10.1001/jamacardio.2018.2009. [PMC free article] [PubMed] [CrossRef] [Google Scholar]
- Ma M., Li Y., Chen R., Huang C., Mao Y., Zhao B. Diagnostic Performance of Fetal Intelligent Navigation Echocardiography (FINE) in Fetuses with Double-Outlet Right Ventricle (DORV) Int. J. Cardiovasc. Imaging. 2020;36:2165–2172.
- Malik P., Pathania M., Rathaur V.K. Overview of Artificial Intelligence in Medicine. J. Fam. Med. Prim. Care. 2019;8:2328–2331. doi: 10.4103/jfmpc.jfmpc_440_19.
- Mathur P., Srivastava S., Xu X., Mehta J.L. Artificial Intelligence, Machine Learning, and Cardiovascular Disease. Clin. Med. Insights Cardiol. 2020;14:117954682092740.
- McCall B. COVID-19 and Artificial Intelligence: Protecting Health-Care Workers and Curbing the Spread. Lancet Digit. Health. 2020;2:e166–e167.
- Kokol P., Završnik J., Blažun Vošner H. Artificial Intelligence and Pediatrics: A Synthetic Mini Review. Pediatr. Dimens. 2017;2
Lakhe A., Sodhi I., Warrier J., Sinha V. Development of Digital Stethoscope for Telemedicine. J. Med. Eng. Technol. 2016;40:20–24.
- Lemaire J.B., Schaefer J.P., Martin L.A., Faris P., Ainslie M.D., Hull R.D. Effectiveness of the Quick Medical Reference as a Diagnostic Tool. CMAJ. 1999;161:725–728. [PMC free article] [PubMed] [Google Scholar]
- Liu Y., Chen S., Zühlke L., Black G.C., Choy M., Li N., Keavney B.D. Global Birth Prevalence of Congenital Heart Defects 1970–2017: Updated Systematic Review and Meta-Analysis of 260 Studies. Int. J. Epidemiol. 2019;48:455–463. doi: 10.1093/ije/dyz009. [PMC free article] [PubMed] [CrossRef] [Google Scholar]
- lo Muzio F.P., Rozzi G., Rossi S., Luciani G.B., Foresti R., Cabassi A., Fassina L., Miragoli M. Artificial Intelligence Supports Decision Making during Open-Chest Surgery of Rare Congenital Heart Defects. J. Clin. Med. 2021;10:5330.
- Lv J., Dong B., Lei H., Shi G., Wang H., Zhu F., Wen C., Zhang Q., Fu L., Gu X., et al. Artificial Intelligence-Assisted Auscultation in Detecting Congenital Heart Disease. Eur. Heart J. Digit. Health. 2021;2:119–124.
- Lytzen R., Vejlstrup N., Bjerre J., Petersen O.B., Leenskjold S., Dodd J.K., Jørgensen F.S., Søndergaard L. Live-Born Major Congenital Heart Disease in Denmark. JAMA Cardiol. 2018;3:829.
- Ma M., Li Y., Chen R., Huang C., Mao Y., Zhao B. Diagnostic Performance of Fetal Intelligent Navigation Echocardiography (FINE) in Fetuses with Double-Outlet Right Ventricle (DORV) Int. J. Cardiovasc. Imaging. 2020;36:2165–2172. doi: 10.1007/
- Ma X.-J., Huang G.-Y. Current Status of Screening, Diagnosis, and Treatment of Neonatal Congenital Heart Disease in China. World J. Pediatr. 2018;14:313–314.
- Mahayni A.A., Attia Z.I., Medina-Inojosa J.R., Elsisy M.F.A., Noseworthy P.A., Lopez-Jimenez F., Kapa S., Asirvatham S.J., Friedman P.A., Crestenallo J.A., et al. Electrocardiography-Based Artificial Intelligence Algorithm Aids in Prediction of Long-Term Mortality after Cardiac Surgery.
- Mayo Clin. Proc. 2021;96:3062–3070. doi: 10.1016/j.mayocp.2021.06.024. [PubMed] [CrossRef]
Narula S., Shameer K., Salem Omar A.M., Dudley J.T., Sengupta P.P. Machine-Learning Algorithms to Automate Morphological and Functional Assessments in 2D Echocardiography. J. Am. Coll. Cardiol. 2016;68:2287–2295.
- Noonan J.A. A History of Pediatric Specialties: The Development of Pediatric Cardiology. Pediatr. Res. 2004;56:298–306. doi: 10.1203/01.PDR.0000132662.73362.96.
- Papoutsidakis N., Heitner S.B., Mannello M.C., Rodonski A., Campbell W., McElheran K., Jacoby D.L. Machine-Assisted Genotype Update System (MAGUS) for Inherited Cardiomyopathies. Circ. Cardiovasc. Qual.Outcomes. 2018;11:e004835.
- Ren Z., Zhu J., Gao Y., Yin Q., Hu M., Dai L., Deng C., Yi L., Deng K., Wang Y., et al. Maternal Exposure to Ambient PM10 during Pregnancy Increases the Risk of Congenital Heart Defects: Evidence from Machine Learning Models. Sci. Total Environ. 2018;630:1–10. doi: 10.1016/j.scitotenv.2018.02.181. [PubMed] [CrossRef] [Google Scholar
- Siontis K.C., Liu K., Bos J.M., Attia Z.I., Cohen-Shelly M., Arruda-Olson A.M., Zanjirani Farahani N., Friedman P.A., Noseworthy P.A., Ackerman M.J. Detection of Hypertrophic Cardiomyopathy by an Artificial Intelligence Electrocardiogram in Children and Adolescents. Int. J. Cardiol. 2021;340:42–47.
- Sreedhar C., Ram M.S., Alam A., Indrajit I. Cardiac MRI in Congenital Heart Disease—Our Experience. Med. J. Armed Forces India. 2005;61:57–62.
- Tandon A., Mohan N., Jensen C., Burkhardt B.E.U., Gooty V., Castellanos D.A., McKenzie P.L., Zahr R.A., Bhattaru A., Abdulkarim M., et al. Retraining Convolutional Neural Networks for Specialized Cardiovascular Imaging Tasks: Lessons from Tetralogy of Fallot. Pediatr. Cardiol. 2021;42:578–589.
- van den Eynde J., Kutty S., Danford D.A., Manlhiot C. Artificial Intelligence in Pediatric Cardiology: Taking Baby Steps in the Big World of Data. Curr. Opin. Cardiol. 2022;37:130–136.
- Wang T., Liu G., Lin H. A Machine Learning Approach to Predict Intravenous Immunoglobulin Resistance in Kawasaki Disease Patients: A Study Based on a Southeast China Population. PLoS ONE. 2020;15:e0237321.
- Xu W., Yu K., Ye J., Li H., Chen J., Yin F., Xu J., Zhu J., Li D., Shu Q. Automatic Pediatric Congenital Heart Disease Classification Based on Heart Sound Signal. Artif. Intell. Med. 2022;126:102257. doi: 10.1016/j.artmed.2022.102257.
- Yao S.-H., Tsai H.-T., Lin W.-L., Chen Y.-C., Chou C., Lin H.-W. Predicting the Serum Digoxin Concentrations of Infants in the Neonatal Intensive Care Unit through an Artificial Neural Network. BMC Pediatr. 2019;19:517. doi: 10.1186/s12887-019-1895-7.
- Zeng X., Hu Y., Shu L., Li J., Duan H., Shu Q., Li H. Explainable Machine-Learning Predictions for Complications after Pediatric Congenital Heart Surgery. Sci. Rep. 2021;11:17244. doi: 10.1038/s41598-021-96721-w. [PMC free article] [PubMed] [

CHAPTER

13

The future of Cardiothoracic surgery in Artificial intelligence

Humans' great and quick technological breakthroughs in the previous decade have undoubtedly influenced how surgical procedures are executed in the operating room. AI is becoming incredibly influential for surgical decision-making to help surgeons make better projections about the implications of surgical operations by considering different sources of data such as patient health conditions, disease natural history, patient values, and finance. Although the application of artificial intelligence in healthcare settings is rapidly increasing, its mainstream application in clinical practice remains limited. The use of machine learning algorithms in thoracic surgery is extensive, including different clinical stages. By leveraging techniques such as machine learning, computer vision, and robotics, AI may play a key role in diagnostic augmentation, operative management, pre-and post-surgical patient management, and upholding safety standards. AI, particularly in complex surgical procedures such as cardiothoracic surgery, may be a significant help to surgeons in executing more intricate surgeries with greater success, fewer complications, and ensuring patient safety, while also providing resources for robust research and better dissemination of knowledge. In this paper, we present an overview of AI applications in thoracic surgery and its related components, including contemporary projects and technology that use AI in cardiothoracic surgery and general care. We also discussed the future of AI and how high-tech operating rooms will use human-machine collaboration to improve performance and patient safety, as well as its future directions and limitations. It is vital for the surgeons to keep themselves acquainted with the latest technological advancement in AI order to grasp this technology and easily integrate it into clinical practice when it becomes accessible. This review is a great addition to literature, keeping practicing and aspiring surgeons up to date on the most recent advances in AI and cardiothoracic surgery.

Artificial intelligence in surgery

Artificial intelligence (AI) can be defined as the study of algorithms that give an ability to reason to a machine and help it to perform cognitive tasks such as problem solving, decision-making, and word recognition .With the blooming of the technological revolution, AI has become the centerpiece of both popular and academic literature. Today where data is key and technology is a major revolutionizing force, there is a shift in productivity like that of the industrial revolution . Surgery stands to benefit from this technological growth as well, with a promising future for AI in surgery. There are four core subfields of AI in surgery namely machine-learning, natural language processing, artificial neural networks, and computer vision .Machine-learning may seem very non-intuitive to the reader at first, as we are accustomed to human learning and machines being operators under human command. Machine learning (ML) basically recognizes patterns in enormous amount of data that may be imperceptible to the human mind, labels the data, and makes accurate predictions . The role ML plays in surgery is evident from its ability to accurately predict surgical site infections and predict lung cancer staging, outperforming approaches based on clinical guidelines to unprecedented levels thought to be unattainable with conventional statistics .Natural language processing (NLP) is a subfield of AI that emphasizes the computer's ability to not only understand human language but also infer meaning and sentiments from unstructured data . In surgical patients, NLP has been able to detect phrases in operative reports that predicted anastomotic leaks after colorectal resection surgeries with sensitivities of 100% . For example, ANN (sensitivity 89% and specificity 96%) have outperformed traditional risk prediction approaches like APACHE II (sensitivity 80% and specificity 85%) for pancreatitis severity 6 h after admission .

Computer vision describes the machine's ability to understand images and videos and has achieved capabilities comparable to human-level understanding in areas such as object and scene recognition . For example, a real time analysis of a laparoscopic video of sleeve gastrectomy has noted missing or unexpected steps to 92.8% accuracy .

Role of AI in diagnostic augmentation

A sub-field of AI called ML can aid in diagnosis, augment surgical performance in the operating room (OR), and skill assessment. There are mainly two imaging-based applications of ML to thoracic surgery: automatic diagnosis of cardiovascular pathology and detection of patterns in imaging to detect thoracic pathologies like the classic chest X-ray example proposed by Wang et al. They used a chest x-ray database of 108,948 frontal view x-ray images from 32,717 unique patients and found out that it was able to distinctively diagnose 8 different pathologies . Kusunose et al. investigated whether deep convolutional neural networks (DCNN) could detect regional wall motion abnormalities on echocardiography and achieved an area under the receiver operating characteristic (AUROC) of 0.99, outperforming physicians at the same task .There are numerous applications of convolutional neural networks (CNN) to thoracic surgery, like detecting aortic diameter and volumetric analysis of the left ventricle to assess cardiac function. Image segmentation plays a pivotal role in assessing the anatomy of moving organs such as the heart and blood vessels by assigning a class label to image voxels so that they can be quantified. Bai W et al. proposed an image sequence segmentation algorithm by combining a fully convolutional network with a recurrent neural network.Experiments of aortic magnetic resonance imaging studies demonstrated that the proposed method significantly improved accuracy and temporal smoothness, compared to a baseline method that only used spatial information. Another example where a video-based deep learning algorithm surpassed human expert performance is the EchoNet-Dynamic algorithm. Human assessment of cardiac function is associated with limited sampling of cardiac cycles and shows a lot of variability between observers but the EchoNet-Dynamic algorithm reported in a study by Ouyang et al. surpassed human performance in assessing for cardiomyopathy and estimation of ejection fraction.These studies show how useful AI can be for a thoracic surgeon's practice in translating to better patient care. Although the tasks of a thoracic surgeon in the OR are highly extensive and making an ML robot that can perform all the actions of a surgeon may be impossible, however, a study by Thananjeyan et al. shows that reinforcement learning (RL) powered robots can perform minor surgical tasks like simple suturing and highly precise surgical incisions . Wijnberge et al. report in a recent randomized controlled trial that ML can detect the intra-operative incidence of hypotension in elective non-cardiac surgery, decreasing the median duration of hypotension from 32.7 min to just 8 min, that is a huge difference .

Human-machine teaming and computer vision in cardiothoracic surgery

Computer vision (CV) is a subdiscipline of AI engineering involved with the study of giving eyes to machines .. Computer vision is a promising AI method that can be used to monitor team dynamics in the OR . Hao Xu et al. recently published a study focusing on the CV analysis of blood stains during thoracoscopic operations. They report that one of the major accidents that occur during thoracoscopic operations is massive bleeding accidents. These accidents lead to increased chances of mortality and prolonged hospital stays . High throughput CV algorithms that could process many thoracic surgical videos were developed. They found a correlation between CV based-proportion of blood pixels (PBP) and bleeding volume by training the CV algorithm with thousands of pixels of either blood or non-blood that were selected randomly and labelled manually. PBP was only computed for some key reference frames but the CV algorithm could detect bleeding volume of whole surgery by just comparing frames from the surgery video with the reference frames of bleeding taught to the algorithm during its training. PBP can help guide postoperative fluid management, anticoagulation strategies, as high PBP values suggest a reduction in anticoagulation and vice versa, and selection of appropriate drainage tubes .Cardiothoracic surgery requires top-notch technical (tying knots, suturing, and putting clamps) and non-technical skills like teamwork, communication, and awareness of the surrounding situation. In such conditions, Avrunin et al. developed Smart checklists. These checklists can help the cardiothoracic surgical team, including surgical, anesthesiology, perfusion, and nursing staff. Smart checklists reduce cognitive load and subsequent procedural errors by reminding the team about the next step in the procedure and by alerting the other team members not to disturb or increase cognitive load on specific members of the team during some high cognitive load scenarios

Communication, coordination, and adaptation are qualities that are critical to human-machine teaming, but machines have not yet fully realized the unique human cognition for effective teaming. The rapid technological advancements in the recent era, especially in the field of AI, have offered new capabilities to machines to maximize their competencies in this regard . According to Seeber et al. rapid technological advancements have enabled machines to acquire transportable teamwork competencies that are critical to teams. For example, machines may leverage a theory of mind reasoning to build a computerized model of their teammates. Using this model, the machine can know what information is available to teammates and what would be the subsequent action of their human teammates, creating better coordination with the human counterparts in a team. This model will also be able to determine when and how best to communicate with teammates, further enhancing ability and trust in machines . Current AI research focuses on specific objectives to be achieved by machines and doesn't incorporate many findings from teaming and human-computer interface literature. For Example, Open AI Five is a five neural network model developed to beat top five human champions in a game, although neural network models performed best when not paired with other machines, they performed worst when partnered with humans. Examining such phenomenon Carroll M et al. found out that the main limiting factor for such behavior of the neural networks was initial machine training in conjunction with other machines .

Role of AI in preoperative performance and safety in cardiothoracic surgery

Chang Junior J et al. studied the role of artificial intelligence and reported that the sheer number of cardiac surgical interventions available for congenital cardiac diseases and the low volume of patients compared with adults make it hard to collect large amounts of data regarding pre-operative safety and efficacy for a single procedure . The random forest model of artificial intelligence can learn from large pools of data and accurately predict individual death risks in patients with congenital heart disease. The findings of this model can assist patients, surgeons, and family members of patients in understanding the risks associated with a cardiac surgical intervention . With the advent and integration of AI into clinical care, the traditional systems are replaced with more efficient and more accurate systems. Using deep and machine learning, AI helps in the pre-operative automation of clerical processes, provides assistance in how patients can be triaged and gives risk predictions during the COVID-19 pandemic where resources were already scarce, and cardiac surgery patients were facing delays in delivery of care . Using machine learning techniques, Yoon et al. devised a new personalized method for prediction of risk both pre- and post-cardiac transplantation. The method is used to classify the heterogeneous cohort of patients and their interactions with each other across different zones of time. The method is so robust that it outperforms the best clinical scores and machine learning methods currently available. The same method can be applied to other fields of medicine and surgery . Pre-operatively, Kwon et al. used the deep learning approach in AI for predicting the mortality of acute heart failure by an algorithm known as deep-learning-based artificial intelligence algorithm for predicting mortality of patients with acute heart failure (DAHF). The deep learning algorithm was so efficient and reliably accurate that it could predict the one-year and three-year mortality of acute heart failure patients more accurately than the existing scores and machine learning methods . A study by Kilic et al. revealed that there is an increase in the use of durable left ventricular assist devices (LVAD) being implanted in the United States but there was no widely used risk stratification tool for LVAD therapy. By utilizing the Interagency Registry for Mechanically Assisted Circulatory Support (INTERMACS) database they studied the 90-day and 1-year mortality rates following primary LVAD implantation using both logistic regression and machine learning approaches and found that machine learning models were both well-calibrated and had improved discriminatory capability as compared to logistic regression Wang et al. developed and validated a machine learning method that can predict the amount of red blood cell transfusions required for a cardiothoracic surgery and showed excellent results Artificial intelligence and virtual reality can give a 3- dimensional view of whole pulmonary anatomy with its intricate parts to the cardiothoracic surgeon to preoperatively get a better insight into the individual patient's anatomy .

Role of artificial intelligence in intra operative performance and safety in cardiac/ cardiothoracic surgery

Humans have made impeccable technological advancements in the past decades, and these advancements have also had an impact on the contemporary OR with artificial intelligence being at the forefront of these technological achievements. Artificial intelligence benefits the surgical team as an augmentation to the normal human cognition in the OR by processing complex computations to provide a meaningful result that helps the surgical team and the patient. Artificial intelligence is used to monitor and assess team as well as individual performance throughout the surgery which can help guide better patient outcomes by addressing the underlying areas of improvement specified by the artificial intelligence system . Goldenberg et al. showed that traditionally, operative quality was assessed by retrospectively reviewing patient medical records, which were inundated with biases like recall bias and non-compliance on the part of the patient. Artificial intelligence allows for a highly sensitive prospective intraoperative approach called the OR black box system, which focuses from major points to the minutiae by collecting and integrating data regarding events that may cause patient harm at a magnitude not feasibly possible by a human . Azari et al. used computer vision to assess individual task performance during an ongoing surgical operation. The computer vision analysis assessed surgeon techniques more reliably and objectively than the individual assessments made by surgical experts Artificial intelligence can accurately predict the risk of hypoxemia during cardiac surgery. Lundberg SM et al. revealed that machine learning can predict the future risk of intraoperative hypoxemia and provide an explanation of the risk factors to an accurate level consistent with literature. Artificial intelligence can amplify the current anesthesiologist's prediction of hypoxemia during surgery by 15%–30%; an almost double when predicting events of hypoxemia . Ali et al. shows in their study that surgeons often either underestimate or overestimate the time required for a surgery, leading to either underutilization of the financial and human resources in the operating room or over-burdening of the resources when time required for a surgery is over-estimated. Artificial intelligence can bridge this gap by accurately predicting surgery duration leading to positive outcomes in the form of proper and commensurate resource utilization . Even now, there is an absence of real-time intraoperative imaging techniques for the right ventricle during cardiac surgery. Muzio L et al. used an AI-based video kinematic evaluation technique for the right ventricle during surgeries for tetralogy of Fallot cases, using a supervised machine learning model to predict the outcome of the intervention and its success upon chest closure .

Role of AI in post-operative management

Using personalized risk factor assessment is a future trend in precision medicine and using the help of AI, especially supervised machine learning can give us a feasible solution to it. Individualized risk assessment by AI models can help us if the results are accurate, predictive, and consistently reproducible each time the assessment is performed. Chang et al. used the Naïve Bayes (NB) - algorithm assisted prediction system to assess the need of patients for high concentration oxygenation, ICU care and the risk of inability to wean-off the ventilator immediately following lung resection surgery with remarkable results of 100% of the patients agreeing that digitalization improved their understanding of the needs and the risks predicted by the NB-algorithm assisted prediction system . Tseng et al. developed and validated machine learning models for 94 pre- and intraoperative features to predict cardiac surgery-associated acute kidney injury (CSA-AKI), which occurs in approximately 22% of cardiac surgery cases. Previous studies and risk scores used categorical division of parameters pertaining to the risk which failed to preserve variability in continuous data. The machine learning method to determine the risk of CSA-AKI was successful and the study also demonstrated that intraoperative time-series and other features are important for acute kidney injury prediction .Fernandes et al. used machine learning methods and also added cardiopulmonary bypass-specific intraoperative hypotension (CBP-specific IOH) as a parameter to the preoperative score leading to results that machine learning methods that incorporated the CBP-specific IOH to demonstrate great predictive ability of post-surgical mortality . Mufti et al. studied different machine learning methods to develop models that could predict the occurrence of delirium after cardiac surgery and found that machine learning methods can help in revealing the hidden patterns in delirium causation and better predicting its occurrence .

Limitations, ethical issues and needs in future

Although AI has shown highly encouraging results in all fields of patientcare, many issues need to be addressed before it can be used in the daily routine of a cardiothoracic surgeon. With the advent of AI, the privacy of patients' data is a big concern . Price et al. argue that overprotection with privacy can lead to a halting or braking in technological innovation, while on the other hand, allowing privacy to drive secrecy can lead to less trust in the technological achievements brought about by it . He et al. argue that transparent and accurate input is required for the AI systems to generate accurate results. Another reason why transparency is related to functioning of the AI system is that if patient care providers can accurately work out how a machine came to a conclusion, this is a way in which it can be tested whether the reasoning is sound. Opaque AI systems do work based on algorithms, but there is no way a patient care provider can know how a system came to such a conclusion. This makes it harder to test for the soundness of its reasoning and integration of a particular a technology into the patient care . Perhaps the biggest shortcoming of ML lies in its lack of interpretability of the produced outcomes. Normal regression techniques can be tested and relationships can be seen such that increasing or decreasing input feature x affects the output feature y in different ways, but AI uncovers non-linear and highly complex associations in and between datasets at a scale so humongous, that it's hard for the human brain to compute. Hence the way AI finds these associations is also a mystery to care providers .

Conclusion

Recent technological advances and diligent research have resulted in intelligent technology by the development of innovative computer algorithms and the augmentation of the application of human cognitive models for AI. AI technologies are becoming increasingly useful and are being integrated into multidisciplinary health-care models, such as perioperative medicine, smart operating theatres, robotic interventions, intraoperative management, maintaining patient safety, identifying risk factors, and postoperative rehabilitation. There is promising future of AI that can open a new world for cardiothoracic surgery, however there are certain barriers to mass-implementation of these novel technologies.

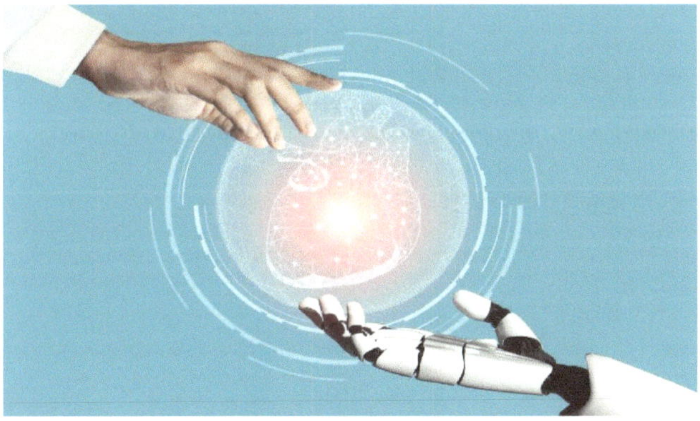

Fig 13.1 Using artificial intelligence (AI) to quantify blood flow in the heart can predict adverse cardiovascular (CV) outcomes over and above other traditional CV risk factors, a new study has shown.

The transparency of patients' data, establishment of secure algorithms, human trials, and ethical concerns regarding involvement of extensive machinery in complex surgeries can limit the growth of this remarkable technology. It is critical for practicing surgeons and aspiring surgeons to stay current on technology advancements in order to better comprehend them and integrate them into clinical practice for improved outcomes and advancement of specialty.

Bibliography and Acknowledgement

- Ali Zahoor, Muhammad Qummer ul Arfeen. 2011. The Role of Machine Learning in Predicting CABG Surgery Duration. [Google Scholar]
  Avrunin, George S., et al. Vol. 2018. 2018. Toward improving surgical outcomes by incorporating cognitive load measurement into process-driven guidance." software engineering in healthcare systems (SEHS) pp. 2–9. (IEEE/ACM International Workshop on). [PMC free article] [PubMed] [CrossRef] [Google Scholar]
- Azari David P., et al. Modeling surgical technical skill using expert assessment for automated computer rating. Ann. Surg. 2019;269(3):574–581. https://doi:10.1097/SLA.0000000000002478 [PMC free article] [PubMed] [Google Scholar]
- Bai W., Suzuki H Qin, Tarroni C., Oktay G., Matthews P.M.O., et al. Medical Image Computing and Computer Assisted Intervention – MICCAI 2018. Springer International Publishing; Cham: 2018. Recurrent neural networks for aortic image sequence segmentation with sparse annotations. [Google Scholar]
- Bellini Valentina, et al. Artificial intelligence in thoracic surgery: a narrative review. J. Thorac. Dis. 2021;13(12):6963–6975. doi: 10.21037/jtd-21-761. [PMC free article] [PubMed] [CrossRef] [Google Scholar]
- Bergquist Savannah L., et al. Machine Learning for Healthcare Conference. PMLR; 2017. Classifying lung cancer severity with ensemble machine learning in health care claims data. [PMC free article] [PubMed] [Google Scholar]
- Carroll M., Shah R., Ho M.K., Griffiths T., Seshia S., Abbeel P., et al. In: Advances in Neural Information Processing Systems 32: Annual Conference on Neural Information Processing Systems 2019, NeurIPS 2019. Wallach H.M., Larochelle H., Beygelzimer A., d'Alché-Buc F.,
- Fox E.A., Garnett R., editors. 2019. On the utility of learning about humans for human-AI coordination; pp. 5175–5186. December 8–14, 2019; Vancouver, BC, Canada. [Google Scholar]
- Chang Junior J., Binuesa F., Caneo L.F., Turquetto A.L.R., Arita E.C.T.C., et al. Improving preoperative risk-of-death prediction in surgery congenital heart defects using artificial intelligence model: a pilot study. PLoS One. 2020;15(9) doi: 10.1371/journal.pone.0238199. [PMC free article] [PubMed] [CrossRef] [Google Scholar]
- Chang Ying-Jen, et al. A real-time artificial intelligence-assisted system to predict weaning from ventilator immediately after lung resection surgery. Int. J. Environ. Res. Publ. Health. 8 Mar. 2021;18(5):2713. doi: 10.3390/ijerph18052713. [PMC free article] [PubMed] [CrossRef] [Google Scholar]
- Char, Danton S., et al. Implementing machine learning in health care - addressing ethical challenges. N. Engl. J. Med. 2018;378(11):981–983. doi: 10.1056/NEJMp1714229. [PMC free article] [PubMed] [CrossRef] [Google Scholar]
- Chen Jonathan H., Steven M Asch. Machine learning and prediction in medicine - beyond the peak of inflated expectations. N. Engl. J. Med. 2017;376(26):2507–2509. doi: 10.1056/NEJMp1702071. [PMC free article] [PubMed] [CrossRef] [Google Scholar
- Dias, Roger D., et al. Artificial intelligence in cardiothoracic surgery. Minerva Cardioangiol. 2020;68(5):532–538. https://doi:10.23736/S0026-4725.20.05235-4 [PMC free article] [PubMed] [Google Scholar]
  Fernandes Marta Priscila Bento, et al. Machine learning models with preoperative risk factors and intraoperative hypotension parameters predict mortality after cardiac surgery. J. Cardiothorac. Vasc. Anesth. 2021;35(3):857–865. doi: 10.1053/j.jvca.2020.07.029. [PubMed] [CrossRef] [Google Scholar]
- Goldenberg Mitchell G., et al. Using data to enhance performance and improve quality and safety in surgery. JAMA surgery. 2017;152(10):972–973. https://doi:10.1001/jamasurg.2017.2888 [PubMed] [Google Scholar
- Gunning D. Aha D.W. DARPA's explainable artificial intelligence program. AI Mag. 2019;40(2):44. [Google Scholar]
- Hashimoto Daniel A., et al. Artificial intelligence in surgery: Promises and Perils. Ann. Surg. 2018;268(1):70–76. doi: 10.1097/SLA.0000000000002693. [PMC free article] [PubMed] [CrossRef] [Google Scholar

- He Jianxing, et al. The practical implementation of artificial intelligence technologies in medicine. Nat. Med. 2019;25(1):30–36. doi: 10.1038/s41591-018-0307-0. [PMC free article] [PubMed] [CrossRef] [Google Scholar]
- Kennedy-Metz, Lauren R., et al. Computer vision in the operating room: opportunities and caveats. IEEE transactions on medical robotics and bionics. 2021;3(1):2–10. doi: 10.1109/tmrb.2020.3040002. [PMC free article] [PubMed] [CrossRef] [Google Scholar]
- Khalsa R.K., Khashkhusha A., Zaidi S., Harky A., Bashir M. Artificial intelligence and cardiac surgery during COVID-19 era. J. Card. Surg. 2021;36:1729–1733. doi: 10.1111/jocs.15417. [PMC free article] [PubMed] [CrossRef] [Google Scholar]
- Kilic A., Dochtermann D., Padman R., Miller J.K., Dubrawski A. Using machine learning to improve risk prediction in durable left ventricular assist devices. PLoS One. 2021;16(3) doi: 10.1371/journal.pone.0247866. [PMC free article] [PubMed] [CrossRef] [Google Scholar]
- Kusunose Kenya, et al. A deep learning approach for assessment of regional wall motion abnormality from echocardiographic images. JACC. Cardiovascular imaging. 2020;13(2 Pt 1):374–381. doi: 10.1016/j.jcmg.2019.02.024. [PubMed] [CrossRef] [Google Scholar]
- Kwon Joon-Myoung, et al. Artificial intelligence algorithm for predicting mortality of patients with acute heart failure. PLoS One. 8 Jul. 2019;14(7) https://doi:10.1371/journal.pone.0219302 [PMC free article] [PubMed] [Google Scholar]
- Lo Muzio, Paolo Francesco, et al. Artificial intelligence supports decision making during open-chest surgery of rare congenital heart defects. J. Clin. Med. Nov. 2021;10(22):5330. doi: 10.3390/jcm10225330. Crossref. [PMC free article] [PubMed] [CrossRef] [Google Scholar]
- Lundberg S.M., Nair B., Vavilala M.S., et al. Explainable machine-learning predictions for the prevention of hypoxaemia during surgery. Nat Biomed Eng. 2018;2:749–760. doi: 10.1038/s41551-018-0304-0. [PMC free article] [PubMed] [CrossRef] [Google Scholar]
- Mofidi Reza, et al. Identification of severe acute pancreatitis using an artificial neural network. Surgery. 2007;141(1):59–66. doi: 10.1016/j.surg.2006.07.022. [PubMed] [CrossRef]
- Mufti, Nabeel Hani, et al. Exploiting machine learning algorithms and methods for the prediction of agitated delirium after cardiac surgery: models development and validation study. JMIR medical informatics. 23 Oct. 2019;7(4) doi: 10.2196/14993.
- Nadkarni Prakash M., et al. Natural language processing: an introduction. J. Am. Med. Inf. Assoc.: JAMIA. 2011;18(5):544–551. doi: 10.1136/amiajnl-2011-000464. [PMC free article] [PubMed] [CrossRef] [Google Scholar]
- Ostberg Nicolai P., et al. Machine learning: principles and applications for thoracic surgery. Eur. J. Cardio. Thorac. Surg.: official journal of the European Association for Cardio-thoracic Surgery. 2021;60(2):213–221.
- Ouyang David, et al. Video-based AI for beat-to-beat assessment of cardiac function. Nature. 2020;580(7802):252–256. doi: 10.1038/s41586-020-2145-8. [PMC free article] [PubMed] [CrossRef] [Google Scholar]
- Price W Nicholson, 2nd, Cohen I Glenn. Privacy in the age of medical big data. Nat. Med. 2019;25(1):37–43. doi: 10.1038/s41591-018-0272-7. [PMC free article] [PubMed] [CrossRef]
- Sadeghi Amir H., et al. Virtual reality and artificial intelligence for 3-dimensional planning of lung segmentectomies. JTCVS techniques. 16 Mar. 2021;7:309–321. https://doi:10.1016/j.xjtc.2021.03.016 [PMC free article] [PubMed] [Google Scholar]
- Seeber Isabella, et al. Machines as teammates: a research agenda on AI in team collaboration. Inf. Manag. 2020;57(2) [Google Scholar]
Soguero-Ruiz Cristina, et al. Support vector feature selection for early detection of anastomosis leakage from bag-of-words in electronic health records. IEEE journal of biomedical and health informatics. 2016;20(5):1404–1415. doi: 10.1109/JBHI.2014.2361688. [PubMed] [CrossRef] [Google Scholar]
- Soguero-Ruiz Cristina, et al. Vol. 2015. AMIA Symposium; 5 Nov. 2015. Data-driven temporal prediction of surgical site infection; p. 1164. (AMIA ... Annual Symposium Proceedings). 73. [PMC free article] [PubMed] [Google Scholar]
- Stowers Kimberly, et al. Improving teamwork competencies in human-machine teams: perspectives from team science. Front. Psychol. 24 May. 2021;12 doi: 10.3389/fpsyg.2021.590290. [PMC free article] [PubMed] [CrossRef] [Google Scholar]
- Sutton Richard S., Barto Andrew G. MIT press; 2018. Reinforcement Learning: an Introduction. [Google Scholar]
- Szeliski Richard. Springer Science & Business Media; 2010. Computer Vision: Algorithms and Applications. [Google Scholar]
- Thananjeyan Brijen, et al. 2017 IEEE International Conference on Robotics and Automation (ICRA) 2017. Multilateral surgical pattern cutting in 2D orthotropic gauze with deep reinforcement learning policies for tensioning; pp. 2371–2378. [Google Scholar]
- Tseng Po-Yu, et al. Prediction of the development of acute kidney injury following cardiac surgery by machine learning. Crit. Care. 31 Jul. 2020;24(1):478. doi: 10.1186/s13054-020-03179-9. [PMC free article] [PubMed] [CrossRef] [Google Scholar]
- Volkov M., et al. IEEE International Conference on Robotics and Automation (ICRA) 2017. Machine learning and coresets for automated real-time video segmentation of laparoscopic and robot-assisted surgery; pp. 754–759. [Google Scholar]
- Wang Z., Zhe S., Zimmerman J., et al. Development and validation of a machine learning method to predict intraoperative red blood cell transfusions in cardiothoracic surgery. Sci. Rep. 2022;12:1355. doi: 10.1038/s41598-022-05445-y. [PMC free article] [PubMed] [CrossRef] [Google Scholar]
- Wang, et al. "ChestX-ray 8: hospital-scale chest X-ray database and benchmarks on weakly-supervised classification and localization of common thorax diseases" arXiv:1705.02315. doi: 10.48550/arXiv.1705.02315.
- Wijnberge Marije, et al. Effect of a machine learning-derived early warning system for intraoperative hypotension vs standard care on depth and duration of intraoperative hypotension during elective noncardiac surgery: the HYPE randomized clinical trial. JAMA. 2020;323(11):1052–1060.
- Xu Hao, Han Tingxuan, Wang Haifeng, Liu Shanggui, Hou Guanghao, Sun Lina, Jiang Guanchao, Fan Yang, Wang Jun, Deng Ke, Zhou Jian. Detection of blood stains using computer vision-based algorithms and their association with postoperative outcomes in thoracoscopic lobectomies. Eur. J. Cardio. Thorac. Surg. 2022 doi: 10.1093/ejcts/ezac154. ezac154. [PMC free article] [PubMed]
- Yoon J., Zame W.R., Banerjee A., Cadeiras M., Alaa A.M., et al. Personalized survival predictions via Trees of Predictors: an application to cardiac transplantation. PLoS One. 2018;13(3) doi: 10.1371/journal.pone.0194985. [PMC free article]

CHAPTER

14

Artificial intelligence in the Diagnosis and Detection of Heart failure-Review

Artificial Intelligence (AI) performs human intelligence-dependant tasks using tools such as Machine Learning, and its subtype Deep Learning. AI has incorporated itself in the field of cardiovascular medicine, and increasingly employed to revolutionize diagnosis, treatment, risk prediction, clinical care, and drug discovery. Heart failure has a high prevalence, and mortality rate following hospitalization being 10.4% at 30-days, 22% at 1-year, and 42.3% at 5-years. Early detection of heart failure is of vital importance in shaping the medical, and surgical interventions specific to HF patients. This has been accomplished with the advent of Neural Network (NN) model, the accuracy of which has proven to be 85%. AI can be of tremendous help in analyzing raw image data from cardiac imaging techniques (such as echocardiography, computed tomography, cardiac MRI amongst others) and electrocardiogram recordings through incorporation of an algorithm. The use of decision trees by Rough Sets (RS), and logistic regression (LR) methods utilized to construct decision-making model to diagnose congestive heart failure, and role of AI in early detection of future mortality and destabilization episodes has played a vital role in optimizing cardiovascular disease outcomes. The review highlights the major achievements of AI in recent years that has radically changed nearly all areas of HF prevention, diagnosis, and management. Artificial Intelligence (AI) possesses the capability to perform human intelligence-dependant tasks such as receiving perspicuity, learning semantics, and formulating an analysis using various algorithms and cognitive computing . AI uses the concept of Learning, which can be classified into supervised, unsupervised, and re-enforcement. Machine Learning (ML) is the core of AI that uses a model based on training data to make decisions, and program algorithms to solve the problem .The commonly utilized classification models include Binary, Multi-class, Multi-label and Imbalanced Classification. Binary classification uses algorithms like Logistic Regression, k-nearest neighbors, decisions tree, support vector machine and naïve bayes to classify two labels' tasks. Multi-class uses algorithms like decisions tree, support vector machine, naïve bayes, random forest, and gradient boosting to classify tasks involving more than two labels. Multi-label classifies tasks that have two or more class labels, where one or more class labels may be predicted for each example, unlike the multi-class where a single class label is predicted for each example. The class labels with unequally distributed tasks are classified using the Imbalanced classification model .The distributions can vary from slightly imbalanced to severely imbalanced. It constitutes a significant challenge in predictive modelling as algorithms used for imbalanced classification are based on assumptions . Class labels are often string values, e.g., "spam", "not spam", which are mapped to numeric values in the process of label encoding . Deep Learning (DL) is a class of the ML algorithm that uses higher level features such as neural networks derived from a model of the human brain which allows a computer system to read, build, and learn complex hierarchical representation It involves the transformation of the input data into a more compounded output data.

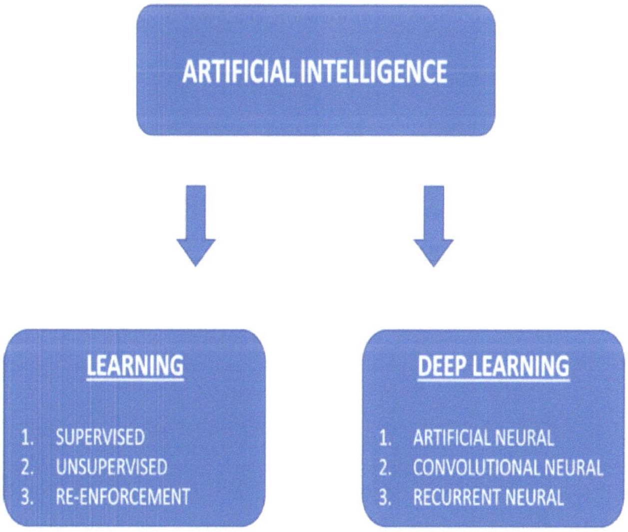

Fig 14.1 Classification of Learning and Deep Learning. The concept of learning can be sub-divided into supervised, unsupervised, and re-enforcement. Deep learning comprises complex features including artificial, convolutional, and recurrent neural networks.

Genetic predisposition is a major factor in the development of cardiovascular diseases such as atherosclerosis and advanced techniques such as the use of DL networks can be used to predict advanced coronary artery calcium through a large-scale genome-wide association study . DL can be further sub-divided into Artificial Neural Network, Convolutional Neural Network, and Recurrent Deep Learning. The evolution in cardiovascular diseases requires advancements in the treatment and diagnostic techniques, thus AI is now being rapidly incorporated in the field of cardiovascular medicine. AI has the potential to revolutionize the medical diagnosis, treatment, risk prediction, clinical care, and drug discovery through the interpretation of vast databases more efficiently as compared to the human brain . The use of DL-based diagnostic modalities such as cardiac angiography, echocardiography, and electrocardiogram (ECG) in the field of cardiovascular medicine has played a pivotal role in revolutionizing the diagnosis of cardiovascular disorders such as heart failure, myocardial infarction, arrhythmia, and valvular heart disease. Paroxysmal Supraventricular Tachycardia (PSVT) is a sporadic, sudden, and recurrent cardiovascular disorder that can worsen the quality of life of the patients Although treatable; the condition is difficult to diagnose due to its instantaneous episodes occurring during normal sinus rhythm. However, the use of DML-based ECG has made the early diagnosis of PSVT possible. The use of diagnostic modalities and other AI-based tools such as medical resonance imaging (MRI), intravascular ultrasound, optical coherence tomography (OCT), and single photon emission computed tomography (SPECT) allows clinicians to make a detailed and faultless diagnosis of potentially fatal cardiovascular diseases . Furthermore, the use of ML-based AI has proven to predict 5-year survival rate in patients with cardiovascular diseases, more accurately (80%) as compared to the clinicians (60%) Heart failure is a major cardiovascular disorder with the mortality following hospitalization being 10.4% at 30 days, 22% at 1 year, and 42.3% at 5 years, despite marked improvement in medical and device therapy . The multifactorial pathophysiology of HF that includes structural and functional abnormalities makes the diagnosis and treatment of HF more difficult. The advent of AI in the field of cardiovascular medicine through diagnostic modalities such as ECG, Echo, angiography, and the use of modern techniques like robotic percutaneous coronary intervention in its management has markedly reduced the mortality of patients with HF. It is unlikely that AI will replace physicians, however, AI can act as an essential tool that can help physicians improve their clinical judgment, and provide a precise diagnosis of diseases like HF. In this study, we aim to discuss the role of AI in the detection and diagnosis of HF. We have also discussed the limitations in the incorporation of AI in cardiovascular medicine, and how it can be further developed.

Table 14.1. Description of various functions of components of artificial intelligence.

TYPE OF AI	DESCRIPTION
SUPERVISED	Usage of a previously labelled database to predict outcomes of future events.
UNSUPERVISED	Identification of previously un-categorised database to predict peculiar relation between the dataset.
RE-ENFORCEMENT	Interaction of a machine with its environment using sensors, camera and GPS. It is typically used for robotic interventions.
ARTIFICIAL NEURAL	Computing system that analyses and processes information in a similar way compared to the human brain
CONVOLUTIONAL NEURAL	Performs analyses of visual images
RECURRENT NEURAL	Functions by developing connections between nodes from a directed graph along a dynamic temporal sequence .

Abbreviations: GPS, global positioning system.

1.The role of AI in the diagnosis of heart failure

According to the European society of cardiology (ESC), nearly 26 million people have been diagnosed with HF worldwide. Furthermore, 3%–5% of hospital admissions have been attributed to HF incidents. Hence, early detection of the disease is of vital importance in shaping the medical and surgical interventions to reduce the high rates of mortality and morbidity. AI has been reported to correct any existing medication errors, and hence can be effectively utilized as an 'assisting resource' on which clinicians can rely, and use in daily clinical practice . Furthermore, AI and human predictive skills have been compared in previous literature. American Heart Association (AHA) and American College of Cardiology (ACC) provide guidelines on primary prevention of cardiovascular disease using risk factors such as nutrition, obesity, physical factors, diabetes, and lipid profile. In a new study, ACC/AHA guidelines were compared with four machine-learning algorithms: random forest, logistic regression, gradient boosting, and neural networks. The results not only indicated NN to predict 7.6% more events than ACC/AHA criteria but also took into account twenty-two more data points including ethnicity, kidney disease, and arthritis which are not part of AHA/ACC guidelines thus demonstrating AI to be of great value in predicting risks . Another study applied NN for the diagnosis of HF on 40 individuals with the dataset comprising age, gender, blood pressure, and smoking history to determine predictors for HF. The model proved to be highly accurate with 85% of the results correctly predicted . The first-line investigation performed in suspected heart problems is usually ECG, after which the diagnosis gets narrowed down, and if HF is suspected, the physicians investigate for cardiac biomarkers such as natriuretic peptides. However, natriuretic peptides are not very specific markers for HF.Instead, they are subjective to factors such as obesity, age, kidney disease amongst others . Heart failure with preserved ejection fraction (HFpEF) is a rapidly emerging global health issue with its prevalence increasing at a rate of 1% per year relative to heart failure with reduced ejection fraction (HFrEF) owing to risk factors including age, gender, weight, and hypertension.

HFpEF is a complex syndrome resulting from structural and functional cardiac disorders rather than one disease entity hence making it difficult to diagnose by clinicians treating HF patients. Kwon et al. . established an adequate tool to screen it reliably and economically. The study developed and validated a DL model (DLM) based on an ensemble NN using 12-, 6-, and single-lead ECG that demonstrated reasonable performance. The DLM was further visualized to determine the characteristics and regions of ECG that were used for HFpEF prediction and confirmed the important variable for the decision in other ML models based on logistic regression (LR), random forest (RF), and convolutional neural network (CNN). A sensitivity map was used to identify where DLM focused on primarily, and it was found to have focused on the R wave in the QRS complex as well as the T wave . The study further showed that in the subgroup of 1412 patients without HFpEF at initial echocardiography, 246 patients developed HFpEF within 24 months. Patients whose DLM was defined as having a higher risk had a significantly higher chance of developing HFpEF than those in the low-risk group (33.6% vs. 8.4%, $p << 0.001$). Hence, the application of DLM to echocardiographic and ECG finding for screening HFpEF proved valuable .AI coupled with ECG findings can also be used to highlight patients with HFrEF. A randomized control trial demonstrated AI to diagnose EF <<50% in greater number of patients (2.1%) compared to usual care (1.6%) . HeartModel is another modern invention that makes use of echocardiography in allowing consultants to determine disease status and treatment options. It is a software package that provides an automated analysis of echocardiographic findings in terms of echocardiographic parameters such as chamber volumes and ejection fractions . A study conducted on the Chinese population compared the results of automated vs. manual echocardiography. It was found that atrial and ventricular volumes were a bit overestimated by the automated echocardiography device in comparison to manual echocardiography, while left ventricular ejection fraction (LVEF) was the same for both employed methods . Statistical results favored the incorporation of automated echocardiography devices in place of manual echocardiography to assess chamber volumes and ejection fraction to diagnose HF .

2. Application of logistic regression (LR), random forest (RF), and support vector machines (SVM)

The LR model of AI has been applied in the diagnosis of congestive heart failure (CHF). Son et al. . included CHF patients presenting with complaints of dyspnea. LR- based decision-making model was used to generate certain decision rules based on predictors of CHF. A decision-relative reduct was selected to generate decision rules using the Rough Set (RS) based decision model. The RS-based model performed much better in the prediction of CHF patients than the LR-based model, with an accuracy of 97.5% and 88.7%, respectively. It was supported by the AUC for the two decision-based models, 97.5 ±± 1.1% and 88.8 ± ± 3.1%, respectively . RF model also provides 100% classification accuracy in detecting CHF.

A study conducted by Masetic et al. made use of long-term ECG findings extracted using the autoregressive Burg method. Various classifiers were tested including SVM, artificial neural network (ANN), and k-nearest neighbors (k-NN) amongst which RF algorithm was selected due to a higher level of accuracy, and specificity for the diagnosis of HF . Detection of HF six months before the actual clinical diagnosis was achieved by Wu et al. 2010 . The Geisinger Clinic's electronic health records were obtained to be used in the model; 179 independent variables were expressed. The authors used SVM, boosting, and LR methods for HF identification. The study demonstrated that HF was detected more than six months before the actual date of clinical diagnosis using the LR model and boosting. SVM demonstrated the poorest performance, possibly owing to imbalanced data .

3. Risk level assessment using decision tree classifiers

Decision-making models involving decision trees have been utilized for the diagnosis of CHF in patients presenting to the emergency department. Rough sets (RS) and LR methods have been used to construct a decision-making model with the RS-based model proved to be more accurate than the LR model . Aljaaf et al. 2015 put forward a 5-risk level assessment (1 = no risk and 5 = extremely high risk) for HF prediction by making use of the C4.5 decision tree classifier . The dataset used for the project was further improved by considering lifestyle factors such as obesity, physical activity, and smoking. The cumulative accuracy for the 5 risk levels was observed to be 86.3% .

4. Least-squares support-vector machines (LS-SVM) application with ML

The heart responds to stimuli from inside and outside the body, which eventually leads to heart rate variability (HRV). The usage of ECG in HRV has limitations because HRV analysis in identifying cardiac problems is usually incomplete. By using linear and nonlinear HRV findings, the accuracy of results can be improved.Linear Autoregressive (AR) makes use of the frequency and time domain. The time-domain makes use of R-R interval, while the frequency domain uses the oscillation analysis of 5-minute ECG recordings or the Holter ECG, which monitors heart rhythm throughout the day. Nonlinear AR takes the humoral, electrophysiological, and hemodynamic variables, etc. into consideration. Support vector machines (SVM) can also be utilized for the detection of CHF as a study demonstrated it to be amongst the top three classification methods with an accuracy rate of nearly 98%. This study analyzed ECGs for normal rhythm, SV arrhythmia, and CHF amongst hundred patients. Vectors were employed for this purpose comprising SVM, artificial neural network (ANN), C4.5 decision tree, and RF which then underwent clustering and classification. Another study was conducted to explore the nonlinear AR in further detail, where the analysis of the spectrum was instead using ML models such as SVM, decision trees, k-NN, and ensemble classifiers. SVM was used with its kernel, enabling it to take data as input and transform it into the required form, i.e., linear, Gaussian, linear base function, and polynomial. This study also reported SVM to demonstrate the highest performance amongst the different methods employed

Finally, Zheng et al. 2015 introduced a computer-assisted system and made use of the least-squares SVM (LS-SVM), which utilized heart sounds and cardiac reverse features. The results showed ANN and Hidden Markov Models to be dominant over the LS-SVM model

5.Expert driven knowledge, ML and DLM

The role of AI in assisting HF specialists in diagnosis can be made easy by potential assistance from Artificial Intelligence-Clinical Decision Support System (AI-CDSS) . It is a hybrid system that contains both expert-driven and ML-driven knowledge to grow the knowledge base with HF . Retrospective cohorts and prospective pilot studies with HF and non-HF patients were carried out to observe the accuracy of AI-CDSS, which was converted into mind maps and then to a decision tree to be assessed by physicians .

Machine-derived learning involved the usage of 5 algorithms that selected LVEF left atrial volume index (LAVI) and left ventricular mass index (LVMI) as contributing factors All algorithms were ranked for accuracy, the number of rules extracted, and the number of attributes involved . The classification and regression tree (CART) algorithm was selected owing to its highest accuracy. Combining the two methods (ED and ML), lead to hybrid knowledge, the clinical knowledge model (CKM), which focused on the physical findings in patients, while a prediction model from ML looked for LVEF. The overall diagnostic accuracy was found to be 90% (expert-driven), 88.5% (ML-driven) and 98.3% (hybrid CDSS) . Direct learning can assess complicated patterns in dataset more than NN, which is why DL is being incorporated more often in the field of medicine . These models have also been studied for diagnosis of HF using chest X-rays. Matsumoto et al. used 952 chest x rays and established a DL model with an accuracy of 82% for HF detection.

6. Modern-day use of sensors in measuring patient vitals and implementation of IoT

Modern and compact implanted sensors are highly efficient in measuring vitals that are highly specific to HF's course and prognosis. These sensors are wireless and battery-less. Raised Left Atrial Pressure (LAP) is the earliest and most specific sign of HF before any symptoms appear. Implantable sensors can now easily record LAP and print a waveform. V-LAP is amongst the first battery-less cardiac monitoring devices which track LAP and provides remote HF care in such patients . With the help of V-LAP, physicians can now continuously monitor a patient's LAP and identify HF even before the onset of HF symptoms .In recent years, pulmonary artery pressure (PAP) measurements at home have been possible through the implantation of pressure sensors in the pulmonary artery. CardioMEMS system is a monitoring device most commonly utilized to measure PAP . It was used in the CHAMPION trial and a 33% decline in cardiac hospitalizations was noted over 18 months . Apart from measuring PAP, devices such as defibrillators and pacemakers have shown inefficacy in preventing hospitalization/rehospitalization in contrast to the CardioMEMS . The level of physical activity determines the course of HF to a great extent. Informative accelerometers are non-invasive devices that can be used to track the physical activity of HF patients which has been found to predict the risk of hospitalization . Remote Dialectic Sensing (ReDS) uses electromagnetic waves to detect the extent of pulmonary congestion which infers lung field concentration, helping in the interpretation of CT scans of lung field concentration .Various objects around us have been incorporated with an electronic software broadly termed the internet of things (IoT). It consists of 3 layers, a sensing layer that is present in the particular sensor used by the patient, a transport layer which is composed of connectors transporting data from sensor to remote device, and an application layer which is the server . Physicians with the help of IoT can now monitor various vitals in their patients and forecast medical emergencies.

This way, patients can now have medical care available at their doorstep, reducing the frequency of hospitalizations. When combined with specific algorithms, IoT can also warn us of heart attacks beforehand . Cardiac resynchronization therapy (CRT) devices can additionally detect intrathoracic impedance, which further helps in predicting hospitalization in HF patients . The MultiSENSE study presented an algorithm based on data from CRT defibrillators which showed 70% sensitivity in hospitalization prediction . To avoid false-positive predictions in HF, the research highlighted this issue and provided that a telephone triage questionnaire can easily eliminate false-positive results . Multisensor Non-invasive Remote Monitoring for Prediction of Heart Failure Exacerbation (LINK-HF) study made use of a non-invasive sensor placed on the patient's chest using adhesive tape. The sensor could record ECG, 3-axis accelerometry, skin impedance, body temperature, and posture . The Bluetooth-enabled connection between the sensor and cellular phone allowed for data transfer. Data-enabled cell phone syncs the transferred data to an encrypted cloud for viewing and storage. Cloud-based data gets converted to similarity-based modeling (SBM), and a baseline model is constructed within 72 hours of hospital discharge. Following this, the sensor on the patient's chest switches to the scrutiny phase and monitors the vitals . Variations in vitals due to normal activities are noted to remove false alarms. This is done by creating a multivariate change index range, from −1 to 1. The change in the patient's physiology would indicate a greater index change, while no change in physiology would be closer to 0. The change in index range (−1 to 1) allows for continuous monitoring of patient's vitals and provides indications for rehospitalizations .

7. Derivation of DEWS using TTS and RRS

To manage and prevent in-hospital cardiac arrest, a track and trigger system (TTS) and rapid response system (RRS) were introduced to identify cardiac arrest. Although TTS proved to be of great help, it was associated with high false alarms and low sensitivity. Single parameter TTS is defined as when anyone's vital sign concerning the heart, i.e., blood pressure, heart rate, respiratory rate, body temperature, and mental status is found to be abnormal . To avoid a high rate of false alarms, a deep learning-based early warning system (DEWS) was introduced. This system has better sensitivity and a low rate of false alarms. The DEWS make use of ML by identifying trends in the dataset, including specific vitals, as mentioned above . The model was used in two hospitals, a cardiovascular teaching hospital, and a community general hospital. Patients who had cardiac arrest had experienced death within 30 minutes of admission, or who were outside the study period were excluded. DEWS is a 3 layered neural network system which makes use of the time series data by going over records to conclude a patient's current state. DEWS was compared with modified early warning score (MEWS) at 3 sensitivities and SPTTS at 1 sensitivity. It was also compared with logistic regression and random forest at 75% sensitivity . The area under the receiver operating characteristic curve (AUROC), the area under the precision-recall curve (AUPRC), and confidence intervals (CIs) were greater for DEWS compared to other models . The specificity, positive and negative predictive value, F measure, MACHP, and net reclassification value were assessed using 75% sensitivity. DEWS was found to be the most accurate amongst all systems, hence DEWs can be used in the RRS to identify cardiac arrest .

8. Classification of HF

Algorithms can be used to classify HF into many types in the same way they have been used to diagnose patients with HF, well beforehand, and prevent hospitalization. Unsupervised ML performs grouping, i.e., observes similarities in the total dataset and compiles similar data in one place whereas supervised ML identifies trends and predictions .A study used model-based clustering (MBC) to classify HF in different phenotypes. HFpEF patients were taken in the study along with their variables such as echocardiography and laboratory results . MBC made use of R in the mclust package. After the application of MBC, classifiers were made to assign patients in their respective groups using Elastic Net, Neural Networks, and Naive Bayes. Resampling was done using cross a validation procedure in which four-fifth of the sample was used in the optimization of the model parameters, while the remaining of the sample was used in the prediction performance assessment, i.e., the ability of the ML model to put samples in the correct phenogroups . Six phenogroups were identified via MBC; phenogroup 1 consisted of young patients with cardiovascular risk factors, including left-sided heart changes along with patients that progressed to chronic kidney disease. Phenogroup 2 patients included severe HF with the highest degree of diastolic dysfunction, and deteriorating right ventricular function. Phenogroup 3 included young patients with milder HF variants. Phenogroup 4 included male patients with hypertension and enlarged left atrium contributing to the risk of atrial fibrillation. Phenogroup 5 and 6 included females with hypertension, atrial fibrillation, and low body mass index (BMI) . After establishing the protocol, a test run was carried out by clustering patients and using Elastic Net to put them into phenogroups accordingly . In another study, unsupervised clustering was used with the addition of CRT devices. The variables including echocardiography values were recorded, and the ML algorithm was used, after which the samples were clustered using the K-algorithm to identify 4 phenogroups undergoing CRT . Phenogroups 1 and 3 involved females with cardiomyopathy and left bundle branch block (LBBB), while phenogroup 1 was found to have prolonged QRS interval in comparison. Phenogroups 2 and 4 involved males with HF, predominantly caused by ischemia but had a lesser percentage of patients with LBBB . Cluster analyses on patients with HFpEF using exercise tolerance have also been performed in published literature. A study included HFpEF patients who underwent echocardiography during rest and following exercise to monitor heart function at both states. Clustering was done of noted variables which lead to the separation of the total dataset into two distinct phenogroups based on data similarities and differences. The first phenotype had a decreased chronotropic/diastolic reserve, ventricular arterial coupling (indicating global heart efficiency), and abnormal longitudinal deformity, while the other phenotype showed a preserved heart rate reserve combined with low left ventricular systolic reserve . Few studies have classified HF using conventional tress and ML classifiers. Classification trees divide the total dataset into many subsets but are found to have questionable accuracy, while ML uses an aggregate of classification trees . Classification trees are simple to use and can utilize binary methods to dividing the dataset into two subsets. The classification of HF has been performed in two parts in a study with all classification techniques used in a manner to keep two classifications as their result, i.e., HFpEF and HFrEF. The bootstrap technique, also known as bagging is a modern technique that has been previously implemented in literature. Multiple bootstraps were applied to the sample size, and a classification/ regression tree was utilized for each bootstrap. The bootstrap samples were compiled with help of majority votes in each sample, and the classification was obtained . Boosting classification technique makes use of multiple weak classifiers and "boosts" their result. A weak classifier has a margin of error slightly better than of guessing . When a classifier puts a subject in the wrong class, the class gets weighted heavier hence at the end when it's all summed up, the samples get correctly classified and placed in subsets . SVM makes use of the hyperplane concept, where the dimensional space gets divided into two distinct planes. Hence two distinct subgroups are made in a single sample. The sample on one side of the hyperplane and the one on the other side are considered as two classifications in a sample .

9.Role of mobile health and internet of things in the early detection and management of heart failure

AI can be of advantage in identifying potential cardiac events faster than a clinician could, using predictive analytics. As described above, ML; the most common application of AI, can recognize patterns in data to improve cardiovascular diagnosis and detection .Mobile health and the internet of things have allowed patients to keep a track of their health parameters, which have been particularly useful for home-based long-term monitoring, detection, and subsequent alertness for abnormal cardiovascular findings, and timely contact with doctors when necessary.

10 MOBILE HEALTH (mHealth)

According to the World Health Organization (WHO)'s Global Observatory for eHealth, Mobile Health (mHealth) is defined as "medical and public health practice supported by mobile devices, such as [cell] phones, patient monitoring devices, personal digital assistants (PDAs), and other wireless devices" . mHealth enables patients to track their health, e.g., in the form of keeping a check on their heart rate, blood glucose levels, medication dosages, and sleep cycles. It also allows for remote consultations and maintaining electronic health records . It has also been used in managing chronic diseases such as diabetes, hypertension, and chronic obstructive pulmonary disease . The mHealth-based interventions have several factors, potentially making them effective for cardiovascular disease; according to Dicianno et al. these factors include: (i) 'interactivity that allows the bidirectional communication and the care delivery, as a form of a personal coach', (ii) 'personalization' that allows for the mHealth interventions to be customized according to the individual's needs, (iii) 'timeliness' which allows for delivery of information within the right time frame, (iv) 'context sensitivity': the ability of interventions to be adapted and modified according to the circumstances and/or the individual's needs, and (v) 'ubiquity and accessibility of the technology to all segments of population'.The advantages of mHealth in the management of HF has been demonstrated . In addition, wearables (e.g., smartwatches, wristbands, patches and sensors) are being used to measure and record a range of parameters, such as heart rate, blood pressure and temperature, and to track diseases such as HF and diabetes.Wearables not only track and transfer biometric data into a shareable and comprehensible user interface but also allow for the continuous monitoring of more than one dozen biometric parameters as reported by several developers of wrist-worn sensors .A study conducted in 2019, under the collaboration of Stanford University and Apple, assessed the ability of a smartwatch to detect atrial fibrillation or atrial flutter using algorithms that use pulse wave data detection of these episodes . According to this study, only 0.52% (2161) of the total participants received an irregular pulse notification. Among those who received an initial notification and returned an ECG patch, it was reported that 84% of their subsequent notifications were confirmed as atrial fibrillation. Moreover, 76% of the participants who received notification were reported to have contacted either a telemedicine provider or a non-study healthcare provider.According to a meta-analysis conducted in 2020 among HF patients (n = 1683), mobile phone-based interventions were associated with a significantly lower rate of all-cause hospital admissions at six months (31% vs. 36%, OR 0.77, 95% CI 0.62–0.97, p = 0.03, I22= 0). A significant difference was also demonstrated for HF admissions (14.0% vs. 18.5%, OR 0.69, 95% CI 0.48 to 0.98, p = 0.04, I22 = 26%) . However, another meta-analysis found mobile monitoring interventions, mostly consisting of a mobile communication device, a blood pressure measuring device, a weighing scale, and an ECG recorder, to be inconclusive for monitoring HF outcomes. It is also difficult to achieve a 100 percent adherence to mHeath based interventions, as seen in many study groups reported by this meta-analysis, with only one study reporting 100% adherence . However, the popularity of mhealth and its potential utilization cannot be undermined since, in the US alone, 91% of adults have been reported to own some kind of cellphone, with 56% reported to be smartphone users . Moreover, a study conducted in 2017 also stated that older individuals had a positive outlook towards the benefits of mHealth and were eager to utilize mhealth interventions, despite facing usability issues with mHealth such as in navigation and visualization, etc.

11 Internet of Things (IoT)

The Internet of Things or IoT is simply a network of different devices in various physical objects or locations, that allows for the exchange and storage of data, using network connectivity . A study conducted in 2017 proposed the structure of an IoT-based system comprising of 3 different layers: the sensing layer, the transport layer, and the application layer, and 4 different modes that could be utilized for heart-disease monitoring. This system could allow for more cost-effective and efficient transmission of data, enabling communication with healthcare practitioners in real-time, in a more structured and systematic way. For cardiovascular management, IoT enables healthcare practitioners to monitor their patients remotely and in real-time, and to collect data, such as blood pressure, pulse rate, oxygen saturation, and ECG simultaneously. This could drastically change the way patients receive medical assistance, making it easier for them to get healthcare at their homes in a timelier fashion, reducing hospital visits concurrently. If IoT is utilized in cohesion with certain real-time algorithms, this could be helpful to alert about potential attacks beforehand . IoT is particularly useful in the detection and diagnosis of certain conditions that may require monitoring throughout the day. To make an accurate diagnosis for arrhythmias, for example, the patient's ECG needs to be monitored for an entire day, at minimum. Hence, making them especially challenging to detect. Moreover, they can be intermittent, so detection and diagnosis can be markedly enhanced by long-term continuous monitoring, using IoT techniques. According to an article published in 2019, mobile cardiac telemetry (MCT) devices that providing real-time monitoring of a patient's heart rhythm over a longer period are essential for AFib detection. MCT devices are the only heart monitoring devices that provide complete arrhythmia detection, with the highest diagnostic yield at 61%, compared to Event monitors at 23% and Holter monitors at 24% . In a study conducted by J. Stehlik et al. it was suggested that non-invasive devices such as wearables may be more useful and cost-effective in predicting and recognizing the risk of rehospitalizations for heart failure.

12 Imaging techniques utilized with AI

ML techniques including supervised and unsupervised networks as well as DL has been incorporated in different cardiac imaging procedures for accurate quantitative and qualitative evaluation of cardiac diseases, particularly, HF.

13 Echocardiography

ML models have been trained to recognize specific images of a wide variety of cardiac diseases . This helps in the interpretation of unused data in three-dimensional imaging, thus leading to faster analysis and better outcomes. Furthermore, DL has been mostly utilized in imaging for segmentation of the ventricles. Chen et al. demonstrated the use of convolutional neural networks (CNN) to segment the ventricle into 5 different 2D views. ANN model was previously used for segmentation which was further extended in studies by Carneiro and Nascimento . Dong et al. and Ghesu et al. also combined DL with traditional methods to segment the left ventricle and the aortic valve. Dezaki et al. utilized electrocardiograms in combination with RNN and CNN to predict end-systolic and diastolic volume.

14 Cardiac MRI

AI and ML algorithms have proved to be of crucial importance in other imaging techniques like Cardiac MRI particularly for ventricular segmentation. Machine learning (ML) can segment the heart chambers from Cardiac MRIs and these segmentations yield imaging biomarkers to predict CHF.

Laser et al. used knowledge-based reconstruction of the right ventricular volumes using images from echocardiography and cardiac MRI and compared them with the gold standard direct cardiac MRI and found that knowledge-based reconstruction has excellent accuracy for right ventricular 3D volumetry. Right ventricle has a complex shape which many times could not be visualized with 2D imaging echocardiography techniques. 3D visualization and cardiac image reconstruction with the help of AI can help in the diagnosis of a variety of similar diseases. Similarly, calculation of left ventricular mass, papillary muscle identification, common carotid artery, and descending aorta measurements with fully automated AI programs have produced far more accurate results. Another study extracted CMRIs from 350 subjects and used CNNs to segment the heart in short and long axis Cardiac MRI. He concluded that cardiac MRI provides a reliable method of extracting indicators for cardiac measurements and function .

15 Cardiac computed tomography (Cardiac CT)

ML based image analysis has been increasingly used for cardiac CT specially for evaluation of coronary artery disease and atherosclerosis. ML models were used for coronary artery calcification scoring and risk stratification. Commandeur et al. used 2 CNNs to segment epicardial and thoracic adipose tissue using cardiac CT images. They evaluated their method in a large cohort of 1638 patients. Multi scale patch-based CNN was also used by Zerik et al. to segment the left ventricle myocardium. Wu et al. used short term memory RNN to label segments of coronary artery tree. Itu et al. and Coenen et al. also used ML models for quantitative analysis of fractional flow reserve in coronary artery disease. The implication of ML models using datasets from Cardiac CT has played a major role in diagnosis of coronary artery stenosis, and risk stratification of future events.

16 Electrocardiogram

ECG is the most widely used diagnostic modality for detection of heart diseases. The application of ML models particularly DL has helped reduce the time taken in diagnosis, and speed up urgent care. Supervised learning models have been used to classify heart rhythm. Algorithms involving unsupervised learning analysis have also been used. In this method, unlabeled data has been grouped according to its ECG phenotype. This was demonstrated by Lyon et al. who classified ECGs with arrhythmia risk factors in patients of cardiomyopathy. Hannum et al used a 34-layer deep NN to classify 12 different types of arrhythmias. Attia et al. used a 6-layer investigators attempted to diagnose asymptomatic left ventricular dysfunction by EKG alone using an AI-based CNN deep learning method. This model proved to be superior to the conventional method of using BNP levels for estimation.

17 Prediction of adverse outcomes

Early detection of future mortality and episodes of destabilization can help provide quality care earlier in the management of the patient and also allow doctors to make crucial clinical decisions when needed. Using statistical analysis, multiple risk calculation scoring systems have been formed for estimation of mortality.

18 Decompensation

Candelieri et al. 2008 used knowledge discovery (KD) models to predict if a patient with HF in a stable phase would decompensate or not. A group of 49 CHF patients was used for the evaluation of the KD approaches. Decision trees, Decision Lists, SVM and Radial Basis Function Networks were used, and the leave-patient-out approach was followed to evaluate the performance. Of the models, decision trees proved to be superior to other models and provided an accuracy of 92.03%, sensitivity 63.64%, and False Positive Rate 6.90%. In 2009 Candelieri et al. used decision trees and SVM on an independent testing. Their results showed that SVM is more reliable in predicting decompensation events with an accuracy of 97.37%, 100.00% sensitivity. This was further extended through the "SVM hypersolution framework" which proved to be more accurate on minority class than Tabu search. Guiti et al. also predicted the frequency of HF decompensation during the year after the first visit using five machine learning techniques (NN, SVM, Fuzzy -Genetic Expert System, Random Forests and CART). CART algorithm proved to be the superior one with 87.6% accuracy.

19 Re-hospitalizations and mortality

Re-hospitalizations add to the burden on the healthcare system and lead to poor quality of life for the patient. Predictive models have been developed to predict the risk of future hospitalization so that adequate monitoring and management can be done to prevent such adverse outcomes. At the same time, mortality can be improved using risk prediction models and discrimination of patients as demonstrated in the studies

Conclusions

HF is associated with poor patient's outcomes, high recurrence rate, mortality rate, and cost burden. Therehas been a major development in the field of cardiovascular medicine with the incorporation of AI in diagnostic modalities, outcome-predictions, and management of HF. Incorporation of AI Deep Learning components particularly ANN and CNN for diagnosis of HF coupled with remote monitoring of at-risk patients via IoT and mHealth can drastically reduce mortality associated with all structural heart diseases, particularly HF. Though AI has the potential to revolutionize medical diagnosis, treatment, risk prediction, clinical care, and drug discovery through interpretation of vast database more efficiently as compared to the human brain, it has its limitations due to the absence of a healthcare system that supports it, as well as a shortage of trained clinicians who can utilize AI models in their clinical decisions, and monitoring of patients. Therefore, it is essential to establish a connection between AI models and clinical practitioners through hybrid expert, and ML-driven systems such as the AI-CDSS to provide more accurate outcomes. AI systems can certainly not replace the expertise of a human brain but it has the potential of revolutionizing accurate diagnosis and prediction of decompensation and mortality of HF patients by acting as a tool of assistance. In the post COVID-19 pandemic era where healthcare systems will be overburdened with HF related hospitalizations, the specialists treating HF patients should make efforts to train themselves in incorporating AI so practice of an AI-dependent medicine can be made more efficient and provide accurate diagnosis in a short span of time

Role of AI in Elucidating HF Pathophysiology, Precision Medicine, and Novel Therapeutics

Currently, HF is broadly characterized by the EF and the presumed etiology contributing to the HF state. Unsupervised ML analytics such as cluster analysis may identify unique HF phenotypes that can then be characterized using traditional statistical methods or supervised learning techniques to determine if identified phenotypes have different prognoses or tolerance of or response to therapies. Such analyses have been performed in patients who have HF with preserved EF (HFpEF) and HFrEF using clinical data as input variables and identified HFpEF and HFrEF phenotypes with different prognoses. It is likely that data beyond clinical features will be needed to further phenotype patients with HF and identify precision or novel HF therapies. Genomic and circulating proteomic data as well as novel clinical data such as microbiome and AI-

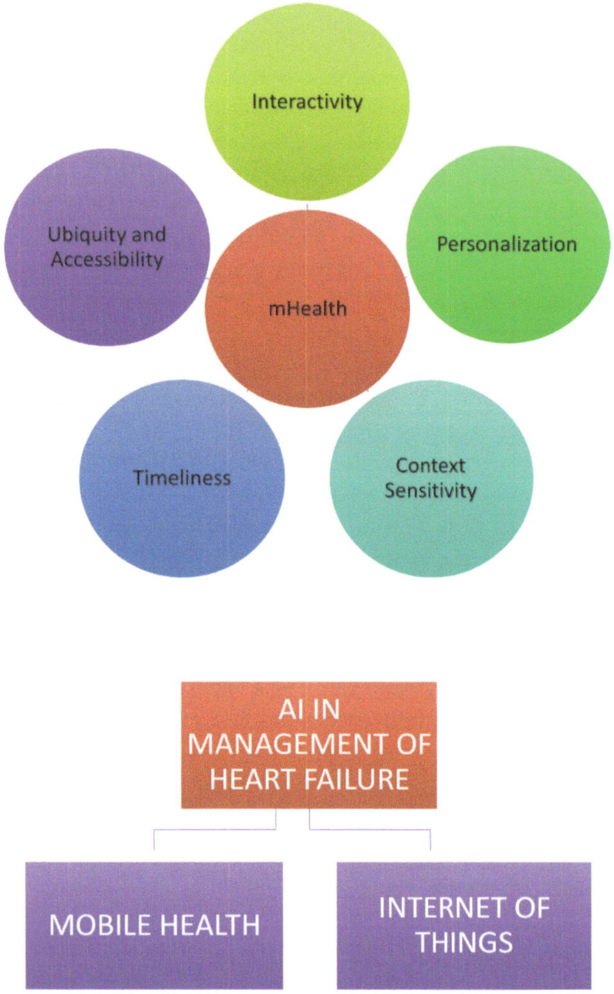

Fig.14.2 The advantages of mHealth in the management of HF. mHealth based interventions has been effective in managing cardiovascular diseases owning to the various benefits including interactivity, personalization, context sensitivity, timeliness, ubiquity, and accessibility,

enabled ECG or image analysis may enable identification of unique pathophysiologic phenotypes with novel therapeutic targets or diagnostic/prognostic biomarkers for testing in clinical trials

Putting AI at the centre of heart failure care

Heart failure (HF) is a global pandemic affecting over 40 million people worldwide and imposing a considerable human and economic burden. At least 1–2% of the global healthcare budget is spent on HF, costs driven primarily by hospitalizations, many of which are regarded as preventable. Worryingly, the prevalence of HF is increasing substantially alongside increases in predisposing diseases and co-morbidities (i.e. diabetes, hypertension, and obesity), a growing 'Western lifestyle' in developing countries, and an ageing population worldwide, together imposing unsustainable demands on our healthcare systems. A new vision of care is required, one that embraces digital technologies to drive fundamental change in HF healthcare.Artificial intelligence (AI), a rapidly evolving field in medicine, especially cardiology, is revolutionizing risk prediction and stratification, diagnostics, precision medicine, workflows, and efficiency. In a strategic paper, we [PAtient Self-care uSing eHealth In chronic Heart Failure (PASSION-HF) consortium] propose using digital therapeutics powered by AI as a personalized approach to HF self-care. 11 PASSION-HF aims to develop a virtual 'doctor at home' system. Being able to pool datasets smartly and extrapolating relevance at an individual level, our AI approach offers huge potential for reducing clinician burden, improving clinical efficacy, and enhancing patient experience and outcomes. AI techniques are transforming cardiovascular diagnosis through interpreting and finding meaning in vast sets of data, faster and more effectively than the human brain. Machine learning, the most common application of AI, is characterized by the ability to learn from data without being explicitly programmed. Through the development of reinforcement learning algorithms, machine learning recognizes patterns in new data to create its own logic to continuously improve cardiovascular disease prediction and diagnosis.Accordingly,AI is able to deal with enormous combinations of multi-markers, essential in the prediction and prevention of deterioration of complex diseases like HF. Even so, such predictive models are largely dependent on high-quality large-scale datasets that are not easily accessible, and datasets of poorer quality may lead to biases with subsequent decrease in the predictive accuracy of models. 12 However, through strategic selection of underlying data and use of sensitivity checks, algorithm developers can mitigate AI bias.This in itself accentuates the need for transparency, reproducibility, and standard reporting guidelines, which have recently been proposed and implemented in AI and machine learning . The ability of AI to mimic the human brain and even overcome bias is fast contributing to the conceptualization of personalized precision medicine. However, overwhelmingly, the focus has been on diagnosis and risk prediction. 15 Evidence demonstrating applications of AI in clinical decision-making are not only lacking but also essential if we are to advance into an era of precision medicine. Only then is AI likely to take over the routine part of a physician's workload, allowing them to spend more quality time with their patients and improve patient engagement.

The future application of AI in HF care offers immense possibilities. For healthcare providers, AI has the potential to decrease risk of adverse events, patient waiting times, and per capita costs whilst increasing accessibility, productivity, and overall patient experience. For clinicians, AI has the capability to reduce workloads and margin of error and improve needs-led patient–doctor interactions and therapeutic decision-making. For patients, AI can empower them through increased knowledge, shared decision-making, and self-efficacy in disease management, ultimately improving their health and well-being Although AI has the ability to overcome many of the key challenges posed by the prevailing HF pandemic, some caution is warranted as it is a rapidly evolving science. Transparency regarding the quality of data, population representativeness, and performance assessment will be imperative. Discussions regarding legal, technical, and regulatory challenges should involve clinicians, informatics and IT experts, regulators, and patients and carers and prioritize ethics and equity. The diversity of AI development teams will mandate interdisciplinary integration to achieve adoption, utility, safety, and inclusion all under the auspices of a new philosophy of care—AI-enabled care. Although the landscape of HF care may be changing, the patient–doctor relationship will not be entirely replaced by AI. However, those who do not use AI will, in all probability, be replaced by those who do.AI is the new tool in the toolbox that is already transforming cardiology. The PASSION-HF consortium see AI as an enabler to personalize medicine and to optimize effective HF self-care in consideration of disease complexity. By adding value and precision to the management of HF, providing equitable and affordable care access, and improving patient expectation and outcomes, AI is transforming HF care.

Artificial Intelligence-Enhanced Smartwatch ECG for Heart Failure-Reduced Ejection Fraction Detection by Generating 12-Lead ECG

Heart failure (HF) is a significant healthcare burden worldwide, with an estimated 64.3 million people living with HF .Despite advances in treatment, HF remains as a high risk of morbidity and mortality and is the most common diagnosis in hospitalized patients aged over 65 years, with a 5-year survival rate of only . In the United States, HF affects ~$30.7 billion total annual costs and projection suggests that by 2030, the total cost of HF will increase by 127%, to $69.8 billion. Patients suffering with HF with reduced ejection fraction (HFrEF) become less active, leading to repeated hospitalization, resulting in a poor quality of life, including a high medical cost burden . Despite its poor prognosis and high economic burden, HFrEF awareness remains relatively low due to its insidious onset, varied presentation, and syndromic nature. Early diagnosis and timely intervention may prevent irreversible HFrEF progression and mortality. Electrocardiography (ECG) is a low-cost test frequently performed for a variety of purposes, especially basic examination and screening for cardiovascular disease . We developed an artificial intelligence (AI)-enabled ECG algorithm, which can increase the diagnosis of HFrEF .However, it is also inconvenient to visit the hospital for a 12-lead ECG

Smart watches have high processing power and sophisticated sensors that can provide new health data, including ECG. In this study, we developed and validated an artificial intelligence-enabled smartwatch ECG for HFrEF detection. As the smartwatch could obtain a single lead ECG, we also developed a deep learning-based model (DLM) for generating a 12-lead ECG from a smartwatch ECG (Lead I and II) to enhance AI performance and detect HFrEF using the generated 12-lead ECG. Moreover, we conducted internal and external validation for the developed AI in this multicenter study. To the best of our knowledge, this is the first study to generate a 12-lead ECG from a smartwatch ECG and detect heart failure. Based on this deep learning model, heart failure with reduced ejection fraction could be detected in daily living by using asynchronous 2-lead ECGs from lifestyle ECG devices, such as smart watches.

Outcomes and Predictive Variables

The primary outcome of this study was the performance of the AI in detecting patients with HFrEF using a standard 10 s 12-lead ECG or smartwatch ECG. HFrEF was defined as an ejection fraction of 40% or less on transthoracic comprehensive echocardiography, which was recorded in the electronic health record database at the time of acquisition, symptom, and signs from medical records . The EF was determined using a biplane approach with the Simpson and 2D methods. If the estimated EF was in a range, we used the middle value as a single EF value. If more than two echocardiographies were obtained within 14 days from the ECG, we used echocardiography that was closest to ECG as index echocardiography. The secondary outcome was the performance of the AI in detecting patients with HF with mildly reduced EF (HFmrEF) to reduced EF (<50%) on echocardiography . Predictive variables were ECG, age, sex, weight, and height

Data Preprocessing

We preprocessed the ECGs for sampling, normalization, and augmentations. Researchers constructed an ECG with 8 s by cropping of 1 s on each side and normalized (z-score) based on the mean and standard deviation. In terms of augmentations, the addition of linear and nonlinear noise causing baseline changes was performed. We also normalized the values of age, weight, and height. We changed the value of sex to one-hot encoding.Development for a Platform Detecting HFrEF Our AI consists of two phases. First phase generates a standard 12-lead ECG. We developed an ECGT2T for generating a 12-lead ECG from an asynchronous 2-lead ECG, ECGT2T is a deep learning model based on a generative adversarial network that synthesizes a 10-lead ECG (III, aVR, aVL, aVF, and V1–6) from an asynchronous 2-lead ECG (leads I and II). It translates source ECGs to reference ECGs by learning the styles of reference ECGs; it first generates a single latent code representing the cardiac condition from two given leads and then reconstructs the other 10 leads by referring to the single latent code based on the single given lead. For ECGT2T development, development data from hospital A were used. We have described the detailed development process of ECGT2T in our previous article

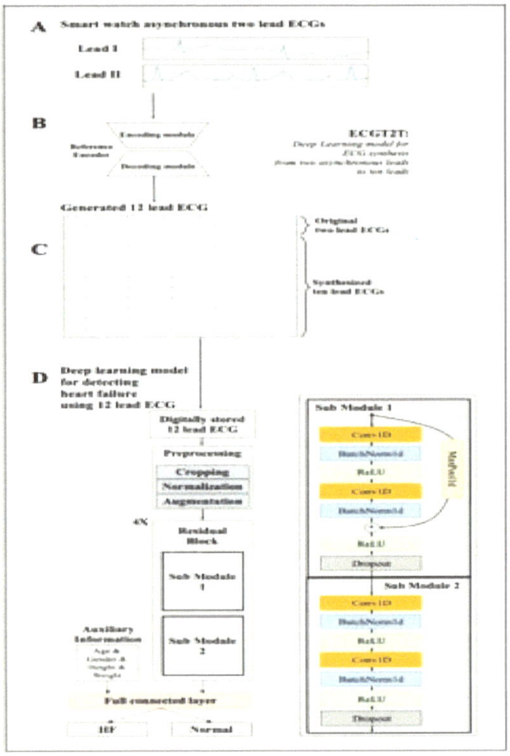

Fig.14.3 Architecture of deep learning model for detecting heart failure. Legend: ECG denotes electrocardiography, ECGT2T ECG synthesis from two-lead to ten-lead, and HF heart failure. (A) Asynchronous two lead ECGs from smart watch. (B) ECGT2T for synthesizing ten lead ECG from two lead ECG. (C) Generated twelve lead ECG which input to final AI model. (D) Deep learning model for detecting heart failure with reduced ejection fraction using generated twelve lead ECG.

Second phase detects a HFrEF. We developed another deep learning model based on four residual blocks for detecting HFrEF using a 12-lead ECG. This model was trained using the development dataset from hospital A. Fig. showed the architecture of the HFrEF detection model. Each residual block contains two submodules, each of which has a one-dimensional convolutional neural network, batch normalization, rectified linear unit activation, and a dropout layer. The difference between both sub modules is the skip connection. The first sub module has only the skip connection. The latent variables passing through all residual blocks are concatenated to auxiliary information including age, gender, height, and weight. Thereafter, the final output was obtained through two fully connected layers. We used the Adam optimizer, which is a popular algorithm in the field of deep learning because it achieves good results fast. Additionally, it was observed that its performance was better than that of SGD, RMSprop, or Adadelta in the pilot study. For parameter settings, we set the learning rate to 1 × 10−4, weight decay to 1 × 10 −5, epsilon to 1× 10−8, beta1 to 0.9, and beta2 to 0.999, respectively.

The study group confirmed the values of parameters by grid search methods. We selected the search space of grid search by using random sampling search of pilot study. We train the models on a high-performance computer composed of 20 DGX servers with 160 NVIDIA A100 graphics processing units. All models were developed using PyTorch and Python.

In one of the studies , there were 137,835 patients from hospital A and after applying exclusion criteria, including 137,673 patients with 458,745 ECG for development dataset for developing ECGT2T

Among 137,673 patients from hospital A, 38,643 adult patients who underwent both 10 s 12-lead ECG and echocardiography within 14 days at hospital A were included to develop model to detect HFrEF using a 10 s 12-lead ECG

For external testing to confirm the performance for detecting HFrEF using smartwatch ECG, 761 patients from hospital B were identified and 6 patients were excluded due to missing values of ECG and echocardiography.

Finally, 755 patients with 1510 ECG dataset (2-lead ECG from smart watch A and B) were included in the external performance test. As described the HFrEF patients were older than the non-HFrEF patients. And HFrEF patients had more prolonged QRS interval and atrial fibrillation or flutter than the non-HFrEF patients.

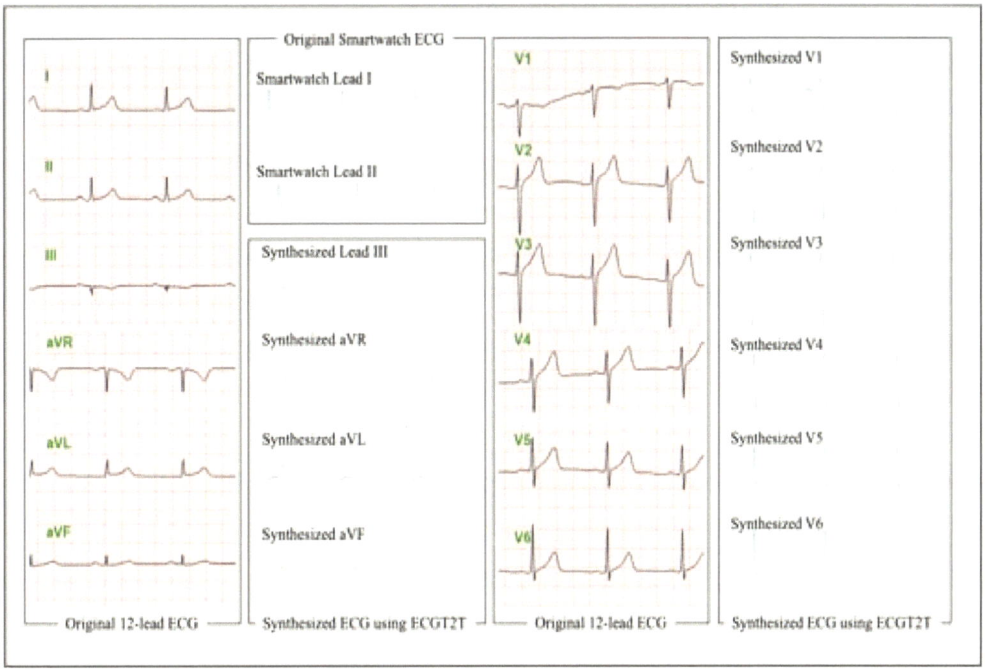

Fig.14.4 12-lead ECG generation using smartwatch ECG based on ECGT2T. Legend: ECG denotes electrocardiography and ECGT2T ECG synthesis from two-lead to ten-lead.

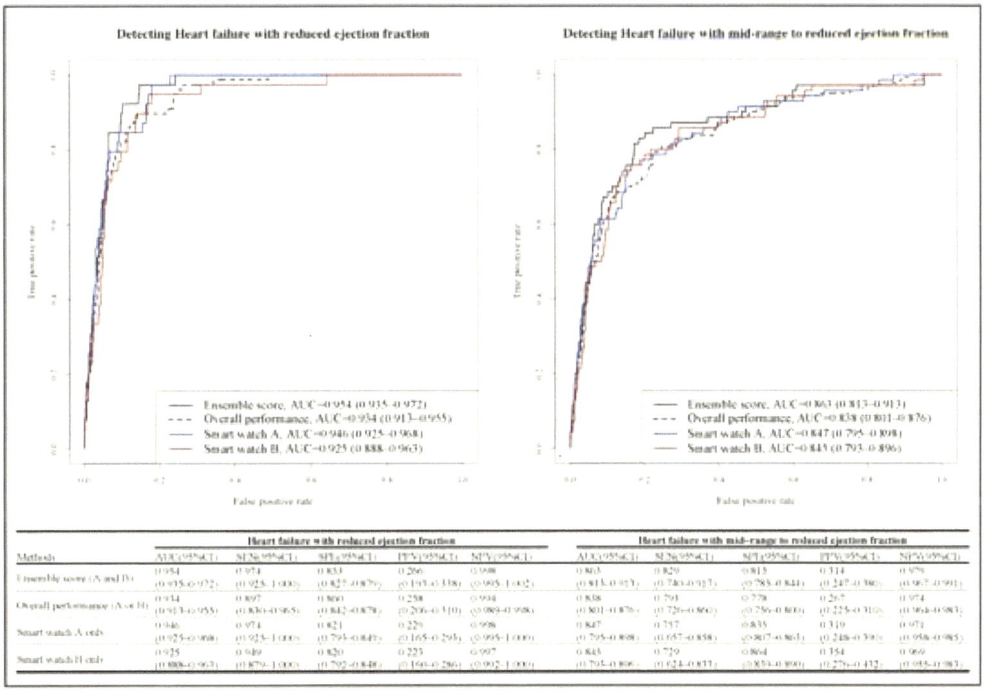

Fig. 14.5 Performance of artificial intelligence for detecting heart failure using smart watch ECG. Legend: AUC denotes area under the receiver operating characteristic curve, CI confidence interval, ECG electrocardiography, NPV negative predictive value, PPV positive predictive value, SEN sensitivity, and SPE specificity

The ECG of each lead is a signal for measuring the electrical flow of the heart in each lead vector. The electrical vector of the heart can be estimated by synthesizing the ECG data of the two leads. A 12-lead ECG can be generated by reconstructing the ECG corresponding to the vector of each lead, determined based on the estimated electrical flow of the heart. ECGT2T is a deep learning model based on this concept and generates an ECG using a generative adversarial network.

Twelve-lead ECG was required for evaluating cardiovascular disease status using diverse vector information of the heart. However, in daily living, 12-lead ECG is not always practical or feasible because it is difficult to place the chest and limb lead at the exact location. In this study, we generated 12-lead ECG and detected heart failure with reduced ejection fraction using only leads I and II, which could be captured by a smart watch in use in daily living. Therefore, this study is a milestone in using ECG to detect cardiovascular disease in daily living. Although previous studies have detected diseases using ECG, studies using 12-lead ECG and other devices have been conducted only in hospital settings. Here, we developed a deep learning methodology that generates ECGs from lifestyle devices and smartwatches. Therefore, our methodology can be used in daily living. The major contribution of this study is to provide a methodology for detecting disease in daily living based on deep learning model using a single lead life style device, such as a smart watch. The increasing prevalence of HF making it among the most costly diseases to Medicare . More than 30% HF patients are seen in the clinic setting, and more than 40% of those recently admitted with decompensation will require a second hospitalization within a year . Early detection of HFrEF offers the opportunity to test and develop an effective lifestyle and life-saving medical therapy The evolution and adoption of digital health technology and mobile health devices may address this issue. Our day-today lives are impacted by technological innovations, and the recent trend of commercial smart wearable devices aims in improving our health. Smart wearables are connected electronic devices designed for everyday use that can be worn on the body as an accessory or integrated into clothing. Smartwatches and wristbands have high processing power and sophisticated sensors that can provide new health information. Wearable health devices are an aspect of medical health that may improve the delivery of HF care by allowing medical data collection outside of a clinician's office or hospital. Wearable devices are externally applied and capture functional or physiological data to monitor and improve patients' health. It could be a cost-effective method to detect HF before it becomes fatal. Personalized patient care has become remote and decentralized owing to the COVID-19 pandemic The cardiovascular community must utilize the commercially available wearable technologies as well as the wide range of clinical applications that they can serve. This technology integration into the clinical workplace, however, is still in its early stages. Per previous medical knowledge, ECGs could be used to detect small coverage diseases, such as arrhythmia and ST-segment elevation myocardial infarction. We could not develop diagnostic criteria and tools using non-linear correlations between diverse diseases and subtle changes based on conventional statistical methods, such as logistic regression. Recently, AI has been adopted to diagnose many diseases and conditions and to predict the development of disease . Most AI for detecting diseases using ECG is based on deep learning. The most important strength of deep learning is the automatic feature extraction . Specifically, deep learning automatically extracts the features of ECG to detect disease, without any human engineering resource needed to define the features for using the model. This has reduced the time and cost of AI development. The importance of automatic feature extraction is that we can extract features and develop a model without human prejudice. AI based on deep learning is based only on information from data, not medical knowledge. This aspect showed the possibility of enhancing the model to detect diverse diseases and show new medical findings over previous medical knowledge. An important pitfall of deep learning is overfitting . Especially, deep learning can be subjugated to the environment in which development data are obtained. Therefore, we should validate the developed AI to other hospitals and environments. The important point of this study was external validation. We confirmed the performance of the AI model using data from other hospitals and other devices in this study. In other word, we developed AI using 12-lead ECG data from hospital A and external validated AI using smartwatch ECG from hospital.

The advantage of AI is that it saves healthcare costs. Using this AI, HFrEF could be screened by a wearable watch without a physician, and it could refer patients at risk to cardiologists for confirmative diagnostic tests. Therefore, this procedure is advantageous for low-income countries to save patients from irreversible disease progression anddeath.

This AI could be used in wearable watches in daily living and HFrEF could be detected and monitored in the early stages without complications. This predictive care solution is essential to reduce healthcare costs.

Bibliography and Acknowledgement

- Adler ED, Voors AA, Klein L, Macheret F, Braun OO, Urey MA, Zhu W, Sama I, Tadel M, Campagnari C, Greenberg B, Yagil A. Improving risk prediction in heart failure using machine learning. Eur J Heart Fail 2020; 22: 139–147. [PubMed] [Google Scholar]
- Beam AL, Manrai AK, Ghassemi M. Challenges to the reproducibility of machine learning models in health care. JAMA 2020; 323: 305–306. [PMC free article] [PubMed]
- Bozkurt, B.; Coats, A.J.; Tsutsui, H.; Abdelhamid, M.; Adamopoulos, S.; Albert, N.; Anker, S.D.; Atherton, J.; Böhm, M.; Butler, J.; et al. Universal Definition and Classification of Heart Failure. J. Card. Fail. 2021, 27, 387–413.
- Braunwald, E. The war against heart failure: The Lancet lecture. Lancet 2015, 385, 812–824. [Google Scholar] [CrossRef] Breiman, L. Statistical Modeling: The Two Cultures. Stat. Sci. 2001, 16, 199–215. [Google Scholar] [CrossRef]
- Cho, J.; Lee, B.; Kwon, J.-M.; Lee, Y.; Park, H.; Oh, B.-H.; Jeon, K.-H.; Park, J.; Kim, K.-H. Artificial Intelligence Algorithm for Screening Heart Failure with Reduced Ejection Fraction Using Electrocardiography. ASAIO J. 2020, 67, 314–321.
- Flint, K.M.; Fairclough, D.L.; Spertus, J.A.; Bekelman, D.B. Does heart failure-specific health status identify patients with bothersome symptoms, depression, anxiety, and/or poorer spiritual well-being? Eur. Hear. J. Qual. Care Clin. Outcomes 2019, 5, 233–241. [Google Scholar] [CrossRef]
- GBD 2017 Disease and Injury Incidence and Prevalence Collaborators. Global, Regional, and National Incidence, Prevalence, and Years Lived with Disability for 354 Diseases and Injuries for 195 Countries and Territories, 1990–2017: A Systematic Analysis for the Global Burden of Disease Study. Lancet 2018, 392, 1789–1858. Available online: http://www.ncbi.nlm.nih.gov/pubmed/30496104 (accessed on 8 October 2021). [CrossRef][Green Version]
- Groenewegen, A.; Rutten, F.H.; Mosterd, A.; Hoes, A.W. Epidemiology of heart failure. Eur. J. Heart Fail. 2020, 22, 1342–1356.Availableonline:http://www.ncbi.nlm.nih.gov/pubmed/32483830 (accessed on 8 October 2021).
- Jackson, S.L.; Tong, X.; King, R.J.; Loustalot, F.; Hong, Y.; Ritchey, M.D. National Burden of Heart Failure Events in the United States, 2006 to Circ. Hear. Fail. 2018, 11, e004873. [Google Scholar] [CrossRef]
- Johnson KW, Soto JT, Glicksberg BS, Shameer K, Miotto R, Ali M, Ashley E, Dudley TD. Artificial intelligence in cardiology. J Am Coll Cardiol 2018; 71: 2668–2679. [PubMed] [Google Scholar]
- Krittanawong C, Zhang H, Wang Z, Aydar M, Kitai T. Artificial intelligence in precision cardiovascular medicine. J Am Coll Cardiol 2017; 69: 2657–2664. [PubMed] [Google Scholar]
- Kwon, J.-M.; Jo, Y.-Y.; Lee, S.Y.; Kim, K.-H. Artificial intelligence using electrocardiography: Strengths and pitfalls. Eur. Hear. J. 2021, 42, 2896–2898. [Google Scholar] [CrossRef] [PubMed]
- Lam, C.S.P.; Gamble, G.D.; Ling, L.H.; Sim, D.; Leong, K.T.G.; Yeo, P.S.D.; Ong, H.Y.; Jaufeerally, F.; Ng, T.P.; Cameron, V.A.; et al. Mortality associated with heart failure with preserved vs. reduced ejection fraction in a prospective international multi-ethnic cohort study. Eur. Heart J. 2018, 39, 1770–1780.
- LeCun, Y.; Bengio, Y.; Hinton, G. Deep learning. Nature 2015, 521, 436–444. Available online: http://arxiv.org/abs/1603.05691 (accessed on 8 October 2021). [CrossRef]
- Lesyuk W, Kriza C, Kolominsky - Rabas P. Cost - of - illness studies in heart failure: a systematic review 2004–2016. BMC Cardiovasc Disord 2018; 18: 74. [PMC free article] [PubMed] , Michalsen A, König G, Thimme W. Preventable causative factors leading to hospital admission with decompensated heart failure. Heart 1998; 80: 437–441. [PMC free article]
- Mishra, T.; Wang, M.; Metwally, A.A.; Bogu, G.K.; Brooks, A.W.; Bahmani, A.; Alavi, A.; Celli, A.; Higgs, E.; Dagan-Rosenfeld, O.; et al. Pre-symptomatic detection of COVID-19 from smartwatch data. Nat. Biomed. Eng. 2020, 4, 1208–1220.
- Murphy, S.P.; Ibrahim, N.E.; Januzzi, J.L. Heart Failure with Reduced Ejection Fraction. JAMA 2020, 324, 488–504.
- Parikh RB, Teeple S, Navathe AS. Addressing bias in artificial intelligence in health care. JAMA 2019; 322: 2377–2378. [Google Scholar]
- Perez, M.V.; Mahaffey, K.W.; Hedlin, H.; Rumsfeld, J.S.; Garcia, A.; Ferris, T.; Balasubramanian, V.; Russo, A.M.; Rajmane, A.; Cheung, L.; et al. Large-Scale Assessment of a Smartwatch to Identify Atrial Fibrillation. N. Engl. J. Med. 2019, 381, 1909–1917. [Google Scholar] [CrossRef]
- Savarese G, Lund LH. Global public health burden of heart failure. Card Fail Rev 2017; 3: 7–11. [PMC free article] [PubMed] [Google Scholar]
- Savarese, G.; Lund, L.H. Global Public Health Burden of Heart Failure. Card. Fail. Rev. 2017, 3, 7–11. [Google Scholar] [CrossRef] Schisterman, E.F.; Perkins, N.J.; Liu, A.; Bondell, H. Optimal Cut-point and Its Corresponding Youden Index to Discriminate Individuals Using Pooled Blood Samples. Epidemiology 2005, 16, 73–81. [Google Scholar] [CrossRef] [PubMed]
- Shafie AA, Tan YP, Ng CH. Systematic review of economic burden of heart failure. Heart Fail Rev 2018; 23: 131–145. [PubMed] [Google Scholar]
- Sharma A, Zhao X, Hammill BG, Hernandez AF, Fonarow GC, Felker GM, Yancy CW, Heidenreich PA, Ezekowitz JA, DeVore AD. Trends in noncardiovascular comorbidities among patients hospitalized for heart failure. Circ Heart Fail 2018; 11: e004646. [PubMed] [Google Scholar]
- Spaccarotella, C.A.M.; Polimeni, A.; Migliarino, S.; Principe, E.; Curcio, A.; Mongiardo, A.; Sorrentino, S.; De Rosa, S.; Indolfi, C. Multichannel Electrocardiograms Obtained by a Smartwatch for the Diagnosis of ST-Segment Changes. JAMA Cardiol. 2020, 5, 1176–1180. [Google Scholar] [CrossRef] [PubMed]
- Tison, G.; Sanchez, J.M.; Ballinger, B.; Singh, A.; Olgin, J.E.; Pletcher, M.J.; Vittinghoff, E.; Lee, E.S.; Fan, S.M.; Gladstone, R.A.; et al. Passive Detection of Atrial Fibrillation Using a Commercially Available Smartwatch. JAMA Cardiol. 2018, 3, 409–416. [Google Scholar] [CrossRef][Green Version]
- Virani, S.S.; Alonso, A.; Benjamin, E.J.; Bittencourt, M.S.; Callaway, C.W.; Carson, A.P.; Chamberlain, A.M.; Chang, A.R.; Cheng, S.; Delling, F.N.; et al. American Heart Association Council on Epidemiology and Prevention Statistics Committee and Stroke Statistics Subcommittee. Heart Disease and Stroke Statistics-2020 Update: A Report from the American Heart Association. Circulation 2020, 141, e139–e596.
- Weber GM. Using artificial intelligence in an intelligent way to improve efficiency of a heart failure care team. J Card Fail 2018; 24: 363–364. [PubMed] [Google Scholar]
- Wolff RF, Moons KGM, Riley RD, Whiting PF, Westwood M, Collins GS, Reitsma JB, Kleijnen J, Mallett S, PROBAST Group . PROBAST: a tool to assess the risk of bias and applicability of prediction model studies. Ann Intern Med 2019; 170: 51–58. [PubMed] [Google Scholar]

Artificial intelligence guidance of advanced heart failure therapies: A systematic scoping review

CHAPTER

15

Advanced heart failure therapies are complex interventions, including mechanical circulatory support (MCS) and heart transplantation (HTx). These treatments can be highly rewarding, restoring quality of life and longevity, however, they are associated with relatively high adverse risk profile. Additionally, the target population is heterogeneous in hemodynamic requirements and risk profile for pre- and post-intervention complications. Ethically such patients are difficult to randomize to therapies when common practice suggests a standard of care. Also, the time lag between innovation, scholarly investigation, and clinical practice significantly limits evidence to guide patient management. Artificial intelligence (AI) has the power and resilience to integrate patient data from several domains and help clinicians navigate the care of the advanced heart failure therapy patient.

As the fields of AI and heart failure therapy both evolve exponentially and in parallel, it remains unclear how AI can integrate in clinical practice and whether these methods are mature enough for clinical application. This scoping review aims to systematically summarize and appraise the literature available in this arena, under the following research question: can AI guide clinicians in personalizing the practice of HTx and MCS to optimize longevity, quality of life, and resource utilization?

Application of Technique

The protocol was performed according to Preferred Reporting Items for Systematic Reviews and Meta-Analyzes extension for Scoping Reviews (PRISMA-ScR) guidelines . Researchers searched Embase, Web of Science, and PubMed databases for published articles containing any of the phrases "artificial intelligence," "machine learning," or "deep learning" and any of the phrases "heart transplantation," "ventricular assist device," or "cardiogenic shock." The latter term was included to target the group on temporary mechanical circulatory support. Search criteria included the above terms anywhere in the title, abstract, or keywords without any filters. Team also excluded review articles, meta-analyzes, conference abstracts, non-English language, animal and ex-vivo studies, non-AI methods, and those whose primary outcome is in the pre-HTx or MCS phase of care. Methodology was considered "AI" based if it fell under the main categories of supervised learning, unsupervised learning, or reinforcement learning . The search was not restricted by the year of publication. However, the number of publications related to AI in medicine has increased exponentially since 2008

Full text review and data extraction of each article were performed by at least one HF and one AI specialist. Conflicts were resolved by a HF specialist (MA). Search results were exported to EndNote (version 20.4.1), where duplicates were automatically identified and removed. The Covidence platform was used for title and abstract screening, full text screening, and data extraction. As this is a scoping review with most studies being first of kind or proof of concept, we have not excluded studies based on quality. Also, the group is heterogenous in methodologies, making objective head–head quality assessment unfeasible. The strength of recommending the AI algorithm for clinical use was categorized based on the message conveyed to the reviewer by the article discussion and conclusion sections.

Study Observations

Our search resulted in 584 publications, of which 17.5% were included in PubMed as many were published via biomedical informatics outlets that are not usually indexed in PubMed. Figure 1 summarizes study screening and exclusion reasons. A total of 31 manuscripts were included in our review, of which data were extracted and summarized from both clinical and informatics perspectives.

Post heart transplant outcome prediction

Reachers found 13 studies that used AI to predict post-HTx outcomes. The most common data sources used for development, training, and validation of AI algorithms

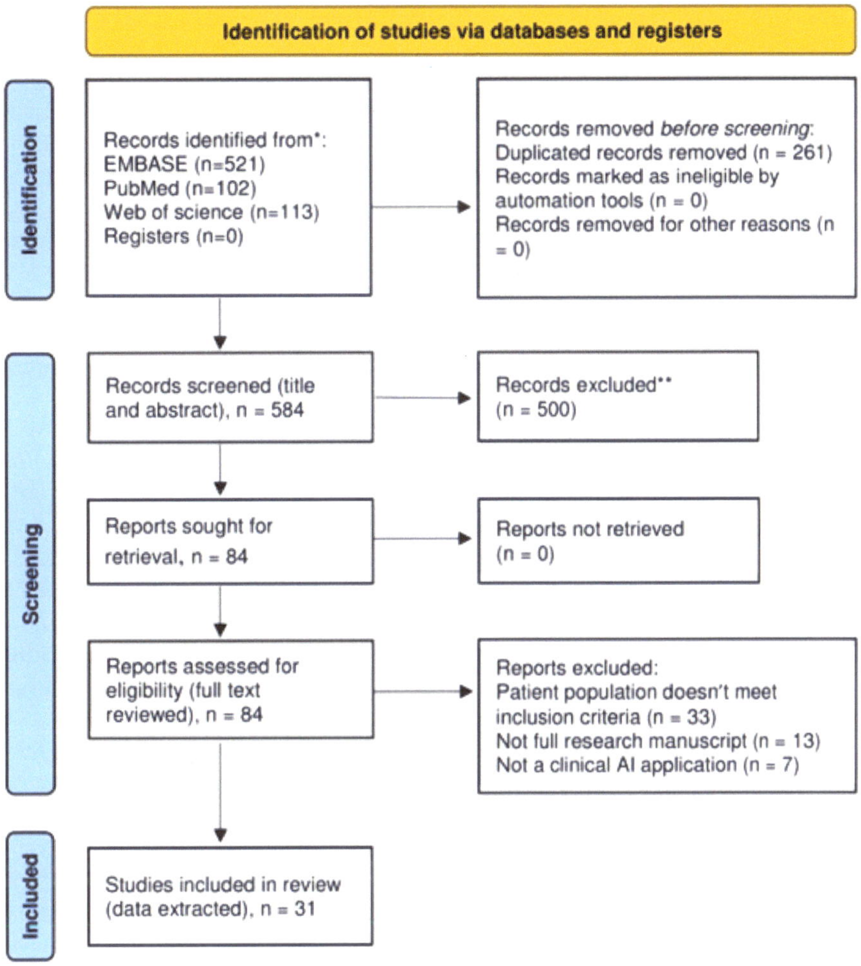

Fig. 15.1 PRISMA 2020 flow diagram for new systematic reviews which included searches of databases and registers only (4). *Consider, if feasible to do so, reporting the number of records identified from each database or register searched (rather than the total number across all databases). **Exclusion criteria included: review articles, meta-analyzes, conference abstracts, non-English language, animal and ex-vivo studies, non-AI methods, and those whose primary outcome is in the phase of care prior to transplantation or mechanical circulatory support.

are the United for Organ Sharing (UNOS) and the International Society of Heart and Lung Transplantation (ISHLT) registry. Both data souces include massive numbers of HTx recipients and donors over four decades with a wide range of relevant donor and recipient variables of relatively high accuracy. While both data sources overcome limitations of generalizability of single center data, special challenges emerged when applying AI algorithms. are the United for Organ Sharing (UNOS) and the International Society of Heart and Lung Transplantation (ISHLT) registry. Both data souces include massive numbers of HTx recipients and donors over four decades with a wide range of relevant donor and recipient variables of relatively high accuracy. While both data sources overcome limitations of generalizability of single center data, special challenges emerged when applying AI algorithms. The main challenge with UNOS data is the high number of missing values, requiring variable elimination and complex data imputation methods . The ISHLT registry, on the other hand, includes the UNOS database plus data from other centers worldwide – recently over 350 entities contributing .The ISHLT registry does not include wait list duration or mortality . In addition, the data reporting varied between regions, centers, and eras. This could introduce systematic difference between training, testing, and validation datasets, thus confounding algorithm development . Algorithms applied to local datasets showed much higher performance upon validation, likely due to better data homogeneity .

Most studies focused on transplantation survival (n = 10 studies), excluding re-transplantation and multiorgan transplantations (n = 9 studies). This is in recognition that these subgroups inherently have low frequency, significant patient heterogeneity, and variable management practices. More recent algorithms addressed specific post HTx complications, such as renal dysfunction and ICU stay .These tools are key as they provide actionable knowledge that can guide multiorgan transplantation, pre-HTx rehabilitation, and perioperative practices to optimize outcomes .

Post heart transplant management guidance

Seven studies were identified utilizing machine learning or AI and management of heart transplant patients .The clinical questions targeted were detection of rejection, cardiac allograft vasculopathy, and guidance of immunosuppression dosing. Models either attempted to automate the steps normally performed by human experts or leverage detailed molecular data to improve sensitivity for early rejection. Two groups described promising AI models for automatic endomyocardial biopsy interpretation; the CRANE model developed by Lipkova and the CACHE-Grader model by Peyster et al., where both reported performance similar to human experts with less variability . The CRANE model offers comprehensive biopsy interpretation (rejection type and grade), and it is adaptable to various populations and camera systems allowing for utilization of multicenter data for research and quality control. The CACHE-grader model, on the other hand, applies transcriptome mapping to identify graft rejection earlier than histopathology. Combining automated histopathologic and transcriptomic data will likely advance the accuracy and efficiency of allograft rejection surveillance to a new level .The study by Chen et al. offered a deep learning algorithm to analyze high resolution coronary optical tomography images looking for vasculopathic changes . Their work offers automatic segmentation of all vessel layers, and it can efficiently detect small changes in coronary architecture on serial measurements. It is novel as it detects vasculopathy early, at a stage where preventative measures might be more effective at avoiding frank graft dysfunction. AI application also allows translation application of molecular markers of graft vasculopathy in the urine, with outcomes nuanced enough to differentiate myocardial injury secondary to rejection vs. vasculopathy

As for medical therapy guidance, two studies developed models to predict cyclosporin and tacrolimus levels . Both models used medication history, hepatic and renal functions, infectious status and risk factors, and patient demographics. AI allows plotting drug pharmacokinetics beyond mere trough level, potentially offering more accurate dosing recommendations. While systems demonstrated good performance, they faced the challenges of inability to determine which factors contributed to the outcome, were overfitted, and missed the opportunity to incorporate genomic and transcriptomic variables

Post mechanical support outcome prediction

A total of 8 studies utilizing AI and MCS outcomes were identified. Of these, one examined VA-ECMO, while all others focused on durable MCS with left ventricular assist devices (LVADs) . All studies evaluated survival or adverse events. Two studies utilized AI to identify adverse event profiles, time sensitive analyzes of adverse events, and phenomapping of patient profiles as it relates to the former in the LVAD population . Grouping of patients facilitates streamlining evaluation and perioperative care pathways that are closely tailored to the patient's particular risk profile The remaining five LVAD studies all evaluated various methods of predicting survival and adverse events post implantation. Consistently, these were determined to have better discriminatory power than human experts given the same task, or conventional risk scoring systems. Collectively, these data suggest that AI techniques can allow for better understanding of patient profiles, timing of MCS related adverse events and can be additive to presently available methods of estimating the risk of post implant mortality. AI also opens new horizons for innovation in device development and surgical techniques, as we can now systematically homogenize study populations to assess the efficacy of each support platform. Ideally, this can then assist in preimplant patient selection as well as post implant monitoring and management to optimize MCS outcomes

Post mechanical support management guidance

Guidance of post MCS care has been targeted by only three algorithms . The InDetector project successfully implemented deep learning to segment driveline pictures for objective detection and grading of driveline infection . This can also be used to follow up response to therapy in the outpatient setting. The algorithm by Maw et al. utilized LVAD log data to diagnose suction events with high success, despite the model overfitting (see below in AI methods. Such physiologic control systems are likely to become more common in the LVAD world, akin to the case of pacemakers, as the large amount of data generated by these devices facilitate AI model training. One study used patient clinical data to guide post-LVAD medical therapy aiming for myocardial recovery . The paucity of similar studies is likely due to the lack of large databanks suitable for AI model development, that follows post MCS management practices along with outcomes. The Interagency Registry for Mechanically Assisted Circulatory Support (INTERMACS) lacks enough granularity on post LVAD care that would be needed for reliable training of AI models to guide medical therapy.

Summary of AI methods

Reseachers noticed a prevalence of utilizing supervised machine learning techniques over unsupervised learning . A major difference between supervised and unsupervised learning is the availability of labels. Only three studies applied unsupervised ML techniques, while the remaining used supervised ML techniques . Each one of these learning techniques encompasses a set of ML algorithms. The choice of the algorithm is governed mostly by the type of data [structured (e.g., medical history), images (e.g., pathology images), longitudinal (e.g., repeated lab measurements), and clinical notes]. The common ML models used to analyze structured data in the reviewed papers were logistic regression, random forest, and eXtreme gradient boosting (XGBoost), likely due to their superior clinical interpretability (see below) . There is a notable underutilization of the treasure trove of clinical notes; none of the reviewed papers analyzed clinical notes. Also, we have not yet seen multidomain data integration, such as combining histopathology, echocardiography, and proteomics to diagnose rejection. These models are expected to emerge in the near future via transferring AI methods being used in other fields into heart failure cardiology. Of note, the clinical natural language processing methods have been increasingly recognized and matured in healthcare over the past years. Utilizing these methods in heart transplant research may provide insightful information beyond the structured electronic health records.

Deep learning models are more common with unstructured data types such as images and videos, due to their superior abilities in automatically extracting important features from raw data that can help in predicting the outcome. Four of the reviewed papers used transfer learning with convolutional neural networks (CNN). For longitudinal data (e.g., lab measurements collected over time and snapshots of pump data), all the reviewed studies manually extracted fixed-dimensional summary statistics (e.g., minimum, maximum, and standard deviation of the laboratory values in each time frame) from the temporal time series before building the ML model.Despite theintuitive need for interpretable AI (explanation of why the decision was made) in medical applications, it is relatively underexplored. Only 15 manuscripts described model interpretability. Two of these papers (Shad et al., Lipkova et al.) used saliency maps to highlight the most contributing region of an image to the predicted outcomes . Zhou et al. and Wang et al. used Shapely Additive exPlanations (SHAP), which quantifies the contribution of each feature (variable) to the predicted outcome related to a specific instance . The rest of the papers used feature importance to explain the outcome of their ML models. Feature importance derivation is done by calculating the model's performance following the permutation of that feature. If the model performance decreases, then the permutated feature is important. While feature importance and SHAP might look similar, the main difference is that feature importance is centered around the decrease in model performance. In contrast, SHAP confers the magnitude contribution of the feature toward the predicted outcome.

Summary of model evaluation methods

The area under the receiver operating characteristic curve (AUC) was the primary performance metric used for model evaluation. Accuracy, sensitivity, and specificity were reported inconsistently between studies. Root mean square error (RMSE), mean percent error, and R2 were commonly reported when evaluating regression models (e.g., continuous outcome). Overall, moderate to high performance was achieved in the studies for survival prediction after heart transplant, likely due to the availability of large training datasets (UNOS and ISHLT registry). That said, biases (e.g., racial and gender bias) in clinical ML is a key constraint and must be addressed to ensure fairness . However, only the study conducted by Nilsson et al. investigated the potential bias of the developed model . The other studies did not have any bias assessment of the developed AI models. Model validation enhances confidence in model generalizability and scalability to other medical systems. K-fold cross-validation was used to evaluate and enhance model performance, in which the dataset is split into K subsets (folds) and the model is trained on K-1 folds and tested on the remaining validation fold. The process is repeated until the algorithm is tested on all folds, and the average performance across all test folds is reported .Three studies, in which sample size was less than 60, used leave-one-out cross-validation in evaluating the model's performance; evaluating the model on one instance / case and training the model using the rest of the cases, iteratively . External validation was only used in the study conducted by Lipkova et al. . ML predictive performance varies across settings, populations, regions, time, potential biases, and practice patterns, and therefore, there is a need of validating on external sources .

Discussion

In this scoping review, we identified 31 studies addressing the implementation of artificial intelligence in the clinical practice of MCS and heart transplantation published between 2005 and 2022. Most publications focused on outcome prediction using large existing databases. However, there is a rising wave of innovation in AI methods to tackle challenging care aspects that currently consume most post-intervention resources. We found the most mature AI applications in this field: the prediction of survival and significant complications, as well as HTx rejection identification. Moreover, early work is being conducted to further leverage AI power by introducing practical concepts (the art of medicine) into AI systems and integrating multiple biodomains (laboratory data, ultrasound, histopathology) into model conclusions. An important area of active investigation is post HTx graft vasculopathy detection, a highly morbid complication. The capabilities of AI methods demonstrated in the current review have the potential to incorporate medical literature into predictive algorithms, providing personalized guidance to medical management and complication surveillance of HTx and MCS .

Electronic health records contain rich sources of historical and current information that span multiple domains (procedures, diagnoses, medication, and demographics). When harnessed appropriately, it is expected to reveal hidden insights that traditional methods are unable to discover . Machine learning (ML) offers flexibility and scalability in assimilating and evaluating large amounts of complex healthcare data. Unlike the traditional statistical methods that focus on inference, ML methods concentrate on prediction by finding patterns in rich and unwieldy data . This is evident in complex data formats such as images, time-resolved data series (e.g., LVAD data logs) or wide data matrices (e.g., genomic array). Even though ML can demonstrate superior capabilities in predict patients' clinical outcomes and risk-stratifying patients according to their clinical and physiological data, it is challenged by the (1) non-explainability of complex algorithms; (2) lack of randomized controlled trials (RCTs) of AI systems, which may not always be feasible; (3) robust evaluation, validation and generalization to various healthcare systems; and (4) identification of biases and unfairness in algorithms. All these factors can hinder the implementation of AI systems in the clinical practice .The domain of Explainable AI (XAI) has emerged as a natural progression to the recent AI developments to increase users' trust and understanding of the ML black-box systems . While some ML models like decision trees, linear models, and attention models are intrinsically explainable, they have

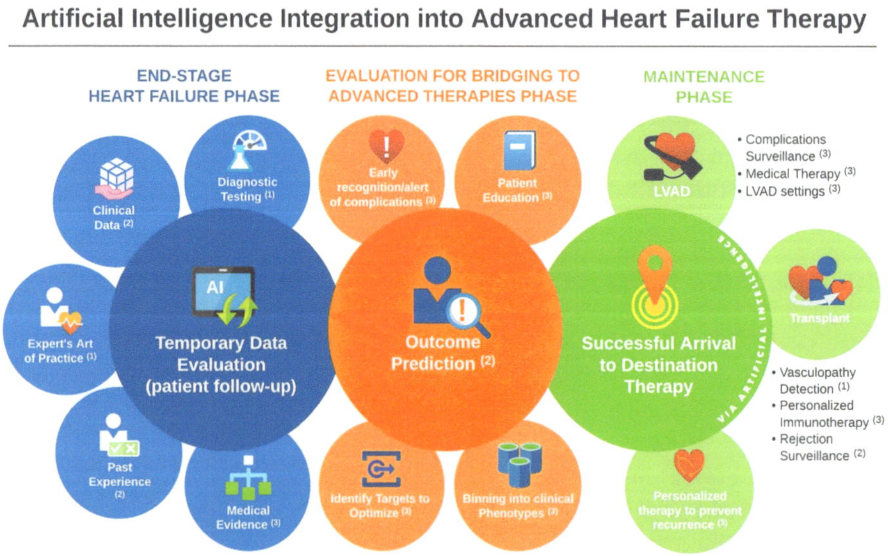

Fig.15.2 Landscape overview of artificial intelligence applications in advanced heart failure practice, with annotations indicative the level of maturity of the available literature of each application; 1Promising, but not yet mature for clinical use. 2Good support, ready for prospective testing. 3Theoretical potential, but no/negligible support.

lower model accuracies compared to more complex ML models like neural network models . However, complex ML models require creating another model to construct explanations, such as using SHAP. The trade-off between intrinsic models and post-hoc models lies between model accuracy and explanation fidelity. Deploying ML in the medical practice requires researchers to put more effort into investigating and evaluating these different explanation techniques to identify which one can best serve health care providers to assess risks and make better decisions. We cannot overlook the demand to improve the trust and transparency of AI systems used in advanced heart failure, as these decisions affect patients' quality of life and longevity. Requiring ML systems to (1) justify their decisions/output, (2) enable healthcare providers to take control to identify errors and correct them, and (3) integrate human expert knowledge into models, can contribute to achieving these demands .In this scoping review, we found several models that, if validated and implemented, can address vital clinical needs. However, validation was limited by the database availability. The UNOS, INTERMACS, and the ISHLT registry databases are the largest databases available. There is a critical need for data sharing infrastructure that is inclusive of multiple biodomains (imaging, clinical text, electronic heart care system entries, and vital outcomes) to enable generation of accurate ML models that can be validated, meet user's expectations, and continuously updated to remain current with the clinical practice. As individual systems emerge and become publicly available, pragmatic evaluation for accuracy, gender and ethnic bias and fairness, and safety for medical application becomes challenging. AI programs are recognized as medical devices by the food and drug administration (FDA), with ongoing efforts to govern their clinical application . As experts specializing in each particular AI method and application are scarce, unbiased external oversight becomes challenging . We have noticed that only one study has external validation. The latter process assures that AI model remain accurate in various settings and are not specifically fitting the population used in the model derivation. "Model waste" can occur where excellent AI models are not clinically applied due to lack of validation . Also, there is possibly a publication bias as there is only one manuscript that suggested limited AI benefit

Limitations

Our scoping review has some limitations. Our search included the 3 major medical databases for feasibility, however, there are many studies published in engineering and bioinformatics journals that may not be indexed in the searched databases. Our results are only up to date as of August 15th, 2022. The search criteria may have missed related studies focusing on cardiogenic shock, cardiac imaging, or heart failure patients not on MCS or post HTx, however, with models transferrable to such populations. Second, the strength of recommending the AI algorithm for clinical use was categorized based on the message conveyed to the reviewer by the article discussion and conclusion, which can be subjective. Despite that papers were reviewed by a multidisciplinary team; a more refined approach could be adopted in the future. Lastly, the outcomes of ML algorithms are subject to systematic errors such as biases. Data sources, mathematical approaches, and results interpretation could introduce these biases into the ML pipeline (56). Given that the nature of this review is to highlight the utilization of AI in the field of heart transplantation, the publication bias assessment was not feasible. However, researchers who aim to implement AI applications in the medical field are warranted to assess these biases.

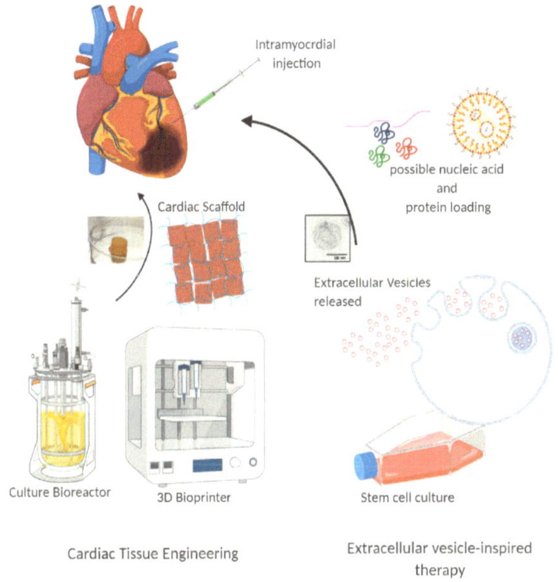

Fig. 15.3 Innovative therapies to treat heart failure includes (1) cardiac tissue engineering, which includes large scale cell culture in bioreactors, 3D bioprinting of constructs and application of cardiac scaffold to the injury. (2) Extracellular-vesicles inspired therapy, which needs large scale cell culture, harvesting of EVs-released by stem cells, possible loading of nucleic acids and proteins, and subsequent intramyocardial injection. (Created with BioRender.com)

CONCLUSION

It is concluded that over the past 2 years have witnessed promising AI models that can guide heart failure cardiologists in HTx donor-recipient matching, allograft surveillance, immunosuppression dosing, and MCS complication screening.

Bibliography and Acknowledgement

- Abdullah TAA, Zahid MSM, Ali W. A review of interpretable ML in healthcare: taxonomy, applications, challenges, and future directions. Symmetry. (2021) 13:2439.
- Agasthi P, Buras MR, Smith SD, Golafshar MA, Mookadam F, Anand S, et al.. Machine learning helps predict long-term mortality and graft failure in patients undergoing heart transplant. Gen Thorac Cardiovasc Surg. (2020) 68:1369–76. doi: 10.1007/s11748-020-01375-6, PMID: [PubMed] [CrossRef]
- Bellavia D, Iacovoni A, Agnese V, Falletta C, Coronnello C, Pasta S, et al.. Usefulness of regional right ventricular and right atrial strain for prediction of early and late right ventricular failure following a left ventricular assist device implant: a machine learning approach. Int J Artif Organs. (2020) 43:297–314.
- Bzdok D, Altman N, Krzywinski M. Statistics versus machine learning. Nat Methods. (2018) 15:233–4. doi: 10.1038/nmeth.4642, PMID: [PMC free article] [PubMed] [CrossRef] [Google Scholar]
- Chen Z, Pazdernik M, Zhang H, Wahle A, Guo Z, Bedanova H, et al.. Quantitative 3D analysis of coronary wall morphology in heart transplant patients: OCT-assessed cardiac allograft vasculopathy progression. Med Image Anal. (2018) 50:95–105. doi: 10.1016/j.media.2018.09.003, PMID: [PMC free article] [PubMed]
- Du M, Liu N, Hu X. Techniques for interpretable machine learning. Commun ACM. (2019) 63:68–77.
- Godown J, Gaies M, Wilkinson JD. Leveraging big data to advance knowledge in pediatric heart failure and heart transplantation. Transl Pediatr. (2019) 8:342–8. doi: 10.21037/tp.2019.07.09, PMID: [PMC free article] [PubMed] [CrossRef] [Google Scholar]
- Hastie T, Tibshirani R, Friedman J. The Eements of Statistical Learning. New York, NY: Springer series in statistics; (2001).
- Jovel J, Greiner R. An introduction to machine learning approaches for biomedical research. Front Med. (2021) 8:771607. doi: 10.3389/fmed.2021.771607, PMID: [PMC free article] [PubMed]
- Kainuma A, Ning YM, Kurlansky PA, Wang AS, Latif F, Sayer GT, et al.. Predictors of 1-year outcome after cardiac re-transplantation: machine learning analysis. Clin Transpl. (2022) 36:e14761. doi: 10.1111/ctr.14761, PMID: [PubMed] [CrossRef]
- Kumar K, Kumar P, Deb D, Unguresan ML, Muresan V. Artificial intelligence and machine learning based intervention in medical infrastructure: a review and future trends. Healthcare. (2023) 11:207.
- Lipkova J, Chen TY, Lu MY, Chen RJ, Shady M, Williams M, et al.. Deep learning-enabled assessment of cardiac allograft rejection from endomyocardial biopsies. Nat Med. (2022) 28:575–82. doi: 10.1038/s41591-022-01709-2, PMID: [PMC free article] [PubMed]
- Maw M, Gross C, Schima H, Moscato F. Development of a suction detection algorithm from patient pump data. Artif Organs. (2017) 41:A50. doi: 10.1016/j.bspc.2021.102910 [CrossRef]
- Miller RJH, Sabovcik F, Cauwenberghs N, Vens C, Khush KK, Heidenreich PA, et al.. Temporal shift and predictive performance of machine learning for heart transplant outcomes. J Heart Lung Transplant. (2022) 41:928–36. doi: 10.1016/j.healun.2022.03.019, PMID: [PubMed] [CrossRef] [Google Scholar]
- Nilsson J, Ohlsson M, Höglund P, Ekmehag B, Koul B, Andersson B. The international heart transplant survival algorithm (IHTSA): a new model to improve organ sharing and survival. PLoS One. (2015) 10:e0118644.
- Oztekin A, Delen D, Kong ZY. Predicting the graft survival for heart-lung transplantation patients: an integrated data mining methodology. Int J Med Inform. (2009) 78:E84–96. doi: 10.1016/j.ijmedinf.2009.04.007, PMID: [PubMed] [CrossRef])
- Page MJ, McKenzie JE, Bossuyt PM, Boutron I, Hoffmann TC, Mulrow CD, et al.. The PRISMA 2020 statement: an updated guideline for reporting systematic reviews. BMJ. (2021) 372:n71
- Piening BD, Dowdell AK, Zhang M, Loza BL, Walls D, Gao H, et al.. Whole transcriptome profiling of prospective endomyocardial biopsies reveals prognostic and diagnostic signatures of cardiac allograft rejection. J Heart Lung Transplant. (2022) 41:840–8. doi: 10.1016/j.healun.2022.01.1377, PMID:
- Puri K, Schweiger M, Rossano JW. The fate of the failing Fontan circulation-no two are alike. J Heart Lung Transplant. (2021) 40:1682–4. doi: 10.1016/j.healun.2021.08.014, PMID: [PubMed] [CrossRef] [Google Scholar]
- Ricci Lara MA, Echeveste R, Ferrante E. Addressing fairness in artificial intelligence for medical imaging. Nat Commun. (2022) 13:4581. doi: 10.1038/s41467-022-32186-3, PMID: [PMC free article] [PubMed] [CrossRef] [Google Scholar]
- Rudin C. Stop explaining black box machine learning models for high stakes decisions and use interpretable models instead. Nat MacH Intell. (2019) 1:206–15. doi: 10.1038/s42256-019-0048-x, PMID: [PMC free article] [PubMed] [CrossRef] [Google Scholar]
- Shad R, Quach N, Fong R, Kasinpila P, Bowles C, Castro M, et al.. Predicting post-operative right ventricular failure using video-based deep learning. Nat Commun. (2021) 12:5192. doi: 10.1038/s41467-021-25503-9, PMID: [PMC free article]
- Tran BX, Vu GT, Ha GH, Vuong QH, Ho MT, Vuong TT, et al.. Global evolution of research in artificial intelligence in health and medicine: a bibliometric study. J Clin Med. (2019) 8:360. doi: 10.3390/jcm8030360, PMID: [PMC free article] [PubMed]
- Wang K, Yan LZ, Li WZ, Jiang C, Wang NN, Zheng Q, et al.. Comparison of four machine learning techniques for prediction of intensive care unit length of stay in heart transplantation patients. Front Cardiovasc Med. (2022) 9:863642. doi: 10.3389/fcvm.2022.863642, PMID: [PMC free article] [PubMed] [CrossRef] [Google Scholar]
- Wei D, Trenson S, Van Keer JM, Melgarejo J, Cutsforth E, Thijs L, et al.. The novel proteomic signature for cardiac allograft vasculopathy. ESC Heart Fail. (2022) 9:1216–27. doi: 10.1002/ehf2.13796, PMID: [PMC free article] [PubMed] [CrossRef] [Google Scholar]
- Weiss ES, Allen JG, Arnaoutakis GJ, George TJ, Russell SD, Shah AS, et al.. Creation of a quantitative recipient risk index for mortality prediction after cardiac transplantation (IMPACT). Ann Thorac Surg. (2011) 92:914–21. doi: 10.1016/j.athoracsur.2011.04.030, PMID: [PubMed] [CrossRef]
- Woillard JB, Labriffe M, Debord J, Marquet P. Tacrolimus exposure prediction using machine learning. Clin Pharmacol Ther. (2021) 110:361–9. doi: 10.1002/cpt.2123, PMID: [PubMed] [CrossRef] [Google Scholar]
- Zhou Y, Chen S, Rao ZQ, Yang D, Liu X, Dong NG, et al.. Prediction of 1-year mortality after heart transplantation using machine learning approaches: a single-center study from China. Int J Cardiol. (2021) 339:21–7. doi: 10.1016/j.ijcard.2021.07.024, PMID: [PubMed] [CrossRef]

Artificial Intelligence and Cardiac Magnetic Resonance Imaging in Myocardial Infarction(CAD)

CHAPTER

16

Cardiovascular magnetic resonance (CMR) is an important cardiac imaging tool for assessing the prognostic extent of myocardial injury after myocardial infarction (MI) as endorsed by the European Society of Cardiology 2017 guidelines and the Society for Cardiovascular Magnetic Resonance 2020 position paper. Within the context of clinical trials, CMR is useful for assessing the efficacy of potential cardioprotective therapies in reducing MI size and preventing adverse left ventricular (LV) remodelling in reperfused MI. It is currently the gold standard imaging modality to quantify MI size,4 and it can delineate subendocardial MI as little as 1 gram in size with a high degree of accuracy.6 Native T1, T2, T2* and post-contrast T1-mapping (to derive extracellular volume [ECV] mapping)7 can also enable deeper insights to be garnered into the pathophysiological processes post MI and their associated prognostic significance. However, manual contouring and analysis can be time-consuming with interobserver and intra-observer variability, which can in turn lead to reduction in accuracy and precision of analysis. There is thus a need to automate CMR scan analysis in MI patients to save time, increase accuracy, increase reproducibility and increase precision.9 In this regard, automated imaging analysis techniques based on artificial intelligence (AI) that are developed with machine learning (ML), and more specifically deep learning (DL) strategies, can enable efficient, robust, accurate and clinician-friendly tools to be built so as to try and improve both clinician productivity and quality of patient care. AI refers to computer algorithm-based techniques that enable machines to perform tasks that resemble human intelligence. ML methods encompass supervised, unsupervised, semi-supervised and reinforcement learning methods, amongst others, to achieve AI.12 DL is a set of advanced ML techniques that are based on artificial neural networks with hidden layers and can be used to detect anddifferentiate patterns in data. DL is currently the most popular ML method for medical image analysis.

Prognostic Implications of Myocardial Infarction Cardiovascular Magnetic Resonance Imaging Biomarkers

The parameters of prognostic importance with clinical implications that may be amenable to automated analysis are volumetric analysis, infarct size, area at risk, presence of microvascular obstruction (MVO) and size of MVO. Historically, left ventricular (LV) ejection fraction (EF) and LV volumes have been the established predictors of mortality in patients with coronary artery disease (CAD) and severe LV dysfunction. Previous studies have shown that LV function and LV end-systolic volume (ESV) were the strongest predictors of cardiac death after MI. MI size refers to the size of the infarcted myocardium and is conventionally demarcated on late gadolinium enhancement (LGE) imaging. Morbidity and mortality post-ST elevation myocardial infarction (STEMI) is closely associated with acute MI size. A meta-analysis of 2,632 patients showed that MI size assessed by CMR or SPECT within 1 month post-primary percutaneous coronary intervention from 10 randomised controlled trials was strongly associated with heart failure hospitalisation and all-cause mortality at 1 year, with a 20% increase in relative hazard ratio for both these clinical outcomes for every 5% increase in MI size. This further adds to the growing body of evidence that acute MI size is prognostic. MVO results from the inability to reperfuse the coronary microcirculation in a previously ischaemic region despite revascularisation of the culprit epicardial vessel. MVO can be identified as a dark hypointense core within areas of hyperenhancement on early gadolinium enhancement imaging.Intramyocardial haemorrhage (IMH) can occur if coronary microvasculature injury is very severe after MI, with resultant damaged vessel integrity and extravasation of red blood cells

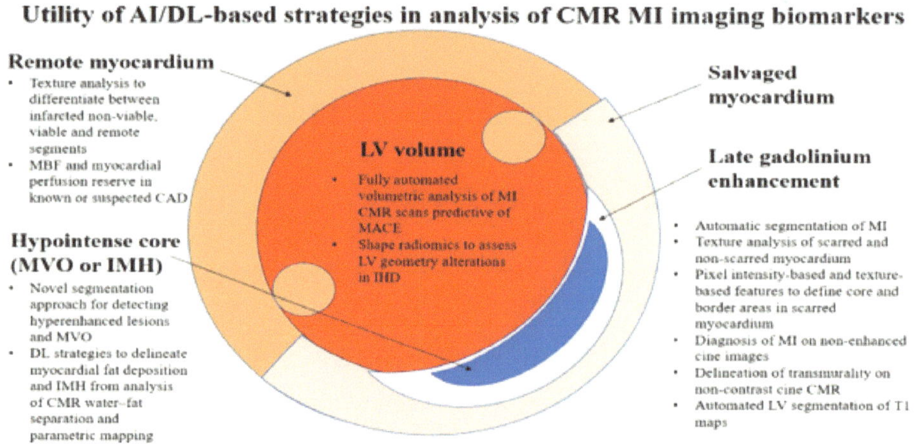

Fig 16.1 Utility of artificial intelligence/deep learning-based strategies in analysis of cardiovascular magnetic resonance myocardial infarction imaging biomarkers.MI: myocardial infarction; CMR: cardiovascular magnetic resonance; AI: artificial intelligence; DL: deep learning; MVO: microvascular obstruction; ML: machine learning; IMH: intramyocardial haemorrhage; LV: left ventricle; MBF: myocardial blood flow; CAD: coronary artery disease; IHD: ischaemic heart disease; MACE: major adverse cardiovascular events; IHD: ischaemic heart disease.

Both MVO and IMH are associated with larger MI size, adverse LV remodelling and overall worse clinical outcomes. In general, prognosis worsens with larger MI size, with patients also more likely to have MVO and IMH with larger MI size. Prognosis for STEMI patients with MVO is worse than those without MVO. Prognosis is worst for patients with MVO and IMH

The area-at-risk (AAR) refers to the myocardial territory supplied by the infarct-related culprit artery that was at risk of infarction and would have infarcted if revascularisation and reperfusion had not taken place to salvage the viable myocardium.The myocardial salvage index (MSI) normalises MI size reduction to AAR and as such is a more sensitive marker compared with MI size alone to assess cardioprotective therapy efficacy. Post-contrast T1-mapping has recently demonstrated promise as an alternative technique to gadolinium enhancement imaging in quantifying MI size.T1-mapping has the potential to complement clinical and imaging parameters and biomarkers to optimise risk stratification in MI patients.8 Oedema, assessed by CMR using T2-mapping, occurs both in the viable and non-viable myocardium during the first week of a reperfused STEMI in the clinical setting. Oedema-based area-at-risk measured by CMR can be used to assess myocardial salvage in clinical cardio-protection studies but the appropriateness of this has been called into question.

Basic Concepts of Machine Learning in Cardiovascular Magnetic Resonance Imaging

Important image characteristics or features such as image contrast, noise characteristics, texture and motion are highlighted as part of a designed feature set to create a ML model that is trained using data. The model training, eg for image segmentation problems, involves using a ML method that allows the model to learn and optimise the parameters of the mathematical model from a set of CMR studies with ground truth segmentations performed by the human expert. The trained model is then used to predict segmentations. The training algorithm extracts the parts of the data that are important for the prediction task and collates the information together to produce the prediction result. ML models can perform either classification or regression tasks. Classification tasks involve discrete labels such as determination of the presence or absence of disease. Regression tasks involve continuous variables such as quantifying the percentage of infarcted myocardium of patients with an acute MI. The training dataset should be sufficiently large with representative variability to optimise performance. A validation dataset is used to evaluate a model's performance and prevent model overfitting It has been challenging to identify optimal discriminative features to create ML systems for a given task. In order to circumvent the need to design these discriminative features, DL methods can be applied that can learn directly (end-to-end learning) from the training dataset. In myocardial contouring for example, DL methods will learn the image features that are most useful for predicting myocardial contour locations. A specific type of DL network known as convolutional neural network (CNN) is often used in image analysis-associated tasks.A typical CNN is made up of multiple layers including convolution layers, pooling layers, fully connected layer, skip layers and

SoftMax layer. Deep CNNs are complex and can contain millions of weights, and although the features resulting from the intermediate layers contain information relevant to the task, it is often difficult to interpret how the predictions are actually made or why the network might have failed to make the accurate prediction. Depending on the availability of reference labels in the training dataset, ML algorithms can be grouped into supervised vs unsupervised learning. In supervised learning, training data of varying pathological status are labelled by human domain experts. In unsupervised learning, hidden structures within the training data are discovered during training. There are different ML methods suited to the varying complexities of the image analysis task. Some of ML methods often encountered in AI literature include linear regression,30 support vector machines (SVM), decision trees, boosting methods, linear discriminant analysis and ensemble method. In linear discriminant analysis for instance, ML model parameters are estimated by assuming a simple functional relationship between the data and the labels to separate data into normal and abnormal categories. The training data is learned and fit to a hyperplane by optimising linear coefficients. However, in complex and multi-dimensional problems involving large amounts of data, more advanced techniques such as support vector machines, random forests (applied to T2 map quantification) and DL CNNs are required.

Applications of Machine Learning in Myocardial Infarction Cardiovascular Magnetic Resonance

Image Segmentation

Manually contouring the borders of the cardiac chambers and myocardium, known as segmentation, is a time-consuming process. In addition, differences in analysis output may still exist between expert readers.In this regard, ML algorithms can help to automate image segmentation and increase productivity, accuracy and reproducibility. This can be achieved through pixel-wise classification or regression-based techniques. Schuster et al showed that fully automated volumetric analysis of MI CMR is feasible and can be equally predictive of major adverse cardiac events when compared with conventional volumetric analysis

Myocardial Tissue Characterisation

Scar volume from LGE CMR imaging is a prognostic quantitative imaging biomarker.Manual delineation methods of scar volume currently used in routine clinical practice are subjective, time-consuming and labour-intensive. In addition, despite using current thresholding techniques for LGE quantification, accuracy and reproducibility is still affected by inter-centre variations, gadolinium kinetics variations and scattered patterns of LGE distribution. A novel, ML-based approach to LGE has been proposed by Fahmy et al using deep CNNs to automatically quantify LV mass and scar volume on LGE images in patients with hypertrophic cardiomyopathy. This could be further extrapolated to quantify infarct size in patients with MI. ML can also be applied to streamline data processing and analysis of cardiac relaxometry.

Infarct Size/Late Gadolinium Enhancement

Chen et al proposed an automatic MI segmentation approach based on CNNs to analyse CMR LGE sequences. Their proposal demonstrated promising segmentation results when compared to the intra-observer and inter-observer variations in manual segmentation, and to automatic segmentation with Gaussian Mixture Model. Engan et al designed an experimental framework for data exploration which involved computing a very large number of features to describe the characteristics of the regions of interest in the images and found that the addition of texture analysis can improve the discriminative power of scarred and non-scarred myocardium to distinguish between patients with high and low risk of serious ventricular arrhythmias post MI. Kotu et al used pixel intensity-based and underlying texture information-based features to define different cardiac segments such as core and border areas in scarred regions of MI. In another study by Kotu et al, the segmentation of scarred and non-scarred myocardium in MI patients is obtained using different features and feature combinations in a Bayes classifier, with segmentation of scarred myocardium being comparable to manual segmentation in all cross-validation cases. Larroza et al aimed to differentiate acute from chronic MI using ML techniques and texture features extracted from CMR imaging scans and they were able to conclude that texture analysis can be used for differentiation of acute from chronic MI on LGE sequences, and standard cine sequences in which the infarction is visually imperceptible in most cases.47 Baessler et al performed a proof-of-concept study whereby stepwise dimension reduction and texture feature selection were performed, enabling the diagnosis of MI on nonenhanced cine images by using LGE imaging as the standard of reference.48 They showed that texture analysis is feasible and allows for the diagnosis of small and large subacute and chronic ischaemic scars on nonenhanced cine CMR images with high accuracy.In another study by Larroza et al, texture analysis was used to differentiate between infarcted nonviable, viable, and remote segments in MI. Zhang et al demonstrated the use of a DL framework on non-contrast cine CMR that can confirm, detect and delineate transmurality and size of chronic MI. This has positive implications particularly for patients with renal impairment who may be precluded from receiving gadolinium contrast but may require myocardial viability assessment on CMR.

Microvascular Obstruction / Intramyocardial Haemorrhage

In another study by Chen et al, they proposed ML-based models to automatically evaluate the severity of MI from physiological, clinical, and paraclinical features. Two types of ML models were investigated for MI assessment: the classification models classify the presence of MI and persistent microvascular obstruction, and the regression models quantify the percentage of infarcted myocardium of patients suspected of having an acute MI in the emergency department.The prediction accuracy for the classification of myocardial state and regression quantification of infarcted myocardium were encouraging. Rosa et al proposed a new automatic method for MI quantification from LGE sequences. Their novel segmentation approach was devised for accurately detecting hyper enhanced lesions and also MVO areas. It also included a myocardial disease detection step which extended the algorithm for working under healthy scans. Goldfarb et al sought to determine the feasibility and performance of CMR water–fat separation and parametric mapping via DL techniques and demonstrated that myocardial fat deposition in chronic MI and IMH in acute MI could be well visualised with DL strategies

T1 Mapping

Farrag et al implemented a DL-based method for automated LV segmentation of T1 maps performed using a shortened modified Look-Locker imaging (shMOLLI) sequence by superimposing prior information from cine CMR images in patients with myocardial fibrosis secondary to MIThis helps to circumvent the issue with delineating endocardial-blood pool borders that conventional algorithmsface in myocardial segmentation of T1-mapping images due to low signal gradients at the endocardial-blood pool boundary. The accurate delineation of myocardial borders will enable quantification of myocardial fibrosis from native (non-contrast) T1 maps.

Myocardial Perfusion

Perfusion mapping uses AI to provide rapid quantification of myocardial blood perfusion by CMR imaging In turn, quantitative myocardial blood flow (MBF) provides important prognostic information in patients with suspected CAD in addition to traditional cardiovascular risk factors Knott et a have shown that in patients with known or suspected CAD, reduced MBF and myocardial perfusion reserve measured automatically inline using AI quantification of CMR perfusion mapping provided robust and independent prediction of major adverse cardiovascular events.

Radiomics

The ability of ML techniques to handle high-dimensional data has led to the development of radiomics, a novel field in which digital medical images are converted into mineable high-dimensional data by extracting a large number of quantitative imaging features based on mathematical and statistical methods. Within the field of radiomics, texture analysis allow for segmentation, analysis and classification of medical images based on underlying tissue textures as opposed to pure visual image interpretation. The application of radiomics to myocardial tissue characterisation may deliver deeper insights into complex tissue changes in association with pathophysiology of cardiovascular disease.

In the area of MI, radiomics and texture analysis have been applied to the segmentation of myocardial scar and the differentiation between acute and chronic MI. Besides MI, texture analysis and radiomics have also been applied to differentiate between causes of myocardial hypertrophy, prognostication in hypertrophic cardiomyopathy patients with systolic dysfunction, T1 mapping-guided discrimination between hypertensive heart disease and hypertrophic cardiomyopathy, and in the assessment of myocardial inflammation. Rauseo et al analysed CMR images from the UK Biobank64 including for patients with history of ischaemic heart disease (IHD) and MI for CMR radiomic signatures and found that shape radiomics such as maximum 2D diameter of the LV and myocardium, myocardial cavity volume and surface area to volume ratio were most relevant in IHD and MI, indicating the tendency for IHD to result in LV geometry alterations.

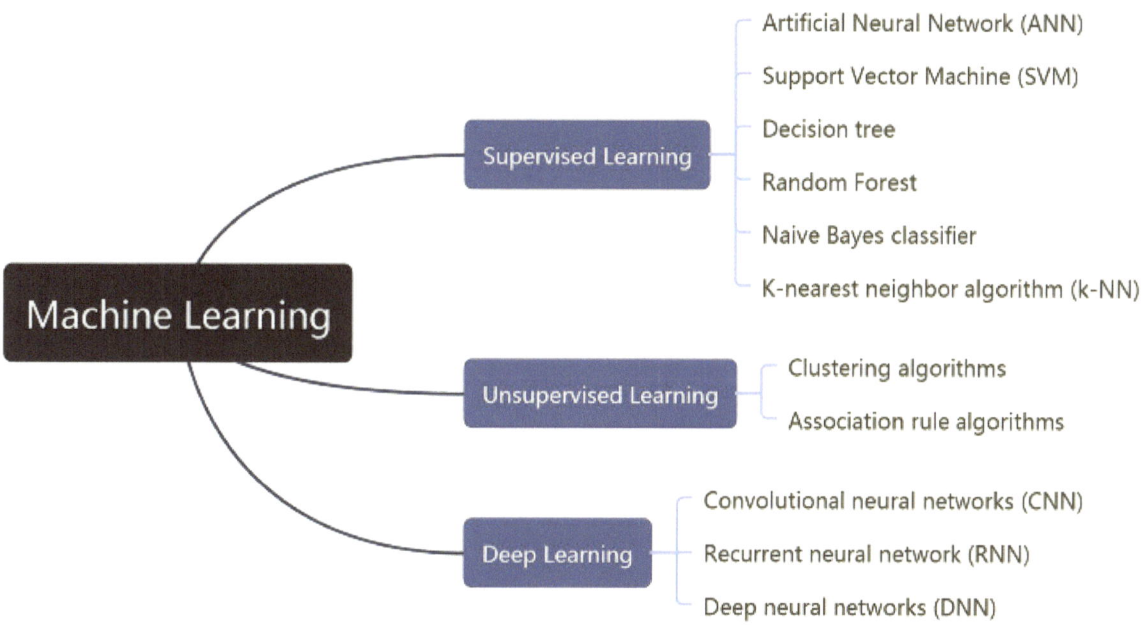

Fig.16.2 The classification of machine learning.

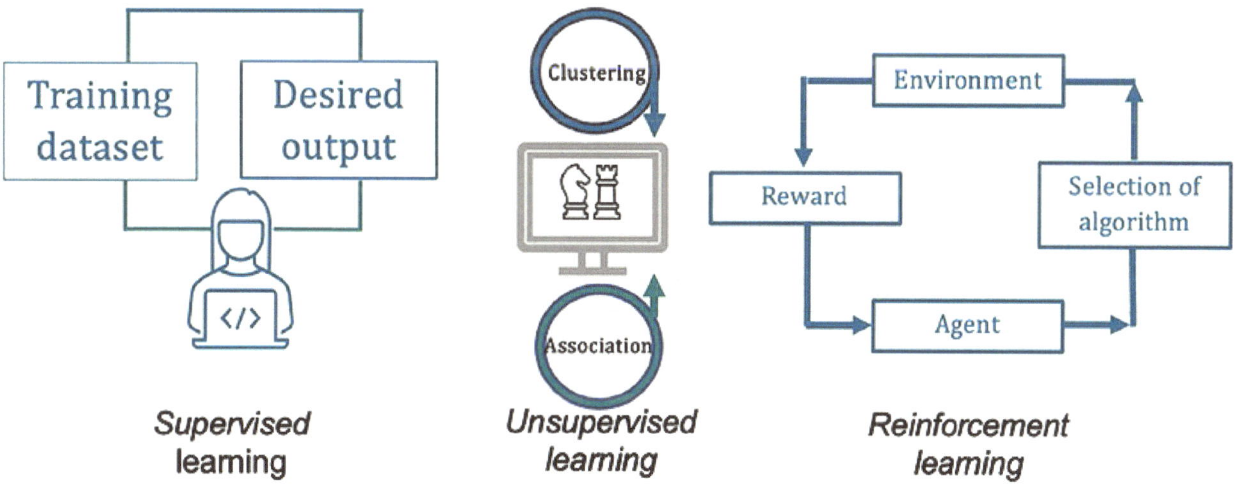

Fig 16.3 Simplified graph describing the three principal machine-learning methods. Supervised learning utilises hand-labelled datasets to design algorithms that predict future events, classify data into defined categories or distinguish the most relevant variables to the output. The predictive model learns through data training and improves over time. In unsupervised learning the software accomplishes the processing of raw data, finding hidden structures in datasets, without prior annotation, identifying meaningful relationships and clusters within the data. Reinforcement learning is a reward-based learning. Its foundation lies in the interactions with an environment, in which positive and negative feedback (reinforcements) contribute to the optimisation of the model.

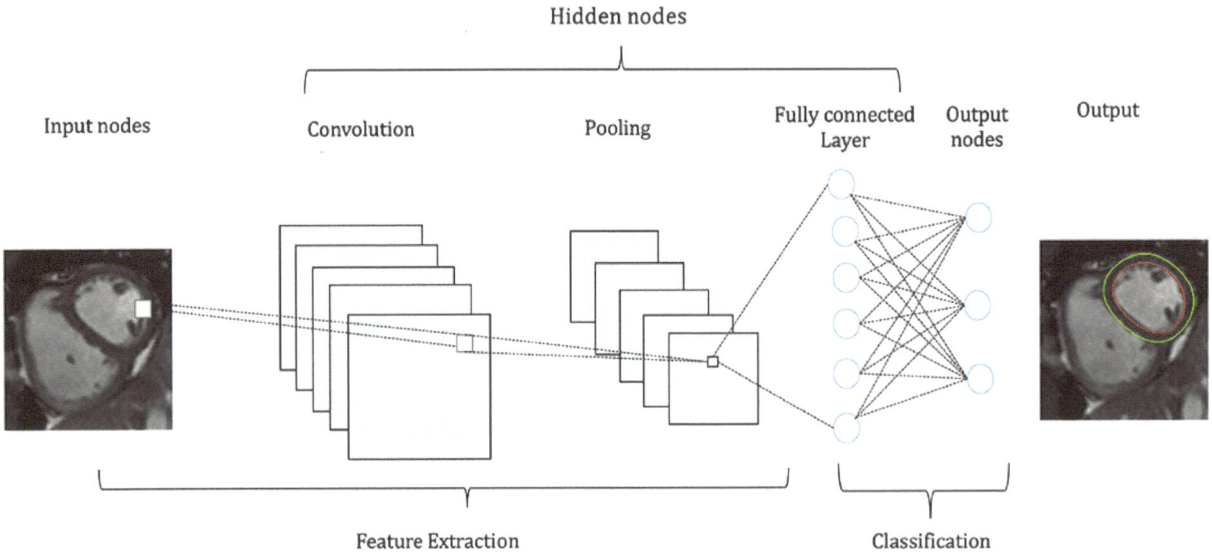

Fig 16.4. Pipeline of a convolutional neural network (CNN). A CMR image functions as input to the CNN. The CNN identifies and classifies the various attributes (features) of the image for analysis in a procedure named Feature Extraction, including a stack of convolutions and pooling operations. In the convolution operation different-level features, such as edges, colour, gradient orientation are extracted from the input image. The pooling layer reduces the dimensionality of the convolved features, in order to decrease the computational requirements. The nodes in the fully-connected layer are connected directly to all nodes in the previous layer. This layer compiles the data extracted by previous layers and applies various filters to form the final output.

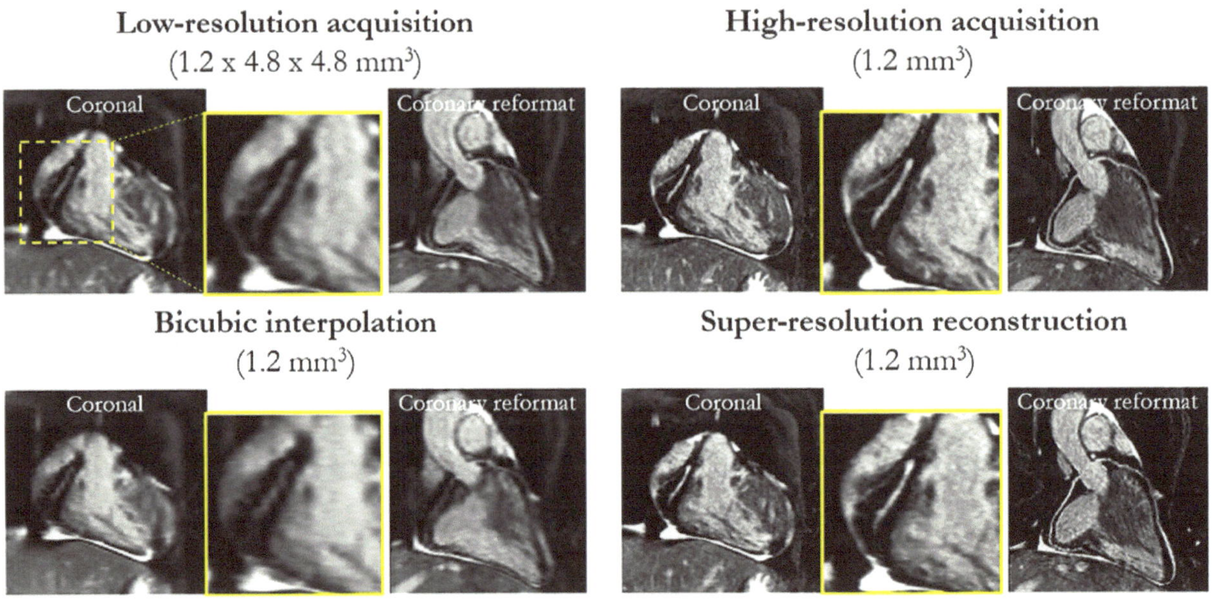

Fig.16.5 Prospective super-resolution reconstruction: coronal and coronary reformat of low-resolution acquisition (1.2 × 4.8 × 4.8 mm3) acquired in ~50 s compared to high-resolution acquisition (1.2 mm3) acquired in ~7 min. Bicubic interpolation (1.2 mm3) and proposed super-resolution reconstruction (1.2 mm3) in a patient with suspected CAD for a prospective acquired low-resolution scan (prospective cohort). Magnified image of RCA shows comparable image quality to the high-resolution acquisition in significantly shorter scan time. Küstner et al. (11). The article is published Open Access under a CC BY licence (https://creativecommons.org/licences/by/4.0/).

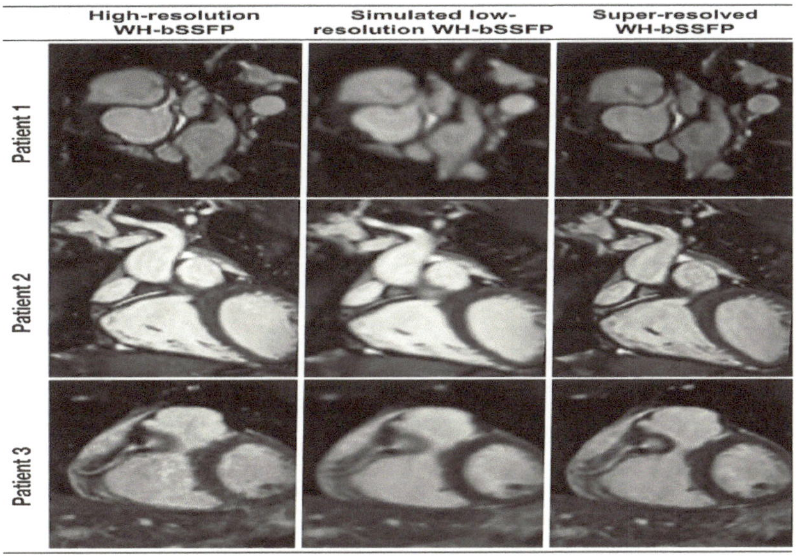

Fig 16.6 Representative image quality of the coronaries from a prospective, clinically integrated study, that utilised a residual U-Net network to facilitate super-resolution reconstruction of rapidly acquired low-resolution three-dimensional whole-heart balanced Steady State Free Precession datasets. Multi-planar reformats of the coronary artery from the respective conventional high-resolution acquisition, low-resolution acquisition, and the corresponding super-resolution reconstruction dataset. Sharpness of vascular borders is enhanced and image distortion is attenuated in the super-resolution reconstruction dataset vs. the low-resolution volume. This is particularly beneficial in the delineation of small vessels, such as the coronary arteries. Qualitative image quality analysis demonstrated no statistically significant differences between the super-resolution and the high-resolution data. Steeden et al. (13).

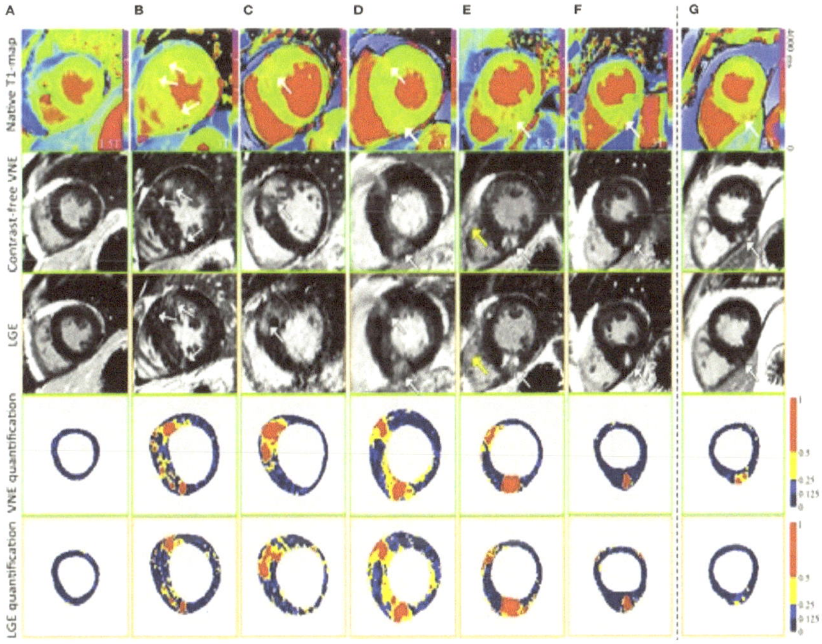

Fig 16.7 Examples to demonstrate the image quality and opticospatial correlation between VNE and conventional LGE images. T1 colormaps (top row) were adjusted to show the T1 signals that pair with the VNE signals. The bottom 2 rows visualise myocardial lesion regions by VNE and LGE using progressive thresholding (full width, at half, a quarter, and eighth maximum) displayed with different colours. In (A–F), high visuospatial agreement was noted between VNE and LGE. White arrows point to the lesions. Yellow arrows point to slightly different depiction of the right ventricular wall in VNE and LGE, suggesting patient movement between acquisitions. (G), An example of VNE displaying subtle changes in the distribution and quantification of the lesion clearer than LGE. LGE, late gadolinium enhancement; VNE, virtual native enhancement. Zhang et al. (16).

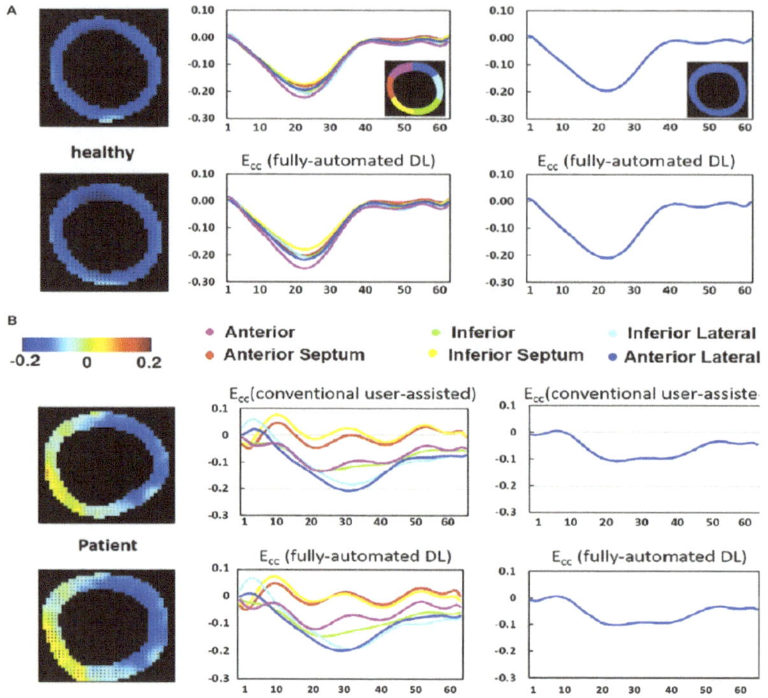

Fig 16.8 DL-based computation of global and segmentalcircumferential strain is compared to the clinician-assisted DENSE analysis. The AI-basedend-systolic circumferential strain (Ecc) maps (left column), segmental (middle column) and global (right column) circumferential strain–time curves for a healthy subject (A) and a heart failure patient (B) demonstrate very close agreement with thconventional segmentation in the depicted mid-ventricular slices. Ghadimi et al. (26). The article is published Open Access under a CC BYlicence(https:creativecommons.org/licenses/by/4.0/).

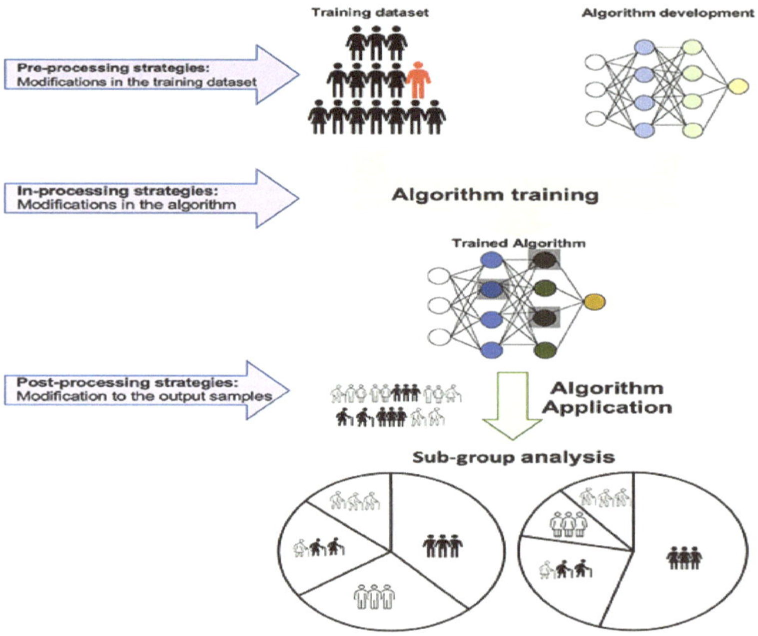

Fig 16.9 Schematic representation of three proposed strategies to introduce fairness in AI algorithms. First, pre-processing modifications in the training dataset can eliminate bias before training. In each training dataset, the data are initially classified by the protected attribute(s) (such as sex, race, ethnic origin, religious and political beliefs, age, socioeconomic background and so forth). Samples are stratified to establish equitable representation of all protected groups in the training. Alternatively, alterations in the AI algorithm can train a model to overcome discrimination and optimise the performance both in the prevalent and unprivileged group(s). The third approach attempts to train distinct models for each protected group.

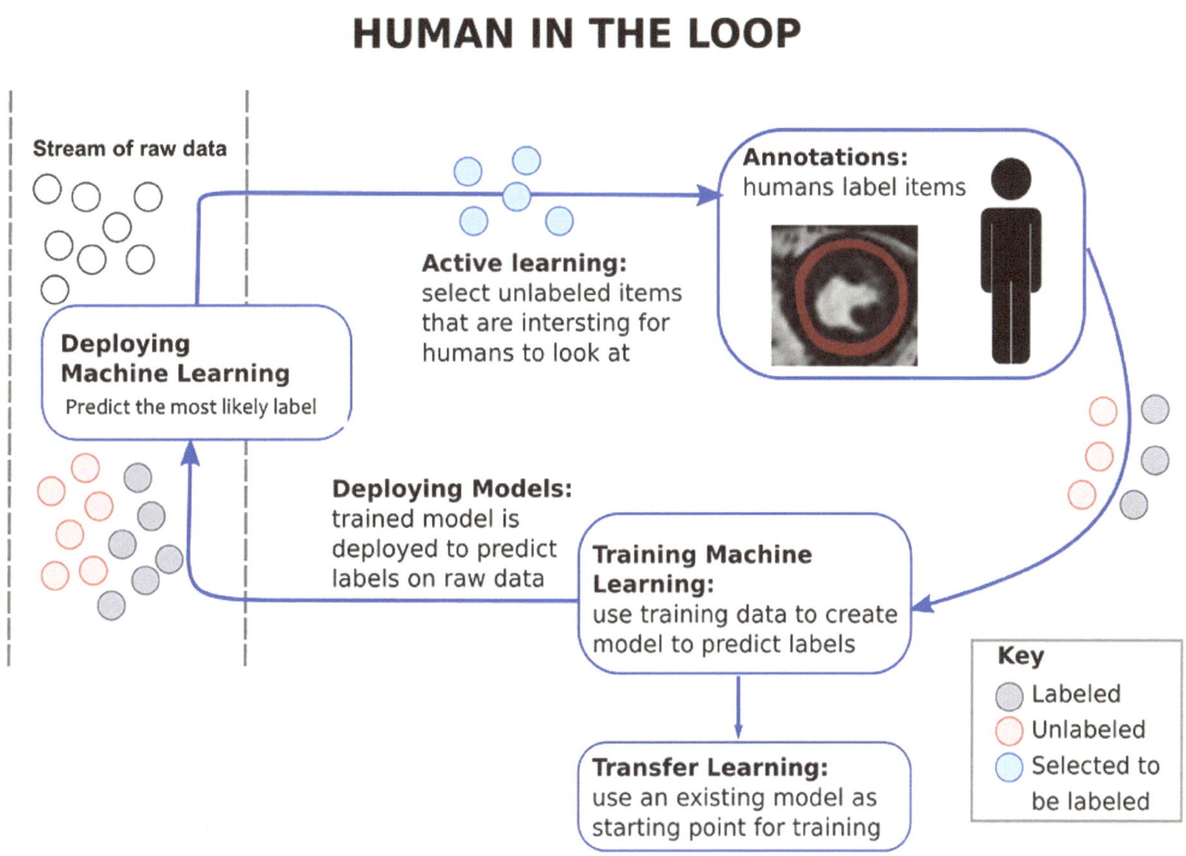

Fig.16.10 Brief chart on the framework of "clinician in the loop." Clinicians are provided with action choices. Data labelled from clinicians contribute to the training of the network.

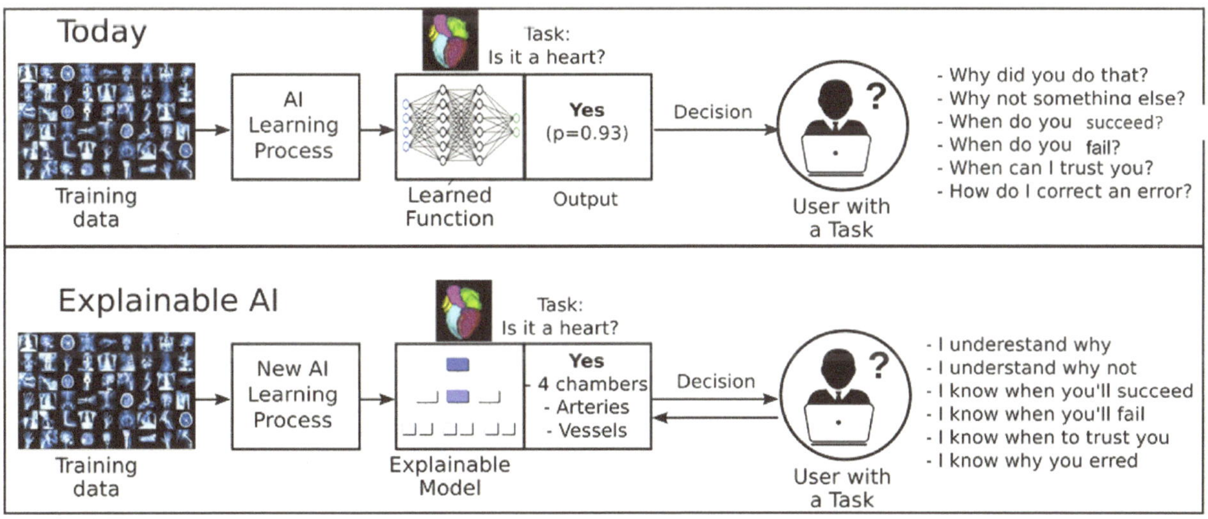

Flig 16.11 An illustrative overview of the explainable MRI concept. The user has insight in the features that influence the decision of the model.

Avard et al used radiomics analysis and feature identification on non-contrast cine CMR images to accurately detect MI, thus presenting a potential alternative diagnostic method to LGE CMR for MI.65 Ma et al have shown that combining radiomic signatures of non-contrast-enhanced T1 mapping and T1 values can provide higher diagnostic accuracy for MVO and radiomic signatures can also provide incremental value in predicting LV longitudinal systolic myocardial contractility at 6 months.

Prognostication

ML is well-suited to handle large amounts of clinical information and to find intrinsic structure within this body of information to predict clinical outcomes. Random survival forests technique has been used to identify the top predictors of each outcome measure in the Multi-Ethnic Study of Atherosclerosis (MESA), and CMR-derived LV structure and function were identified as one of the top predictors of incident heart failure. Information maximising component analysis, a supervised feature extraction method, has been used to determine more efficient and sensitive indices of overall remodelling between patients with MI and asymptomatic volunteers from the MESA study. Supervised ML of CMR imaging scans has been used to predict occurrence of cardiac arrhythmia in patients with MI from image-derived scar texture features, size and location of scar

Barriers to Implementation

One limitation of ML techniques is the black-box nature of DL algorithms, where it is often unclear what information is used or what interactions between nodes and layers have occurred to derive a certain successful or unsuccessful classification or result.The lack of transparency and explainability could affect user trust which can restrict the use of AI in healthcare. ML models for CMR imaging analysis also need to be robust and portable between scanners, sequences, imaging parameters and centres. Radiomic analysis in particular, is highly dependent on image acquisition parameters that can affect texture and histogram-based intensity values. Heterogenous datasets from different centres should be evaluated to check the validity of proposed ML algorithms on a large scale. Large, publicly available CMR datasets also need to be developed so that different algorithms can be objectively compared for their performance.

Governance and Quality Control

Open source publication of computational processes, codes and datasets can help to mitigate the unpredictable failures of ML algorithms that may occur.Current ML and DL methods can be vulnerable to adversarial attacks that can influence results and render models unsafe for clinical use. To ensure top quality of labelled training data, ground truth must be rigorously reviewed, particularly in clinical reporting where clinicians from different centres may disagree in reporting style and findings Controlled trials are required to evaluate the application of ML methods across multiple centres and varied patient groups. Validation should be performed using data from the same cohort as well as from other cohorts at different centres and using different acquisition devices. For continued advancement of the field, algorithms should be published in open-source repositories to enable cross-checking, benchmarking, replication and improvement by international groups. In addition, although large cohort data sets have been used for ML training, these applications must be extended with care to specific patient groups with various pathologies and with fair representation so that variations between age, sex and ethnicities can also be accounted for.

Future Applications and Directions

Conclusion

AI, ML and more specifically DL can improve efficiency, reproducibility, precision and accuracy in the assessment of important prognostic imaging biomarkers in MI CMR scans through the development of automated CMR analysis strategies. Global collaboration through open-source publication of codes and datasets will help to further advance the field and improve governance, safety and quality control through knowledge sharing. Future directions include the incorporation of automated analysis within clinical trials that assess clinical outcomes, and the extension of existing ML applications to heterogenous patient cohorts

Bibliography and Acknowledgement

- Alzubaidi L, Zhang J, Humaidi AJ, Al-Dujaili A, Duan Y, Al-Shamma O, et al. Review of deep learning: concepts, CNN architectures, challenges, applications, future directions. J Big Data. (2021) 8:53. doi: 10.1186/s40537-021-00444-8
- Bello GA, Dawes TJW, Duan J, Biffi C, de Marvao A, Howard LSGE, et al. Deep Bratt A, Kim J, Pollie M, Beecy AN, Tehrani NH, Codella N, et al. Machine learning derived segmentation of phase velocity encoded cardiovascular magnetic resonance for fully automated aortic flow quantification. J Cardiovasc Magn Reson. (2019) 21:1.
- Brocklehurst P, Field D, Greene K, Juszczak E, Keith R, Kenyon S, et al. Computerised interpretation of fetal heart rate during labour (INFANT): a randomised controlled trial. Lancet. (2017) 389:1719–29.
- Chen C, Qin C, Qiu H, Tarroni G, Duan J, Bai W, et al. Deep learning for cardiac image segmentation: a review. Front Cardiovasc Med. (2020) 7:25. doi: 10.3389/fcvm.2020.00025
- Collins GS, Dhiman P, Andaur Navarro CL, Ma J, Hooft L, Reitsma JB, et al. Protocol for development of a reporting guideline (TRIPOD-AI) and risk of bias tool (PROBAST-AI) for diagnostic and prognostic prediction model studies based on artificial intelligence. BMJ Open. (2021) 11:e048008. doi: 10.1136/bmjopen-2020-048008
- Collins GS, Reitsma JB, Altman DG, Moons KG. Transparent reporting of a multivariable prediction model for individual prognosis or diagnosis (TRIPOD): the TRIPOD statement. BMJ. (2015) 350:g7594. doi: 10.1136/bmj.g7594
- Dawes TJW, de Marvao A, Shi W, Fletcher T, Watson GMJ, Wharton J, et al. Machine learning of three-dimensional right ventricular motion enables outcome prediction in pulmonary hypertension: a cardiac MR imaging study. Radiology. (2017) 283:381–90. doi: 10.1148/radiol.2016161315
- Diller GP, Orwat S, Vahle J, Bauer UMM, Urban A, Sarikouch S, et al. Prediction of prognosis in patients with tetralogy of Fallot based on deep learning imaging analysis. Heart. (2020) 106:1007–14.
  Ding M. A second generation of the neural network model for predicting weighted mean temperature. GPS Solutions. (2020) 24:1–6. doi: 10.1007/s10291-020-0975-3
- Duan J, Bello G, Schlemper J, Bai W, Dawes TJW, Biffi C, et al. Automatic 3D Bi-ventricular segmentation of cardiac images by a shape-refined multi- task deep learning approach. IEEE Trans Med Imaging. (2019) 38:2151–64. doi: 10.1109/TMI.2019.2894322
- Erickson BJ, Korfiatis P, Akkus Z, Kline TL. Machine learning for medical imaging. Radiographics. (2017) 37:505–15. doi: 10.1148/rg.2017160130
- Fahmy AS, El-Rewaidy H, Nezafat M, Nakamori S, Nezafat R. Automated analysis of cardiovascular magnetic resonance myocardial native T1 mapping images using fully convolutional neural networks. J Cardiovasc Magn Reson. (2019) 21:7. doi: 10.1186/s12968-018-0516-1
- Fahmy AS, Rausch J, Neisius U, Chan RH, Maron MS, Appelbaum E, et al. Automated cardiac MR scar quantification in hypertrophic cardiomyopathy using deep convolutional neural networks. JACC Cardiovasc Imaging. (2018) 11:1917–8. doi: 10.1016/j.jcmg.2018.04.030
- Fuin N, Bustin A, Kustner T, Oksuz I, Clough J, King AP, et al. A multi-scale variational neural network for accelerating motion-compensated whole-heart 3D coronary MR angiography. Magn Reson Imaging. (2020) 70:155–67. doi: 10.1016/j.mri.2020.04.007
- Genin K, Grote T. Randomized controlled trials in medical AI a methodological critique. Philos Med. (2021) 2. doi: 10.5195/philmed.2021.27
- Ghadimi S, Auger DA, Feng X, Sun C, Meyer CH, Bilchick KC, et al. Fully-automated global and segmental strain analysis of DENSE cardiovascular magnetic resonance using deep learning for segmentation and phase unwrapping. J Cardiovasc Magn Reson. (2021) 23:20. doi: 10.1186/s12968-021-00712-9
- Hao Z, Shyam RBA, Rathinam A, Gao Y. Intelligent spacecraft visual GNC architecture with the state-of-the-art AI components for on-orbit manipulation. Front Robot AI. (2021) 8:639327. doi: 10.3389/frobt.2021.639327
- Holzinger A, Biemann C, Pattichis C, Kell D. What do we need to build explainable AI systems for the medical domain? arXiv preprint arXiv:1712.09923. (2017).
- Huang B, Ji Z, Zhai R, Xiao C, Yang F, Yang B, et al. Clock bias prediction algorithm for navigation satellites based on a supervised learning long short-term memory neural network. GPS Solutions. (2021) 25:80. doi: 10.1007/s10291-021-01115-0 Intell. (2019) 1:95–104. doi: 10.1038/s42256-019-0019-2
- Karimi-Bidhendi S, Arafati A, Cheng AL, Wu Y, Kheradvar A, Jafarkhani H. Fullyautomated deeplearning segmentation of pediatric cardiovascular magnetic resonance of patients with complex congenital heart diseases. J Cardiovasc Magn Reson. (2020) 22:80. doi: 10.1186/s12968-020-00678-0
- Keane PA, Topol EJ. With an eye to AI and autonomous diagnosis. NPJ Digit Med. (2018) 1:40. doi: 10.1038/s41746-018-0048-y
- Keenan NG, Captur G, McCann GP, Berry C, Myerson SG, Fairbairn T, et al. Regional variation in cardiovascular magnetic resonance service delivery across the UK. Heart. (2021). doi: 10.1136/heartjnl-2020-318667
- Knott KD, Seraphim A, Augusto JB, Xue H, Chacko L, Aung N, et al. The prognostic significance of quantitative myocardial perfusion: an artificial intelligence-based approach using perfusion mapping. Circulation. (2020) 141:1282–91. doi: 10.1161/CIRCULATIONAHA.119.044666
- Kotu LP, Engan K, Borhani R, Katsaggelos AK, Orn S, Woie L, et al. Cardiac magnetic resonance image-based classification of the risk of arrhythmias in post-myocardial infarction patients. Artif Intell Med. (2015) 64:205–15. doi: 10.1016/j.artmed.2015.06.001
- Kustner T, Fuin N, Hammernik K, Bustin A, Qi H, Hajhosseiny R, et al. CINENet: deep learning-based 3D cardiac CINE MRI reconstruction with multi-coil complex-valued 4D spatio-temporal convolutions. Sci Rep. (2020) 10:13710. doi: 10.1038/s41598-020-70551-8
- Kustner T, Munoz C, Psenicny A, Bustin A, Fuin N, Qi H, et al. Deep-learning based super-resolution for 3D isotropic coronary MR angiography in less than a minute. Magn Reson Med. (2021) 86:2837–52. doi: 10.1002/mrm.28911

- Leiner T, Rueckert D, Suinesiaputra A, Baessler B, Nezafat R, Isgum I, et al. Machine learning in cardiovascular magnetic resonance: basic concepts and applications. J Cardiovasc Magn Reson. (2019) 21:61. doi: 10.1186/s12968-019-0575-y
- Lin H, Li R, Liu Z, Chen J, Yang Y, Chen H, et al. Diagnostic efficacy and therapeutic decision-making capacity of an artificial intelligence platform for childhood cataracts in eye clinics: a multicentre randomized controlled trial. EClinicalMedicine. (2019) 9:52–9. doi: 10.1016/j.eclinm.2019.03.001
- MacGregor RM, Guo A, Masood MF, Cupps BP, Ewald GA, Pasque MK, et al. Machine learning outcome prediction in dilated cardiomyopathy using regional left ventricular multiparametric strain. Ann Biomed Eng. (2021) 49:922–32. doi: 10.1007/s10439-020-02639-1
- Mancio J, Pashakhanloo F, El-Rewaidy H, Jang J, Joshi G, Csecs I, et al. Machine learning phenotyping of scarred myocardium from cine in hypertrophic cardiomyopathy. Eur Heart J Cardiovasc Imaging. (2021) jeab056. doi: 10.1093/ehjci/jeab056. [Online ahead of print].
- Menacho K, Ramirez S, Segura P, Nordin S, Abdel-Gadir A, Illatopa V, et al. INCA (Peru) study: impact of non-invasive cardiac magnetic resonance assessment in the developing world. J Am Heart Assoc. (2018) 7:e008981.
- Neisius U, El-Rewaidy H, Nakamori S, Rodriguez J, Manning WJ, Nezafat R. Radiomic analysis of myocardial native T1 imaging discriminates between hypertensive heart disease and hypertrophic cardiomyopathy. JACC Cardiovasc Imaging. (2019) 12:1946–54. doi: 10.1016/j.jcmg.2018.11.024
- Ng M, Guo F, Biswas L, Petersen SE, Piechnik SK, Neubauer S, et al. Estimating Uncertainty in Neural Networks for Cardiac MRI Segmentation: A Benchmark Study 2020
  Puyol-Anton E, Chen C, Clough JR, Ruijsink B, Sidhu BS, Gould J, et al. Interpretable deep models for cardiac resynchronisation therapy response prediction. Med Image Comput Comput Assist Interv. (2020) 2020:284–93.
- Puyol-Antón E, Ruijsink B, Harana JM, Piechnik SK, Neubauer S, Petersen SE, et al. Fairness in cardiac magnetic resonance imaging: assessing sex and racial bias in deep learning-based segmentation.medRxiv.(2021).
- Ravi D, Wong C, Deligianni F, Berthelot M, Andreu-Perez J, Lo B, et al. Deep Learning for Health Informatics. IEEE J Biomed Health Inform. (2017) 21:4–21. doi: 10.1109/JBHI.2016.2636665
- Ruijsink B, Puyol-Anton E, Oksuz I, Sinclair M, Bai W, Schnabel JA, et al. Fully automated, quality-controlled cardiac analysis from CMR: validation and large-scale application to characterize cardiac function. JACC Cardiovasc Imaging. (2020) 13:684–95. doi: 10.1016/j.jcmg.2019.05.030
- Saito T, Rehmsmeier M. The precision-recall plot is more informative than the ROC plot when evaluating binary classifiers on imbalanced datasets. PLoS ONE. (2015) 10:e0118432. doi: 10.1371/journal.pone.0118432
- Scannell CM, Veta M, Villa ADM, Sammut EC, Lee J, Breeuwer M, et al. Deep-learning-based preprocessing for
- quantitative myocardial perfusion MRI. J Magn Reson Imaging. (2020) 51:1689–96. doi: 10.1002/jmri.26983Shah NH, Milstein A, Bagley DS. Making machine learning models clinically useful. JAMA. (2019) 322:1351–2. doi: 10.1001/jama.2019.10306
- Sinclair M, Peressutti D, Puyol-Anton E, Bai W, Rivolo S, Webb J, et al. Myocardial strain computed at multiple spatial scales from tagged magnetic resonance imaging: Estimating cardiac biomarkers for CRT patients. Med Image Anal. (2018) 43:169–85. doi: 10.1016/j.media.2017.10.004Singh A, Sengupta S, Lakshminarayanan V. Explainable deep learning models in medical image analysis. J Imaging. (2020) 6:52. doi: 10.3390/jimaging6060052
- Sony S, Dunphy K, Sadhu A, Capretz M. A systematic review of convolutional neural network-based structural condition assessment techniques. Engineering Structures. (2021) 226:11137. doi: 10.1016/j.engstruct.2020.111347
- Steeden JA, Quail M, Gotschy A, Mortensen KH, Hauptmann A, Arridge S, et al. Rapid whole-heart CMR with single volume super-resolution. J Cardiovasc Magn Reson. (2020) 22:56. doi: 10.1186/s12968-020-00651-x
- Sudlow C, Gallacher J, Allen N, Beral V, Burton P, Danesh J, et al. UK Biobank: an open access resource for identifying the causes of a wide range of complex diseases of middle and old age. PLoS Med. (2015) 12:e1001779. doi: 10.1371/journal.pmed.1001779
- Tang S, Modi A, Sjoding M, Wiens J. Clinician-in-the-loop decision making: reinforcement learning with near-optimal set-valued policies. In: Hal D, Aarti S, editors. Proceedings of the 37th International Conference on Machine Learning; Proceedings of Machine Learning Research. (2020). p. 9387–96.
- Tao Q, Yan W, Wang Y, Paiman EHM, Shamonin DP, Garg P, et al. Deep learning-based method for fully automatic quantification of left ventricle function from cine MR images: a multivendor, multicenter study. Radiology. (2019) 290:81–8. doi: 10.1148/radiol.2018180513
- Wang J, Yang F, Liu W, Sun J, Han Y, Li D, et al. Radiomic analysis of native T1 mapping images discriminates between MYH7 and MYBPC3-related hypertrophic cardiomyopathy. J Magn Reson Imaging. (2020) 52:1714–21.
- Winther HB, Hundt C, Schmidt B, Czerner C, Bauersachs J, Wacker F, et al. ν-net: deep learning for generalized biventricular mass and function parameters using multicenter cardiac MRI data. JACC Cardiovasc Imaging. (2018) 11:1036–8. doi: 10.1016/j.jcmg.2017.11.013

Artificial Intelligence / Machine learning For Predicting Cardiac Events What Does The Future Hold?

CHAPTER

17

Cardiovascular diseases (CVD) accounted for nearly 900,000 deaths in 2016 in the US alone , and it is well known that the CVD burden will rise because of the aging population. Researchers have created prediction models from existing data to identify individuals who are at risk for cardiovascular events using statistical methods. Statistical analysis is heavily dependent on data sampling methods, their distribution, and the types of tests used before elucidating statistical inferences at the population level using representative sampling. With machine learning (ML), it is possible to make individual-level predictions about cardiovascular diseases and events. ML is a form of artificial intelligence (AI) that uses complex algorithms and does not require any assumption about the sample or population – unlike statistical methods. Statistical methods are useful for drawing inferences, while ML methods are better suited to make predictions . ML can aid clinicians in providing individualized predictions and tailoring treatment plans for their patients. we will succinctly discuss how machine learning works, followed by a review of how machine learning has been utilized to predict cardiovascular events such as major adverse cardiovascular events, heart failure and arrhythmias. We will also focus on how various machine learning algorithms compare to existing statistical-based models for predicting cardiovascular events.

Machine learning

The concept of artificial intelligence emerged around 1950 s. One of the seminal papers published by Alan Turing about "Can machines think? in 1950 created a platform for future work for computer scientists. Over the next few decades, the field suffered from 'AI winter' before its revival and tremendous growth in algorithms and technology. There are many ML algorithms exist, however, a simplest form of ML algorithm we know is logistic regression. But, its inability to process data as an ML algorithm may limit its utilization on big data and in complex data analysis. There are three approaches through which the 'machine' can be trained: supervised learning, unsupervised learning, and reinforcement learning. In supervised learning, the input datasets and desired outcomes are labeled. For example, let us say that we would like the machine to identify cases of heart failure. First, we train it with known (labeled) variables, such as biomarkers, imaging and clinical exam findings that are associated with the outcome (heart failure). In unsupervised learning, data points (biomarkers, imaging and clinical assessment findings) are entered into the algorithm, and we ask the machine to identify patterns or clusters within the population without a prespecified outcome. In this case, the algorithm is not asked to identify heart failure patients; rather, it creates clusters of variables that are closely related to heart failure.

Neither of these approaches involves any feedback mechanism. In reinforcement learning, the algorithm is challenged to reanalyze the data and optimize the predictive model based on feedback given for falsely identified cases. For example, crackles could be present in patients without heart failure. Patients without heart failure can have crackles, and they are relabeled as non-heart failure cases. The machine 'relearns' that the presence of crackles does not equate to heart failure. Thus, we can say that reinforcement learning is a hybrid form of supervised and unsupervised learning. Supervised learning is the most common method used in ML.summarizes the steps taken to create a predictive model using ML.

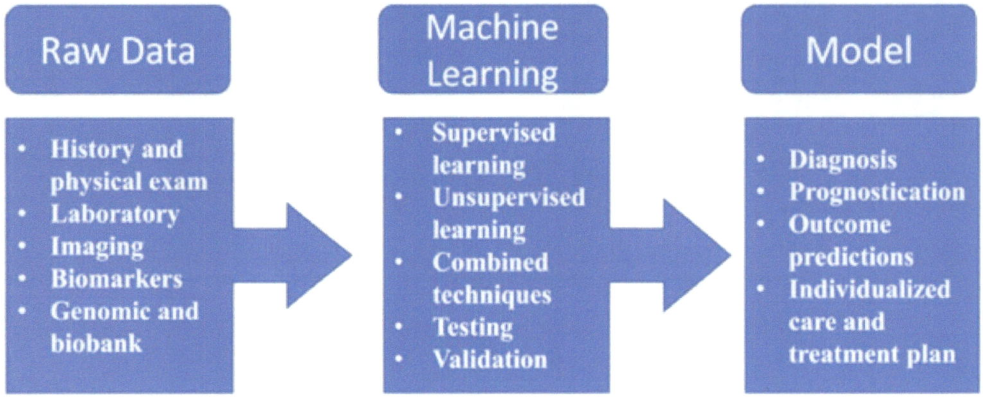

Fig.17.1 Generalized diagram of the steps in machine learning used to create models.

Predicting cardiovascular events

In the remainder we will discuss specific cardiovascular events than can be predicted by ML and how it has performed in comparison to statistical methods in the recent literature .

Major adverse cardiovascular events and myocardial infarction

Ischemic heart disease accounts for more than 9 million deaths globally, with a downward trend in mortality in Western countries. This phenomenon is attributed to advanced therapy and a strong emphasis on prevention [5]. It is essential to identify high-risk patients with readily available and pragmatic predictive models.

Simple EKG-based predictive models using neural networks have been used to detect myocardial infarction with an accuracy of more than 95% [6]. The availability of electronic health records and the incorporation of data from various cardiac imaging modalities allow us to create better predictive models. Prior studies have focused on regression-based models such as the Framingham risk score (FRS), thrombolysis in myocardial infarction (TIMI) and the Global Registry of Acute Coronary Events (GRACE) for risk assessment of initial, short-term and long-term major adverse cardiovascular events (MACE), respectively [7–10]. However, regression-based models do not address the complex interactions between clinical variables existing in the

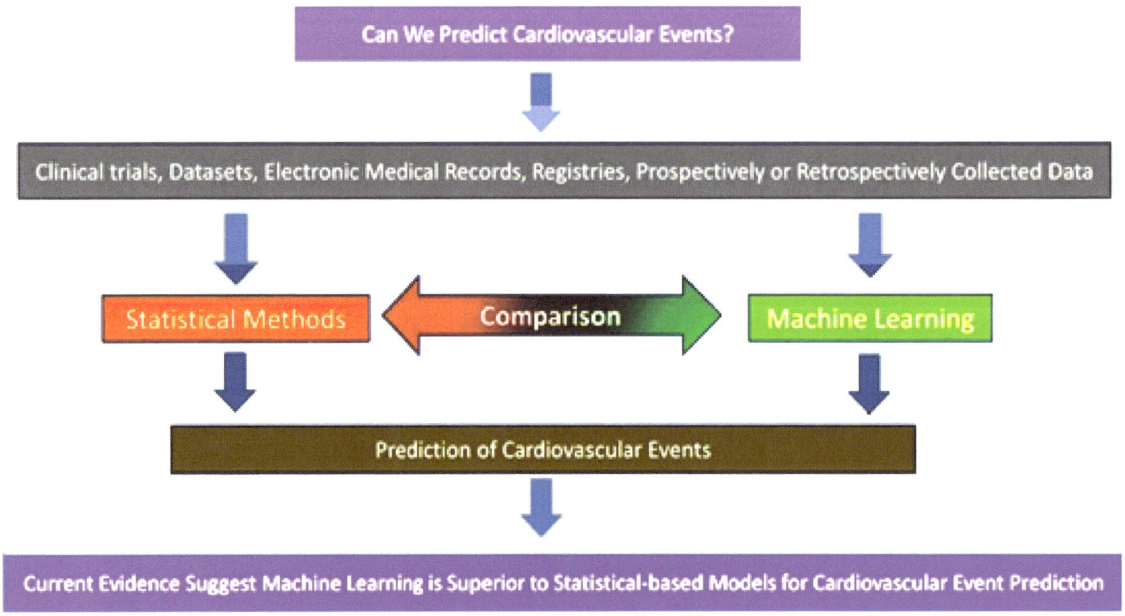

Fig 17.2. Central theme of literature reviewed in this review chapter

Table 17.1. Summary for predicting cardiovascular events.

Major Adverse Cardiovascular Events (MACE) and Myocardial Infarction (MI)

1. Machine learning (ML) is more accurate in predicting short-,intermediate and long-term mortality after index the myocardial infarction event
2. In comparison to Global Registry of Acute Coronary Events (known as GRACE) risk score, ML based models are better predictors of MACE
3. The combination of clinical, demographics and nuclear imaging findings have better predictive ability for MACE using ML algorithms.
4. Coronary computed tomography angiography plus clinical variables have better predictive values with ML algorithms than Framingham Risk Score for all-cause mortality.

Heart Failure

1. Traditional statistics-based models such as Get With the Guideline-Heart Failure and MAGGIC risk scores were outperformed by ML models for short- and long-term mortality in acute heart failure patients.
2. Using ML models, a simple risk score in diabetic patients, WATCH-DM was created. This model requires patient's age, presence of hypertension, creatinine and high-density lipoprotein levels, QRS duration, history of MI and coronary artery bypass surgery. A unit increase indicated 24% increased risk of heart failure.
3. The risks of mortality and hospitalization in diastolic heart failure patients were better predicted by ML algorithms. Kansas City Cardiomyopathy Questionnaire (KCCQ) score and body mass index were the best predictors of mortality, while BUN and hemoglobin levels, KCCQ score and previous heart failure admissions were the best indicators for rehospitalization.
4. The ML algorithms can predict 30-risk of readmissions and post-discharge outcomes with decent accuracy.

Arrhythmia

1. The future prediction of developing atrial fibrillation is made possible by ML models.
2. ML can predict the risk of sudden cardiac death (SCD) from heart rate variability.
3. In-hospital risk of cardiac arrest was developed using ML from patients' body temperature, heart and respiratory rate, which outperformed Modified Early Warning Score (MEWS)
4. The risk of SCD in hypertrophic cardiomyopathy patients can be more accurately predicted by ML models.
5. A shockable rhythm detection on automated external defibrillators improvisation has been proposed with ML derived algorithm.

studies. ML can reveal complex interactions among variables and provide accurate, predictive models for future outcomes.To predict outcomes after myocardial infarction, various machine learning algorithms have been tested for their predictive ability. Using the Hungarian Myocardial Infarction Registry, researchers studied 47,391 patients who were hospitalized for acute myocardial infarction. They compared the relative performance of decision tree, neural network and logistic regression models for short-term (30-day) and long-term (1-year) mortality post-myocardial infarction. The decision tree, neural network and logistic regression models had areas under the receiver operating characteristic curves (AUCs) of 0.788, 0.837 and 0.834 for 30-day mortality and 0.754, 0.819 and 0.819 for 1-year mortality, respectively. Although the neural network was not superior to logistic regression, it was significantly superior to the decision tree model in this study. Another registry-based (KAMIR: Korea Acute Myocardial Infarction Registry) ML model was superior to regression-based models in predicting outcomes up to one year post-myocardial infarction.More than 14,000 acute myocardial infarction patients were included in the registry. The primary goal was to predict MACE using 51 variables, such as demographic information, clinical presentation variables and other variables. For this project, three ML algorithms, a deep neural network

(DNN), a generalized linear model (GLM) and a gradient-boosting model (GBM) were developed, and the accuracy of traditional regression-based GRACE model was also tested. For the 1-, 6-, and 12-month follow-ups, the AUCs for predicting MACE were as follows: 0.97, 0.94, and 0.96 for the DNN; 0.96, 0.95, and 0.96 for the GBM; 0.76, 0.67, and 0.72 for the GLM; and 0.75, 0.72 and 0.76 for GRACE, respectively. In fact, the DNN had a > 95% accuracy for the prediction of MACE, and thus, ML far outperformed the regression-based GRACE model. Nevertheless, in an Israeli study, ML-derived models did not outperform GRACE.The study included 2,782 patients and 54 variables. The objective of this study was to predict 30-day mortality after ST-elevation myocardial infarction. Six different ML models were compared, along with GRACE and TIMI. The GRACE risk score outperformed that of TIMI, but the ML models were not superior to GRACE. Interestingly, the performance of the algorithm plateaued with 15 variables, which means that only certain variables are necessary to predict such outcomes; creatinine level, Killip class on admission, blood pressure, glucose and age were among the important predictors.Patients with angina or its equivalent symptoms often undergo stress testing. In nuclear cardiology, ML has shown improved detection of myocardial ischemia . It is possible to combine clinical variables and stress test data to predict cardiovascular outcomes. Betancur and colleagues studied 2,619 consecutive patients who underwent exercise or pharmacologic stress myocardial perfusion imaging (MPI) . The goal was to study the combined value of MPI and clinical variables to predict 3-year MACE, including nonfatal myocardial infarction. As expected, the combined ML model predicted with better accuracy than the imaging ML model (AUC 0.81 vs. 0.78, respectively, $p < 0.01$). While there is value in incorporating MPI data, better predicting models are needed to identify short- and long-term MACE.

Computer Computed Tomography

(CCTA) has been studied to predict long-term outcomes. CCTA is an invaluable tool in both diagnosing and excluding coronary artery disease [16]. Data from the CONFIRM registry was used to predict 5-year all-cause mortality by combining 44 CCTA variables and 25 clinical variables .The study included more than 10,000 patients with suspected coronary artery disease and had at least 5 years of follow-up data. They utilized the iterative LogitBoost algorithm, which is an ensemble boosting algorithm. Compared to FRS (AUC: 0.61) as well other CCTA-based risk models [segment stenosis score (AUC: 0.64), segment involvement score (AUC: 0.64)], the ML model combining CCTA and clinical variables (AUC: 0.79) was far better in predicting 5-year all-cause mortality. With ML, it is possible to predict MACE. A large-scale, registry-based analysis in the United Kingdom has shown the superiority of ML-based predictive modeling . Similar analyses using US registries are needed. The accuracy of models heavily relies on the selected algorithm, clinical variables and heterogeneity of the population. Based on the available data, ML methods seem to perform better when combining clinical variables with cardiac imaging modalities.

Heart Failure

Acute heart failure (AHF) leads to more than one million hospital admissions representing 1 to 2% of all hospitalizations. The condition has been associated with morbidity and mortality as well as financial burden. Nearly 26 million patients worldwide carry a diagnosis of heart failure..The overall survival rate from heart failure has improved with improved diagnostic tools and new drug therapies, but 2–17% of individuals admitted with heart failure die while hospitalized .

Risk models (GWTG-HF, MAGGIC, ADHERE, LAPS2, EFFECT, Premier) to identify individuals at high risk for mortality have been developed for inpatient and outpatient settings .These models require commonly collected variables in typical heart failure patients. However, the complexity of inter-variable interactions are not be well defined with statistical methods used to create these predictive models.

Traditional mortality models for heart failure patients were compared to machine learning models in a Korean study . The source of data was hospitalized patients at two Korean hospitals (test data set) and the KorAHF registry (validation dataset). They analyzed more than 8,000 patients for testing and validation purposes. When the GWTG-HF and MAGGIC risk models were compared to ML models to predict in-hospital, 12- and 36-month mortality in AHF patients, the ML models significantly outperformed the other two models. The AUCs for in-hospital mortality were 0.88 [deep learning (DL) algorithm] and 0.73 for the ML and GWTG-HF models, respectively.

Similarly, the AUCs for 12-month and 36-month mortality were 0.78 and 0.81 (deep learning) and 0.72and 0.73 (MAGGIC score), respectively. In fact, the deep learning algorithm also outperformed the random forest, support vector machine, Bayesian network and logistic regression models for all three time points.

Machine learning is also able to predict HF better than the Cox-based method in diabetic patients [26]. Data from ACCORD (Action to Control Cardiovascular Risk in Diabetes) and ALLHAT (Anti-hypertensive and Lipid-lowering Treatment to Prevent Heart Attack Trial) were analyzed to compare a random survival forest (RSF) model and the Cox-based method for HF events (death or hospitalization). The RSF model had a better AUC of 0.77 vs. 0.73 for the Cox-based model. Using the best predictors from the RSF algorithm, the WATCH-DM model was created. Weight, age, hypertension, creatinine, high-density lipoprotein level, QRS duration, myocardial infarction and coronary artery bypass surgery were the prediction variables in the model. An increase of 1 unit was associated with a 24% increased risk of HF.

In the most recent analysis of TOPCAT (Treatment of Preserved Cardiac Function Heart Failure with an Aldosterone Antagonist), Angraal and colleagues demonstrated that ML had a better predictive ability than logistic regression for HF-related hospitalization or mortality . Among the studied algorithms (logistic regression, gradient boosting, random forest and support vector machine), the random forest model had the best predictive ability, with AUCs of 0.72 and 0.76 for mortality and HF hospitalizations over 3 years of follow-up, respectively. The analysis also showed that blood urea nitrogen (BUN) and alkaline phosphatase levels, Kansas City Cardiomyopathy Questionnaire (KCCQ) score and body mass index were the best predictors for mortality, while hemoglobin and BUN levels, KCCQ score and previous HF-related admissions were the best predictors for HF hospitalizations over 3 years of follow-up. Readmission is another issue burdening our healthcare system. The Hospital Readmission Reduction Program was intended to reduce hospital admissions for certain conditions, including heart failure. Despite its best efforts, readmission rates for heart failure-related readmission remain approximately 20% nationwide. Several studies have tried to identify high-risk patients, and a better prediction model is still needed. Mortazavi and colleagues used data from Tele-HF to compare a machine learning model to a logistic regression model to predict heart failure-related readmissions They analyzed the 30-day post-discharge readmission data from 1,001 patients. The majority of patients had a left ventricle ejection fraction <40%. The ML-based algorithms had better C-statistics (AUCs) than the logistic regression model. The random forest algorithm (vs. logistic regression) had the highest C-statistic of 0.68 (vs. 0.54) for readmission at 30 days. Additional supporting data to predict 30-day HF readmission risk using ML (vs. traditional models) comes from a retrospective analysis of 11,510 patients (out of 27,334 admissions). Among the logistic regression, gradient boosting, deep unified network (DUN) and max-out network models, the DUN model was the best prediction model for 30-day risk of readmission, with an AUC of 0.71 vs. 0.66 for logistic regression. A similar finding was also observed in another study, in which ML-based algorithms (deep neural network and random forest models) outperformed logistic regression models for the 30-day risk of readmission .

To predict post-discharge outcomes (readmissions and deaths), enhanced machine learning, multilayer perceptron (MLP) technique is even superior to traditional ML or regression-based modeling. In MLP, there is input, hidden and output layers. All input layers directly connect to nodes in the hidden layer(s), which also receive output from the output layer(s). This creates a higher level of non-linear transformation for learning. Using the Western Australia Data Linkage System, Awan and colleagues studied a cohort of 10,757 patients, among whom 23.6% were readmitted or died within 30 days of the index discharge .They created a multilayer perception (MLP) model, which is a model derived from a neural network. They also formed models using other ML algorithms used in the other studies described above. The MLP model has the best AUC (0.63) vs. 0.55 for the LR model or 0.53 for the weighted random forest model. The MLP model had an improved sensitivity (48%) compared to the other models. This study highlighted intra-ML model variability to predict post-HF discharge outcomes. It is important to consider various ML algorithms before creating a final predictive model.

For HF patients, machine learning algorithms are superior to conventional statistical-based models for predicting HF-related readmissions and mortality in multiple studies. However, data on model-based decision making and interventions to avert readmissions or improve outcomes are not well defined.

Arrhythmia

The dynamic and transient nature of arrhythmias make them unpredictable in a clinical setting.

Limited epidemiologic data have shown that the worldwide burden of arrhythmia and sudden cardiac death is rising. This phenomenon is probably due to better detection methods, an aging population and an increased incidence of risk factors . While there are tools available to detect arrhythmias as they are occurring, predictive tools for arrhythmia before the onset are lacking. Atrial fibrillation (AF) is well known to be independently associated with thromboembolic events such as stroke . In the SMART (The Stroke and Monitoring for PAF in Real Time) study, AF was detected in 1 out of 9 cryptogenic stroke patients with a 30-day event monitor . This finding means that AF can be transient and clinically unknown unless patients are monitored for a long time. However, the goal should be to identify patients who are likely to develop AF so that they are promptly treated. With this question in mind, a large study involving 180,000 patients in normal sinus rhythm (SR) was carried out by Attia and colleagues . The authors developed a convolutional neural network (CNN) using AI-enabled EKGs to predict AF in patients in sinus rhythm. For this study, both AF and atrial flutter (AFL) were labeled as AF. More than 450,000 EKGs from 126,526 patients, 64,340 EKGs from 18,116 patients, and 130,802 EKGs from 36,280 patients were used for training, internal validation and testing, respectively. The model predicted AF from a single EKG with an area under the curve (AUC) of 0.89(0.86–.88) and 0.90 (0.90–0.91) when the EKGs with the highest risk score were used. The sensitivity and specificity of the model were 79% and 79.5%, respectively. Since AF affects many individuals and such data can influence treatment, validation using an external dataset and optimization of the model is necessary.

EKG signals have been studied to predict sudden cardiac death (SCD). Heart rate variability (HRV) was studied by Ebrahimzadeh and colleagues using various ML algorithms to predict SCDs . In this study, the authors analyzed EKGs from 70 patients (35 who had experienced SCD and 35 healthy subjects) with a sampling rate of 256 Hz. They found that the two-minute interval before an SCD can be prognostically important to identify high-risk patients. The multilayer perceptron (MLP) neural network showed superiority to the k-nearest neighbor (k-NN) algorithm. The MLP model had an 84% SCD prediction rate of vs. 81.5% for the k-NN model 4 minutes before the event. EKG signals and various ratios calculated from EKG, such as the timing of the T-wave relative to the QT interval, have been shown to predict SCDs by means of ML-based models with greater than 97% accuracy (the maximum accuracy for the random forest model was 99.49%). More than 200,000 in-hospital cardiac arrest events occur in US hospitals .For early detection, at-risk patients are admitted to hospitals, but accurate prediction is essential to divert appropriate resources to these patients. Using only blood pressure, heart and respiratory rates and body temperature, Kwon and colleagues developed deep and machine learning models to predict in-hospital cardiac arrest . The DL-based early warning system outperformed the Modified Early Warning Score (MEWS) significantly (AUC of 0.85 vs. 0.60). Random forest and LR models were also better than MEWS with AUCs of 0.78 and 0.61, respectively. Importantly, the DL- and ML-based algorithms reduced the number of early warnings without compromising sensitivity. In essence, DL and ML models predicted cardiac arrest significantly better than the currently adopted MEWS. Likewise, ML has been used to accurately predict out-of-hospital cardiac arrest via data obtained from emergency calls with medical dispatchers. Heart failure (HF) patients are susceptible to fatal arrhythmias and sudden cardiac deaths (SCDs). Implantable cardioverter defibrillators (ICDs) are associated with a greater than 50% risk reduction in SCD in selected patients .Patients with reduced systolic function (≤ 35%) are susceptible to fatal ventricular arrhythmias and can benefit from an ICD. A study was designed to create a predictive model based on existing data from a retrospective, multicenter registry of Chinese patients with HF . The primary goal of this study is to predict all-cause sudden cardiac deaths. Various ML algorithms and Cox proportional hazards regression models will be utilized to create a predictive model for SCD in HF patients with low systolic function. Hypertrophic cardiomyopathy patients are at increased risk for sudden cardiac death. An ML-based model (HCM-VAr-Risk) was created to predict ventricular arrhythmias in hypertrophic cardiomyopathy patients . The goal was to detect at least one episode of sustained ventricular tachycardia or fibrillation .

The baseline logistic regression model had an AUC of 0.80, and a 0.80 false-negative rate, the HCM-VAr-Risk model had an AUC of 0.83 and a 0.27 false-negative rate. Out of 93 clinical variables, twenty-two variables (11 positively and 11 negatively) predicted the risk of arrhythmia.

There are currently 10 known variables in the HCM-Risk-SCD model (AUC > 0.69) developed by the American College of Cardiology and American Heart Association but the HCM-VAr-Risk model identified 12 new variables that increased the predictive ability; blood pressure before exercise, early diastolic strain rate, body mass index and statin use were among the new variables.

Furthermore, ML and DL algorithms have been utilized to optimize automated external defibrillators (AEDs). These devices notify the operator whether the rhythm is shockable or not (for ventricular tachycardia or fibrillation). Minimum standards for arrhythmia analysis algorithms for AEDs have been published . To further enhance the accuracy, an ML-derived algorithm using a convolutional neural network has been proposed. The algorithm had an accuracy of 99.26%, with a sensitivity of 97.07% and a specificity of 99.44% .Ideally, a sensitivity of 100% is preferable to avoid artificial sudden cardiac arrest, but the current work promises future development for further optimization. The application of ML seems very promising for detecting arrhythmias using simple clinical variables and EKGs. In the era of wearable devices such as those used in the Apple Heart Study and improved algorithms, the ability to predict arrhythmias before their occurrence in the near future is very plausible.

Bayesian statistics

Regression-based models lack the ability to predict outcomes at an individual level, while Bayesian statistical-based modeling can overcome this hurdle. The majority of current risk-predicting models are regression based (or frequentist statistics). Fundamentally, , Bayesian statistics uses prior knowledge, data or belief to construct a probability distribution, while frequentist statistics does not take any prior knowledge of an event into account. Individualized risk prediction and learning from prior data are similar features in Bayesian statistics and ML. Risk prediction models using Bayesian statistics have been created for cardiovascular events .Regression-based models can be incorporated in the Bayesian methods; similarly, Bayesian theory is also utilized in ML algorithms. But, a comparative study for various ML algorithms that includes Bayesian theory to predict cardiovascular event is lacking. Future work should focus on comparing various ML modeling that includes Bayesian machine learning approach.

Discussion With Expert Personels

Enormous amounts of data are generated by electronic health records, registries, research studies, and genomic and biospecimens. The complexity and size of the data poses challenges for data scientists to process, analyze, interpret and put them into clinical contexts. Although AI is not a new concept, its popularity has grown tremendously in the last decade. Machine learning is a part of AI and addresses complex data and 'trains' itself through mathematical models. By 2020, the US healthcare industry is expected to generate a trillion megabytes of data, with an annual growth of 36–48% [50]. To process even a fraction of these data, advanced modeling and statistical analysis techniques are necessary. Due to fast computing power, ML methods allow us to look at the data in unforeseeable ways.

Machine learning-based models have a better predictive ability than statistical-based models. Nonlinear modeling, complex calculations, and a higher dimension of data analysis are unique characteristics that set ML apart from statistical analysis. Further analysis should focus on the implementation of a prediction model for altering clinical outcomes. If an EKG-based algorithm can detect the future risk of developing atrial fibrillation, then trials should evaluate whether early treatment with anticoagulation reduces the risk of future cardiovascular events. Indeed, atrial fibrillation is detected in 10–30% of patients after an index cryptogenic stroke

Similarly, algorithm-based at-risk detection for HF or myocardial infarction can possibly alter outcomes and save healthcare costs. Duration of dual-antiplatelet therapy, identifying ideal candidates for implantable cardioverter defibrillators or cardiac resynchronization therapy and advanced heart failure treatments are among several topics and issues that ML can help us to further delineate. The role of ML in structural heart disease and interventions can be paramount. The application of ML in genome-based projects has been shown to predict advanced coronary artery calcium, which is a known risk factor for future cardiovascular events [52]. Studies focusing on incorporating genomic-level data into existing large datasets are quintessential to predict cardiovascular events. Future studies focusing on cost-saving strategies using ML algorithms are also needed as healthcare costs are skyrocketing.

Our ongoing work is focused on the reclassification and clustering of patients for specific diseases and outcomes using patient similarity analysis. In a patient similarity analysis, patients are presented as nodes, and they are connected by edges that represent similarities among the patients. This analysis reveals a heterogeneous relationship among the patients and represents the data in network and graphical format. In a recent publication, we showed the two main pathways of how patients with severe aortic stenosis progress were able to demonstrate how each region predicted MACE. For example, patients with increased filling pressure and increased left atrial volume index will have an increased risk of cardiovascular events, and then, the patients can be treated to have these parameters within the normal range. Thus, the application of AI can aid the analysis of data in unique ways that can aid clinicians in identifying and predicting individual-level risk.

One of major caveat in understanding of ML based prediction model is the 'black box'. Lack of clear understanding how information journeys from input variables to outcomes predictors create uncertain trusts in the implantation of ML based decision making. Improper and undertested models can create a huge public health risk. Creating testing and validation datasets requires utmost accuracy and confidence as much as implementing the model prospectively. An applicability of data interpretation is not as widely common as statistical based research among clinicians, and therefore, the systemwide integration of predictive models are not practical in every hospital or clinic at present time. AI-based modeling is largely driven by data scientists. Mastering the complexity of programming, data management, and application of appropriate algorithms can be a daunting task for clinicians. We therefore recommend establishing a team approach in which clinicians, statisticians and data scientists are included. Although AI is widely popular among commercialized industries, it is still lagging in the medical field. We strongly believe that AI can transform the medical industry and deliver precision medicine

Conclusion

Machine learning-based algorithms are superior to traditional statistical methods for predicting cardiovascular events. Certain algorithms, such as deep neural networks, are superior to other ML algorithms for certain outcomes. Further studies evaluating the applicability of such algorithms in the real world are needed

Key Points

- Machine learning (ML), a branch of artificial intelligence, is widely utilized in cardiovascular medicine
- Thus far, predictive models for cardiovascular events are based on statistical-based methods
- Evidence favors ML as a better predictive tool for cardiovascular events
- Future research showing applications of ML to prevent cardiovascular events is needed

Bibliography and Acknowledgement

- Acharya UR, Fujita H, Oh SL, et al. Application of deep convolutional neural network for automated detection of myocardial infarction using ECG signals. Inf Sci 2017. November 01;415–416:190–198. [Google Scholar]Alaa AM, Bolton T, Di Angelantonio E, et al. Cardiovascular disease risk prediction using automated machine learning: a prospective study of 423,604 UK biobank participants. Plos One. 2019;14(5):e0213653. [PMC free article] [PubMed][GoogleScholar]
- Ambrosy AP, Fonarow GC, Butler J, et al. The global health and economic burden of hospitalizations for heart failure: lessons learned from hospitalized heart failure registries. J Am Coll Cardiol. 2014. April 01;63(12):1123–1133. [PubMed] [Google Scholar] Angraal S, Mortazavi BJ, Gupta A, et al. Machine learning prediction of mortality and hospitalization in heart failure with preserved ejection fraction. JACC Heart Fail. 2019. October 5;8(1):12–21. [PubMed][GoogleScholar]
- Antman EM, Cohen M, Bernink PJLM, et al. The TIMI risk score for unstable angina/non–ST elevation MIA method for prognostication and therapeutic decision making. JAMA. 2000;284(7):835–842.
- Aro AL, Chugh SS, ESC CardioMed. Epidemiology and global burden of arrhythmias. Oxford, UK: Oxford University Press; 2018. Attia ZI, Noseworthy PA, Lopez-Jimenez F, et al. An artificial intelligence-enabled ECG algorithm for the identification of patients with atrial fibrillation during sinus rhythm: a retrospective analysis of outcome prediction. Lancet. 2019. September 7;394(10201):861–867. [PubMed] [Google Scholar]•• This paper used EKG as tool to predict one of the most common arrhythmia, atrial fibrillation. This project created an opportunity many researchers to use EKG as a tool topredictvariouscardiovascularevents.
- Awan SE, Bennamoun M, Sohel F, et al. Machine learning-based prediction of heart failure readmission or death: implications of choosing the right model and the right metrics. ESC Heart Fail. 2019. April;6(2):428–435. [PMC free article] [PubMed] [Google Scholar]
- Betancur J, Otaki Y, Motwani M, et al. Prognostic value of combined clinical and myocardial perfusion imaging data using machine learning. JACC Cardiovasc Imaging. 2018;11(7):1000–1009. [PMC freearticle][PubMed]
- Bhattacharya M, Lu D-Y, Kudchadkar SM, et al. Identifying ventricular arrhythmias and their predictors by applying machine learning methods to electronic health records in patients with hypertrophic cardiomyopathy (HCM-VAr-risk model). Am J Cardiol. 2019;123(10):1681–1689. [PubMed] [Google Scholar]
- Blomberg SN, Folke F, Ersbøll AK, et al. Machine learning as a supportive tool to recognize cardiac arrest in emergency calls. Resuscitation. 2019;138:322–329. [PubMed] [Google Scholar] Bridge F, Thijs V. How and when to screen for atrial fibrillation after stroke: insights from insertable cardiac monitoring devices. J Stroke. 2016. May;18(2):121–128. [PMC free article] [PubMed] [Google Scholar]
- Budoff MJ, Dowe D, Jollis JG, et al. Diagnostic performance of 64-multi-detector row coronary computed tomographic angiography for evaluation of coronary artery stenosis in individuals without known coronary artery disease: results from the prospective multicenter ACCURACY (Assessment by Coronary Computed Tomographic Angiography of Individuals Undergoing Invasive Coronary Angiography) trial. J Am Coll Cardiol. 2008. November 18;52(21):1724–1732. [PubMed] [Google Scholar]

- Bzdok D, Altman N, Krzywinski M. Statistics versus machine learning. Nat Methods. 2018. April 03 online;15:233. [PMC free article] [PubMed] [Google Scholar] C, Roth GA, Johnson CO, et al. Global Burden of CardiovascularDiseases
- Casaclang-Verzosa G, Shrestha S, Khalil MJ, et al. Network tomography for understanding phenotypic presentations in aortic stenosis. JACC Cardiovasc Imaging. 2019;12(2):236–248.[PubMed][GoogleScholar]
- D'Agostino RB, Vasan RS, Pencina MJ, et al. General cardiovascular risk profile for use in primary care. Circulation. 2008;117(6):743–753. [PubMed] Ebrahimzadeh E, Pooyan M, Bijar A. A Novel Approach to Predict Sudden Cardiac Death (SCD) Using Nonlinear and Time-Frequency Analyses from HRV Signals. Plos One. 2014;9(2):e81896.
- Flint AC, Banki NM, Ren X, et al. Detection of paroxysmal atrial fibrillation by 30-day event monitoring in cryptogenic ischemic stroke. Stroke. 2012;43(10):2788–2790. [PubMed]] Fox KAA, Dabbous OH, Goldberg RJ, et al. Prediction of risk of death and myocardial infarction in the six months after presentation with acute coronary syndrome: prospective multinational observational study (GRACE). BMJ. 2006;333(7578):1091.
- Futoma J, Morris J, Lucas J. A comparison of models for predicting early hospital readmissions. J Biomed Inform. 2015. Aug;56:229–238. [PubMed] [Google Scholar] Golas SB, Shibahara T, Agboola S, et al. A machine learning model to predict the risk of 30-day readmissions in patients with heart failure: a retrospective analysis of electronic medical records data. BMC Med Inform Decis Mak. 2018. June 22;18(1):44. [PMC free article] [PubMed]
- Huang W, FitzGerald G, Goldberg RJ, et al. Performance of the GRACE risk score 2.0 simplified algorithm for predicting 1-year death after hospitalization for an acute coronary syndrome in a contemporary multiracial cohort. Am J Cardiol.2016;118(8):1105–1110.
- Juarez-Orozco LE, Martinez-Manzanera O, Storti AE, et al. Machine learning in the evaluation of myocardial ischemia through nuclear cardiology. Curr Cardiovasc Imaging Rep. 2019.Feb09;12(2):5.
- Kim YJ, Saqlian M, Lee JY. Deep learning–based prediction model of occurrences of major adverse cardiac events during 1-year follow-up after hospital discharge in patients with AMI using knowledge mining. Pers Ubiquitous Comput. 2019. July 04. [Google Scholar]•• In this study, the authors studied various ML algorithms to compare them with GRACE score, to predict long-term outcomes after acute myocardial infarction. They were able to show the ML algorithms outformed GRACE score in predicting cardivascularevents.
- Kwon J, Lee Y, Lee Y, et al. An algorithm based on deep learning for predicting in-hospital cardiac arrest. J Am Heart Assoc. 2018;7(13):e008678. [PMC free article]
- Lai D, Zhang Y, Zhang X, et al. An automated strategy for early risk identification of sudden cardiac death by using machine learning approach on measurable arrhythmic risk markers. IEEE Access. 2019. July 01;1:94701–94716
- Merchant RM, Yang L, Becker LB, et al. Incidence of treated cardiac arrest in hospitalized patients in the United States. Crit Care Med. 2011. November;39(11):2401–2406. [PMC free article] Lai D, Zhang Y, Zhang X, et al. An automated strategy for early risk identification of sudden cardiac death by using machine learning approach on measurable arrhythmic risk markers. IEEE Access. 2019. July01;1:94701–94716.
- Merchant RM, Yang L, Becker LB, et al. Incidence of treated cardiac arrest in hospitalized patients in the United States. Crit Care Med. 2011. November;39(11):2401–2406. Mortazavi BJ, Downing NS, Bucholz EM, et al. Analysis of machine learning techniques for heart failure readmissions. Circ Cardiovasc Qual Outcomes. 2016;9(6):629–640. [PMC free article][PubMed][GoogleScholar]
- Nguyen MT, Nguyen BV, Kim K. Deep feature learning for sudden cardiac arrest detection in automated external defibrillators. Sci Rep. 2018. November 21;8(1):17196. [PMC free article] [PubMed] [Google Scholar] Nowbar AN, Gitto M, Howard JP, et al. Mortality from ischemic heart disease. Circulation Cardiovasc Qual Outcomes. 2019;12(6):e005375. [PMC free article] [PubMed] [Google Scholar]
- Perez MV, Mahaffey KW, Hedlin H, et al. Large-scale assessment of a smartwatch to identify atrial fibrillation. N Engl J Med. 2019. November 14;381(20):1909–1917. [PMC free article] [PubMed] [Google Scholar]
- Piros P, Ferenci T, Fleiner R, et al. Comparing machine learning and regression models for mortality prediction based on the hungarian myocardial infarction registry. Knowledge-Based Syst. 2019. September 01;179:1–7. [Google Scholar]
- Segar MW, Vaduganathan M, Patel KV, et al. machine learning to predict the risk of incident heart failure hospitalization among patients with diabetes: the WATCH-DM risk score. Diabetes Care. 2019. September 13;42:2298–2306. [PMC free article] [PubMed] [Google Scholar]
- Shouval R, Hadanny A, Shlomo N, et al. Machine learning for prediction of 30-day mortality after ST elevation myocardial infraction: an acute coronary syndrome israeli survey data mining study. Int J Cardiol. 2017;246:7–13. [PubMed] [Google Scholar] Simeone O A very brief introduction to machine learning with applications to communication systems. IEEE
- Trans Cognit Commun Networking. 2018;4(4):648–664. [Google Scholar]The burden of cardiovascular diseases among US States, 1990–2016. JAMA Cardiol. 2018. May 1;3(5):375–389. [PMC free article] [PubMed] [Google Scholar] Thompson ME, Dulin MF. Leveraging data analytics to advance personal, population, and system health: moving beyond merely capturing services provided. N C Med J. 2019. July–Aug;80(4):214–218. [PubMed] [Google Scholar]
- Weng SF, Reps J, Kai J, et al. Can machine-learning improve cardiovascular risk prediction using routine clinical data? Plos One. 2017;12(4):e0174944. [PMC free article] [PubMed]
- Wolf PA, Abbott RD, Kannel WB. Atrial fibrillation as an independent risk factor for stroke: the Framingham study. Stroke. 1991;22(8):983–988. [PubMed] [Google Scholar]
- Yousuf O, Chrispin J, Tomaselli GF, et al. Clinical management and prevention of sudden cardiac death. Circ Res. 2015. June 5;116(12):2020–2040. [PubMed] [Google Scholar]

CHAPTER

18

Artificial Intelligence-Based Smart Comrade Robot for Elders Healthcare.

Technology is a trend that affects human existence in every part of the world. Robots are an exciting example of what the future of technology holds. Robotics has enhanced human life and industry significantly, thanks to the technology . Adults with autism are already a regular thing in many industries, including healthcare, military service, and domestic assistance. The global population is growing, therefore making the requirements of this demographic an increasingly significant issue for health providers, government officials, caretakers, and families. Due to these reasons, buddy robots (which serve as aids to elderly people) are often seen as having an authoritarian function in helping individuals do their caring duties without assistance. An increased old population is often brought up as a method of dealing with the rising number of senior persons. Actually, robots are becoming more prevalent in the senior care sector. We should have been aware of certain ethical issues that have recently been brought to light as a result of these advances. Artificial intelligence approaches are applicable for various fields of utility. Digital smart systems, medical data analysis, healthcare system, and other applications are possible with AI model. Specifically, disease diagnosis with deep learning, radiology model with ML, automatic systems, and so forth are the most utilized healthcare systems of AI.

A rising need for new technology has emerged for older adults because of the greying of our current generation. The primary reasons in favour of this are that there are too few hospital workers and many individuals want to live as independently as possible rather than be placed in an institution . Additionally, we will need an adequate supply of healthcare professionals together with the use of cutting-edge technology. Robotics is playing a significant role in helping older people these days. A household use robot that is particularly intended for use at home may be regarded as a level of service robot. The business of making robots specifically for the house is expanding from scientific and commercial standpoints. In order for Comrade robot to be the most effective in the house, it should be able to carry out several activities such as home monitoring, gadget management, personal assistance, and entertaining.

When more and more robots are developed to engage with a human being to give the sort of care that is often provided by a licensed therapist, the lack of healthcare and the standard of living for the elderly will both improve . Designing a providing assurance "robotic arm" to supervise the old person is the method being used. The overall aim is to create a low rental Comradeship robot to assist an elderly person with daily home automation.

In the end, the house robot could traverse the usual home settings without any human assistance, carrying out duties such as senior citizens monitoring devices, home gadget management, and security and stability sensing, as well as in the case of an attack. This document has two distinct sections. One is a Comrade robot, while the other is a health monitoring band. A Comrade robot does so in the form of "making itself helpful"; that is, it is capable of assisting people in a household setting. The old person is constantly being kept under constant supervision by the Comrade robot . With the sensors incorporated in the design, the leaving comments industrial vehicle ensures both safe and secure environment in the family environment. Trespassers, gas leaks, and fire are all on the list. In the creative and emotional realm, Comrade robots and emotional synthetic avatars have now been created for graduate training. It may be difficult to extract a ministry of planning from both materials; therefore, teams that want to build Comrade robots must create their own website from scratch. Of course, there are many representations of structure for Comrade robot, but it is also tough to locate how the actual ones operate. Most articles concern themselves with how well an overall behavior performs, with little emphasis on the detailed architecture needed for replication.

The RoboCare program is dedicated to creating distributed applications where programming and autonomous agents all work together to accomplish an overall objective, which is to provide a supply of services that are ready for use in settings where people may need help and direction.

While we are also interested in supporting endangered elderly individuals to enjoy an inclusive environment in their own homes, our primary focus is on bringing the concept to market. According to recent data, Europe and Japan are gradually growing older. In order to increase public attention to this matter of "independence" and "ageing at home," new ways of supporting the seniors and persons with disabilities have been created.

This is why when it comes to RoboCare, most of the study deals with two potential situations, which are referred to as the RoboCare Household Atmosphere and the Quality of Life Institution setting . Robotic frameworks, wearable devices, activity monitoring in complicated settings, and human relationships are the main components of strong reliance for the future of robotic care. Here we will give the reader a short summary of the key findings that we have discovered so far and many lessons we have learnt from those efforts to custom-tailor AI for assisted living. Remote sensing data-based applications, image processing, video and audio recognition system, security system, and so forth are the applications of this research field. The major objective is to improve the performance state of medical data analysis and the robot model construction with efficient analysis is designed. This research contributes to improving the robot technology and availability of AI in medical healthcare system. Comrade robot model with AI utility helps to obtain a better performance result.

Why Robotic Help Would Be Required In Future?

Lifespans across the globe are rising, and therefore the percentage of the people in retirement ages is growing (Moyle et al. As visual acuity in older adults diminishes, this necessitates the provision of more services and has a larger impact on budgets for healthcare provision. The older population needs more research to help them retain emotional human fellow. Robotic technology may be used to assist both rehabilitative and sociable robots in relieving strain on social care facilities. Large data processing, overlapping issue, and feature set analysis difficulties are the major problem of conventional work.You may also look into Comradeship robotics, which are little robots that are made to look and behave like animals (Pu et al]). They aid creatures during rodent therapy by decreasing the dangers for the mammals individually. In general, Schrödinger, the mechanical seal, is a famous example. The advantages of getting to know Paro, a simulated nursing care Comrade for elderly people, include decreased irritation as well as depressive disorder in cognitive impairment, better immune responses, less burden on care providers, and enhanced affect and information exchange among both elderly people and their day care providers.. Furthermore, paracetamol may help to minimize the need for hallucinogenic and analgesia medications and may help to lower cholesterol levels.

The authors in and others examine the main methodologies, including designation as well as learning algorithms, which are essential in the development of developing quantum computing, as well as designation and learning algorithms, and computational efficiency that are applicable in the field of growing artificial intelligence and intricate their use .Research methods employed in data security, personal computing, and cloud services provide better findings, as diverse assessment criteria are taken into consideration.

The impact of robot animals upon autonomous older adults was examined in a clinical trial (Abubshait et al.) and also the researchers reported that robotic dogs may offer social enjoyment and relationships. While practical assistance was very attractive, the fact that the robot looked and felt more like a human created a conflict. People preferred soft fur and recommended play elements, such as plush toys, as potential improvements for the Comrade robots that are presently available. When new, brightly colored, child-oriented dogs were used, this restricted the kind of impressions respondents might create. Note that although older persons and individuals with memory are incorporated throughout Comrade robot creation, they are seldom, if ever, offered the opportunity to be engaged. Interaction typically happens in the project design whenever healthcare services are engaged.

It was recommended that the construction of something like an everyone around collapse detection technique be undertaken (Celis et al.). Utilizing just one aeration rate, an innovative wearable gadget for the detection of falls was created. Ubiquitous computing Remote Monitoring for the Old capable of detecting an individual's fall as maintaining the health of the patients. An Intelligent Home Security System based on GSM and ARM Architectural design: Industrial robots have lately been created utilizing a range of technologies, including the Web, wireless communications, wirelessly, and speech recognition.

Robotic Over Review In General

The word robot was originally derived from the Czech word robot, which means forced labor. Karel Capek, the Czech writer, introduced the term robot in his play "R.U.R." Capek used the term robotic in a series called "Rossum's Universal Robots" that premiered in Prague in 1921. The robots in R.U.R were built by man, and they were supposed to work for humanity. Thus, from generations to generations, human people have made use of robots to do various jobs. However, there is just no generally accepted definition for robots Despite this disagreement, the University of the Robot Society still sees a robot as a multipurpose fully programmable tool that is used to transfer credible commitments, tools, or optical disks in various ways using preprogrammed movements. This concept differentiates robots from other automated machines, because they are programmable. A robot may be described as an upgradeable, complex nervous, sentient, and transportable machine that uses energy to do work. Regardless of its form and size, a robot has seven major elements. This collaboration serves a particular goal. Figure 1 depicts the parts of a robot.

1. Controller

The commander is in charge of coordinating the robot's movements. The operational environment refers to the area within which a robot may operate . The microcontroller is also in charge of collecting input first from surrounding environment via the use of its sensing.

2. Power Conversion Unit

The fusion reactor supplies the robot's controls. Electricity, combustible materials, and battery storage are all commonplace power stations in robots . Most of the electricity that is provided to a building comes from the grid, and, in order to power the building, the system uses an AC/DC electrical power converter to change the AC electricity into DC electricity.

• Sensors

Robots may now have the sensor take a specific measurements of the surroundings, with the sensing' data helping to shape the robot's behaviors. To guarantee the robot's security, this is often done. Devices utilize a robot to respond to environmental variations.

• Actuator

In most of the robots, the actuators are often known as the muscles of the robot. The conversion takes place by using the energy that drives your robot's mobility.

• Control and Task Program

A collection of commands from the manufacturers of the robot's controller are known as the management plan, while a sequence of questions typically supplied by the user are called the task programme . To accomplish a particular job, the manipulator must carry out the movements task programmed by the task programme.

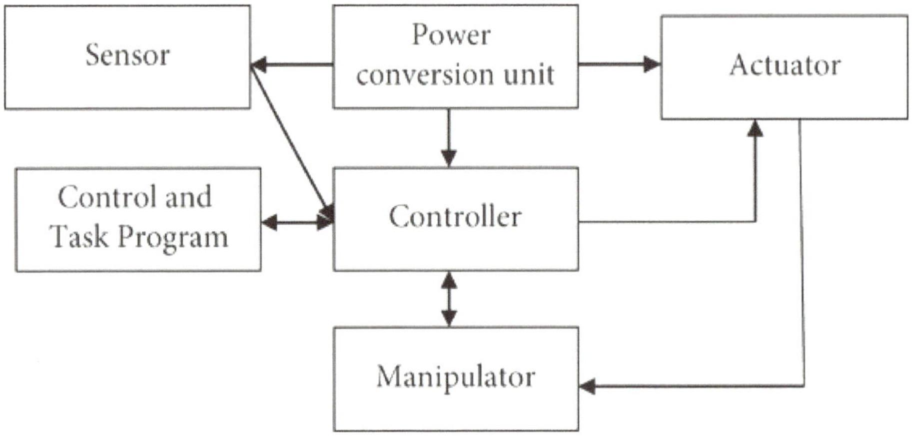

Fig. 18.1 Components of a robot.

3. Manipulator

The robotics have had the capacity to pick up, alter, and blow things up. The robot's manipulation imitates outstretched arm of something like a human individual. Manipulators typically refer to the joints connecting the arms with the upper arms, elbows, and wrists. Joints tend to be either rotational or sliding . Reaction kinetics refer to the way wherein the joints are arranged to define the potential stepper motor.

4. End Effector

The final part of the system, which connects to the input device, is known as the manipulation link. The instrument handle's link is known as an actuation. It imitates the mechanical arm, mimicking the results obtained.

Development Of Comrade Robot Structure

To develop up with a proper Comrade robot structure, we also must research the many needs that Comrade robots may have. Just one "perfect" Comrade robot might fulfill all these criteria. Meanwhile, theoretically speaking, the need of a Comrade robot does not quite apply; in reality, one is still required . The specifications for a given robot rely on a variety of different variables, including the kind of intended application and also the particular hardware components that are required.Here we provide a comprehensive list of all potential criteria an engineer should consider while designing a generic structure. The main task of the Comrade robot is to sense the environment around it, including hearing, seeing, and touching. Intercultural competence calls for synchronizing data; thus, various kinds of data need attention

In addition, inputs processing may be programmed to target specific sensor data, in response to predictions from a mixing process. Significance must be verified on every piece of data received, and all information collected must also be classified before it can be kept.

The Comrade robot was able to have a classroom discussion with the user. What this implies is not just to create effective sentences and also to take fundamental principles of communicating into consideration . A Comrade robot should constantly be likely to preserve the dialogue flowing in order to sustain a strong connection. The usage of live interaction also incorporates elements like this; for instance, in order to prevent boring or misunderstanding the user, lengthy pauses should not be present in a discussion. It should be able to communicate across all modalities and should do so in a logical and reasonable manner. Speech would overlap with proper lip motions, which have been prioritized about the present face animations and the robot dealing with the lips both of it. We illustrate the construction of a Comrade robot and address the specifications outlined above. However, observe that perhaps the design is abstracted from the specifics of various kinds of friend robotics, allowing its application to diverse kinds of robot Comrades. We are emphasizing again here that it was for a Comrade robot that also has an "overall" personality; nevertheless, you may build various parts without putting any content into them. Initial set of data processing uses dialogue engine and reasoning engine. Depending on the goals, rules, memory unit, and emotion recognitions are taken with heuristics approach. After that, the input and output processing states are determined with facial recognition with animation approach. Dataset uses source from camera, sound, and so forth and the speech recognition and facial recognition data are synchronized. With the low-level behavior, the animation controls are processed. Here this conflict scheduler, the performance of output state is determined.

AI and Robotic Technology in Elder Healthcare

By building a framework that incorporates current state-of-the-art AI technologies from an off way, RoboCare aims to help service providers fully appreciate the kind of assistance resources available . The difficult part is to find out whether the methods listed above might help create educational software parts that can be purchased off market. Robotic systems now provide us the ability to create robotic system with very accurate survival skills. We have effectively implemented these systems in both the home and hospital facility settings thanks to a variety of methods.

The professional diagnosis and management Comrade robot is able to provide guidance on prevention and prognosis by collecting data like clinical findings, a client's medical records, and previous medical instances. The robot was created by the robotics and artificial intelligence, that is, related to clinical texts, two million clinical data, and many individual instances The hospital is conducting a pilot programme in which people participate to evaluate the robot. When interacting with a client all through physical diagnosis, the robot "pays attention" to the dialogue and takes the sensor readings along with source information to help the clinician diagnose and prescribe medication . The clinician then collects information to interact with the clinician. It is anticipated that the robot would assist doctors to come to a conclusion about the cause of the patient's symptoms quicker and cut down on mistakes.

The Health System Mechanism, shown in Figure 3, is made up of several AI industrial robots.

To arrive at a prognosis, the speech based EHR system and image natural antibiotic are both utilized. Comrade proposes a diagnosis and therapy in which all relevant information is collected.

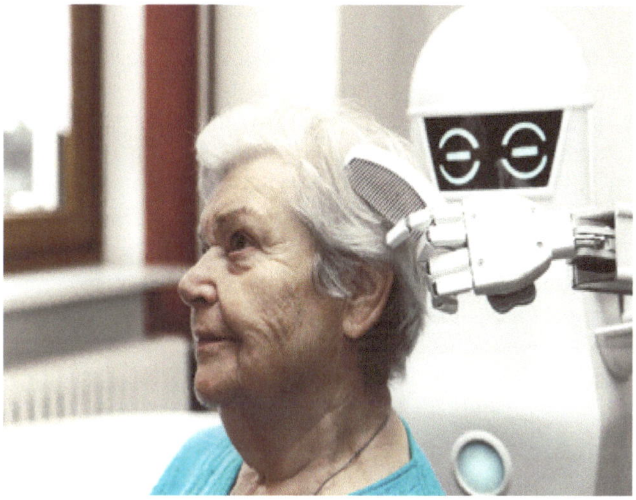

Fig.18.2 AI chatbots can help fill the void by providing some companionship

Thanks to advancements in technology, it is now possible to provide ambient independent living solutions to help seniors in their dwellings . The multidisciplinary approach that is required for robotics technology problems includes knowledge from fields like building, fashion, psychological, law, and ethics, as well as technology, computer programming, science, and medicine. In order to benefit everyone, robots and information and communication technology (ICT) must be made accessible across the populace at school, in hospitals, in home languages, and in smart neighborhoods. A high degree of acceptance and usefulness for the users may be achieved by integrating these approaches in the development of the surroundings.

Some basic suggestions for social order, together with technological and legal troubles, may be discovered through the applying load with actual customers in some kind of a contemporary context

Society Centered Design

Robotic technologies should be planned, manufactured, and

deployed to assist people in the day-to-day tasks in a societal architecture.The intelligent machines must be able to go from a user-centered design process to a social system design process, at which development process is properly considered and is further integrated with the society's requirements . Many of the ideas shown in the previous sections included users throughout the whole development process, starting with the study of end-users' requirements and leading all the way through the assessment of the prototype system for valuable suggestions..

Stakeholder Readiness

It is also essential to consider the speed to market in evaluating integrated services. That level of readiness indicates how soon the individuals and organizations are prepared to take and spread the technologies. The gap among study and implementation is the only problem with this topic.

Low Cost

Considering that personalized robotics are meant to be used by the individual, the price must be in line with their financial capability, in place to encourage for broad service usage. Robotic alternatives incur a reduced cost for the sake of a costing system , they are costly owing to the increased components they employ, but then on the other hand they are less costly for the public health system. Cloud automation solution models may enable a new breed of personalized robots for businesses.

Customizability, Flexibility, and Modularity

The requirements of the users will fluctuate. Having provided component services, it is essential to offer one that can respond to customer requirements and competences that vary.

Robustness, Dependability, Safety, and Security

Because the test equipment is expected to engage with those who are vulnerable and aged, it must have been secure and dependable.

Autonomy

Robotics institutions are expected to move independently and make choices based on the needs of consumers. They ought to be capable of identifying errors that users have made or they have made and make corrections on their own when required.

Social Informatics of Knowledge Embodiment

Our study has significance that are present in the system; it is applied to other comparable systems. Nonetheless, in order to validate our results, further research with healthcare practitioners in the field is required. In our research of AI-infused autonomous vehicles, we disregarded electronic archives, too. The usage of other things, like computers, may be affected by AI industrial robotics; however, in our research paper, we have not seen this. The possibility of further study includes research that compares cognitive manifestation in various entities in order to learn about how they support or replace one another.Lastly, we have not investigated the nature of senior executives' interest in, or usage of, AI machines. Understanding the four forms of information embodiment as a generative framework for finding motivators may be the most useful. Mechanistic explanation of cognitive immersion should rely on knowing the motive. From a social bioinformatics viewpoint, AI technology is relevant in the context.

It is vital to understand the sociospatial relationships AI has with people in order to fully comprehend its true worth. STIN analytic approach is particularly helpful, since it offers a paradigm for incorporating various social actors' perspectives while considering technologies. An excellent illustration of our findings is that, in contrast to the robots that were intended to make people's job and emphasizing, the AI humanoid systems that operate as rivals and magisters encounter greater opposition from economic systems than those that work as collaboration and guild mates.

This STIN study also showed that the automation technologies supplier has a minimal but nonetheless significant impact on the market. Requiring timely deployment of AI mobile robots for skilled employees, the supplier highlighted the technologies' complimentary and nonconfrontational character to help people gain confidence. This research confirms that our awareness of the use of AI industrial robotics in intellectual work requires a social information systems viewpoint.

By using powerful computers like AI robotic systems, researchers are showing that they can behave as an independent social actor in addition to just being a tool for humans. When humans and robots interact more naturally and intuitively, the difference between the humanity and the machine may become obsolete. Further refinement of the notion of interconnections in social bioinformatics as interpersonal relations and living organism connection converge may be required in order to help more people have social networks.

A manifestation of information changes understanding labor, and the introduction of new privacy practices is probable. Since making scientific have yet to comprehend the consequences of artificial intelligence, it is possible that the necessary training activities may need new methods of collecting, analyzing, and displaying data at employment. Social and community customers frequently need to work with machines, as well. Because of the resulting shift in the organization, in other words, the dissemination of materials is most likely to be caused. and shows major module utilizing expansion, emancipation, equipping, and expediting. Speech data with knowledge analysis, human cognition, augmentation, and AI robot are analyzed in expansion set. Actuation and competitor design of emancipation is determined. Assistance and automation model uses the procedural knowledge and final declaration.

Methodology Employed

Robotic systems that utilize the making plans, observation, concurrence, and successive cognitive orientations review process acquire questionnaire questions from guardians and carry out the intellectual orienting examination control and experimental group. The robot then engages in a discussion with the user and gathers feedback. When the robot has finished evaluating the responses, it reports back to those same caregivers with the results .This section describes the cognitive assessment method and the communication mechanisms platform. Our Friend Robotic, a 3D-printed desk device, is fitted with a cognition assessment process. The capacitive touch screen is linked to an ARM-based microcomputer executing Android platform, and the interaction is shown on it. In addition to having a 3D camera, this robot is equipped with a vision circuit composed of an RGB-D camera for image recognition and four loudspeakers that help with sound localization. We have also included voice and physical movement detection in our robot arm.The cognitive orientation assessment method has seven critical features: a development tool, inquiry and response creation, agreement between two parties, excessive screen, Internet computer vision, answer appraisal, and intelligence score .An online dataset and native databases are required for the relational database. In the public cloud, Q&A worksheets containing users' accounts and summaries of memory score are stored, along with cognitive orientations evaluations. These may be revised and checked by a caretaker. The personal dataset provides the user's focus strategy, test timetables, and Q&A answers.

Modeling and Formulations of Comrade Robots

The study of bending moment enables one to approach performs of large masses. According to the current motion, one may see the position, orientations, and higher incidence as having evolved through time. Dynamics in robotics are used to build up basic equations of controls, with the dynamic transfer function for deceivers acting as the explanation governing motion. Torque is the mechanism that is responsible for producing the dynamic movement of both manipulating arms in a robot's arm .. Dynamic modeling is involved in the development of the differential equations of the manipulation as a function of something like the displacements acting on it. In dynamic modeling, the robotics manipulator's components are constrained to a set of forces and; as a result, the locations, velocities, and deceleration are determined:(i)People who have torque needed to achieve certain end-effector movements are all determined by this calculation (the direct dynamic problem) (ii)The elastic scattering issue is modeled mathematically, and there are a variety of control methods which use the model(iii)It enables the calculation of the real manipulation to be done usinga control scheme equations and manipulate Lagrange's movement. Joint characteristics and characteristics of the manipulation define the motion. A communication model with overall energy K and gravitational potential V is shown as follows. Lagrange refers to. It is a simple procedure using the Lagrangian differential equation derived. The general force that corresponds to the generalized coordinate qi is referred to as Qi. Connection I has kinetic and potential energy provided. A second-order linear evolution equation may be used to describe the Lagrangian equations of motion for the n-th links manipulators.where

Evaluation Process

Google has published a new open software speech recognition processing framework, known as SyntaxNet, to the public. Syntax Net's main purpose is to find out the words and phrases, and each word is clearly shown in phrase. A parser is capable of determining the morphological purpose of any single phrase, including conjunctions, in the phrase. In addition to providing an also before the model named Parse McParseface, Goggling also offers a grammar models, known as Parsey McParseface, that is developed. No matter how complicated the root of a phrase may be, SyntaxNet is able to recognize it is able to trace out the connection between the word meaning and each individual word in the phrase. This study aimed to use SyntaxNet, so that the customer's voice communication may be processed genuinely.

To illustrate, a phrase will be spoken, at which point the voice activation component will transform textual content, which is then processed by SyntaxNet for deeper comprehension. To put a POS on a word, SyntaxNet examines the whole phrase as well as the word's semantics. Similarly, since SyntaxNet can correctly predict the calculated value used when a machine evaluates the provided response with the right answer, assessing answers that utilize math is quite simple. The capabilities of SyntaxNet may also be utilized to detect whether there is negativity in the word but when the phrase has a pejorative perception.The programming language we use to describe paragraph characteristics is called SyntaxNet. Step one is answering the question, and step two is evaluating the response. Next, the input is examined and processed using SyntaxNet to identify both user responses and right answers. Long computational network and right answer structure are created from the interpreted results. Those trees stand for the concept of a "pos" and how words relate to one other . The second step in the algorithm is to connect two trees, and the saplings are compared using a mating Canadian land. A compatibility score is given for these tree trunks, depending on their resemblance.

The robot gives a score of 1 to a right answer tree and a score of 0 to an erroneous solution tree. A partial number may be given if the answer matches both trees; however, the progress and achievement are used to evaluate the two trees. To determine the user's cognitive score, the participant's characteristics and a caregiver-determined criterion are utilized.

Recognition state of robot has various questionnaires, which translates the audio data to text data. Depending on the availability of given response, the NLP is performed and messages are taken with NLP analysis model. The parsed text is extracted with the feature set of given database. These correlated results are analyzed and desired answers are taken for the task accomplishment. Feedbacks are saved; then the respective description database assessment result is produced.

In conlusion ,Artificial intelligence is a rapidly expanding area of research, which has implications in many sectors, such as medical services, and to provide pharmaceutical aid. It is well established that the area of healthcare is a dynamic market for AI. In this article, a robotics framework is created which uses human messages between a human and a robot to carry out cognitive orientation evaluation. SyntaxNet, which enables the robots to comprehend programming knowledge naturally, helped carry out natural language processing. The Comrade robot was created from the ground up to handle this entire ecosystem. We do not need outside assistance in order to conduct a cognitive orientation evaluation, since the system is capable of doing it. This research sought to elicit tasks where a certain robot aids with increasing the quality of life (QoL) and assisting with an autonomous, healthy ageing. This research presents occupations that are an important component of the lives of older people in all the secondary classrooms. This study demonstrates that it is possible to use technologies with an eye on improving the quality of life for older people. At a profound level, elderly people need robots to do more complex tasks. In the future, the research work may be adopted with big data analysis, image processing, and statistical analysis reviewed with comparative analysis of machine learning approach.

AI Robots- the future of technology

Artificial intelligence (AI) is the simulation of human intelligence in machines that programmed to think and act like humans. The machine associated with a human mind such as learning and problem-solving. The ideal characteristic of artificial intelligence is its ability to take action for the best chance of achieving a specific goal. The goals of artificial intelligence are based on learning, reasoning, and perception. Machines use a cross-disciplinary approach based on mathematics, computer science, linguistics, psychology, and more. Key points are as;-

- AI is the simulation of human intelligence in machines.
- The aim of artificial intelligence includes learning, reasoning, and perception.
- AI is used across different industries including finance and healthcare.
- Weak AI tends to be single-task oriented and strong AI is more complex and human-like.

AI Robots

Robotics is a domain in artificial intelligence with the study of creating intelligent and efficient robots. Robots are the artificial agents for the real-world environment. Robots manipulate the objects by perceiving, picking, moving, modifying the physical properties of objects, destroying it, or having an effect thereby freeing manpower from doing repetitive functions without getting bored, distracted, or exhausted. It is a branch of AI composed of Electrical Engineering, Mechanical Engineering, and Computer Science for designing, construction, and application of robots. The robots have mechanical construction designed to accomplish a particular task with power and control of the machinery. They contain some level of a computer program that determines what, when, and how a robot doing things.

Difference in Robot System and AI Program

Here is the difference between the two –

- AI programs operate in computer-simulated worlds. The input of the AI program is in symbols and rules. They need general-purpose computers to operate the programs.
- Robots operate in the real physical world. The Inputs to robots is in analog signal in the form of speech waveform or images. They function with special hardware with sensors and effectors

Robot Locomotion

Locomotion is the mechanism where the robot is capable of moving in its environment. There are various types of locomotions

Legged

This type of locomotion consumes more power while doing walk, jump, trot, hop, climb up or down, etc. It requires several motors to accomplish a movement. It is suited for rough and smooth terrain wherein irregular or too smooth surface it consumes more power for wheeled locomotion. Sometimes it is a little difficult to implement because of stability issues. It comes with a variety of legs that is two, four, or six legs. Leg coordination is necessary for locomotion which has multiple legs. Gaits is a periodic sequence of lift and release events for each of the total legs. The total number of possible gaits where a robot travel depends upon the number of its legs. If a robot has k legs, then the number of possible events N = (2k-1)!. There are six possible different events –

- Lifting the Left leg
- Releasing the Left leg
- Lifting the Right leg

- Releasing the Right leg
- Lifting both the legs together
- Releasing both the legs together

In the case of k=6 legs, there are 39916800 possible events. Hence, the complexity of robots is directly proportional to the number of legs.

Wheeled Locomotion

It requires fewer number of motors to complete a movement. It is easy to implement with less stability issues in case if there is more number of wheels. It is more efficient as compared to legged locomotion. The Standard wheel rotates around the wheel axle and the contact. The Castor wheel rotates around the wheel axle and the offset steering joint. Swedish 45o and Swedish 90o wheels rotate around the contact point, around the wheel axle, and the rollers. Ball or spherical wheel is the Omnidirectional wheel which is difficult to implement technically.

Slip/Skid Locomotion

The robot is steered by moving the tracks with different speeds in the same or opposite direction. It has stability because of the large contact area of track and ground.

Components of a Robot

Robots are constructed with the following –

- Power Supply – The robots are powered by batteries, solar power, hydraulic
- Actuators – It converts energy into movement.
- Electric motors (AC/DC) – Motors are required for rotational movement.
- Pneumatic Air Muscles contract almost 40% when air is sucked in them.
- Muscle Wires contract by 5% when an electric current is passed through them.
- Piezo Motors and Ultrasonic Motors are the best for industrial robots.
- Sensors provide knowledge of the real-time information on the task environment

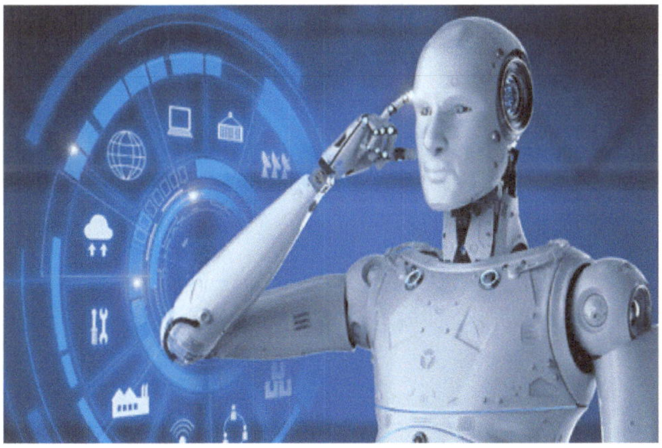

Fig.18.3 Showing the features of a Robot in use

Computer Vision

This is a technology of AI in which the robots can see. Vision plays a crucial role in the domains of safety, security, health, access, and entertainment. It automatically extracts, analyzes, and comprehends useful information from a single image or an array of images. This process accomplishes automatic visual comprehension.

Hardware of Computer Vision System

This involves Power supply, Image acquisition devices such as camera, processor, software, a Display device, accessories such as camera stands, cables, and connectors

Tasks of Computer Vision

- Optical Character Reader is a software to convert scanned documents into editable text, which accompanies a scanner.
- Face Detection comes with this feature, which enables to read the face and take the picture of perfect expression.
- Object Recognition is installed in supermarkets, cameras, high-end cars such as BMW, GM, and Volvo.
- Estimating the Position of an object to the camera as in the position of the tumor in the human body.

Application of Computer Vision

- Agriculture
- Autonomous vehicles
- Biometrics
- Character recognition
- Forensics, security, and surveillance
- Industrial quality inspection
- Face recognition
- Gesture analysis
- Geoscience
- Medical imagery
- Pollution monitoring
- Process control
- Remote sensing
- Robotics
- Transport

Applications of Robotic. The robotics has been instrumental in the various domains such as –

- Industries – Robots are used for handling material, cutting, welding, color coating, drilling, polishing, etc.
- Military – It reaches inaccessible and hazardous zones during the war. A robot named Daksh, developed by DRDO used to destroy life-threatening objects safely.
- Medicine – These robots carry hundreds of clinical tests simultaneously, rehabilitating permanently disabled people, and performing complex surgeries such as brain tumors.
- Exploration – These robots used for space exploration, underwater drones used for ocean exploration.
- Entertainment – Disney's have created hundreds of robots for animated movies.

Using AI to Help Care for Senior Citizens

- Providing Companionship
- Helping Seniors Live Securely and Independently in Their Homes
- Pose Detection for Preventive Care
- Trust Mindy Support for Your Medical Data Annotation Needs

As the world's population gradually becomes older, there is an increasing need to develop new technology to help provide better care for them. In fact, according to a report by the United Nations, there are 703 million people aged 65 and older, a number that is expected to more than double by 2050. Since the population of older adults is growing at such a rapid speed, there are various social, economic, and health challenges that must be addressed. This is an area where AI can be of great assistance since it can help the healthcare system deal with the increased demand for senior healthcare services. In this article, we will take a look at some of the ways AI is helping senior citizens take better care of themselves and maintain their independence.

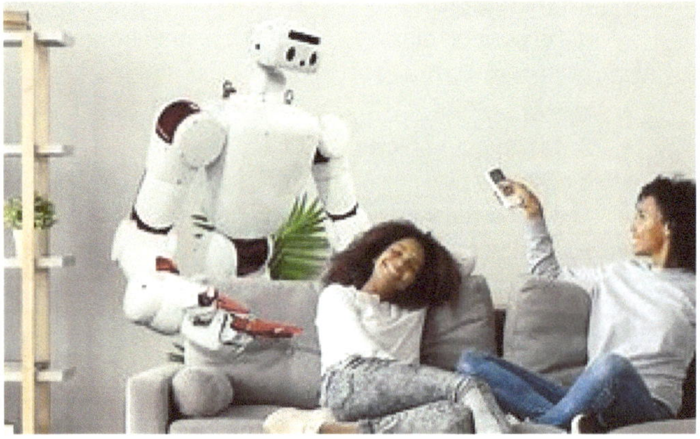

Fig. 18.4 Personal AI-based robots as lifetime human companions

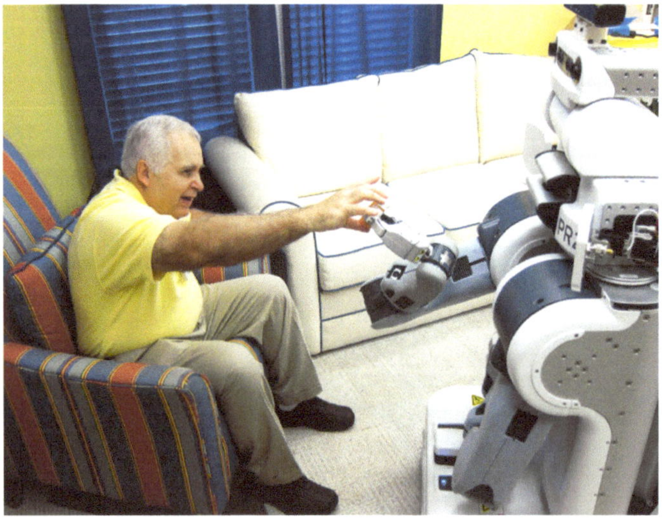

Fig, 18.5 Scientists have created a robot that could help elderly people with dementia and other limitations live independently in their own homes

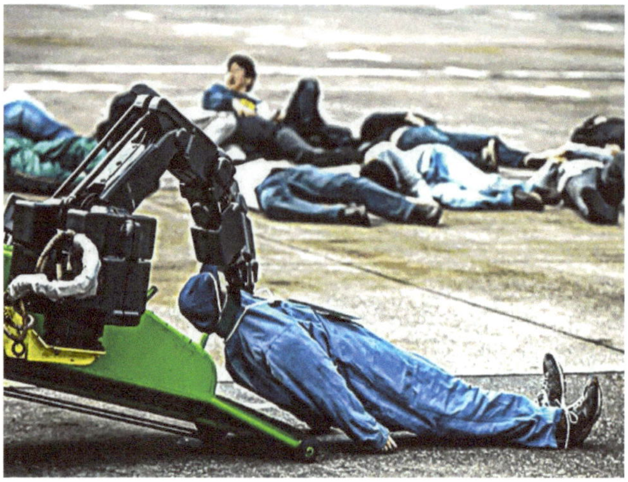

Fig.18.6 Robot is doing rescue-job

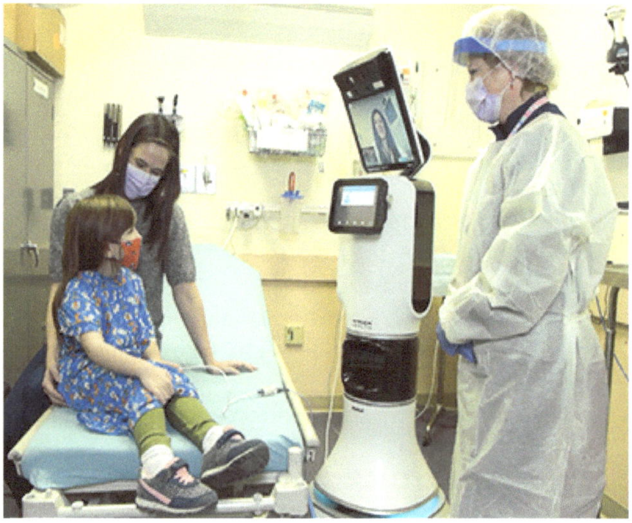

Fig.18.7 New robot helps care for kids in the emergency room

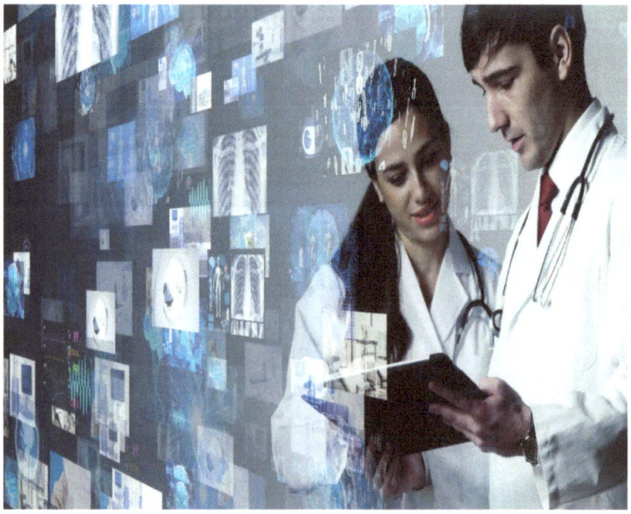

Fig. 18.8 Using AI to Efficiently Diagnose and Reduce Medical Errors

Pose Detection for Preventive Care

Falls are a leading cause of unintentional injuries and can result in devastating disabilities and fatalities when left undetected and not treated in time. In fact, worldwide, falls are a leading cause of unintentional injuries in adults older than 65 years old, with 37.3 million falls requiring medical attention and 646,000 resulting in deaths annually. Human pose detection can play a key role in elderly care for fast responses and preventing seniors from falling. A lot of studies have been done in Japan to create such pose detection software. For example, researchers at the Toyohashi University of Technology have done extensive research into estimating human poses using deep learning with depth data from twin camera systems in elderly care robots. The technology was able to generate data using computer graphics and motion capture technologies various poses that could signal a potential fall within acceptable reliability levels.

While fall prevention products are still being perfected, there are other products on the market, such as For example, in Canada there is a very useful tool called the AltumView's Cypress Smart Home Care Alert System that can call for help if a fall does occur. It can also provide a heat map of an area where falls have frequently occurred. This allows the caregiver to take measures, such as removing certain obstacles or blocking access to that location, to prevent similar accidents from happening again.

Trust Mindy Support for Your Medical Data Annotation Needs

Regardless of whether or not your dataset requires trained medical professionals to do the annotation or such work can be done without a medical background, Mindy Support can assemble a team for you to get the job done. Thanks to our skills and expertise, we can help you actually even the most daring and imaginative products. Contact us today to learn more about how we can help you.

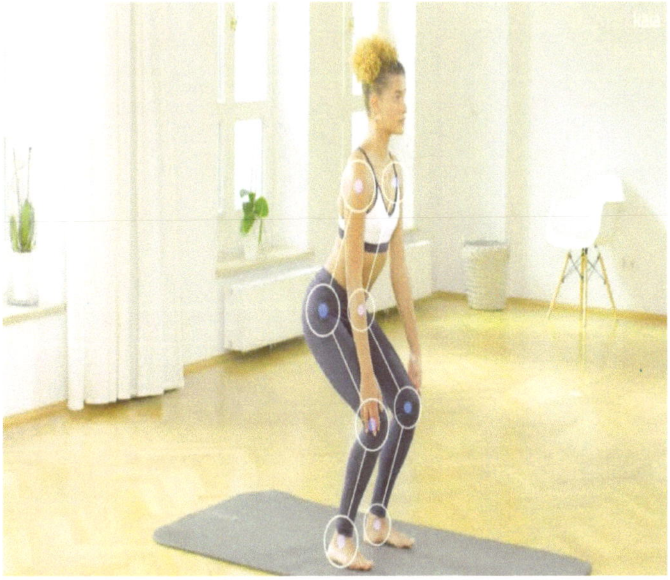

Fig. 18.9 AI Pose Estimation Technology and How You Can Use It

Helping Seniors Live Securely and Independently in Their Homes

According to a report from the AARP, 90% of seniors want to stay in their homes as they age. However, the homes of senior citizens often cannot accommodate their individual needs, posing many risks to their safety and wellness. This is why a lot of seniors in the US us various smart home devices to maintain their independence. This includes activity-based sensors that are connected to a smart security system and can trigger alarms and send help for potential break-ins, fires, and unsafe levels of carbon monoxide.

Another interesting feature is using machine learning to understand a senior's patterns and behaviors. If the system detects a change in their routine, such as the sensor on a medicine cabinet not being triggered when it's time to take a scheduled prescription, the AI spots this break in the pattern and notifies interested parties via email, text, and/or push notifications.

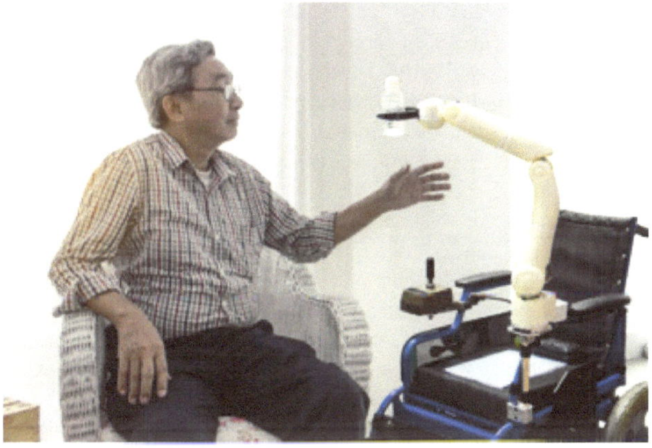

Fig. 18.10 AI Helping Seniors Live Securely and Independently in Their Homes

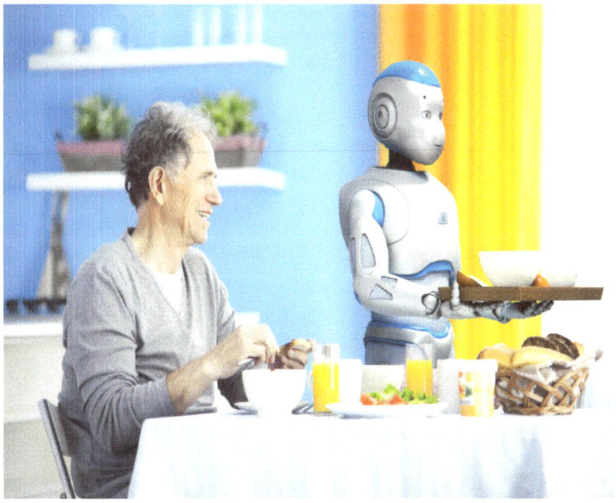

Fig. 18.11 AI Romeo-An Intelligent French Robot To Help Elderly With Daily Tasks

Bibliography and Acknowledgement

- Abubshait, E. Wiese, and Y. L. Human, "You look human, but act like a machine: agent appearance and behavior modulate different aspects of Human-Robot interaction," Frontiers in Psychology, vol. 8, 2017.
- B. Kartal, E. Nunes, J. Godoy, and M. Gini, "Monte Carlo tree search with branch and bound for multi-robot task allocation symposium conducted at the meeting of the the IJCAI-16 workshop on autonomous mobile service robots," vol. 30, no. 1, 2016.
- B. Zohuri and M. Moghaddam, "Neural network driven supper artificial intelligence based on internet of things and big data," Business Resilience System (BRS), vol. 1, 2018.
- D. SverreSyrdal, J. Saunders, and K. DautenhahnK. L. Koay and N. Burke, ""Teach me–show me""'—"end-user personalization of a smart home and comrade robot"," IEEE transactions on Human Machine Systems, vol. 46, no. 1, 2016.
  Davison, Introduction to Robotics, Department of Computing, Imperial College, London, UK, 2016.
- F. Al-Turjman and J. P. Lemayian, "Intelligence, security, and vehicular sensor networks in internet of things (IoT)-enabled smart-cities: an overview," Computers & Electrical Engineering, vol. 87, Article ID 106776, 2020.
- G. Viejo, D. D. Torrico, F. R. Dunshea, and S. Fuentes, "Development of artificial neural network models to assess beer acceptability based on sensory properties using a robotic pourer: a comparative model approach to achieve an artificial intelligence system," Beverages, vol. 5, 2019.
- G. Yang, Z. Pang, M. J. Deen et al., "Homecare robotic systems for healthcare 4.0: visions and enabling technologies," IEEE Journal of Biomedical and Health Informatics, vol. 24, pp. 2535–2549, 2020.
- H. Ashrafian, A. Darzi, and T. Athanasiou, "A novel modification of the Turing test for artificial intelligence and robotics in healthcare," International Journal of Medical Robotics and Computer Assisted Surgery, vol. 11, pp. 38–43, 2015.
- H. BozU. Kose, "Emotion extraction from facial expressions by using artificial intelligence techniques," Broad Research in Artificial Intelligence and Neuroscience, vol. 8, pp. 5–16, 2017.
- H. Manoharan, Y. Teekaraman, P. R. Kshirsagar, S. Sundaramurthy, and A. Manoharan, "Examining the effect of aquaculture using sensor-based technology with machine learning algorithm," Aquaculture Research, vol. 51, no. 11, pp. 4748–4758, 2020.
- J. Celis, S. Castro, and D. Guevara, "Voice processing with Internet of Things for a home automation system," in Proceedings of the International conference on Electronics, Electrical engineering and computing, pp. 8–10, IEEE, Lima, Peru, August 2018.
- J. Cowie, "Evaluation of a digital consultation and self-care advice tool in primary care: a multi-methods study," Inter. Jour.of Environ Res Public Health, vol. 15, 2018.
- J. Sensmeier, "Harnessing the power of artificial intelligence," Nursing Management, vol. 48, no. 11, pp. 14–19, 2017.
- K. Hameed, I. S. Bajwa, S. Ramzan, W. Anwar, and A. Khan, "An intelligent IoT based healthcare system using fuzzy neural networks," Scientific Programming, vol. 2020, Article ID 8836927, 15 pages, 2020.
- L. Pu, W. Moyle, C. Jones, and M. Todorovic, "The effectiveness of social robots for older adults: a systematic review and meta-analysis of randomized controlled studies," Gerontologist Jan, vol. 59, no. 1, pp. e37–51, 2019.
- M. M. A. D. Graaf, S. B. Allouch, and J. A. G. M. V. Dijk, "Why would I use this in my home? a model of domestic social robot acceptance," Human-Computer Interaction, vol. 34, pp. 115–173, 2019.
- M. Mortazavi, F. Aminiazad, H. Parsaei, and M. A. Mosleh-Shirazi, "An artificial neural network-based model for predicting annual dose in healthcare workers occupationally exposed to different levels of ionizing radiation," Radiation Protection Dosimetry, vol. 189, 2020.
- M. Sg, T. Ak, A. St, S. Sv, and O. Mj, "Role of artificial intelligence in health care," Biochemistry Ind Journal, vol. 11, no. 5, pp. 1–14, 2017.
- Mesko, "The role of artificial intelligence in precision medicine," Expert Rev Precis Med Drug Dev, vol. 2, pp. 239–241, 2017.
- P. R. Kshirsagar, H. Manoharan, F. Al-Turjman, and K. Kumar, "Design and testing of automated smoke monitoring sensors in vehicles," IEEE Sensors Journal, vol. 1, p. 1, 2020.
- P.-P. C. F. Rudzicz and S. Raimondo, "Ludwig: a conversational robot for people with alzheimer's," The Journal of the Alzheimer's Association, vol. 13, 2017.
- R. Bhatnagar and D. Batra, "Robotic process automation in healthcare-a review," International Robotics & Automation Journal, vol. 5, 2019.
- S. Montani, R. Bellazzi, A. Riva, C. Larizza, L. Portinale, and M. Stefanelli, "Artificial intelligence techniques for diabetes management: the T-IDDM project. ECAI," in Proceedings of the 14th European conerence on Artificial Intelligence, pp. 1–5, Berlin, Germany, August 2000.
- W. Moyle, C. Jones, L. Pu, and S. C. Chen, "Applying user-centred research design and evidence to develop and guide the use of technologies, including robots, in aged care," Contemporary Nurse, vol. 54, pp. 1–3, 2018.
- W. Yu, A. Kapusta, J. Tan, C. C. Kemp, G. Turk, and C. K. Liu, "Haptic simulation for robot-assisted dressing," in Proceedings of the IEEE International Conference on Robotics and Automation, pp. 6044–6051, Singapore, May 2017

CHAPTER

19

Emerging Role of Artificial Intelligence in Cardiac Electrophysiology

The 1956 Dartmouth Summer Research Project on Artificial Intelligence introduced the term "artificial intelligence" (AI) on the assumption that human intelligence "can be so precisely described that a machine can be made to simulate it . The term "machine learning" (ML) was defined in 1959 by Arthur Samuel, who stated, "Programming computers to learn from experience should eventually eliminate the need for much of this detailed programming effort. In ML, AI systems "learn" from the data that they are provided, complementing the original ideas of encoding "intelligence" into the AI system.

The ML process may be "supervised" or "unsupervised" .In supervised learning, the machine is provided a set of labeled images as a source of truth, for instance electrocardiograms (ECG) labeled as sinus rhythm or atrial fibrillation (AF). For this approach to succeed, the right number of image features need to be identified, to accurately distinguish between right and wrong answers while not overfitting the model (being too specific) to this image set.This task of feature extraction can be prone to incompleteness or error. In contrast, unsupervised learning methods build the feature set by themselves, surfacing whatever they find of significance. For instance, the machine model may organize itself to find clinical factors in patient history that lead to a greater propensity for sudden cardiac death (SCD). These processes can be further refined by reinforcement learning, where the machine interacts with the environment and attempts to find an optimal way to achieve a desired goal. For instance, a drug treatment regimen model interacts with the "environment" (patient sub-phenotypes based on prior treatment regimens) to optimize treatments for individual patients. The efficiency of this model is improved by dimensionality reduction, which reduces the number of input factors to the most significant set in predicting desired outcomes. For example, to predict risk of AF, the model may start with multiple clinical factors, and finally identify only a few factors that are most important. This can make the model more user friendly.

Deep learning (DL) employs artificial neural networks inspired by the structure and functioning of the human brain. It is especially useful where the data are "unstructured"—such as images and text. Each layer (effectively, a step in a series) in the network performs a task, which is propagated to the next layer in the network . There can be feedback to each layer from its downstream layer, to make adjustments. Iterations continue until the output has reached an acceptable level of accuracy. The number of processing layers through which data must pass is what inspired the term DL. For example, DL may be used to train AI models to recognize cardiac chambers or areas of abnormal cardiac tissue like myocardial scar or fibrosis from cardiac magnetic resonance imaging (MRI). Both ML and DL techniques depend on ingesting large amounts of data and employing statistical and predictive modeling techniques. A basic tenet of AI models is that even within 1 form of modeling, there may be many methods available. A collaboration with data scientists may help select the most appropriate model for the existing setting (eg, rare conditions with sparse data, or complex conditions or time to diagnosis in underserved communities). They may potentially even combine predictions from several models into 1 prediction using specialized techniques

Cardiac electrophysiology (EP) presents a unique opportunity where device industry has a vast amount of patient data. Clinical providers are now forming partnerships that allow such data to be combined with the rest of the clinical records. Analyzing such big data in innovative ways can potentially provide insights and help make superior predictions about the behavior of complex systems, such as progression of AF or risk of SCD in a patient. While employing this general AI methodology, it is important to ensure that the data themselves are representative of the patient population where the AI models are to be deployed.

AI framework in EP

AI and ML have a huge potential in the field of cardiac EP, where current patient data including ECG; information from wearables, smart devices, and implantable devices; and cardiac imaging may improve our understanding of

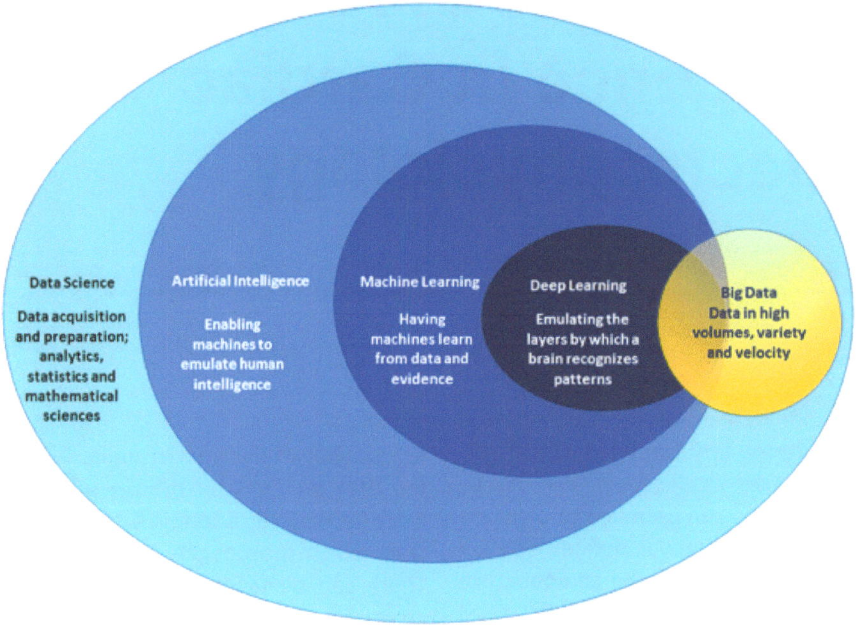

Fig. 19.1 Positioning of disciplines commonly associated under the rubric of "AI." This includes data science, artificial intelligence, machine learning, deep learning, and big data. Data velocity refers to the speed in which data are generated, distributed, and collected.

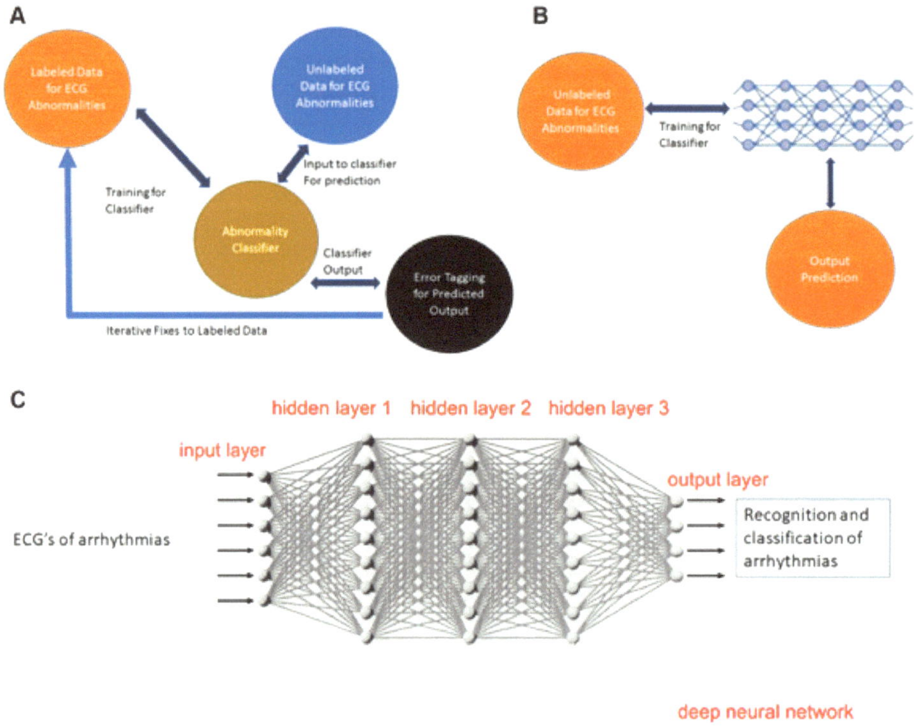

Fig.19.2 A: Supervised learning: The data for electrocardiogram (ECG) abnormality is labeled with human oversight and then used to train a classifier. Unlabeled data can then be classified by the classifier and the errors in classification can be measured with human oversight. Additional labeled data may be added to augment the Training Data to reduce error. An example would be classification of an abnormal rhythm (atrial fibrillation) from wearable devices using photoplethysmography in real time, after having been trained on labeled simulated signals. B: Unsupervised learning: The data for ECG is not labeled; many layers of the deep learning system iteratively learn the features and keep iteratively reducing the error with each run. C: Deep learning: ECGs of arrhythmias go through many layers of the deep learning system, which iteratively learns the features of arrhythmias and keeps reducing the error with each run to recognize and classify arrhythmias appropriately.

, risk prediction, and personalized treatment for arrhythmias like AF.Advanced imaging and mapping techniques can be used to accurately identify ablation targets and improve invasive and noninvasive treatment of arrhythmias. Multifactor data, with suitable computing and AI support, provide models for clinical and surgical decision support. The assembled data need human annotations to be AI-ready, especially in medical applications, where supervised learning dominates. Over time and with more data, the machine learns and classifies data patterns much better with the annotations. A critical challenge in an emerging AI domain like EP is that only a few institutions have systematically collected sufficient data to create rich, robust models for clinical EP applications. Traditionally, such data have not been shared among centers owing to HIPAA compliance and preserving patient privacy. This creates an opportunity for EP to establish data-sharing standards and build relationships to create a new future for AI-enabled clinical medicine. AI models are much more difficult to create, and less impactful, when they are built on multiple small islands of data that are not co-located. Federated learning has emerged as an alternative where models learn from data that are distributed and shared in a restrictive way, so that patient privacy is maintained

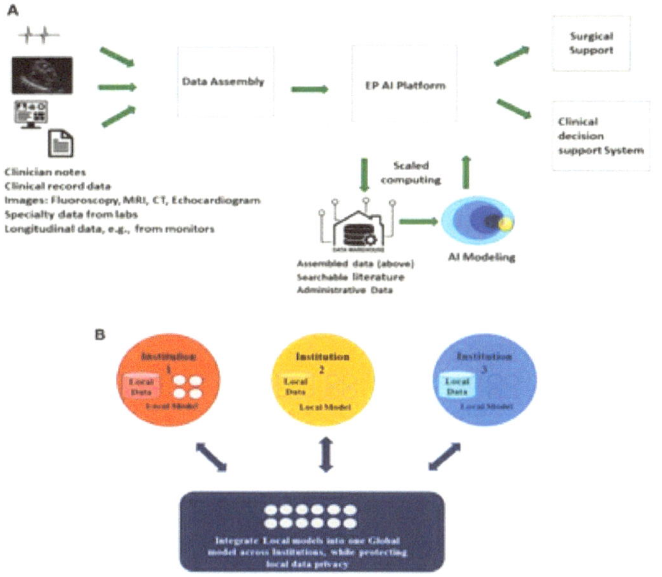

Fig.19.3 A: An artificial intelligence (AI) framework for clinical decision support in electrophysiology. Data from multiple sources are assembled, annotated, and processed by advanced computing and AI platform to generate models for clinical and surgical/procedural decision support. B: Federated data and modeling. In order to overcome restrictions on sharing of patients' private data between institutions, models learn in a distributed fashion from data that are distributed and shared in a restrictive way.

AI and ECG

Although the ECG itself is nearly a century old, advances in computing power and the availability of digital ECG data with clinical linkage have fostered a renaissance for this humble diagnostic test. In general, the application of AI to the ECG can be seen as serving 2 main goals: (to create workflow efficiencies by performing human-like tasks in ECG interpretation (standard ECG annotation), or to add value to the ECG through extending human capability by using the physiologic signal for risk stratification, disease screening, or detection of noncardiac conditions. Toward the former goal, the AI "sees" discernible patterns on the ECG in order to help cardiologists perform routine tasks; in the latter, the AI "sees beyond" human capability. The capacity for AI to perform human-like ECG interpretation has been demonstrated by several groups on single-lead and 12-lead ECG interpretation at times outperforming standard analog software. The ability to "see beyond" the human eye has been demonstrated by models that can detect patient sex or age, or even detect diseases that may not have a pathognomonic ECG signature, such as cardiac amyloidosis, pulmonary hypertension, aortic stenosis, hypertrophic cardiomyopathy, AF risk, concealed long QT syndrome, COVID- or low ejection fraction. Some of these models have been tested in prospective trials, while others are in earlier stages of development. As the clinical utility of these models becomes better established, next phases include validating them across multicenter datasets and integrating them into systems to make them available at the at the point of care. These models may be integrated intoan "AI-ECG dashboard" that is linked from within the system's electronic health record. This dashboard allows real-time AI analysis of all existing ECG data

AI and arrhythmia detection/prediction with wearables and smart devices

Technological innovations in mobile technology, including the production of wearables and smart devices, have created opportunities to measure physiologic data relevant to heart rhythm health. The widespread access to and consumer appeal of these devices has created a plethora of available data broadly accessible to the healthcare enterprise, including optical sensor–derived photoplethysmography (PPG) signals, ECGs, and accelerometers that enable measurement of physical activity. AI has potentially several clinical uses when applied tophysiologic data from wearables or smart devices—classification of physiological data into clinically interpretable information, identification of disease states and prediction of future diseases, and clinical decision support. Examples of classification of physiologic data include the analysis of pulse waveform data from PPG that can infer the presence of an irregular heart rhythm,21 which has been studied most extensively for AF to date.22 Software operating on devices can further enable linkage of individuals to the healthcare enterprise. Algorithms coupled with PPG and pedometer data have been validated in a few studies for detecting AF.23,24 Newer active contact-free facial and fingertip plethysmography on smartphone cameras have shown potential for AF screening and diagnosis.

AI algorithms applied to ECG data exhibit high discrimination for cardiac rhythms, including those measured using single-lead ECG patch monitors26 or mobile cardiac telemetry.27 Translating these exciting discoveries into improvements in clinical outcomes requires rigorous validation of algorithms, integration of data with the healthcare system, augmentation of existing clinical workflows, and robust access by patients. For consumer technology in particular, some aspects remain challenging, including ensuring that patients can effectively communicate results with providers28 as well as providing healthcare providers with formal guidance on the clinical use of mobile technology results with clinical care. AI incorporation has reached new horizons with the start of the COVID-19 pandemic. Recent innovations such as the TeleCheck-AF project, home antiarrhythmic drug loading with smartphone tracings, and smartphone ECG surveillance are a few great examples.AI algorithms that are applied to individual tracings, obtained from an ECG or PPG, for instance, examine only a small fraction of the available clinical data. It is likely that with time, broader models will be developed to aggregate data from multiple sensors as well as structured and unstructured data from the electronic health record, or other sources. In a recent study, AF prediction was significantly improved with the combination of clinical risk factors and AI-based ECG analysis

AI in the management of cardiac implantable devices

Pacemakers and implantable cardioverter-defibrillators (ICDs) contain a wealth of therapeutic and diagnostic features. In particular, cardiac resynchronization therapy (CRT) devices and ICDs track variables that are known to correlate with worsening heart failure. Further, many patients with these devices are at risk for atrial and ventricular arrhythmias. The ability to predict and manage arrhythmias and heart failure events has significant implications for patients' care, and the volume and complexity of the data makes it a prime area to benefit from AI.In a successful risk factor model, 37 electrogram-based parameters from ICD data were successfully used to predict the risk of electrical storm.33 Although this is useful for only short-term prediction of ventricular tachycardia (VT) storm events, it is an important example of how the high-value data cardiovascular implantable electronic devices generate can be harnessed by ML, even in the absence of clinical parameters.Remote monitoring has been shown to be as effective as in-clinic device checks for patients with pacemakers and ICDs and has shown to reduce shocks, facilitate early detection of device malfunction, and improve mortality. It is challenging for programs to manage the large volume of data that these systems generate.In addition to the high burden and quality of the data, different manufacturers have distinct algorithms and institutions have various mechanisms for collecting and managing these data, which makes this another important area to benefit from AI. Rosier and colleagues were able to show that a system that integrated patient's medical history with pacemaker alert notifications was able to reduce the notification workload by 84%. Another study demonstrated that application of a 2-part AI filter to implantable loop recorder AF alerts was able to reduce the false-positive rate by more than 60%.Work is ongoing to devise ways to use AI to manage heart failure alerts more effectively.

There has been considerable work to create ML models to predict response to CRT. Using the data from the major CRT trials, successful supervised learning and unsupervised learning models have been created. While many of these are complex to employ, a naïve Bayesian classifier that predicts CRT response using 9 variables led to the design of publicly available calculator and can be used in shared decision-making.

AI in ablation and mapping

During an ablation procedure, there is an exceptionally high information input: patient history, previous recordings, real-time navigation, electrograms, ablation parameters, ablation impact, and clinical follow-up. Historical description of intracardiac electrograms has been mono- or pauci-parametric: voltage amplitude, frequency, number of deflections, visually recognizable morphologies, or sequences. There is significant interobserver variation in the interpretation and significance of individual electrograms. While good targets are nearly impossible to describe with mono-parametric linear models, the ML/DL multiparametric nonlinear models are ideally suited to find outcome-relevant targets and treat patients. Multicenter randomized clinical trials are needed to demonstrate the usefulness of such analytical tools on the long-term outcomes of arrhythmia ablation. For example, one study is testing the hypothesis that the catheter ablation (CA) of ML/DL-adjudicated electrogram locations in addition to pulmonary vein isolation (PVI) is superior to PVI alone for patients in persistent AF .

In order to develop such AI capabilities for mapping and ablation, it is important for centers to pool data and help train expert systems using information about the patient (age, sex, race, and comorbidities), centers (multiple practices and operators), and equipment (mapping systems, recording systems, and catheters). AI and ML can establish outcome prediction models for arrhythmia interventions such as AF CA. Recently, AI was used to study the prognostic potential of left atrial wall stress in AF recurrence after CA . A DL model using preablation pulmonary vein computed tomography predicted AF trigger origins with good reliability. Beyond atrial arrhythmias, ML has been applied to the detection and mapping of ventricular arrhythmias and to predicting the outcomes of cardiovascular implantable electronic device therapies.

ML algorithms were shown to have excellent sensitivity and specificity for premature ventricular contraction detection and reliable localization of VT. Prediction of complications of arrhythmias can also benefit from AI owing to its ability to establish 3-dimensional structural models such as the left atrial appendage. A statistical shape analysis can provide further quantitative assessment of left atrial appendage shape and its association with stroke risk in AF patients. Lastly, novel intracardiac mapping modules incorporating ML were also reported in recent years to accurately reconstruct left atrial and pulmonary vein anatomy during AF ablation.

Synergistic application of ML and personalized computational modeling in arrhythmias and EP

The application of ML in arrhythmia and EP requires typically large datasets curated for specific applications. There are several practical obstacles to collecting and making medical data available to the AI community, including legal and ethical issues. Personalized computational modeling offers an attractive alternative to overcome these challenges and limitations. In contrast to traditional ML, in this form of AI, computer systems construct a personalized virtual-heart model (also referred to as a digital twin of the patient's heart) that is unique to the patient and requires only 1 clinical scan. This model is used to assess the arrhythmogenic propensity of the patient's disease-remodeled substrate. It is typically based on cardiac imaging that visualizes the individual geometry and disease remodeling of the heart, such as the distribution of scar and fibrosis in the ventricles and atria. Patient data can be combined with the results of computational modeling of patients' arrhythmogenic propensity, as such results, when generated by personalized computational models of patients' hearts, can be inexpensive to obtain. Furthermore, including results of computational modeling imparts mechanistic underpinning to the resulting AI model. As an application, computational modeling has been used for noninvasive prediction of the targets of ablation of VT and persistent AF, and for assessing arrhythmia risk in patients with ischemic cardiomyopathy and repaired tetralogy of Fallot. Mechanistic computational modeling of the heart in an AI model presents novel precision technologies to predict risk of ventricular arrhythmias in patients with cardiac sarcoidosis54 and risk of AF recurrence following PVI in patients with paroxysmal AF . A supervised multivariable classifier learned both from the results of mechanistic modeling and from clinical and imaging biomarkers to predict clinical outcome. For instance, in the cardiac sarcoid study by Shade and colleagues,54 the mechanistic computational model was a novel MRI–positron emission tomography fusion model that assessed the arrhythmogenic propensity of the remodeled substrate incorporating fibrosis infiltration and inflammation. The combination with ML resulted in the creation of the Computational Heart and Artificial Intelligence (CHAI) Risk Predictor for patients with cardiac sarcoidosis

and risk of AF recurrence following PVI in patients with paroxysmal AF.55 A supervised multivariable classifier learned both from the results of mechanistic modeling and from clinical and imaging biomarkers to predict clinical outcome. For instance, in the cardiac sarcoid study by Shade and colleagues, the mechanistic computational model was a novel MRI–positron emission tomography fusion model that assessed the arrhythmogenic propensity of the remodeled substrate incorporating fibrosis infiltration and inflammation. The combination with ML resulted in the creation of the Computational Heart and Artificial Intelligence (CHAI) Risk Predictor for patients with cardiac sarcoidosis. Personalized heart models of arrhythmogenesis were constructed using late gadolinium-enhanced MRI and positron emission tomography scans of the patient, and validated with clinical ablation data. Once the model was validated, features extracted from simulation results were combined with those extracted from imaging and other clinical data and fed into CHAI. In a cohort of 45 patients, the predictor achieved a balanced sensitivity and specificity and an excellent area under the receiver operating characteristic curve. In this proof-of-concept study, the CHAI results demonstrate that the technology outperformed clinical metrics in predicting risk of SCD in these patients.

A similar approach was used in a study predicting preprocedurally the risk of AF recurrence post-PVI in paroxysmal AF patients, where personalized atrial models were constructed from late gadolinium-enhanced MRI scans, and results of simulations of AF inducibility were used in a classifier together with other clinical data. These recent studies illustrate how the 2 approaches can be used synergistically and to overcome concerns over clinical decisions being informed by "black-box" algorithms that lack explainability. Such technologies pave the way for the use of integrative approaches in precision medicine that predict adverse events in complex diseases with a high degree of accuracy and mechanistic underpinning.

AI in precision medicine

Next-generation sequencing technologies have greatly increased the availability of whole genome sequencing and high-resolution array genotyping and led to improvements in our understanding of the genetic basis for cardiovascular and arrhythmia disorders. The fulfillment of the promise of precision medicine to deliver patient-specific treatment for arrhythmias requires the synthesis and interpretation of data from multiple sources, including medical history, lifestyle and mobile health data, and rhythm monitoring data, as well as genomics, proteomics and metabolomics.56 The complexity and speed of this data accumulation makes it impractical for human-based analysis, particularly in the field of EP. ML is particularly suited to handle the tasks of integrating this wealth of clinical data with genetic data to inform disease classification, diagnosis, and treatment. Genomics, which seeks to correlate genotype and phenotype, identify biomarkers for patient stratification, and predict gene function, has become a dominant application for DL in healthcareThe range of potential applications of AI to drive precision medicine in EP is broad. For example, ML algorithms have been applied to identify abnormal calcium transient profiles in induced pluripotent stem cell–derived cardiomyocytes harboring mutations in genes associated with catecholaminergic polymorphic VT, long QT syndrome, and hypertrophic cardiomyopathy with classification accuracies of up to 87%.59 This could enhance efforts not only on genotype-phenotype correlation, but also on rapid examination of drug effects to guide treatment. Schmitz and colleagues61 examined the utility of 15 different ML algorithms that integrated both clinical and genetic parameters for the prediction of positive left ventricularremodeling with CRT. An optimal rule-based decision tree algorithm that incorporated clinical data and genotypes of genetic loci (eg, GNB3 rs5443 allele) predicted CRT response with >82.5% accuracy. Similar efforts to integrate genetic information to predict efficacy of antiarrhythmic drug therapy and CA procedures for arrhythmia therapy may be enhanced with ML. AF, which is often the end result of a complex interplay between genetic, clinical, and environmental factors, is one disease that may be best poised to be managed with the aid of ML-derived deep phenotyping and treatment optimization.

AI and SCD prediction

It is well recognized that the current risk stratification models for SCD risk are very limited in determining ICD candidacy in patients with both structurally normal and abnormal hearts.

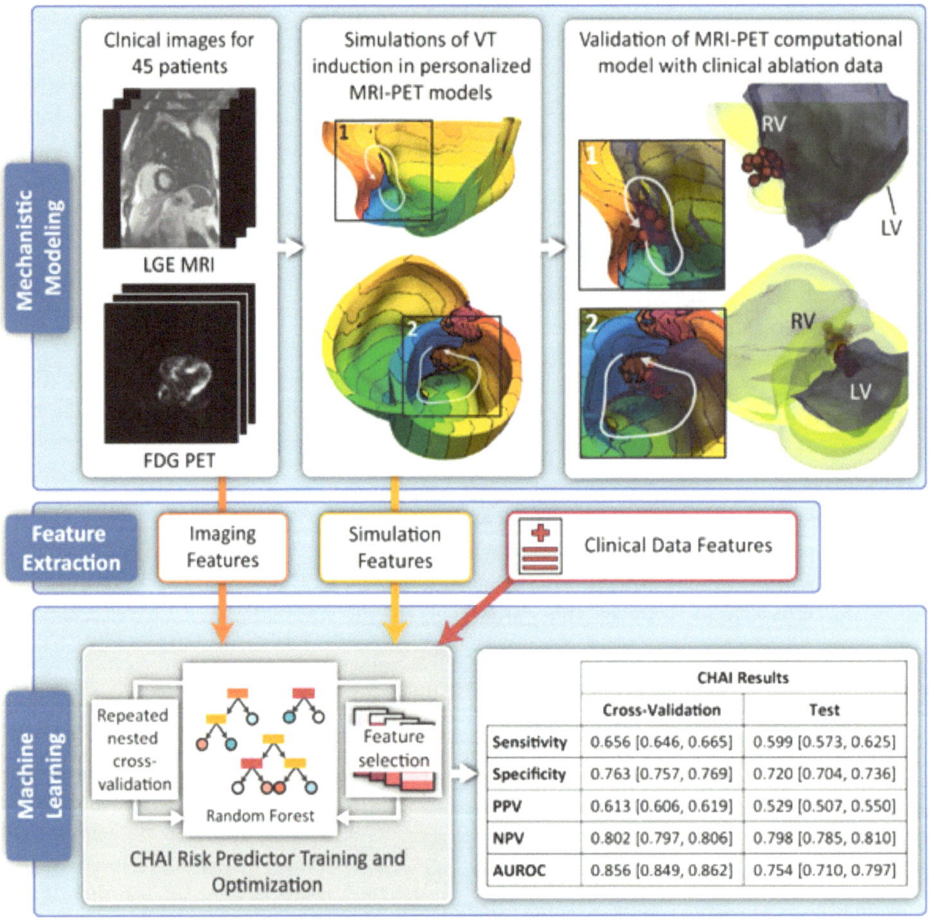

Fig.19.4 Overview of Computational Heart and Artificial Intelligence (CHAI) Risk Predictor Study. Top panel, left: Magnetic resonance imaging–positron emission tomography (MRI-PET) fusion models were created for 45 patients. Each model incorporates patient-specific ventricular geometry and spatial distributions of fibrosis and inflammation. Top panel, middle: Simulations of ventricular tachycardia (VT) induction were performed in each model. Isochrone lines represent activation times; line spacing is 22.5 ms. White arrows indicate reentry pathways. Top panel, right: Electroanatomic geometry (gray) is registered to computational model geometry (green) with clinical ablation lesions (red circles); insets show reentry pathways and ablation lesions. Bottom panel, left: Features from imaging, simulations, and clinical data are used as input to a supervised random forest classifier to predict risk of clinical VT. Bottom panel, right: Cross-validation and test results are aggregated over 560 iterations of nested cross-validation. Results are presented as mean [95% confidence interval]. AUROC = area under the receiver operation characteristic curve; FDG PET = 18[F]-fluorodeoxyglucose positron emission tomography; LGE-MRI

There has been significant interest in developing better risk stratification models for risk of SCD using AI algorithms to harvest large population datasets.

Various ML algorithms have been developed by different groups to predict the risk of SCD in individuals using clinical and demographic variables, ECG and Holter parameters, intracardiac electrogram characteristics derived from ICDs imaging parameters from echocardiograms, MRIs and nuclear cardiac imaging, and even cellular phenotypes such as ventricular monophasic action potentials.67 The models use these parameters solely, or in different combinations as a multivariable classifier for SCD risk prediction, and have achieved variable successes with a wide range of areas under thecurve .

Apart from SCD risk prediction for individuals, there have also been attempts to use AI algorithms to temporally predict a higher risk of SCD in populations using complex meteorological and chronological data, showing that risk of SCD was higher with sudden temperature drops and on certain days of the week.Many of these algorithms serve as a proof of concept, demonstrating the capability of advanced computing and AI algorithms to derive patterns from extremely complex data. However, they are not close to clinical adoption at this time and require further prospective studies to pave the way for AI-guided risk stratification for SCD and determination of ICD candidacy.

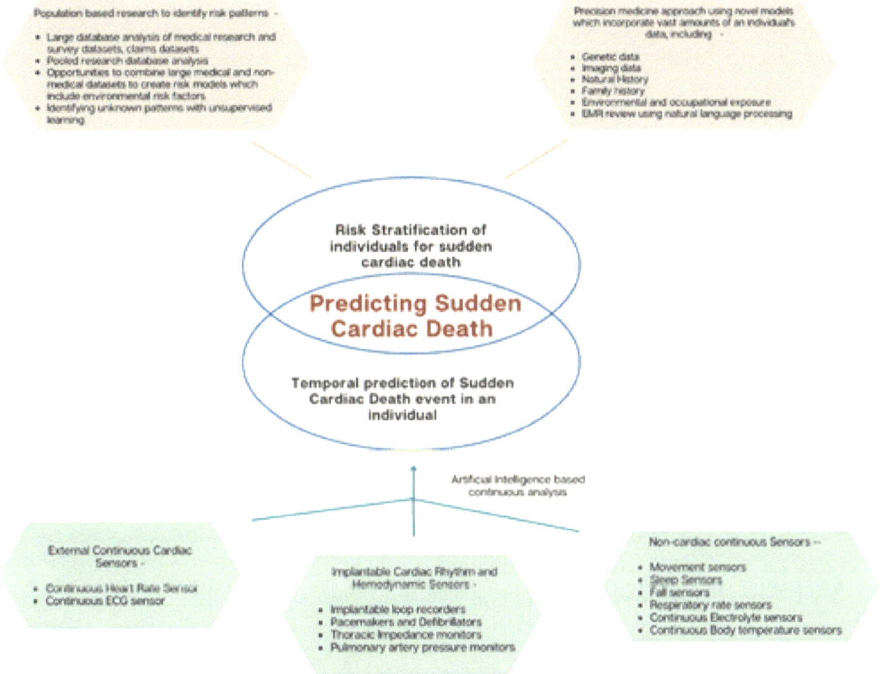

Fig.19.5 Artificial intelligence model for prediction of sudden cardiac death using multiple inputs. ECG = electrocardiogram; EMR = electronic medical records.

Regulatory framework and challenges for AI in EP

AI has the potential for significant impact on diagnosis and treatment of heart rhythm disorders and democratized care, but only if devices and software using AI can successfully navigate the US regulatory process. The Division of Digital Heath works interactively with the device-specific offices and stakeholders to discuss and develop policy and guidelines to support review of Software as a Medical Device (SaMD) submissions, including AI and ML. The US Food & Drug Administration's (FDA) AI/ML SaMD Action Plan includes novel proposals like software precertification, predetermined change control, good ML practices, and real-world performance monitoring. Important FDA guidance has been issued for Clinical Decision Support software and Mobile Medical Applications.Within the EP space, diagnostic software most commonly uses AI, and these products are primarily regulated as Class II SaMD devices. The pathway to market is either a 510(k) submission or de novo request.. Developers may tune their Indications For Use, clinical utility claims, and patient population to optimize the regulatory process and level of evidence required to support a marketing application. Staged development strategies and presubmission interactions with the FDA are recommended.Training and validation of data sources is a big challenge. The FDA expects studies to represent the US population, cover the intended patient group, have independent training/validation sources, and include prespecified analysis and endpoints.

Table 19.1 Important challenges/obstacles to translating artificial intelligence to clinical practice and suggestions for overcoming them

Challenges and obstacles	Potential approaches
1. Lack of transparency (black box analyses) inhibits clinician uptake	Correlation analyses can sometimes help improve transparency. Use of new approaches, such as gradient-weighted class activation mapping, can help provide a level of interpretability.
2. Lack of validation and reproducibility in independent data sets	As the main reason behind this challenge is lack of access to independent data sets, any approaches that facilitate consistent data sharing would help alleviate the problem. For example, journals could require data be made public and provide a unified service that is HIPAA compliant and gives authorized users access.
3. Implementation in the EHR may be inhibited by regulatory requirements for clinical use	FDA review and advances mayacilitate approval steps.
4.Need for strong technical teams, including data scientists, computer scientists, analysts; attracting skilled personnel to academics and medicine can be difficult, as industry offers	Increase training pipelines. Provide institutional incentives for multidisciplinary approaches. Create and facilitate access to AI consulting services within each institution. Incorporate AI in medical training.
5 Need for large, harmonized quality data sets with representation of normal and abnormal examples and representation of data from diverse populations to avoid bias; HIPAA and need to preserve patient privacy can inhibit availability of large data sets for development	FDA National Evaluation System for health technology initiative – aims to establish accessible data networks, including device registries, EHR, claims databases, and patient-generated health data.

AI = artificial intelligence; EHR = electronic health records.

Solutions include the FDA's National Evaluation System for Health Technology initiative, which is working to establish accessible data networks, including device registries, electronic health records, claims databases, and patient-generated health data. Coordination, cooperation, and linking of data sources by all EP SaMD stakeholders in an open and accessible network could accelerate the development and regulatory approval of EP SaMD incorporating AI. Limitations of AI in cardiac EP Despite unparalleled advancement in AI across numerous healthcare domains, a number of limitations are present . Large and diverse data sets with representation of normal and abnormal examples are required to increase both accuracy and generalizability of working models. The quality of the data is critical and the input data must reflect some level of heterogeneity to promote an iterative process. ML can also have errors or unexpected results. One of the more difficult concerns with AI in clinical EP is that algorithms can perform quite well during a test fit (training period) but when applied to the actual test set there is poor generalizability. This concept of "overfitting" within these very complex computational algorithms can be addressed by providing high-quality data at the time of training, careful monitoring of the training, and ensuring anoptimal balance on the bias-variance trade-off curve. Furthermore, these complex computer results are mired by a certain level of opaqueness or black-box nature where it is challenging to understand how the result was generated. To achieve clinical usefulness and adoption of these algorithms for patient care, the development of explainable AI models, larger-scale multicenter controlled studies and thorough external validation of these algorithms are needed. Another limitation, especially in DL, relates to the challenge of integrating often complementary but separately obtained data on the same patient.

How can MRI, nuclear testing, ECG, and imaging all be used in a large data set to create a functioning algorithm when the data points were obtained at varying time points? Large data sets should also bridge institutions, as the more complete and versatile data sets entered will establish better models. As always, AI should serve as an aid rather than a mandated voice to change clinical course. Clinicians should cautiously embrace the paradigm shift toward AI while striving to improve the computational models. No data set is valid and ready for AI without the right balance of data from diverse populations. It is well known that demographics, socioeconomics, genetics, and case histories can have an impact on the patient's situation. The ethical collection and use of data are fundamental tenets of AI in medicine

Table. 19.2 Future directions of artificial intelligence in electrophysiology and proposed studies to advance toward these future directions

Future directions	Approaches
1. Centralized global data collection, collation, and access to improve the accuracy and efficiency of many algorithms and processes	Greater collaboration and coordination among clinician scientists, professional societies, medical institutions, research organizations, and regulatory bodies, driven by governments and appropriate legislations to promote easy and open data exchange
2. Upstream primary prevention and downstream secondary prevention models for disease management using genetic, molecular, demographic, clinical, and environmental data	Consider focusing on individual diseases with a broader interlinking as one makes incremental progress in unlocking the pathophysiology and disease evolution
3. Creation of robust infrastructure that facilitates open, accessible platform	Interlinking of electronic medical records and epidemiological data with appropriate regulatory oversight

Future directions of AI clinical electrophysiology

We stand at the precipice of a digital revolution that will forever change the landscape of EP. Although significant progress has been made in diagnostics and therapeutics, there are many gaps in our understanding of pathophysiology, risk stratification, and prevention. As outlined earlier in this manuscript, the medical field needs more collaboration in centralized global data collection, collation, and access to improve the accuracy and efficiency of many algorithms and processes. Upstream primary prevention and downstream secondary prevention models for disease management using genetic, molecular, demographic, clinical, and environmental data is an important directive for the future. This provides a real opportunity for basic scientists, clinicians, epidemiologists, computer scientists, and regulators to work together in creating robust infrastructure that facilitates open, accessible platforms for further creative development. This infinite journey has to be mapped and staged in multiple progressive segments with continued appraisal of the precision, efficiency, and reliability of the prevailing AI/ML engines. Clinicians should consider focusing on individual diseases with a broader interlinking as one makes incremental progress in unlocking the secrets of pathophysiology and disease evolution. We live in a world of data silos. Interlinking electronic medical records and epidemiological data with appropriate regulatory oversight will be an important first step in the right direction.

Conclusion

AI and ML have revolutionized the field of EP from detection and diagnosis of arrhythmia to risk prediction and management. Prediction of future diseases and outcomes based on current patient data including ECG, information from wearables/smart devices, and patient genomics offers a chance to provide personalized precision care to our patients. Advances in imaging, computational models for arrhythmia propensity, and accurate identification of ablation targets will improve invasive and noninvasive treatment of arrhythmias. Further advancement of this field is, however, dependent on availability of quality data, which may sometimes be challenging owing to HIPAA compliance and patient privacy. There are significant regulatory requirements that need to be navigated carefully. These are exciting times for the field of EP, where close collaboration between the clinicians, scientists, epidemiologists, and policy makers is the key to use technology for enhancing care of patients with cardiac arrhythmia.

Bibliography and Acknowledgement

- Acharya U.R., Fujita H., Lih O.S., Hagiwara Y., Tan J.H., Adam M. Automated detection of arrhythmias using different intervals of tachycardia ECG segments with convolutional neural network. Information Sciences. 2017;405:81–90. [Google Scholar]
- Arevalo H.J., Vadakkumpadan F., Guallar E. Arrhythmia risk stratification of patients after myocardial infarction using personalized heart models. Nat Commun. 2016;7 [PMC free article] [PubMed] [Google Scholar]
- Ashburner J.M., Lee P.R., Rivet C.M., et al. The implementation and acceptability of a mobile application for screening for atrial fibrillation at home. Telemed J E Health. 2021;27:1305–1310. [PubMed]
- Attia Z.I., Friedman P.A., Noseworthy P.A., et al. Age and sex estimation using artificial intelligence from standard 12-lead ECGs. Circ Arrhythm Electrophysiol. 2019;12
- Attia Z.I., Kapa S., Dugan J., et al. Rapid exclusion of COVID infection with the artificial intelligence electrocardiogram. Mayo Clin Proc. 2021;96:2081–2094. [PMC free article] [PubMed] [Google Scholar]
- Attia Z.I., Kapa S., Lopez-Jimenez F., et al. Screening for cardiac contractile dysfunction using an artificial intelligence-enabled electrocardiogram. Nat Med. 2019;25:70–74. [PubMed] [Google Scholar]
- Au-Yeung W.T., Reinhall P.G., Poole J.E., et al. SCD-HeFT: use of R-R interval statistics for long-term risk stratification for arrhythmic sudden cardiacdeath.HeartRhythm. 2015;12:2058–2066
- Bieging E.T., Morris A., Chang L., Dagher L., Marrouche N.F., Cates J. Statistical shape analysis of the left atrial appendage predicts stroke in atrial fibrillation. Int J Cardiovasc Imaging. 2021;37:2521–2527. [PMC freearticle][PubMed][GoogleScholar]
- Bos J.M., Attia Z.I., Albert D.E., Noseworthy P.A., Friedman P.A., Ackerman M.J. Use of artificial intelligence and deep neural networks in evaluation of patients with electrocardiographically concealed long QT syndrome from the surface 12-lead electrocardiogram. JAMA Cardiol. 2021;6:532–538. [PMC free article] [PubMed] [Google Scholar]
- Boyle P.M., Zghaib T., Zahid S., et al. Computationally guided personalized targeted ablation of persistent atrial fibrillation. Nat Biomed Eng. 2019;3:870–879. [PMC free article] [PubMed] [Google Scholar]
- Bumgarner J.M., Lambert C.T., Hussein A.A., et al. Smartwatch algorithm for automated detection of atrial fibrillation. J Am Coll Cardiol. 2018;71:2381–2388.
- Cikes M., Sanchez-Martinez S., Claggett B., et al. Machine learning-based phenogrouping in heart failure to identify responders to cardiac resynchronization therapy. Eur J Heart Fail. 2019;21:74–85. [PubMed]
- Cohen-Shelly M., Attia Z.I., Friedman P.A., et al. Electrocardiogram screening for aortic valve stenosis using artificial intelligence. Eur Heart J. 2021;42:2885–2896.[PubMed][GoogleScholar]
- Dainis A.M., Ashley E.A. Cardiovascular precision medicine in the genomics era. JACC Basic Transl Sci. 2018;3:313–326. [PMC free article] [PubMed][GoogleScholar]
- de Marvao A., Dawes T.J.W., O'Regan D.P. Artificial intelligence for cardiac imaging-genetics research. Front Cardiovasc Med. 2019;6:195. [PMCfreearticle][PubMed][GoogleScholar]
- Feeny A.K., Chung M.K., Madabhushi A., et al. Artificial intelligence and machine learning in arrhythmias and cardiac electrophysiology. Circ Arrhythm Electrophysiol. 2020;13 [PMC free article] [PubMed] [Google Scholar]
- Feeny A.K., Richard J., Patel D., et al. Machine learning prediction of response to cardiac resynchronization therapy: improvement versus current guidelines. Circ Arrhythm Electrophysiol. 2019;12 [PMC free article][PubMed][GoogleScholar]
- Gawalko M., Duncker D., Manninger M., et al. The European TeleCheck-AF project on remote app-based management of atrial fibrillation during the COVID-19 pandemic: centre and patient experiences. Europace. 2021;23:1003–1015. [PMC free article] [PubMed] [Google Scholar]
- Giudicessi J.R., Schram M., Bos J.M., et al. Artificial intelligence-enabled assessment of the heart rate corrected QT interval using a mobile electrocardiogram device. Circulation. 2021;143:1274–1286.

- Hannun A.Y., Rajpurkar P., Haghpanahi M., et al. Cardiologist-level arrhythmia detection and classification in ambulatory electrocardiograms using a deep neural network. Nat Med. 2019;25:65–69. [PMC free article] [PubMed] [Google Scholar]
- Juhola M., Penttinen K., Joutsijoki H., Aalto-Setälä K. Analysis of drug effects on iPSC cardiomyocytes with machine learning. Ann Biomed Eng. 2021;49:129–138. [PMC free article] [PubMed]
- Kalscheur M.M., Kipp R.T., Tattersall M.C., et al. Machine learning algorithm predicts cardiac resynchronization therapy outcomes. Circ Arrhythm Electrophysiol. 2018;11 [PMC free article] [PubMed] [GoogleScholar]
- Kashou A.H., Ko W.Y., Attia Z.I., et al. A comprehensive artificial intelligence–enabled electrocardiogram interpretation program. Cardiovasc Digit Health J. 2020;1:62–70. [PMC free article] [PubMed] [Google Scholar
- Lee J.H., Kwon O.S., Shim J., et al. Left atrial wall stress and the long-term outcome of catheter ablation of atrial fibrillation: an artificial intelligence-based prediction of atrial wall stress. Front Physiol. 2021;12 [PMC free article] [PubMed] [Google Scholar]
- Liu C.M., Chang S.L., Chen H.H., et al. The clinical application of the deep learning technique for predicting trigger origins in patients with paroxysmal atrial fibrillation with catheter ablation. Circ Arrhythm Electrophysiol. 2020;13 [PubMed] [Google Scholar]
- Mascarenhas D.A.N., Mudumbi P.C., Kantharia B.K. Outpatient initiation of dofetilide: insights from the complexities of atrial fibrillation management during the COVID-19 lockdown. J Interv Card Electrophysiol. 2021;63:21–28. [PMC free article] [PubMed] [Google Scholar]
- Maurizi N., Fumagalli C., Cecchi F., Olivotto I. Use of Smartphone-operated ECG for home ECG surveillance in COVID-19 patients. European Heart Journal - Digital Health. 2021;2:175–178. [Google Scholar]
- Mittal S., Oliveros S., Henry C., et al. An artificial intelligence-based solution to reduce false positive detection of atrial fibrillation in by an implantable loop recorder. Heart Rhythm. 2021;17(Suppl 5):S67–S68.
- Nakashima T., Ogata S., Noguchi T., et al. Machine learning model for predicting out-of-hospital cardiac arrests using meteorological and chronological data. Heart. 2021;107:1084–1091. [PMC free article] [PubMed] [Google Scholar]
  Nguyen M.T., Nguyen B.V., Kim K. Deep feature learning for sudden cardiac arrest detection in automated external defibrillators. Sci Rep. 2018;8 [PMC free article] [PubMed] [Google Scholar]
- O'Sullivan J.W., Grigg S., Crawford W., et al. Accuracy of smartphone camera applications for detecting atrial fibrillation: a systematic review and meta-analysis. JAMA Netw Open. 2020;3 [PMC free article] [PubMed] [Google Scholar]
- Pereira T., Tran N., Gadhoumi K., et al. Photoplethysmography based atrial fibrillation detection: a review. NPJ Digit Med. 2020;3:3. [PMC free article] [PubMed] [Google Scholar]
- Perez M.V., Mahaffey K.W., Hedlin H., et al. Large-scale assessment of a smartwatch to identify atrial fibrillation. N Engl J Med. 2019;381:1909–1917. [PMC free article] [PubMed] [Google Scholar
- Piccini J.P., Mittal S., Snell J., et al. Impact of remote monitoring on clinical events and associated health care utilization: A nationwide assessment. Heart Rhythm. 2016;13:2279–2286. [PubMed] [Google Scholar]
- Popescu D.M., Shade J.K., Lai C., et al. Arrhythmic sudden death survival prediction using deep learning analysis of scarring in the heart. Nat Cardiovasc Res. 2022;1:334–343. [PMC free article] [PubMed] [Google Scholar]
- Prakosa A., Arevalo H.J., Deng D., et al. Personalized virtual-heart technology for guiding the ablation of infarct-related ventricular tachycardia. Nat Biomed Eng. 2018;2:732–740. [PMC free article] [PubMed] [Google Scholar]
- Rogers A.J., Selvalingam A., Alhusseini M.I., et al. Machine learned cellular phenotypes in cardiomyopathy predict sudden death. Circ Res. 2021;128:172–184. [PMC free article] [PubMed] [Google Scholar]
- Rosier A., Mabo P., Temal L., et al. Presonalized and automated remote monitoring of atrial fibrillation. Europace. 2016;18:347–352. [PubMed] [Google Scholar]
- Schwartz A.L., Chorin E., Mann T., et al. Reconstruction of the left atrium for atrial fibrillation ablation using the machine learning CARTO 3 m-FAM software. J Interv Card Electrophysiol. 2022;64:39–47. [PubMed] [Google Scholar]
- Shade J.K., Ali R.L., Basile D., et al. Preprocedure application of machine learning and mechanistic simulations predicts likelihood of paroxysmal atrial fibrillation recurrence following pulmonary vein isolation. Circ Arrhythm Electrophysiol. 2020;13:617–627. [PMC free article] [PubMed] [Google Scholar
- Shade J.K., Cartoski M.J., Nikolov P., et al. Ventricular arrhythmia risk prediction in repaired tetralogy of Fallot using personalized computational cardiac models. Heart Rhythm. 2020;17:408–414. [PMC free article] [PubMed] [Google Scholar]
- Shakibfar S., Krause O., Lund-Andersen C., et al. Predicting electrical storms by remote monitoring of implantable cardioverter-defibrillator patients using machine learning. Europace. 2019;21:268–274. [PubMed] [Google Scholar]
- Siontis K.C., Liu K., Bos J.M., et al. Detection of hypertrophic cardiomyopathy by an artificial intelligence electrocardiogram in children and adolescents. Int J Cardiol. 2021;340:42–47. [PubMed] [Google Scholar]
- Tison G.H., Zhang J., Delling F.N., Deo R.C. Automated and interpretable patient ECG profiles for disease detection, tracking, and discovery. Circ Cardiovasc Qual Outcomes. 2019;12 [PMC free article] [PubMed] [Google Scholar]
- Wasserlauf J., You C., Patel R., Valys A., Albert D., Passman R. Smartwatch performance for the detection and quantification of atrial fibrillation. Circ Arrhythm Electrophysiol. 2019;12 [PubMed] [Google Scholar]
- Willcox M.E., Compton S.J., Bardy G.H. Continuous ECG monitoring versus mobile telemetry: A comparison of arrhythmia diagnostics in human- versus algorithmic-dependent systems. Heart Rhythm O2. 2021;2:543–559. [PMC free article] [PubMed] [Google Scholar]
- Xiong Z., Stiles M., Zhao J. Robust ECG signal classification for detection of atrial fibrillation using a novel neural network. Computing in Cardiology. 2017;1–4 [Google Scholar]
- Yao X., Attia Z.I., Behnken E.M., et al. Batch enrollment for an artificial intelligence-guided intervention to lower neurologic events in patients with undiagnosed atrial fibrillation: rationale and design of a digital clinical trial. Am Heart J. 2021;239:73–79. [PubMed] [Google Scholar]
- Yao X., Rushlow D.R., Inselman J.W. Artificial intelligence-enabled electrocardiograms for identification of patients with low ejection fraction: a pragmatic, randomized clinical trial. Nat Med. 2021;27:815–819. [PubMed] [Google Scholar]
- Yu J., Wang X., Chen X., Guo J. Automatic premature ventricular contraction detection using deep metric learning and KNN. Biosensors (Basel) 2021;11:69. [PMC free article] [PubMed] [Google Scholar]
- Zou F., Brahier M., Migliarese F., et al. A machine learning-derived recurrence risk model for atrial fibrillation after catheter ablation. Heart Rhythm. 2021;18:S219–S220. [Google Scholar]

CHAPTER

20

New AI Can Automatically Detect a Serious Heart Condition

Utilizing Intravascular Optical Coherence Tomography Images, A New Technique Made It Easier To Identify Plaque Eosion

Researchers have created a brand-new artificial intelligence (AI) technique that uses optical coherence tomography (OCT) images to automatically detect plaque erosion in the arteries of the heart. Monitoring arterial plaque is crucial because, if it disintegrates, it may obstruct blood flow to the heart, triggering a heart attack or other dangerous problems.

"If cholesterol plaque lining arteries starts to erode it can lead to a sudden reduction in blood flow to the heart known as acute coronary syndrome, which requires urgent treatment," said research team leader Zhao Wang from the University of Electronic Science and Technology of China. "Our new method could help improve the clinical diagnosis of plaque erosion and be used to develop new treatments for patients with heart disease."

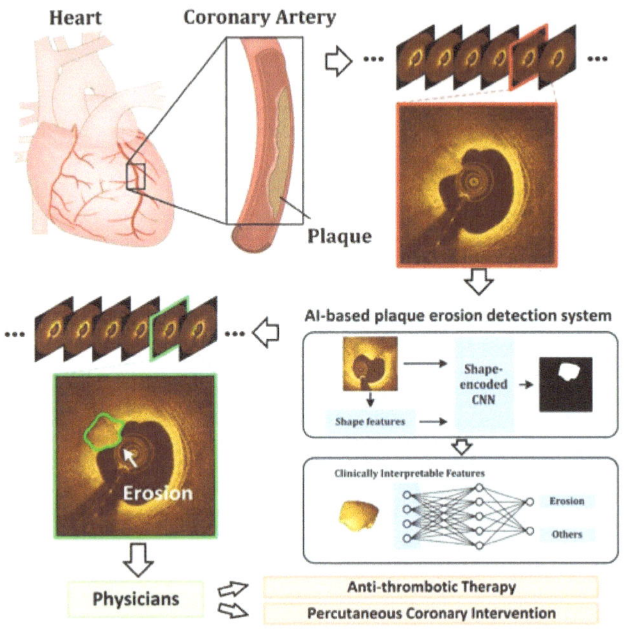

Fig.20.1 Researchers have developed a new AI method that can automatically detect plaque erosion in arteries using OCT images. This type of erosion can block blood flow to the heart, leading to a heart attack or other serious conditions. Credit: Zhao Wang, University of Electronic Science and Technology of China

OCT is an optical imaging technique with micron-scale resolution that may be utilized within blood vessels to produce 3D pictures of the coronary arteries, which carry blood to the heart. Although intravascular OCT is being used by doctors more frequently to check for plaque erosion, there is a substantial level of interobserver variability because of the volume of data generated and the difficulty of visually interpreting the images.

In order to address this issue, Wang collaborated with a team of engineers from his institution and medical professionals from The 2nd Affiliated Hospital of Harbin Medical University under the direction of Bo Yu to create an automated, objective method that uses AI to identify plaque erosion based on OCT images. They explain the new method in the Optica Publishing Group journal Biomedical Optics Express and demonstrate that it is accurate enough to possibly serve as the foundation for clinical diagnosis.

"Our new AI-based method can automatically detect the presence of plaque erosion using the original OCT images without any additional input," said Wang. "The ability to detect plaque erosion objectively and automatically will reduce the laborious manual assessment associated with diagnosis."

Application of AI

The new method consists of two primary steps. First, an AI model known as a neural network uses the original image and two pieces of shape information to predict regions of possible plaque erosion. The initial prediction is then refined with a post-processing algorithm based on clinically interpretable features that mimic the knowledge professional physicians use to make a diagnosis.

"We had to develop a new AI model that incorporates explicit shape information, the key feature used to identify plaque erosion in OCT images," said Wang. "The underlying intravascular OCT imaging technology is also crucial because it is currently the highest resolution imaging modality that can be used to diagnose plaque erosion in living patients."

When OCT is used for intravascular imaging, the imaging probe is automatically pulled backward inside a catheter, producing hundreds of images for each pullback. The researchers tested their method using 16 pullbacks of 5,553 clinical OCT images with plaque erosion and 10 pullbacks of 3,224 images without plaque erosion.

The automated method correctly predicted 80 percent of the plaque erosion cases with a positive predictive value of 73 percent. They also found that diagnoses based on the automated method matched well with those from three experienced physicians.

"Although further safety validation and regulatory approval are needed for stand-alone clinical use in patients, the technique could be used to facilitate diagnosis of plaque erosion," said Wang. "This would involve physicians making a final check of the algorithm's finding and then determining the cause of acute coronary syndrome and the best treatment strategies."

Studying new treatments

The method could also be useful for analyzing the massive amounts of existing OCT data by eliminating the time-consuming and tedious process of manual image analysis. This could help scientists improve the identification and treatment of plaque erosion. For example, a stent is often used to recover reduced blood flow in patients with acute coronary syndrome, but recent studies suggest that some medications might offer a less-invasive alternative.

"Intravascular imaging, accompanied with AI technologies, can be an extremely valuable tool for diagnosis of coronary artery disease and treatment planning," said Wang. "In the future, this new approach could help physicians develop individualized treatment strategies for optimal management of patients with acute coronary syndrome."

The researchers are now working to improve their new technique by better incorporating 3D information and incorporating more unlabeled data to improve the AI model's performance. In the future, they also plan to use a larger dataset that includes a global population for training and evaluating the algorithm. They also want to explore how it might be used in various clinical situations to further demonstrate its potential utility and value.

Reference:

"In vivo detection of plaque erosion by intravascular optical coherence tomography using artificial intelligence" by Haoyue Sun, Chen Zhao, Yuhan Qin, Chao Li, Haibo Jia, Bo Yu and Zhao Wang, 16 June 2022, Biomedical Optics Express.
DOI: 10.1364/BOE.459623

AI may accurately detect heart valve disease and predict cardiovascular risk

(American Heart Association Scientific Sessions 2023, Abstracts Mo3070 and 306)

Research Highlights:

- Artificial intelligence (AI) and deep learning models may help to predict the risk of cardiovascular disease events and detect heart valvular disease, according to two preliminary research studies.
- One study found that artificial intelligence analyzing sound data of the heart recorded from a digital stethoscope was able to more accurately detect heart valve disease than a health care professional who listened to the heart with a traditional stethoscope.
- In a study evaluating data from the UK Biobank, an artificial intelligence/deep learning program effectively analyzed and sorted eye images of people with prediabetes and Type 2 diabetes to determine their risk of cardiovascular disease events.

Real World Evaluation of an Artificial Intelligence Enabled Digital Stethoscope for Detecting Undiagnosed Valvular Heart Disease in Primary Care (Abstract 306)

A study conducted at three different primary care clinics in the U.S. compared the ability of a medical professional using a standard stethoscope to detect potential heart valve disease vs. the ability of an artificial intelligence program using sound data from a digital stethoscope to do the same.

Each study participant had a physical exam that included a primary care professional, either a physician or nurse practitioner, listening to their heart and lungs with a traditional stethoscope for unusual sounds or murmurs plus an exam with a digital stethoscope that recorded heart sounds. All participants also received an echocardiogram at a follow-up appointment 1-2 weeks later to determine if heart valve disease was present, though the results were not shared with the clinician or the patient.

The analysis found:

The AI method with the digital stethoscope detected 94.1% of cases of valvular heart disease compared to the standard stethoscope used by primary care professionals, which detected only 41.2% of cases.

The AI method identified 22 people with previously undiagnosed moderate-or-greater heart valve disease, and the professionals using the standard stethoscopes identified 8 previously undiagnosed people with heart valve disease.

"The implications of undiagnosed or late diagnosis of valvular heart disease are dire and pose a significant cost to our health care system," said lead author Moshe Rancier, M.D., senior medical director of Mass General Brigham Community Physicians in Lawrence, Massachusetts. "This study demonstrates that health care professionals can screen patients for valvular heart disease more effectively and quickly using a digital stethoscope paired with high-performing AI that could detect cardiac murmurs associated with significant valvular heart disease."

The study's limitations include the small sample size of the study group, which prevents analyses of differences between subsets of participants (based on characteristics such as gender, race, ethnicity and age). Additionally, while the AI method had greater sensitivity to sounds detected with the digital stethoscope, medical professionals using a standard stethoscope were able to be more specific in their diagnosis, 95.5% versus 84.5% for the AI method, which may reduce the potential for false positives and/or additional tests or screenings for valvular heart disease. However, this study only evaluated the accuracy of the digital stethoscope in comparison to a traditional stethoscope. Rancier noted researchers plan to evaluate six-month patient follow-up data to review more closely the clinical outcomes and additional diagnostic tests and treatments.

Study background and details:

- The study included 369 adults, all ages 50 and older, and 61% of participants identified as female.
- None of the participants had a prior diagnosis of heart valve disease or a history of a heart murmur.
- The health care professionals who performed their standard exam on their patients were not aware of the AI results or the echocardiogram results, making it a blind study.
- Participants were enrolled from June 2021 through May 2023. Data collection and analysis are ongoing.
- The health care clinics where patients received care were located in Queens, New York, and Lawrence and Haverhill, Massachusetts.
- The study participants self-identified their race or ethnicity: 70% identified as white adults, 18% were Hispanic or Latino adults, 9% were Black adults and 2% identified as Asian adults; with 1% of participants identified as other.

"We saw here that the AI-based stethoscope did extraordinarily well, it predicted nearly 90% of the of the valve disease diagnoses that were ultimately there. I see that as an emerging technology — using an AI-enabled stethoscope and perhaps combining it with other imaging modalities, like an AI-enabled echocardiogram built into your stethoscope," Roden said. "Use of these new tools to detect the presence of valvular disease as well as the extent of valvular disease and the extent of other kinds of heart disease will likely help to transform CVD care."

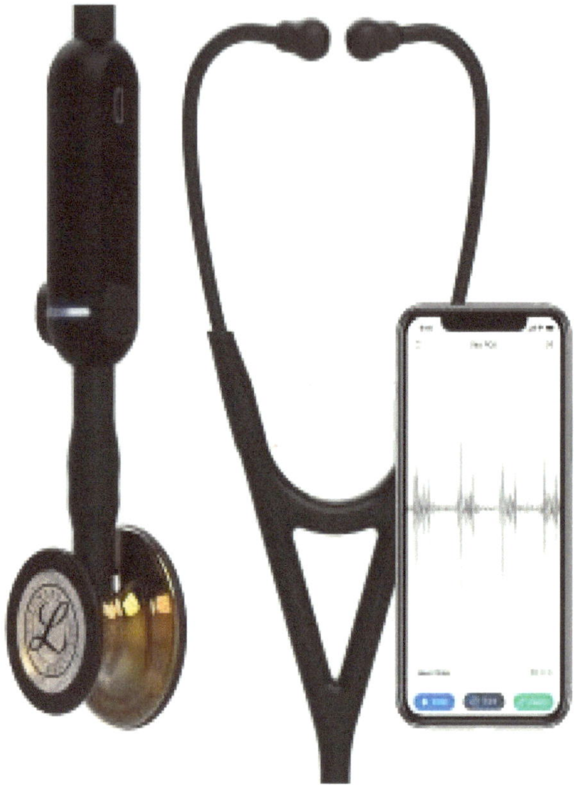

Fig.20.2 3M Littmann CORE Digital Stethoscope . Digital Stethoscope is innovation you never knew you needed. It is suitable for pediatric and adult patients, allowing doctors to get even more accurate heartbeat readings per time. Feel free to switch between the stethoscopes analog and digital modes whenever you like. 3M has also thrown in several impressive features, including active noise cancellation and a tunable chest piece. With these features - and much more - you will find that getting heartbeat sounds and recording readings will be more simple than you imagined. The stethoscope also lasts very long, so you can rest assured that this will be an impressive investment.

Deep Learning-Based Retinal Imaging for Predicting Cardiovascular Disease Events in Prediabetic and Diabetic Patients: A Study Using the UK Biobank (Abstract Poster Mo3070)

Using data from the UK Biobank, a second study by another research group evaluated the effectiveness of using pictures of the retina at the back of the eye that were analyzed by a deep-learning algorithm tool to predict the risk of cardiovascular disease events, defined as heart attack, ischemic stroke, transient ischemic attack or death due to heart attack or stroke.

Deep learning is a method of artificial intelligence that trains computers to analyze multiple layers of data and gives computers the ability to "learn" by evolving their model independent of human intervention based on new information presented to it – a process challenged by the requirement of both large amounts of computing power and data. Previous research had successfully developed a deep learning algorithm to predict cardiovascular disease events by analysis of retinal images and coronary artery calcium scores.

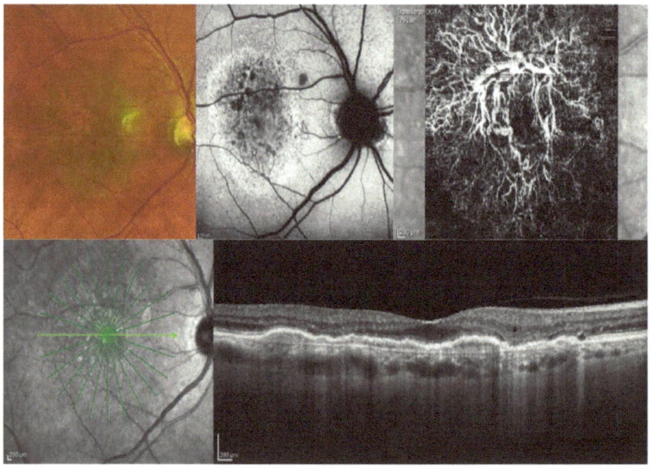

Fig.20.3 Retinal imaging is an emerging helpful tool in cardiovascular disease risk assessment. Note: Image does not necessarily depict an individual at risk for heart attack. Photo: Jessica Haynes, OD, James Williamson, OD, and Mohammad Rafieetary, OD. Click image to enlarge.

Researchers used the deep-learning algorithm to categorize retinal images of 1,101 people with prediabetes or Type 2 diabetes into low-risk, moderate-risk and high-risk groups for likelihood of cardiovascular disease. They then measured the number of cardiovascular disease events among participants over a median period of 11 years.

The analysis found:

8.2% of participants in the low-risk group, 15.2% of participants in the moderate-risk group and 18.5% of participants in the high-risk group had experienced cardiovascular disease events by the end of the study period of 11 years.

After accounting for demographic and other potential CVD risk factors, such as age, gender, high blood pressure medication use, cholesterol medication use and smoking history, people in the moderate-risk group were 57% more likely to experience a cardiovascular event compared to people in the low-risk group; and people with high-risk scores were 88% more likely to experience a cardiovascular event compared to those in the low-risk group.

"These results show the potential of using AI analysis of retinal imaging as an early detection tool for heart disease in high-risk groups such as people who have prediabetes and Type 2 diabetes," said study lead author Chan Joo Lee, M.D., Ph.D., an associate professor at Yonsei University in Seoul, Korea. "This could lead to early interventions and better management of these patient groups, ultimately reducing the incidence of heart disease-related complications."

Study background and details:

- The UK Biobank is a large biomedical database and research resource with health records of about 500,000 adults — enrolled from 2006 until 2010 — who receive care through the United Kingdom's National Health Service. The researchers accessed the data in March 2023 and analyzed health records through June 2023.
- Participants were 59 years old, on average; 45.5% were female and predominantly identified as white race (85.5%).
- Of the 1,101 adults with prediabetes or Type 2 diabetes, 550 people were in the low-risk group, 276 were in the moderate-risk group and 275 were in the high-risk group.
- At the end of the study period, 138 (12.5%) of the participants had experienced cardiovascular events: 45 were from the low-risk group; 42 were from the moderate-risk group; and 51 were from the high-risk group.

The researchers tested the ability of the imaging to predict cardiovascular disease using a large dataset of people, however, this population was noted as primarily white race, which means the researchers' findings may not be applicable to other populations. Additional follow-up studies among people from diverse races and ethnicities are needed."These systems learn from big data sets, and they only learn from the data we give them to learn from. In the UK Biobank, for example, 93% of the participants are of European ancestry, so we have no sense of whether the approaches derived in the UK Biobank are relevant or meaningful to people who are not of European ancestry," Roden said.

"Another question is: does the retinal scan do a better job of predicting coronary artery disease than the pooled risk equations, or a polygenic risk score for coronary artery disease, or coronary calcium measurements? Those are all questions that need to be answered because as we develop more tools to predict events like coronary artery disease, we want to make sure that we use the right ones and the right combinations, rather than complicating care with alternate tools that have not been validated."

Co-authors, disclosures and funding sources are listed in the manuscript.

Statements and conclusions of studies that are presented at the American Heart Association's scientific meetings are solely those of the study authors and do not necessarily reflect the Association's policy or position. The Association makes no representation or guarantee as to their accuracy or reliability. Abstracts presented at the Association's scientific meetings are not peer-reviewed, rather, they are curated by independent review panels and are considered based on the potential to add to the diversity of scientific issues and views discussed at the meeting. The findings are considered preliminary until published as a full manuscript in a peer-reviewed scientific journal.

Additional Resources:

- *https://newsroom.heart.org/news/ai-may-accurately-detect-heart-valve-disease-and-predict-cardiovascular-risk?preview=efd38ca812ee8da96c70d95ab3027201*
- *After Nov. 6, view Abstract Poster Mo3070 and Abstract 306 in the AHA Scientific Sessions 2023 Online Program Planner*
- *AHA news release: Artificial intelligence-enhanced ECGs may speed heart failure diagnosis and treatment (August 2020)*
- *AHA news release: CAROL Act will prioritize research on heart valve disease (December 2022)*
- *AHA health information: Diabetes Tools and Resources*
- *About Scientific Sessions 2023*
- *For more news at AHA Scientific Sessions 2023, follow us on X (formerly known as Twitter) @HeartNews,#AHA23*

CHAPTER

21

Applications of ChatGPT In Medical Practice, Education and Research

ChatGPT, which can automatically generate written responses to queries using internet sources, soon went viral after its release at the end of 2022. The performance of ChatGPT on medical exams shows results near the passing threshold, making it comparable to third-year medical students. It can also write academic abstracts or reviews at an acceptable level. However, it is not clear how ChatGPT deals with harmful content, misinformation or plagiarism; therefore, authors using ChatGPT professionally for academic writing should be cautious. ChatGPT also has the potential to facilitate the interaction between healthcare providers and patients in various ways. However, sophisticated tasks such as understanding the human anatomy are still a limitation of ChatGPT. ChatGPT can simplify radiological reports, but the possibility of incorrect statements and missing medical information remain. Although ChatGPT has the potential to change medical practice, education and research, further improvements of this application are needed for regular use in medicine

ChatGPT (OpenAI, San Francisco, CA, USA) is an AI chatbot which was introduced in November 2022 and soon after went viral. ChatGPT has the ability to respond to various kinds of queries, automatically generating responses using internet sources. People across different fields, generations and continents started using ChatGPT, leading to a continuous increase in its popularity. Medicine is a field in which simplifying artificial intelligence (AI)-based technologies are highly important. It is obvious that applications such as ChatGPT have the potential to change medicine, with uses ranging from the automated extraction of electronic medical records to the development of sophisticated treatment plans. This article presents an overview of the early applications of ChatGPT in medicine.

ChatGPT in medical education

A recent study evaluated the performance of ChatGPT on the United States Medical Licensing Examination (USMLE). The study revealed that ChatGPT passed all three exams (Step 1, Step 2 CK, Step 3) near the passing threshold without any previous training. On the other hand, Gilson et al state that there is a significant decrease in performance with an increased difficulty of the questions.

However, the authors compare the performance of ChatGPT to a third-year medical student. Antaki et al tested ChatGPT for use in two multiple-choice question banks for the Ophthalmic Knowledge Assessment Program (OKAP) exam. The authors found similar results, with ChatGPT achieving 55.8% and 42.7% accuracy in the exams. Another study from Korea aimed at directly correlating the knowledge of ChatGPT to that of medical students on the topic of parasitology. The authors revealed that the performance of ChatGPT was lower than medical students and concluded that ChatGPT's ability is not yet at an entirely acceptable level.

Academic writing

Gao et al tested ChatGPT's ability to write academic abstracts. They included 50 abstracts from five high-impact medical journals and asked ChatGPT to produce research abstracts using provided titles and journal requirements. The authors concluded that all ChatGPT-derived abstracts were acceptably written, but only 8% of them respected the formatting requirements of the journals. 68% of the generated abstracts by ChatGPT were correctly identified by the reviewers due to the 'vaguer' and more 'formulaic' type of writing. An AI output detector showed similar results in detecting the ChatGPT-derived abstracts.

In a recent article by Guo et al, the main attributes of ChatGPT's writing style are identified. The authors mention that ChatGPT writes in an organised manner and prefers a straightforward concept in the questions. Its answers are long and detailed, it shows less harmful information, and refuses to answer when it has no information about topics. However, it might 'fabricate facts' to give an answer, which should make users cautious regarding the professional use of ChatGPT. The authors observed that the main difference between ChatGPT's writing style and human writing is that the human writer is more subjective, colloquial and emotional, giving human abstracts a personal note.9 OpenAI warns that ChatGPT could sometimes 'responds to harmful instructions

A recent study evaluated ChatGPT's ability to generate a literature review on the concept of the 'digital twin' in

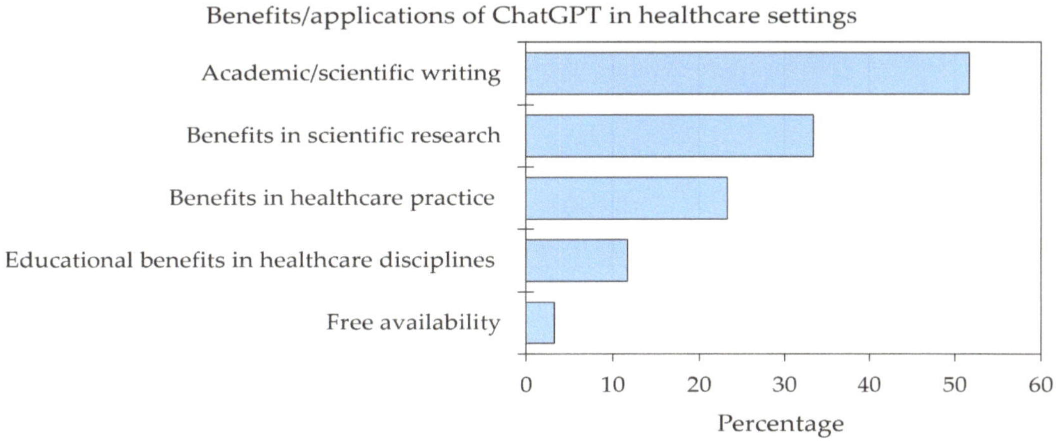

Fig. 21.1 Summary of benefits/applications of ChatGPT in health care education, research, and practice based on the included records.

healthcare, asking it to paraphrase selected literature from 2020 to 2022. Although the results were promising, the iThenticate plagiarism detection tool identified many plagiarism matches.

Interaction with Patients and Radiological Reporting

Thurzo et al reviewed AI-based applications, including ChatGPT, in the dental field. They concluded that ChatGPT could facilitate the interaction between healthcare providers and patients in various ways, from analysing patient messages to personalising the communication between healthcare professionals and patients. However, they found that ChatGPT has limitations in relation to sophisticated tasks such as understanding the human anatomy. Nov et al tested ChatGPT against healthcare providers' responses to patients. They found that ChatGPT had a similar rate of correct answers compared to the providers. In a case study conducted by Jeblick et al, radiologists had the task of evaluating the quality of simplified radiology reports generated with ChatGPT. The results showed that the reports were 'correct, complete, and not potentially harmful to patients'. However, incorrect statements and missing medical information that could potentially have led to harmful conclusions were also detected. Although this case study comprises small sample numbers, the authors emphasise the great potential of ChatGPT in radiology while also mentioning the need for further improvements.

The far-reaching consequences of ChatGPT among other LLMs can be described as a paradigm shift in academia and health care practice. The discussion of its potential benefits, future perspectives, and importantly, its limitations, appear timely and relevant . Therefore, the current review aimed to highlight these issues based on the current evidence.

The following common themes emerged from the available literature.

Benefits of ChatGPT in Scientific Research

ChatGPT, as an example of other LLMs, can be described as a

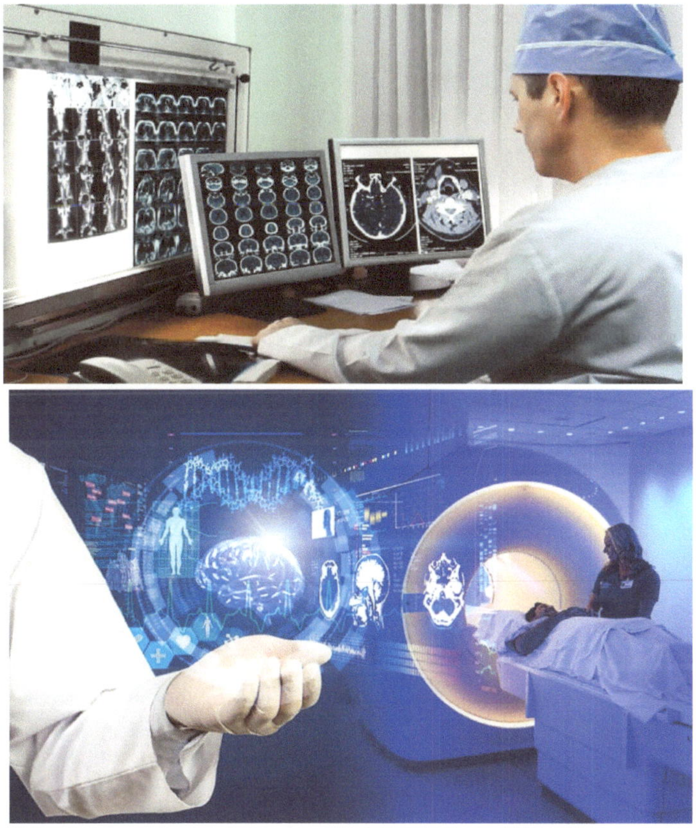

Fig.21.2 A Radiology Information System (RIS) is a sophisticated EHR system designed specifically for use in a radiology practice. A radiology information system (RIS) is a networked software system for managing medical imagery and associated data. A RIS is especially useful for tracking radiology imaging orders and billing information, and is often used in conjunction with PACS to manage image archives, record-keeping and billing.

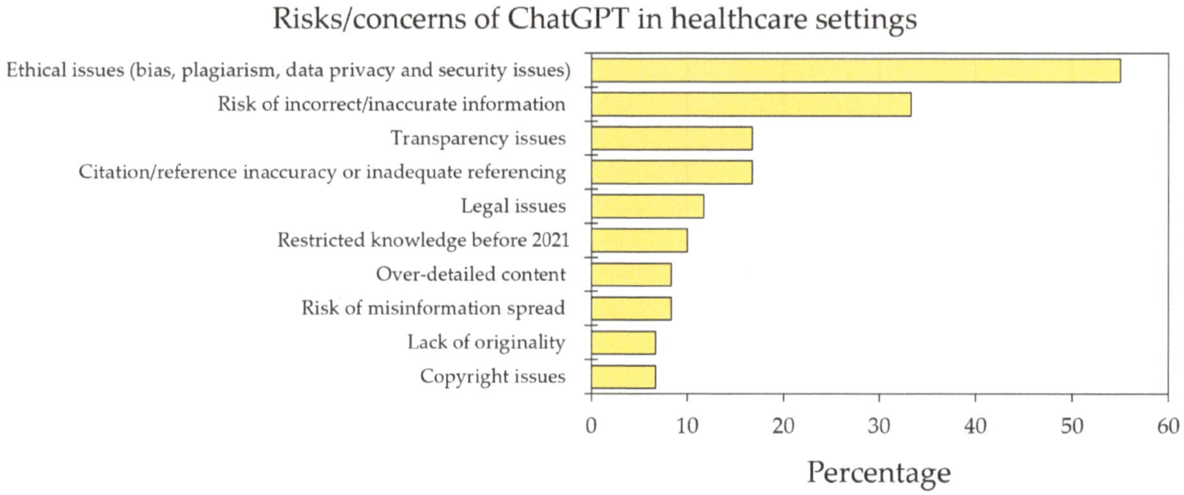

Fig.21.3 Summary of risks/concerns of ChatGPT use in health care education, research, and practice based on the included records

a promising or even a revolutionary tool for scientific research in both academic writing and in the research process itself. Specifically, ChatGPT was listed in several sources as an efficient and promising tool for conducting comprehensive literature reviews and generating computer codes, thereby saving time for the research steps that require more efforts from human intelligence (e.g., the focus on experimental design) . Additionally, ChatGPT can be helpful in generating queries for comprehensive systematic review with high precision, as shown by Wang et al., despite the authors highlighting the transparency issues and unsuitability for high-recall retrieval . Moreover, the utility of ChatGPT extends to involve an improvement in language and a better ability to express and communicate research ideas and results, ultimately speeding up the publication process with the faster availability of research results . This is particularly relevant for researchers who are non-native English speakers .Such a practice can be acceptable considering the already existent English editing services provided by several academic publishers. Subsequently, this can help to promote equity and diversity in research .

Limitations of ChatGPT Use in Scientific Research

On the other hand, the use of ChatGPT in academic writing and scientific research should be conducted in light of several limitations that could compromise the quality of research as follows.

First, superficial, inaccurate, or incorrect content was frequently cited as a shortcoming of ChatGPT use in scientific writing . The ethical issues including the risk of bias based on training datasets and plagiarism were also frequently mentioned, aside from the lack of transparency regarding content generation, which justifies the description of ChatGPT, on occasions, as a black box technology . Importantly, the concept of ChatGPT hallucination could be risky if the generated content is not thoroughly evaluated by researchers and health providers with proper expertise . This comes in light of the ability of ChatGPT to generate incorrect content that appears plausible from a scientific point of view .

Second, several records mentioned the current problems regarding citation inaccuracies, insufficient references, and ChatGPT referencing to non-existent sources .This was clearly shown in two recently published case studies with ChatGPT use in a journal contest . These case studies discouraged the use of ChatGPT, citing the lack of scientific accuracy, the limited updated knowledge, and the lack of ability to critically discuss the results . Therefore, the ChatGPT generated content, albeit efficient, should be meticulously examined prior to its inclusion in any research manuscripts or proposals for research grants.

Third, the generation of non-original, over-detailed, or excessive content can be an additional burden for researchers who should carefully supervise the ChatGPT-generated content This can be addressed by supplying ChatGPT with proper prompts (text input), since varying responses might be generated based on the exact approach of prompt construction .

Fourth, as it currently stands, the knowledge of ChatGPT is limited to the period prior to 2021 based on the datasets used in ChatGPT training . Thus, ChatGPT cannot be used currently as a reliable updated source of literature review . Nevertheless, ChatGPT can be used as a motivation to organize the literature in a decent format, if supplemented by reliable and up-to-date references .

Fifth, the risk of research fraud (e.g., ghostwriting, falsified or fake research) involving ChatGPT should be considered seriously ,as well as the risk of generating mis-

or disinformation with the subsequent possibility of infodemics,

Sixth, legal issues in relation to ChatGPT use were also raised by several records including copyright issues .

Finally, the practice of listing ChatGPT as an author does not appear to be acceptable based on the current ICMJE and COPE guidelines for determining authorship, as illustrated by Zielinski et al. and Liebrenz et al. This comes in light of the fact that authorship entails legal obligations that are not met by ChatGPT . However, other researchers have suggested the possibility of ChatGPT inclusion as an author in some specified instances .

A few instances were encountered in this review, where ChatGPT was listed as an author that can point to the initial perplexity of a few publishers regarding the role of LLM including ChatGPT in research . The disapproval of including ChatGPT or any other LLM in the list of authors was clearly explained in Science, Nature, and the Lancet editorials, which referred to such practice as scientific misconduct, and this view was echoed by many scientists . In the case of ChatGPT use in the research process, several records advocated the need for the proper and concise disclosure and documentation of ChatGPT or LLM use in the methodology or acknowledgement sections. A note worthy and comprehensive record by Borji can be used as a categorical guide for the issues and concerns of ChatGPT use, especially in the context of scientific writing .

Benefits of ChatGPT in Health Care Practice

From the health care practice perspective, the current review showed a careful excitement vibe regarding ChatGPT applications. The ability of ChatGPT to help in streamlining the clinical workflow appears promising, with possible cost savings and increased efficiency in health care delivery . This was illustrated recently by Patel and Lam, highlighting the ability of ChatGPT to produce efficient discharge summaries, which can be valuable to reduce the burden of documentation in health care .Additionally, ChatGPT, among other LLMs, can have a transforming potential in health care practice via enhancing diagnostics, prediction of disease risk and outcome, and drug discovery among other areas in translational research . Moreover, ChatGPT showed moderate accuracy in determining the imaging steps needed in breast cancer screening and in the evaluation of breast pain, which can be a promising application in decision making in radiology . ChatGPT in health care settings also has the prospects of refining personalized medicine and the ability to improve health literacy by providing easily accessible and understandable health information to the general public . This utility was demonstrated by ChatGPT responses, highlighting the need to consult health care providers among other reliable sources on specific situations .

Concerns Regarding ChatGPT Use in Health Care Practice

On the other hand, several concerns regarding ChatGPT use in health care settings were raised. Ethical issues including the risk of bias and transparency issues appeared as recurring major concerns Additionally, the generation of inaccurate content can have severe negative consequences in health care; therefore, this valid concern should be cautiously considered in health care practice . This concern also extends to involve the ability of ChatGPT to provide justification for incorrect decisions .

Other ChatGPT limitations including the issues of interpretability, reproducibility, and the handling of uncertainty were also raised, which can have harmful consequences in health care settings including health care research . In the area of personalized medicine, the lack of transparency and unclear information regarding the sources of data used for ChatGPT training are important issues in health care settings considering the variability observed among different populations in several health-related traits [69]. The issue of reproducibility between the ChatGPT prompt runs is of particular importance, which can be a major limitation in health care practice .

Medico-legal and accountability issues in the case of medical errors caused by ChatGPT application should be carefully considered . Importantly, the current LLMs including ChatGPT are unable to comprehend the complexity of biologic systems, which is an important concept needed in health care decisions and research [52,68]. The concerns regarding data governance, health care cybersecurity, and data privacy should draw specific attention in the discussion regarding the utility of LLMs in health care .

Other issues accompanying ChatGPT applications in health care include the lack of personal and emotional perspectives needed in health care delivery and research . However, ChatGPT emulation of empathetic responses was reported in a preprint in the context of hepatic disease . Additionally, the issue of devaluing the function of the human brain should not be overlooked; therefore, stressing the indispensable human role in health care practice and research is important to address any psychologic, economic, and social consequences that could accompany the application of LLM tools in health care settings .

Benefits and Concerns Regarding ChatGPT Use in Health Care Education

In the area of health care education, ChatGPT appears to have a massive transformative potential. The need to rethink and revise the current assessment tools in health care education comes in light of ChatGPT's ability to pass reputable exams (e.g., USMLE) and possibility of ChatGPT misuse, which would result in academic dishonesty .

Specifically, in ophthalmology examination, Antaki et al. showed that ChatGPT currently performed at the level of an average first-year resident . Such a result highlights the need to focus on questions involving the assessment of critical and problem-based thinking . Additionally, the utility of ChatGPT in health care education can involve tailoring education based on the needs of the student with immediate feedback .. Interestingly, a recent preprint by Benoit showed the promising potential of ChatGPT in rapidly crafting consistent realistic clinical vignettes of variable complexities that can be a valuable educational source with lower costs .Thus, ChatGPT can be useful in health care education including enhanced communication skills given proper academic mentoring . However, the copyright issues should be taken into account regarding the ChatGPT-generated clinical vignettes, aside from the issue of inaccurate references . Additionally, ChatGPT availability can be considered as a motivation in health care education based on the personalized interaction it provides, enabling powerful self-learning as well as its utility as an adjunct in group learning.

Other limitations of ChatGPT use in health care education include the concern regarding the quality of training datasets that could result in biased content and inaccurate information limited to the period prior to the year 2021. Additionally, other concerns include the current inability of ChatGPT to handle images as well as its low performance in some topics (e.g., failure to pass a parasitology exam for Korean medical students), and the issue of possible plagiarism .Despite ChatGPT versatility in the context of academic education , the content of ChatGPT in research assignments was discouraged, being currently insufficient, biased, or misleading .

Future Perspectives

As stated comprehensively in a commentary by van Dis et al., there is an urgent need to develop guidelines for ChatGPT use in scientific research, taking into account the issues of accountability, integrity, transparency, and honesty . Thus, the application of ChatGPT to advance academia and health care should be carried out ethically and responsibly, taking into account the potential risks and concerns it entails .

More studies are needed to evaluate the content of LLMs including its potential impact to advance academia and science with a particular focus on health care settings .In academic writing, a question arises as to whether authors would prefer an AI-editor and an AI-reviewer considering the previous flaws in the editorial and peer review processes . A similar question would also arise in health care settings involving the personal preference of emotional support from health care providers, rather than the potential efficiency of AI-based systems.

In health care education, more studies are needed to evaluate the potential impact of ChatGPT on the quality and efficiency of both educational content and assessment tools. ChatGPT utility to help in refining communication skills among health care students is another aspect that should be further explored as well as the applications of LLMs in the better achievement of the intended learning outcomes through personalized and instantaneous feedback for the students.

Conclusions

The imminent dominant use of LLM technology including the widespread use of ChatGPT in health care education, research, and practice is inevitable. Considering the valid concerns raised regarding its potential misuse, appropriate guidelines and regulations are urgently needed with the engagement of all stakeholders involved to ensure the safe and responsible use of ChatGPT powers. The proactive embrace of LLM technologies with careful consideration of the possible ethical and legal issues can limit the potential future complications. If properly implemented, ChatGPT, among other LLMs, have the potential to expedite innovation in health care and can aid in promoting equity and diversity in research by overcoming language barriers. Therefore, a science-driven debate regarding the pros and cons of ChatGPT is strongly recommended and its possible benefits should be weighed with the possible risks of misleading results and fraudulent research .

Based on the available evidence, health care professionals could be described as carefully enthusiastic regarding the huge potential of ChatGPT among other LLMs in clinical decision-making and optimizing the clinical workflow. "ChatGPT in the Loop: Humans in Charge" can be the proper motto to follow based on the intrinsic value of human knowledge and expertise in health care research and practice . An inspiring example of this motto could be drawn based on the relationship between the human character Cooper and the robotic character TARS from Christopher Nolan's movie Interstellar .

However, before its widespread adoption, the impact of ChatGPT from the health care perspective in a real-world setting should be conducted (e.g., using a risk-based approach) . Based on the title of an important perspective article "AI in the hands of imperfect users" by Kostick-Quenet and Gerke ,the real-world impact of ChatGPT among other LLMs should be properly evaluated to prevent any negative impact of its potential misuse. The same innovative and revolutionary tool can be severely deleterious if used improperly. An example to illustrate such severe negative consequences of ChatGPT misuse can be based on Formula 1 racing, as follows. In the 2004 Formula 1 season, the Ferrari F2004 (the highly successful Formula 1 racing car) broke several Formula 1 records in the hands of Michael Schumacher, one of the most successful Formula 1 drivers of all time. However, in my own hands —as a humble researcher without expertise in Formula 1 driving— the same highly successful car would only break walls and be damaged beyond repair.

Bibliography and Acknowledgement

- Aczel, B.; Wagenmakers, E. Transparency Guidance for ChatGPT Usage in Scientific Writing. PsyArXiv, 2023; Preprint. [Google Scholar] [CrossRef]
- Ahn, C. Exploring ChatGPT for information of cardiopulmonary resuscitation. Resuscitation 2023, 185, 109729. [Google Scholar] [CrossRef] [PubMed]
- Akhter, H.M.; Cooper, J.S. Acute Pulmonary Edema After Hyperbaric Oxygen Treatment: A Case Report Written With ChatGPT Assistance. Cureus 2023, 15, e34752. [Google Scholar] [CrossRef] [PubMed]
- Alberts, I.L.; Mercolli, L.; Pyka, T.; Prenosil, G.; Shi, K.; Rominger, A.; Afshar-Oromieh, A. Large language models (LLM) and ChatGPT: What will the impact on nuclear medicine be? Eur. J. Nucl. Med. Mol. Imaging, 2023; Online ahead of print. [Google Scholar] [CrossRef]
- Bašić, Ž.; Banovac, A.; Kružić, I.; Jerković, I. Better by You, better than Me? ChatGPT-3 as writing assistance in students' essays. arXiv, 2023; Preprint. [Google Scholar] [CrossRef]
- Benoit, J. ChatGPT for Clinical Vignette Generation, Revision, and Evaluation. medRxiv, 2023; Preprint. [Google Scholar] [CrossRef]
Biswas, S. ChatGPT and the Future of Medical Writing. Radiology 2023, 223312. [Google Scholar] [CrossRef]
- Borji, A. A Categorical Archive of ChatGPT Failures. arXiv 2023, arXiv:2302.03494. [Google Scholar] [CrossRef]
Brown, T.; Mann, B.; Ryder, N.; Subbiah, M.; Kaplan, J.D.; Dhariwal, P.; Neelakantan, A.; Shyam, P.; Sastry, G.; Askell, A. Language models are few-shot learners. Adv. Neural Inf. Process. Syst. 2020, 33, 1877–1901. [Google Scholar] [CrossRef]
- Cahan, P.; Treutlein, B. A conversation with ChatGPT on the role of computational systems biology in stem cell research. Stem. Cell. Rep. 2023, 18, 1–2. [Google Scholar] [CrossRef]
- Cascella, M.; Montomoli, J.; Bellini, V.; Bignami, E. Evaluating the Feasibility of ChatGPT in Healthcare: An Analysis of Multiple Clinical and Research Scenarios. J. Med. Syst. 2023, 47, 33. [Google Scholar] [CrossRef] [PubMed]
- Chatterjee, J.; Dethlefs, N. This new conversational AI model can be your friend, philosopher, and guide ... and even your worst enemy. Patterns 2023, 4, 100676. [Google Scholar] [CrossRef] [PubMed]
- D'Amico, R.S.; White, T.G.; Shah, H.A.; Langer, D.J. I Asked a ChatGPT to Write an Editorial About How We Can Incorporate Chatbots Into Neurosurgical Research and Patient Care. Neurosurgery 2023, 92, 993–994. [Google Scholar] [CrossRef]
- De Angelis, L.; Baglivo, F.; Arzilli, G.; Privitera, G.P.; Ferragina, P.; Tozzi, A.E.; Rizzo, C. ChatGPT and the Rise of Large Language Models: The New AI-Driven Infodemic Threat in Public Health. SSRN, 2023; Preprint. [Google Scholar] [CrossRef]
- Deng, J.; Lin, Y. The Benefits and Challenges of ChatGPT: An Overview. Front. Comput. Intell. Syst. 2023, 2, 81–83. [Google Scholar]
- Domingos, P. The Master Algorithm: How the Quest for the Ultimate Learning Machine Will Remake Our World, 1st ed.; Basic Books, A Member of the Perseus Books Group: New York, NY, USA, 2018; p. 329. [Google Scholar]
- Fijačko, N.; Gosak, L.; Štiglic, G.; Picard, C.T.; John Douma, M. Can ChatGPT Pass the Life Support Exams without Entering the American Heart Association Course? Resuscitation 2023, 185, 109732.
Gilson, A.; Safranek, C.W.; Huang, T.; Socrates, V.; Chi, L.; Taylor,
- R.A.; Chartash, D. How Does ChatGPT Perform on the United States Medical Licensing Examination? The Implications of Large Language Models for Medical Education and Knowledge Assessment. JMIR Med. Educ. 2023, 9, e45312. [Google Scholar] [CrossRef] [PubMed] Gordijn, B.; Have, H.t. ChatGPT: Evolution or revolution? Med. Health Care
- Philos. 2023, 26, 1–2. [Google Scholar] [CrossRef]
- Hallsworth, J.E.; Udaondo, Z.; Pedrós-Alió, C.; Höfer, J.; Benison, K.C.; Lloyd, K.G.; Cordero, R.J.B.; de Campos, C.B.L.; Yakimov, M.M.; Amils, R. Scientific novelty beyond the experiment. Microb. Biotechnol. 2023; Online ahead of print. [Google Scholar] [CrossRef]
- Harzing, A.-W. Publish or Perish. Available online: https://harzing.com/resources/publish-or-perish (accessed on 16 February 2023).
- Hisan, U.; Amri, M. ChatGPT and Medical Education: A Double-Edged Sword. Researchgate, 2023; Preprint. [Google Scholar] [CrossRef]
- Jeblick, K.; Schachtner, B.; Dexl, J.; Mittermeier, A.; Stüber, A.T.; Topalis, J.; Weber, T.; Wesp, P.; Sabel, B.; Ricke, J.; et al. ChatGPT Makes Medicine Easy to Swallow: An Exploratory Case Study on Simplified Radiology Reports. arXiv 2022, arXiv:2212.14882. [Google Scholar] [CrossRef]
- Johnson, K.B.; Wei, W.Q.; Weeraratne, D.; Frisse, M.E.; Misulis, K.; Rhee, K.; Zhao, J.; Snowdon, J.L. Precision Medicine, AI, and the Future of Personalized Health Care. Clin. Transl. Sci. 2021, 14, 86–93. [Google Scholar] [CrossRef] [PubMed]
- Jordan, M.I.; Mitchell, T.M. Machine learning: Trends, perspectives, and prospects. Science 2015, 349, 255–260. [Google Scholar] [CrossRef]
- Khan, A.; Jawaid, M.; Khan, A.; Sajjad, M. ChatGPT-Reshaping medical education and clinical management. Pak. J. Med. Sci. 2023, 39, 605–607. [Google Scholar] [CrossRef]
- Kim, S.G. Using ChatGPT for language editing in scientific articles. Maxillofac. Plast. Reconstr. Surg. 2023, 45, 13. [Google Scholar] [CrossRef] [PubMed]
- Kitamura, F.C. ChatGPT Is Shaping the Future of Medical Writing but Still Requires Human Judgment. Radiology 2023, 230171.
- Korteling, J.E.; van de Boer-Visschedijk, G.C.; Blankendaal, R.A.M.; Boonekamp, R.C.; Eikelboom, A.R. Human- versus Artificial Intelligence. Front. Artif. Intell. 2021, 4, 622364. [Google Scholar] [CrossRef] [PubMed]
- Kostick-Quenet, K.M.; Gerke, S. AI in the hands of imperfect users. Npj Digit. Med. 2022, 5, 197. [Google Scholar] [CrossRef] [PubMed]
Kumar, A. Analysis of ChatGPT Tool to Assess the Potential of its Utility for Academic Writing in Biomedical Domain. Biol. Eng. Med. Sci. Rep. 2023, 9, 24–30. [Google Scholar] [CrossRef]
- Kung, T.H.; Cheatham, M.; Medenilla, A.; Sillos, C.; De Leon, L.; Elepaño, C.; Madriaga, M.; Aggabao, R.; Diaz-Candido, G.; Maningo, J.; et al. Performance of ChatGPT on USMLE: Potential for AI-assisted medical education using large language models. PLOS Digit. Health 2023, 2, e0000198. [Google Scholar] [CrossRef]
- Liebrenz, M.; Schleifer, R.; Buadze, A.; Bhugra, D.; Smith, A. Generating scholarly content with ChatGPT: Ethical challenges for medical publishing. Lancet Digit. Health 2023, 5, e105–e106.
- Lin, Z. Why and how to embrace AI such as ChatGPT in your academic life. PsyArXiv, 2023; Preprint. [Google Scholar]
- Lubowitz, J. ChatGPT, An Artificial Intelligence Chatbot, Is Impacting Medical Literature. Arthroscopy, 2023; in press. [Google Scholar]
- Lund, B.; Wang, S. Chatting about ChatGPT: How may AI and GPT impact academia and libraries? Library Hi. Tech. News, 2023; ahead-of-print. [Google Scholar] [CrossRef]
- Mann, D. Artificial Intelligence Discusses the Role of Artificial Intelligence in Translational Medicine: A JACC: Basic to Translational Science Interview With ChatGPT. J. Am. Coll. Cardiol. Basic Trans. Sci. 2023, 8, 221–223. [Google Scholar] [CrossRef]
- Manohar, N.; Prasad, S.S. Use of ChatGPT in Academic Publishing: A Rare Case of Seronegative Systemic Lupus Erythematosus in a Patient With HIV Infection. Cureus 2023, 15, e34616. [Google Scholar]

- Marchandot, B.; Matsushita, K.; Carmona, A.; Trimaille, A.; Morel, O. ChatGPT: The Next Frontier in Academic Writing for Cardiologists or a Pandora's Box of Ethical Dilemmas. Eur. Heart J. Open 2023, 3, oead007. [Google Scholar] [CrossRef]
- Margalida, A.; Colomer, M. Improving the peer-review process and editorial quality: Key errors escaping the review and editorial process in top scientific journals. PeerJ. 2016, 4, e1670. [Google Scholar] [CrossRef] [Green Version]
- Mavrogenis, A.F.; Quaile, A.; Scarlat, M.M. The good, the bad and the rude peer-review. Int. Orthop. 2020, 44, 413–415. [Google Scholar] [CrossRef] [Green Version]
- Mbakwe, A.B.; Lourentzou, I.; Celi, L.A.; Mechanic, O.J.; Dagan, A. ChatGPT passing USMLE shines a spotlight on the flaws of medical education. PLoS Digit. Health 2023, 2, e0000205. [Google Scholar] [CrossRef]
- McCarthy, J.; Minsky, M.L.; Rochester, N.; Shannon, C.E. A Proposal for the Dartmouth Summer Research Project on Artificial Intelligence, August 31, 1955. AI Mag. 2006, 27, 12. [Google Scholar] [CrossRef]
  Mijwil, M.; Aljanabi, M.; Ali, A. ChatGPT: Exploring the Role of Cybersecurity in the Protection of Medical Information. Mesop. J. CyberSecurity 2023, 18–21. [Google Scholar] [CrossRef]
- Moher, D.; Liberati, A.; Tetzlaff, J.; Altman, D.G. Preferred reporting items for systematic reviews and meta-analyses: The PRISMA statement. PLoS Med. 2009, 6, e1000097. [Google Scholar]
- Nachshon, A.; Batzofin, B.; Beil, M.; van Heerden, P.V. When Palliative Care May Be the Only Option in the Management of Severe Burns: A Case Report Written With the Help of ChatGPT. Cureus 2023, 15, e35649. [Google Scholar] [CrossRef] [PubMed]
- Nisar, S.; Aslam, M. Is ChatGPT a Good Tool for T&CM Students in Studying Pharmacology? SSRN, 2023; Preprint.
  Nolan, C. Interstellar; 169 minutes; Legendary Entertainment: Burbank, CA, USA, 2014. [Google Scholar]
- O'Connor, S. Open artificial intelligence platforms in nursing education: Tools for academic progress or abuse? Nurse Educ. Pract. 2023, 66, 103537. [Google Scholar] [CrossRef]
- Ollivier, M.; Pareek, A.; Dahmen, J.; Kayaalp, M.E.; Winkler, P.W.; Hirschmann, M.T.; Karlsson, J. A deeper dive into ChatGPT: History, use and future perspectives for orthopaedic research. Knee Surg. Sports Traumatol. Arthrosc. 2023;
- OpenAI. OpenAI: Models GPT-3. Available online: https://beta.openai.com/docs/models (accessed on 14 January 2023).
- Paranjape, K.; Schinkel, M.; Nannan Panday, R.; Car, J.; Nanayakkara, P. Introducing Artificial Intelligence Training in Medical Education. JMIR Med. Educ. 2019, 5, e16048. [Google Scholar] [CrossRef]
- Patel, S.B.; Lam, K. ChatGPT: The future of discharge summaries? Lancet Digit. Health 2023, 5, e107–e108. [Google Scholar] [CrossRef]
- Polonsky, M.; Rotman, J. Should Artificial Intelligent (AI) Agents be Your Co-author? Arguments in favour, informed by ChatGPT. SSRN, 2023; Preprint. [Google Scholar] [CrossRef]
- Quintans-Júnior, L.J.; Gurgel, R.Q.; Araújo, A.A.S.; Correia, D.; Martins-Filho, P.R. ChatGPT: The new panacea of the academic world. Rev. Soc. Bras. Med. Trop. 2023, 56, e0060.
- Rajpurkar, P.; Chen, E.; Banerjee, O.; Topol, E.J. AI in health and medicine. Nat. Med. 2022, 28, 31–38. [Google Scholar] [CrossRef]
- Rao, A.; Kim, J.; Kamineni, M.; Pang, M.; Lie, W.; Succi, M.D. Evaluating ChatGPT as an Adjunct for Radiologic Decision-Making. medRxiv 2023. [Google Scholar] [CrossRef]
- Sallam, M.; Salim, N.A.; Al-Tammemi, A.B.; Barakat, M.; Fayyad, D.; Hallit, S.; Harapan, H.; Hallit, R.; Mahafzah, A. ChatGPT Output Regarding Compulsory Vaccination and COVID-19 Vaccine Conspiracy: A Descriptive Study at the Outset of a Paradigm Shift in Online Search for Information. Cureus 2023, 15, e35029.
- Sallam, M.; Salim, N.A.; Barakat, M.; Al-Tammemi, A.B. ChatGPT applications in medical, dental, pharmacy, and public health education: A descriptive study. Narra J. 2023, 3, e103. [Google Scholar] [CrossRef]
- Sanmarchi, F.; Bucci, A.; Golinelli, D. A step-by-step Researcher's Guide to the use of an AI-based transformer in epidemiology: An exploratory analysis of ChatGPT using the STROBE checklist for observational studies. medRxiv, 2023; Preprint.
- Sarker, I.H. AI-Based Modeling: Techniques, Applications and Research Issues Towards Automation, Intelligent and Smart Systems. SN Comput. Sci. 2022, 3, 158. [Google Scholar] [CrossRef] [PubMed]
- Shahriar, S.; Hayawi, K. Let's have a chat! A Conversation with ChatGPT: Technology, Applications, and Limitations. arXiv 2023, arXiv:2302.13817. [Google Scholar] [CrossRef]
- Sharma, G.; Thakur, A. ChatGPT in Drug Discovery. ChemRxiv, 2023; Preprint. [Google Scholar] [CrossRef]
- Shen, Y.; Heacock, L.; Elias, J.; Hentel, K.D.; Reig, B.; Shih, G.; Moy, L. ChatGPT and Other Large Language Models Are Double-edged Swords. Radiology 2023, 230163. [Google Scholar] [CrossRef]
- Smith, R. Peer review: A flawed process at the heart of science and journals. J. R. Soc. Med. 2006, 99, 178–182.
  Stokel-Walker, C. AI bot ChatGPT writes smart essays—Should professors worry? Nature, 9 December 2022.
- Stokel-Walker, C. ChatGPT listed as author on research papers: Many scientists disapprove. Nature 2023, 613, 620–621. [Google Scholar]
- Stokel-Walker, C.; Van Noorden, R. What ChatGPT and generative AI mean for science. Nature 2023, 614, 214–216.
- Taecharungroj, V. "What Can ChatGPT Do?"; Analyzing Early Reactions to the Innovative AI Chatbot on Twitter. Big Data Cogn. Comput. 2023, 7, 35. [Google Scholar] [CrossRef]
- Tai, M.C. The impact of artificial intelligence on human society and bioethics. Tzu Chi. Med J. 2020, 32, 339–343. [
- Thorp, H.H. ChatGPT is fun, but not an author. Science 2023, 379, 313.
  Tobore, T.O. On Energy Efficiency and the Brain's Resistance to Change: The Neurological Evolution of Dogmatism and Close-Mindedness. Psychol. Rep. 2019, 122, 2406–2416.
- van Dis, E.A.M.; Bollen, J.; Zuidema, W.; van Rooij, R.; Bockting, C.L. ChatGPT: Five priorities for research. Nature 2023, 614, 224–226.
- Wang, S.; Scells, H.; Koopman, B.; Zuccon, G. Can ChatGPT Write a Good Boolean Query for Systematic Review Literature Search? arXiv 2023, arXiv:2302.03495. [Google Scholar] [CrossRef]
- Wogu, I.A.P.; Olu-Owolabi, F.E.; Assibong, P.A.; Agoha, B.C.; Sholarin, M.; Elegbeleye, A.; Igbokwe, D.; Apeh, H.A. Artificial intelligence, alienation and ontological problems of other minds: A critical investigation into the future of man and machines. In Proceedings of the 2017 International Conference on Computing Networking and Informatics (ICCNI), Lagos, Nigeria, 29–31 October 2017; pp. 1–10. [Google Scholar]
- Zielinski, C.; Winker, M.; Aggarwal, R.; Ferris, L.; Heinemann, M.; Lapeña, J.; Pai, S.; Ing, E.; Citrome, L. Chatbots, ChatGPT, and Scholarly Manuscripts WAME Recommendations on ChatGPT and Chatbots in Relation to Scholarly Publications. Maced J. Med. Sci. 2023, 11, 83–86. [Google Scholar] [CrossRef

CHAPTER 22

Educating Future Physicians in Artificial Intelligence. Will AI Eventually Replace Doctors?

As medicine and the delivery of healthcare enters the age of Artificial Intelligence (AI), the need for competent human–machine interaction to aid clinical decisions will rise. Medical students need to be sufficiently proficient in AI, its advantages to improve healthcare's expenses, quality, and access. Similarly, students must be educated about the shortfalls of AI such as bias, transparency, and liability. Overlooking a technology that will be transformative for the foreseeable future would place medical students at a disadvantage. However, there has been little interest in researching a proper method to implement AI in the medical education curriculum. This study aims to review the current literature that covers the attitudes of medical students towards AI, implementation of AI in the medical curriculum, and describe the need for more research in this area.

Trends in Healthcare

The United States is projected to see a growth in healthcare expenditure at a rate of 5.4% to reach $10 trillion by 2022 thereby constituting 9% of gross domestic product.. The expansion of healthcare has permeated many aspects of medical practice. For physicians, there are many concerning trends in healthcare including the growth of information and information technology. Ten years ago it was predicted that the doubling time of medical knowledge in 1950 was 50 years; in 1980, 7 years; and in 2010, 3.5 years, and in 2020 it was projected to be 0.2 years—just 73 days. At the given rate, entering medical students will experience a doubling of medical knowledge 5 times in their first year alone. Already strained under a regular medical school curriculum, accumulating dynamically changing information without proper aid will present an unprecedented challenge in medical education and medical careers.

Rise of AI

Artificial Intelligence (AI) is defined as the ability of a machine to imitate human intelligence. From its inception, AI has permeated everyday life, business and in particular, AI is increasingly applied to healthcare. The technology has the potential to impact many aspects of both institutionalized and private healthcare, from diagnosis to treatment options and from benchwork research to pharmaceutical design. AI is being tested in healthcare to assist and replace repetitive tasks such as image recognition in diagnosis and augmentation of images in radiology. AI is expected to augment healthcare workflow through automated triage, improve the productivity of individual physicians, reduce human errors, discover better patterns of patient care, defray medical costs, perform minimally invasive surgery, and reduce mortality rates Ultimately, physicians roles are changing due to the superior efficacy of AI in dealing with many established physician practices, chemical synthesis planning, and drug discovery.

The Need to Adapt

In the past, as with the introduction of robotics, physicians roles were under similar pressure from change. 16 In response, physicians adapted their roles to best match their tools to further advance patient care. However, with the rapid advancement of AI, physicians face an unprecedented stress to learn entire new skill sets and to manage an exponential growth of medical knowledge. Fortunately, solving the challenge of learning about AI can provide a useful solution to the issue of expanding medical knowledge. AI has the ability to equip physicians with an alternative to efficiently deal with and translate medical knowledge into practice.

Transforming Education

Healthcare is advancing and along with it is the necessity to improve medical education. As the rate of discovery of medical knowledge grows, physicians will have trouble managing, organizing, and retaining information.

Technologies such as AI are needed to enable healthcare professionals to effectively use this knowledge to practice medicine. As medicine and the delivery of healthcare enters the age of AI, the need for competent human–machine interaction for the use of data to aid clinical decision making will rise.

Medical students need to be sufficiently proficient in understanding the fundamental concepts of how AI functions, its advantages to improve expenses, increase quality, and ease access to healthcare..Similarly, students must be educated about the shortfalls of AI such as transparency and liability. Finally, overlooking a technology that will be transformative for the foreseeable future would place medical students at a disadvantage.

Goals

We aim to provide an extensive literature review of previous studies describing the role of teaching AI in medical education as a curriculum subject. This includes teaching AI as a concept, tools, principles, methodologies, implications, risks, and applications. Medical students should be able to use, interpret, and explain the results of an AI output. Although teaching medical students with AI tools is meaningful and important, that is beyond the scope of this paper. This paper also aims to further transition from a call to teach medical students about AI to an advanced path of implementation. In this paper, we summarize recent relevant papers in the field of medical education that have addressed the main topics of interest in this paper, particularly the curricular, cultural, and attitudinal changes required to successfully incorporate the teaching of AI contents in undergraduate medical education (UME).

Design and Search

An integrative review approach was chosen to identify the past and current literature from different types of research. Integrative review is a unique approach to combining different approaches to research including experimental and nonexperimental. The sequential approach to integrative review is problem identification, literature search, data evaluation, data analysis, and presentation. The problem identified was to understand the lack of AI implementation in medical education.

A search design was agreed upon by all authors. The designed strategy was to search Pubmed, Medline (Ovid), GoogleScholar, and Web of Science. Key terms searched were ("AI" or "artificial intelligence" or "machine learning") AND ("medical education" or "undergraduate medical education") AND ("curriculum" or "learning" or "teaching"). Resulting article lists were saved, reviewed, and analyzed for selection criteria on Excel.

Exclusion and Inclusion Criteria

This study included national and international experimental and nonexperimental studies published in English. We selected articles dating from 2010 in order to include the period before the major growth in electronic health records and digital information. Article inclusion criteria included studies discussing the need for AI to be incorporated in the medical curriculum either at undergraduate level. We included literature reviews, studies that repeated prior speculative suggestions of curriculum reform, dissertations, letters, opinions, perspectives, and commentaries. We included articles with at least speculative suggestions of curriculum reform, medical student and faculty attitude towards AI, planned out curriculum changes, reports of implemented changes, and institutional level programs to train students in AI.However, we excluded research that did not mention the need for education of AI in medical school or provide new educationalstrategies or insight into the actual progression of AI in medical education. Additionally, we excluded research focusing on incorporation of AI tools to enhance medical learning as this was not the purpose of our study. Finally, we excluded research on graduate level medical education or continued medical education.

Data Selection

Using Excel functions, duplicate research studies were screened out. The authors went through each match and analyzed manuscript title and abstract based on predetermined inclusion and exclusion criteria for relevance. Two of the authors independently screened the articles for inclusion and exclusion criteria. They discussed their results and resolved any discrepancies using the third author. Individual articles were then reanalyzed for inclusion criteria accuracy based on article content in the same manner.

Relevance Grading

Articles were then coded according to relevance for this integrative review. Relevance was scored on a 4-point scale: 1— articles call for change with speculative reform, 2—determining student and faculty attitudes, 3—thorough plans for a curriculum change, 4—reports of implemented curriculum change or institutional programs. This was determined through careful reading of the full manuscript and determining the best fit category. The scores were then verified by another author who had no previous exposure to the previous values scored. Any discrepancies were discussed holistically and rescored jointly.

What is the Best way Forward?

In order to anticipate changes and challenges in medical education environments, this review integrated the opinions, studies, and reported changes of implementation of AI in medical education. The results of our systematic review show that no institutional comprehensive studied and researched initiatives were conducted. Among the 2 reports of implemented changes, there were no previous reported studies researching what students hope to gain from such changes or what methods would be most effective.36,47 Similarly, among the 6 articles with proposed changes to medical curriculum, there was no evidence-based method backing these proposals.40,54 The detailed programs introduced in this study could be useful for medical educators in the development of curricula. Further research is required to integrate the educational trends into graduate and continuing medical education, and to investigate the status or effects of innovative educational programs in each medical school.Going forward, we propose a longitudinal study searching for a comprehensive understanding of how to conduct a large and unparalleled change by incorporating AI in the medical education curriculum.

Call for Research of AI in Medical Education

The exposure of gaps in medical faculty knowledge of AI is in the process of research but is likely to conclude that there is a need to restructure faculty positions to bridge these gaps; these gaps may be inhibiting learners who have an active interest in AI applications but lack exposure to knowledgeable faculty to help them understand, access, and apply them.A 2015 publication noted that 30% of US medical students surveyed had interest in clinical informatics, but were not able to identify training opportunities to help. These knowledge gaps, however, should not be solely characterized in a negative fashion, as they also present important opportunities for new faculty development into the medical education environment. Employing a new cohort of educators with skills in new areas is necessary but also innovative. The AMA Council on Medical Education wrote that institutional leaders and academic deans must proactively accelerate their inclusion of nonclinicians, such as data scientists and engineers, onto their faculty rosters The proper plan should incorporate a longitudinal model to study AI across the medical education continuum. This study should begin with national surveys of medical students and educators on the attitudes and expectations of learning AI in medical school. These surveys should identify the realistic goals and expectations of what future physicians should expect and what faculty members need to meet these expectations. These surveys should be measurable and have interpretable data to advance the implementation of AI in UME. A concerted multi institutional study is a logical approach to achieve thesegoals.Thereafter, multidisciplinary research, collaboration, training, and learning about the role of AI in medicine should be incorporated through previously proven methods in similar drastic curricular changes.

Barriers to Change

As the push for AI in medical education continues to make advancements, it is not without challenges and barriers. Change is met with resistance from faculty and physicians ill equipped for such an evolution of clinical practice. Fear of eventual physician replacement by machine may prevent these opportunities. Furthermore, misunderstanding and lack of background in AI can create skepticism in the trustworthiness of a machine learning prediction.

This is compounded by the regular difficulties in organizing large curricular change. Further research on how best to incorporate these changes is warranted.

Moving Forward

A school wishing to keep up with the technologies and advances in healthcare should heed the warnings of numerous physicians about the role of AI as a partner in medicine. Not doing so would disadvantage the future generation of physicians and place them at the mercy of catching up to technology.Physicians should be trained to understand the technological capabilities and limitations of AI so that they can properly employ it as a safe tool in practice. Physicians need the ability to interpret the results and communicate a recommendation to the patients.

Furthermore, physicians should be exposed to the emerging ethical challenges that AI will bring to the workplace. How can a physician untrained in the field of AI expect to navigate ethical scenarios such as if a computer algorithm predicts a high chance of death for a patient.

The implementation of AI in medicine will change the way care is delivered going forward. Medicine is headed along with most other fields, into the age of information technology. Using the Normalization Process Theory, we perceive that AI will become embedded in society both individually and collectively and ultimately will be a necessity in the daily routine of a physician. 53 However, this process can be accelerated in extreme circumstances that call upon the need for AI. During COVID-19, medicine changed and it was accelerated by AI and other advanced technologies. We saw entire practices and hospitals switch over to telehealth and this exemplifies the need to train doctors in advanced healthcare technology. The future of medical education and medicine is uncertain after the pandemic resolves but an AI-centric future is likely to be the disruptive change that will guide the future of learning and medicine.Some of the large problems in healthcare, such as patient wait times, cost of healthcare, and insufficient care may find AI to be extremely helpful. But the costs of misusing AI may be equally problematic. These advantages and liabilities call for future physicians to begin to be properly trained in AI's uses and pitfalls.

Our study has its limitations including a limited amount of databases searched and limited search queries. We accounted for this by looking through the resulting included studies' references for possible missed studies. Additionally, we tried to limit bias in the relevance and scoring process by using a third author opinion and discussing all discrepancies.

There is little doubt among the literature we reviewed that AI will be the future of medicine. In order to continue to efficiently train physicians to be able to handle today and tomorrow, a national and multiinstitutional initiative is warranted.

Will AI Eventually Replace Doctors?

Maybe not entirely. But the doctor–patient relationship is likely to change dramatically. Based on the research of ***David Dranove Craig Garthwaite.***

The year is 2070. You walk into an urgent care clinic feeling unwell, and an Alexa-esque device asks you to describe your symptoms. The computer takes down your information, retrieves details from your past electronic health records, and suggests diagnostic tests for a human technician to perform. After getting the test results, the software program prescribes a medication to treat your condition.This futuristic scenario is one example of how AI might become part of healthcare. In fact, AI systems are already being developed to read medical scans and tissue samples to determine if a patient has a disease.Future software could analyze patterns across thousands of health records to pinpoint the most effective treatment for a particular patient—for instance, which cancer therapy might work best given their genetic makeup.

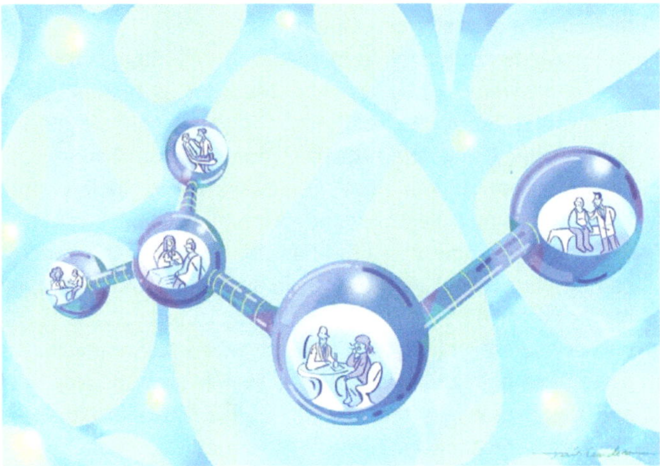

Fig.22.1 Showing a patient would be managed by the doctor with AI.

In a recent paper, David Dranove and Craig Garthwaite, professors of strategy at Kellogg, explored the implications of incorporating AI into healthcare—in particular, how such software would affect the central role of the physician.

For now, the need for human interaction in healthcare is likely to keep AI on the sidelines as a complement, rather than a substitute, for doctors, Dranove says. But perhaps in a few decades, patients will be comfortable interacting with computers and even trust them as their main source of medical guidance. "Maybe in the long run, that will change," he says.

Mixed evidence

Proponents of this new technology believe that AI could help in two main ways.

The first area where AI could make inroads is treatment plans informed by data mining. The software could extract patterns from electronic records of previous patients' characteristics, genetic variations, symptoms, treatment, and health outcomes. Based on a new patient's similarities to past cases, the AI program then might be able to predict the most effective drugs to prescribe or surgery to perform.

The second area is in diagnosis, particularly in the fields of radiology and pathology. A computer could be given a large set of images from previous patients with known diagnoses. The software program could then be trained on those images to recognize features that indicate a positive or negative result.Some studies suggest that AI can perform such tasks fairly well—and sometimes pick up on signs of disease that doctors miss. For instance, one team reported that an AI program detected breast cancer in mammograms—particularly, invasive cancers in the early stages—more accurately than did radiologists.

Other studies have explored whether it's better for AI to complement or replace physicians' expertise when it comes to making diagnoses. But this research has come to conflicting conclusions, Dranove says. In some cases, such as the breast-cancer study, doctors who were given guidance from AI made less-accurate decisions than AI alone.

But in other cases, the combination of physician expertise and AI was the best option. For example, one team tested AI software trained to detect hip fractures in radiographs. Two experienced radiologists who incorporated the AI program's output into their evaluations performed better than the software by itself.

"The evidence is mixed," Dranove says.

A need for compassion

But, even if the evidence ends up showing that AI can do as well or better than doctors in some situations, will AI actually replace physicians? The answer depends partly on how critical human interaction is, Dranove says. For instance, physicians elicit information from patients, explain why a procedure is necessary, and provide instructions for follow-up care. Dranove believes that most older adults today, and perhaps younger adults as well, still want to hear from a human being about their health.

"There's a need for compassion in communication that AI is unable to contribute," he says.

Healthcare organizations might decide that a lower-paid medical professional, such as a nurse or physician assistant, can play that role, with their decisions guided by AI. But that too will depend on whether doctors' tasks can be boiled down to standardized questions and responses, or whether greater nuance and expertise is required, Dranove says. For example, a physician might be more adept at helping the patient feel comfortable discussing their health condition and determining how much a disease is truly affecting a person's quality of life.

"I think we're going to see a patchwork quilt where AI gets implemented."—David Dranove

Even in radiology, one of the specialties that seems the most threatened by AI, the job still involves substantial human interaction. Dranove and Garthwaite examined a list of tasks for which radiologists bill; these included services such as X-ray scans, CT scans, ultrasound examinations, mammography, and so on. At first glance, radiologists appeared to be largely spending their days using technology.

But a more comprehensive list of tasks, from the Occupational Information Network, showed that the job also involved many interpersonal exchanges. For instance, radiologists need to discuss results with other medical staff and explain risks, benefits, and treatment options to patients. "It's not just reading a film and writing a report," Dranove says.

Who gets the profits?

The researchers also considered what would happen to the value chain in healthcare if AI were to become a complement to physicians, rather than a substitute. The value chain includes all the parties who contribute to and benefit from it: the patient, doctor, nurse, healthcare system, drug company, insurance company, and so on. As with the production of any good or service, healthcare can create value—including better health for patients, wages for providers, and profits for companies—and incur costs. Because physicians play such a central role, they often capture a large portion of the value in the form of very high salaries. If AI took over diagnosis and treatment decisions, one might expect doctors to become less valued and for their wages to sink accordingly. On the other hand, might doctors end up receiving even higher salaries, if they can issue faster or more-accurate medical decisions with AI's help?

Although doctors may become more productive, they won't necessarily reap financial benefits, Dranove says. Instead, the healthcare system is more likely to capture the additional value through higher profits. For example, the organization might improve its healthcare quality metrics and thus argue to an insurance company that they should be paid more."Doctors will not be replaced by AI, but they may not directly profit from it either," Dranove says. And it's not clear if even the healthcare organization will get monetary rewards. Medical care in the United States is often based on a fee-for-service model. If AI reduces overtreatment and leads to fewer procedures, "you're losing money," he says. Organizations therefore might not have a strong financial motivation to develop and use AI, even if it improves patient outcomes. The exception would be self-contained systems such as the Veterans Health Administration; if they save money, they reap all the benefits.

A patchwork quilt

Incorporating AI into healthcare faces many other hurdles. One of the biggest is lack of access to data. "You can't outperform a physician based on reams and reams of data if you don't have lots and lots of patients on which to train the computer," Dranove says. In the United States, medical records are scattered across healthcare systems, and HIPAA restricts the ability to share information. As a result, most AI development so far has occurred within medical organizations that are using only their own patients' records. This means that large healthcare systems have an advantage over smaller ones, which might not have enough data to train the software effectively. "I think we're going to see a patchwork quilt where AI gets implemented," he says. While it's possible that these large organizations could share their trained software with others, they might hesitate to do so. "From a societal standpoint, I should share that information" because it could improve health outcomes for patients elsewhere, Dranove says. But the organization's perspective might be, "why would I give away for free something that makes my system that much more valuable?" Without a federal law requiring data or software sharing, he says, "I think this is going to be a highly fragmented process for a long time."That doesn't mean that large healthcare organizations should be held back from developing AI, he says. But a coordinated approach will distribute the benefits of AI more equally."If data can be shared, then everybody will have that opportunity," he says.

5 Reasons why Artificial Intelligence won't replace physicians --Another view

There is a lot of concern and fear surrounding Artificial Intelligence taking over jobs in medicine. Will physicians become obsolete? Will AI replace most medical professionals? We look into this throughout this article and set the record straight: here are the 5 main reasons why artificial intelligence won't take the place of physicians.

The medical community should take no notice of the fearmongering around A.I.

While we await the industrial revolution, digitization and automation are drastically changing the job market. Lots of professionals dear that AI, robots, and automation will take their jobs without any alternative. These very same worries emerge in medicine when AI is talked about. Especially in the radiology field, with robots surpassing the skills of surgeons.

One of the most renowned speakers in tech, Kai-Fu Lee, who is the founder of Sinovation Ventures, was noted to say that AI will be much larger than any other tech revolution, and robots are likely to replace around 50% of all jobs within the next decade. Another prominent voice, Vinod Khosla said that machines will substitute around 80% of doctors in medicine in the future and that healthcare will be run by entrepreneurs and not medical experts. Prof Geoffrey Hinton said in 2016 that it's "quite obvious that we should stop training radiologists." This all comes about as the AI algorithms are showing themselves to be better than humans. But is all of this true?

Not in the slightest, they are all completely wrong. Perhaps there are indeed many signs suggesting that AI will completely take over the world of healthcare, and yes, there are many technologies that are transforming the industry. However, fear-mongering and staring that medical professionals will disappear is simply irresponsible. For instance, it could very well scare off medical students from beginning a career in radiology. Curtis Langlotz, stated in a presentation recently, that one of his students sent him an email suggesting that he was thinking about going into the field of radiology, but he wasn't sure whether it's a viable profession any longer.

Healthcare will always need humans in the future

There is a suggestion that investors like Vinod Khosla don't really understand the medical sector, and therefore his suggestion isn't really based on proper knowledge. A report by Carl Benedikt Frey and Michael A. Osborne from the University of Oxford suggested that medical records, medical transcriptionists, and health information technicians, and medical secretaries are the most likely jobs to be computerized in the future. It suggested that physicians had around a 0.42% chance of their profession becoming automated.That isn't to suggest, however, that AI will appear in healthcare in the next 10-15 years. For instance, many believe that in 10 years' time, AI will be routinely used in NHS practices. And others suggest that within three years, we could see a lot of machine learning algorithms being used in clinical pilot testing and being approved by the US.

Furthermore, AI will totally change the meaning of what it means to become a doctor. Of course, some tasks will change, others will go away entirely. But, there will never ever be a scenario where automation via a robot or an algorithm will replace a doctor. Here are the reasons why

1.Robots cannot replace empathy

The world of technology has a vast array of excellent solutions, but it would be hard for any of them to embody empathy. Why? That's because empathy is all about building trust, listening intently to the other person, paying attention to their feelings and needs, and being compassionate and responsive in a manner that the other person feels understood.

At the moment, no one would trust a robot of an AI algorithm with a life-threatening decision or even a decision whether to take a form of medicine or not. For example, the NHS undertook an experiment to ease the burden on their health lines by using chatbots. Those taking part in the trial suggested that they would use the system to get an appointment with the doctor quicker instead of using the chatbot's recommendations. This could all change in the future, however, as patients take better care of their health and have more responsibility in their own care, but still, we simply cannot imagine a healthcare system without empathy. Doctors will always be needed to hold our hands and tell us about a life-altering diagnosis, and we will need them to guide us through therapy and provide support. No algorithm or robot could ever replace that. Period.

2. Physicians have changing working methods

One of the episodes in House M.D., showed a team trying to figure out how a small boy might have been poisoned. They thought about many options, food, drugs, pesticide poisoning, etc. And for each possible diagnosis, they came up with a different treatment choice. Every option made the patient feel worse, until they finally figured out, by accident, that the child had phosmet, a kind of insecticide from the jeans he was wearing that he purchased from a street vendor. The child hadn't washed the clothes before wearing them, and his skin absorbed the poison.There is no possible algorithm that could have made the diagnosis. Even though data, measurements, and analytics are a huge part of a doctor's job, they will become even more so in the future, but finding a diagnosis and setting up a treatment plan are not linear processes. A doctor's job requires creativity and problem-solving abilities, something that robots and algorithms will never have.

There are many kinds of patients, each with different lifestyles. And, diseases have the same feature. Therefore, no two cases are the same, each one is entirely different and requires human physicians. Before the evolution of digital solutions and complex technology, physicians used basic medical devices to make healthcare decisions. This process won't change in the future, there will just be more complex technology involved.

3. Complex digital technology requires competent professionals

With a lot more advanced digital health solutions available, there will be a need for competent, qualified medical professionals, whether it's about robotics or AI or not. For example, let's consider the surgical robot, the da Vinci Surgical System. The robot has a magnified 3D high-definition vision system and tiny instruments that can rotate and bend much further than any human hand. But, surgeons will need to learn how to operate it, and to master, this will take practice.

Similarly, there is IBM Watson. A program for oncologists that is very unique. It provides clinicians with evidence-based treatment choices. Regardless of this though, only doctors and their patients will choose the treatment, and only physicians can assess whether the algorithm's suggestion was useful or not. There is no algorithm or robot that will be able to deal with such complex, multi-layered challenges. They may provide the data, but the interpretation of such will always remain with humans.

4.There will always be tasks algorithms and robots can never complete

Doctors, nurses, and lots of other medical staff members have lots of monotonous, cumbersome, and repetitive tasks that they undertake each day. In the US, a study suggested that the average doctor has to spend 8.7 hours each week on admin tasks. Psychiatrists spend the largest proportion of their day on paperwork (20.3%), followed by internists (17.3%), and then family GPs (17.3%). All of these kinds of procedures and tasks could be and should be, automated.

But, there will always be duties and responsibilities that technology cannot do. Although IBM Watson can work through millions of pages of a document in seconds, it won't ever be able to perform the Heimlich maneuver. So there will always remain tasks that humans can do much quicker, much more reliably, and much cheaper than technology can.

5. It has never been about tech vs. human

The view that many have, and the constant enemy building image needs to stop once and for all. It's never been a case of technology vs. humans. There is no them versus us, after all,

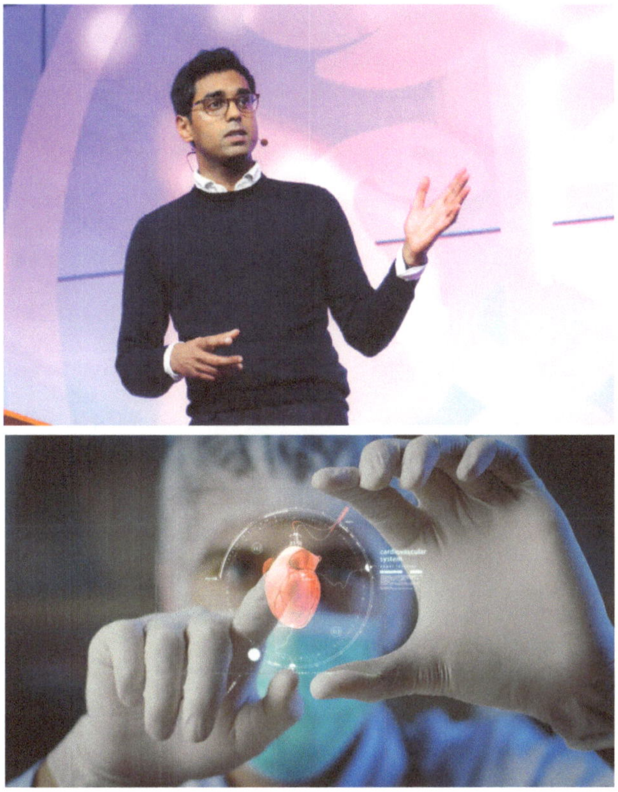

Fig.22.2 AI Won't Replace Doctors, It Will Augment Them

technology is there to help people. We are all on the same team. Whether it's AI, AR or VR, or robots, we must all accept that technology plays a huge part in the way our healthcare works, and we must start utilizing their powers. Imagine what could be capable in healthcare when we have the problem-solving skills and creativity combined with the computing power and cognitive resources of technology.

The ultimate response is the collaboration between humans and technology. A recent study that used deep learning to identify metastatic breast cancer showed something similar. When the findings of the deep learning system were combined with the pathologist's diagnoses, the tumor localization score, and the image classification, significantly increased. Furthermore, the error rate for hums was reduced by 85%. When cooperating, the outcome of AI and humans can be the most potent.

Many believe that technology will help medical professionals to become more efficient, less prone to error and mistakes, and more seamless. Perhaps in the future, we could have an occurring answer to this fear of AI taking over healthcare and look at it in a more positive light

Bibliography and Acknowledgement

- Alrassi J, Katsufrakis PJ, Chandran L. Technology can augment, but not replace, critical human skills needed for patient care. Acad Med. 2021;96(1):37–43.
- American Medical Association. Medical education, professional development and credentialing. Published online 2020.
- Aungst TD, Patel R. Integrating digital health into the curriculum—considerations on the current landscape and future developments. J MedEducCurricDev.2020;7:238212051990127.
- Banerjee R, George P, Priebe C, Alper E. Medical student awareness of and interest in clinical informatics. J Am Med Inform Assoc. 2015;22(e1):e42–e47. doi: 10.1093/jamia/ocu046. [PMC free article] [PubMed][CrossRef][GoogleScholar]
- Barbour AB, Frush JM, Gatta LA, et al. Artificial intelligence in health care: insights from an educational forum. J Med Educ Curric Dev. 2019;6:2382120519889348. 10.1177/2382120519889348 [PMC free article] [PubMed] [CrossRef] [Google Scholar]
- Briganti G, Le Moine O. Artificial intelligence in medicine: today and tomorrow. Front Med. 2020;7(February):1–6. doi: 10.3389/fmed.2020.00027. [PMC free article] [PubMed] [CrossRef] [Google Scholar]
- Brouillette M. AI Added to the curriculum for doctors-to-be. Nat Med. 2019;25(12):1808–1809. doi: 10.1038/s41591-019-0648-3. [PubMed][CrossRef][GoogleScholar]
- Carin L. On artificial intelligence and deep learning within medical education. Acad Med. Published online August 4, 2020. 10.1097/ACM.0000000000003630 [PubMed] [CrossRef] [Google Scholar]
- Chan KS, Zary N. Applications and challenges of implementing artificial intelligence in medical education: integrative review. J Med Internet Res. 2019;21(6). doi: 10.2196/13930. [PMC free article] [PubMed][CrossRef][GoogleScholar]
- Chen J. Playing to our human strengths to prepare medical students for the future. Korean J Med Educ. 2017;29(3):193–197. 10.3946/kjme.2017.65 [PMC free article] [PubMed]
- Davenport T, Kalakota R. The potential for artificial intelligence in healthcare. SSRN Electron J. 2020;6(2):94–98. doi: 10.2139/ssrn.3525037.. [PMC free article] [PubMed]
- Densen P. Challenges and opportunities facing medical education. Trans Am Clin Climatol Assoc. 2011;122(319):48–58. [PMC free article][PubMed][GoogleScholar]
- Ellaway RH. Medical education and the war with the machines. Med Teach. 2014;36(10):917–918. 10.3109/0142159X.2014.955088 Fan KY, Hu R, Singla R. Introductory machine learning for medical students: a pilot. Med Educ. 2020;54(11):1042–1043.
- Gallix B, Chong J. Artificial intelligence in radiology: who's afraid of the big bad wolf? Eur Radiol. 2019;29(4):1637–1639. 10.1007/s00330-018-5995-9 [PubMed] [CrossRef] [Google Scholar]
- Guo J, Li B. The application of medical artificial intelligence technology in rural areas of developing countries. Heal Equity. 2018;2(1):174–181. doi: 10.1089/heq.2018.0037. [PMC free article]
- Han ER, Yeo S, Kim MJ, Lee YH, Park KH, Roh H. Medical education trends for future physicians in the era of advanced technology and artificial intelligence: an integrative review. BMC Med Educ. 2019;19(1). doi: 10.1186/s12909-019-1891-5.
- Hasan Sapci A, Aylin Sapci H. Artificial intelligence education and tools for medical and health informatics students: systematic review. JMIR Med Educ. 2020;6(1).

- Imran N, Jawaid M. Artificial intelligence in medical educationare we ready for it? Pakistan J Med Sci. 2020;36(5):857–859. doi: 10.12669/pjms.36.5.3042. [PMC free article] [PubMed] [CrossRef] [Google Scholar]
- James C, Wheelock K, Woolliscroft J. Machine learning: the next paradigm shift in medical education. Acad Med. 2021;Publish Ah. doi: 10.1097/ACM.0000000000003943. [PubMed] [CrossRef] [Google Scholar]
- Kang J, Thompson RF, Aneja S, et al. National cancer institute workshop on artificial intelligence in radiation oncology: training the next generation. Pract Radiat Oncol. Published online June 13, 2020. 10.1016/j.prro.2020.06.001 [PMC free article] [PubMed] [CrossRef] [Google Scholar]
- Khurana. M. Keeping Pace: The Need for Digital Health Education in Medical Schools. Acad Med. 2020;95(11):1629–1630. doi: 10.1097/ACM.0000000000003672 [PubMed] [CrossRef] [Google Scholar]
- Kolachalama VB, Garg PS. Machine learning and medical education. npj Digit Med. 2018;1(1):2–4. doi: 10.1038/s41746-018-0061-1. [PMC free article] [PubMed] [CrossRef] [Google Scholar]
- Lang J, Repp H. Artificial intelligence in medical education and the meaning of interaction with natural intelligence – an interdisciplinary approach. GMS J Med Educ. 2020;37:Doc59. doi: 10.3205/zma001352. [PMC free article] [PubMed] [CrossRef] [Google Scholar]
- Lanza F, Seidita V, Chella A. Agents and robots for collaborating and supporting physicians in healthcare scenarios. J Biomed Inform. 2020;108:103483. doi: 10.1016/j.jbi.2020.103483. [PMC free article] [PubMed] [CrossRef] [Google Scholar]
- Li D, Kulasegaram K, Hodges BD. Why we needn't fear the machines: opportunities for medicine in a machine learning world. Acad Med. 2019;94(5):623–625. doi: 10.1097/ACM.0000000000002661. [PubMed] [CrossRef] [Google Scholar]
- Masters K. Artificial intelligence developments in medical education: a conceptual and practical framework. MedEdPublish. 2020;9(1):1–20. doi: 10.15694/mep.2020.000239.1. [CrossRef] [Google Scholar]
- McCoy LG, Nagaraj S, Morgado F, Harish V, Das S, Celi LA. What do medical students actually need to know about artificial intelligence? npj Digit Med. 2020;3(1):2–4. doi: 10.1038/s41746-020-0294-7. [PMC free article] [PubMed] [CrossRef] [Google Scholar]
- Meskó B, Hetényi G, Győrffy Z. Will artificial intelligence solve the human resource crisis in healthcare? BMC Health Serv Res. 2018;18(1):545. 10.1186/s12913-018-3359-4 [PMC free article] [PubMed] [CrossRef] [Google Scholar]
- Murdoch TB, Detsky AS. The inevitable application of big data to health care. JAMA. 2013;309(13):1351–1352.
- O'Doherty D, Dromey M, Lougheed J, Hannigan A, Last J, McGrath D. Barriers and solutions to online learning in medical education – an integrative review. BMC Med Educ. 2018;18(130). [PMC free article] [PubMed] [Google Scholar]
- Papanicolas I. Health Care Spending in the United States and Other High-Income Countries. The Commonwealth Fund. Published 2018. https://www.commonwealthfund.org/publications/journal-article/2018/mar/health-care-spending-united-states-and-other-high-income
- Paranjape K, Schinkel M, Panday RN, Car J, Nanayakkara P. Introducing artificial intelligence training in medical education. J Med Internet Res. 2019;21(12). doi: 10.2196/16048. [PMC free article]
- Park SH, Do KH, Kim S, Park JH, Lim YS. What should medical students know about artificial intelligence in medicine? J Educ Eval Health Prof. 2019;16:16–21. doi: 10.3352/jeehp.2019.16.18.
- Randhawa GK, Jackson M. The role of artificial intelligence in learning and professional development for healthcare professionals. Healthc Manag Forum. 2020;33(1):19–24.
- Robeznieks A. 3 ways medical AI can improve workflow for physicians. American Medical Association. 2018 [Google Scholar]
- Sanal MG, Paul K, Kumar S, Ganguly NK. Artificial intelligence and deep learning: the future of medicine and medical practice. J Assoc Physicians India. 2019;67(4):71–73. https://login.ezproxy.fau.edu/login?url=https://search.proquest.com/docview/2258734066?accountid=10902. [PubMed] [Google Scholar]
- Scantlebury A, Sheard L, Watt I, Cairns P, Wright J, Adamson J. Exploring the implementation of an electronic record into a maternity unit: a qualitative study using normalisation process theory. BMC Med Inform Decis Mak. 2017;17(1):4. doi: 10.1186/s12911-016-0406-0. [PMC free article] [PubMed] [CrossRef] [Google Scholar]
- Sit C, Srinivasan R, Amlani A, et al. Attitudes and perceptions of UK medical students towards artificial intelligence and radiology: a multicentre survey. Insights Imaging. 2020;11(1):7–12. doi: 10.1186/s13244-019-0830-7. [PMC free article] [PubMed] [CrossRef] [Google Scholar]
- Srivastava TK, Waghmare L. Implications of artificial intelligence (AI) on dynamics of medical education and care: a perspective. J Clin Diagnostic Res. Published online 2020:2019–2020. doi: 10.7860/jcdr/2020/43293.13565. [CrossRef] [Google Scholar]
- Topol EJ. High-performance medicine: the convergence of human and artificial intelligence. Nat Med. 2019;25(1):44–56. doi: 10.1038/s41591-018-0300-7. [PubMed] [CrossRef] [Google Scholar]
- van der Niet AG, Bleakley A. Where medical education meets artificial intelligence: 'does technology care?'. Med Educ. 2021;55(1):30–36. doi: 10.1111/medu.14131. [PubMed] [CrossRef] [Google Scholar]
- Walsh K. Artificial intelligence and healthcare professional education: superhuman resources for health? Postgrad Med J. 2020;96(1133):121–122. doi: 10.1136/postgradmedj-2019-137132 [PubMed] [CrossRef] [Google Scholar]
- Wang JK, Roy SK, Barry M, Chang RT, Bhatt AS. Institutionalizing healthcare hackathons to promote diversity in collaboration in medicine. BMC Med Educ. 2018;18(1):269. 10.1186/s12909-018-1385-x [PMC free article] [PubMed] [CrossRef] [Google Scholar]
- Wang Z, Majewicz Fey A. Deep learning with convolutional neural network for objective skill evaluation in robot-assisted surgery. Int J Comput Assist Radiol Surg. 2018;13(12):1959–1970. doi: 10.1007/s11548-018-1860-1. [PubMed] [CrossRef] [Google Scholar]
- Wartman SA, Combs CD. Reimagining medical education in the age of AI. AMA J Ethics. 2019;21(2):146–152. doi: 10.1001/amajethics.2019.146.. [PubMed] [CrossRef] [Google Scholar]
- Wartman SA, Donald Combs C. Medical education must move from the information age to the age of artificial intelligence. Acad Med. 2018;93(8):1107–1109. doi: 10.1097/ACM.0000000000002044. [PubMed] [CrossRef] [Google Scholar]
- Wartman SA. The empirical challenge of 21st-century medical education. Acad Med. 2019;94(10):1412–1415. doi: 10.1097/ACM.0000000000002866. [PubMed] [CrossRef] [Google Scholar]
- Weng SF, Vaz L, Qureshi N, Kai J. Prediction of premature all-cause mortality: a prospective general population cohort study comparing machine-learning and standard epidemiological approaches. PLoS One. 2019;14(3):1–22. doi: 10.1371/journal.pone.0214365. [PMC free article] [PubMed] [CrossRef] [Google Scholar]
- Whittemore R, Knafl K. The integrative review: updated methodology. J Adv Nurs. 2005;52(5):546–553. doi: 10.1111/j.1365-2648.2005.03621.x. [PubMed] [CrossRef] [Google Scholar]
- Wiljer D, Hakim Z. Developing an artificial intelligence-enabled health care practice: rewiring health care professions for better care. J Med Imaging Radiat Sci. 2019;50(4 Suppl 2):S8–S14. 10.1016/j.jmir.2019.09.010 [PubMed] [CrossRef] [Google Scholar]

CHAPTER 23

Artificial Intelligence Advancements in the Cardiovascular Imaging of Coronary Atherosclerosis

The application of AI in cardiology has increased exponentially annually, specifically in the diagnosis of coronary artery disease (CAD). These novel approaches may enhance future implementation of the new 2021 American College of Cardiology/American Heart Association Chest Pain Guideline that elevate the role of imaging to Class I recommendation in both acute and stable chest pain in intermediate risk patients. Current investigations aim to augment and enhance current risk-based approaches through the analysis of multiomic data sets, while also recently showing promise in the direct image interpretation of cardiac and coronary structures through a myriad of approaches. Between 2001 and 2015 the proportion of AI/ML related articles in relevant journals per month was 0.1% in relation to the total number published in the journals. This increased to 16.2% per month by 2020 . Literature search was completed on PubMed and EMBASE databases by searching "artificial intelligence" or "machine learning" AND various terminology related to cardiology such as "cardiac," "cardio," "cardiology," "infarct," "valve," "cardiosurgical," etc. . Over the past 5 years there were over 3,000 papers published in Pubmed related to AI/ML learning in cardiovascular medicine . In cardiovascular imaging specifically, there's been increases in non-invasive coronary imaging including applications of coronary artery plaque, automated calcium scoring, perivascular fat attenuation and machine learning based image enhancement as well in the application of nuclear imaging, and myocardial perfusion to large data sets to improve risk enhancement. This review chapter serves to summarize the recent advancements of Artificial Intelligence in respect to coronary artery disease (CAD) and imaging.

Coronary Artery Disease Risk Prediction

Current prevention guidelines incorporate the use of the pooled cohort equation for adults aged 40–75 with non-traditional cardiovascular risk factors to determine a 10 year risk of cardiac events The pooled cohort equation creates a simplified risk score with a finite number of variables; however the simplification of the approach may overestimate cardiovascular risk in certain populations

Multiple studies have sought to enhance the risk prediction model. AI has been particularly impactful in the area of improved cardiovascular risk prediction. Nakanishi et al. demonstrated that ML using logistic regression modeling that incorporate multiple clinical and cardiac computed tomography (CT) variables was superior in predicting 10 year coronary artery disease death [area under the curve (AUC) = 0.86] than clinical data alone (AUC = 0.835), coronary artery calcium (CAC) alone (AUC = 0.816), or ML CT (AUC = 0.827) . This model used a total of 77 variables [46 clinical such as atherosclerotic cardiovascular disease (ASCVD) risk score, sex, age] and 31 CT variables from CAC scan to train the machine learning algorithm. Similarly, Motwani et al. demonstrated that ML incorporating 25 clinical and 44 coronary computed tomography angiography (CCTA) parameters better predicted 5 year mortality than current clinical or imaging metrics. This study involved 10,030 patients, and ML exhibited a higher AUC compared with Framingham Risk Score (FRS) (ML 0.79 vs. FRS 0.61) or CCTA severity scores such as segment stenosis score (SSS) (ML 0.79 vs. SSS 0.64) . Al'Aref studied 13,054 patients in The Coronary CT Angiography Evaluation For Clinical Outcomes (CONFIRM) registry. ML with CAC performed the best in predicting obstructive CAD on CCTA (AUC 0.881) compared to ML alone (AUC = 0.682) and CAD consortium clinic score +CACS (0.866) (3). These models demonstrate the potential to improve predictive models. By incorporating numerous variables, both clinical and imaging, these machine learning algorithms can better predict cardiovascular mortality. Therefore, in addition to current tools such as the 10-year ASCVD risk, CAC score, and CCTA, these models can prove to add invaluable information in assessing a patient's cardiovascular risk.

Coronary Stenosis

The recent 2021 American Heart Association/American College of Cardiology/Multisociety Guideline for the Evaluation and Diagnosis of Chest Pain redefines the presence of coronary artery disease as obstructive (≥50% stenosis) and non-obstructive (<50%) stenosis). In the realm of invasive and non-invasive coronary angiography (via CCTA), the evaluation of coronary artery stenosis requires visual analysis by a trained provider.

However, there can be inter-provider variability in interpretation of these studies in real world practice. Lu et al. showed in the analysis of the Prospective Multicenter Imaging Study for Evaluation of Chest Pain (PROMISE) trial, coronary CTA scans read by both core laboratory and local site readers, 41% of the scans were in discordance regarding the presence of significant stenosis (defined as stenosis ≥50%). There remains great interest in identifying solutions that allow for improved reproducibility. AI has shown promising advancements in the detection of obstructive CAD. In 2015, Kang et al. demonstrated that machine learning algorithms allowed for the detection of both obstructive (≥50% stenosis) and non-obstructive (<50% stenosis) lesions with an AUC of 0.94. In addition, Freiman et al. used a deep sparse autoencoder—mixed structure regularization approach in 90 subjects and observed an AUC that ranged from 0.78 to 0.94 for discrimination of mild stenosis <30% to severe stenosis ≥70%. More recently, the CT Evaluation by Artificial Intelligence for Atherosclerosis, Stenosis and Vascular Morphology (CLARIFY) multi-center study compared AI to level 3 (L3) readers in detecting coronary artery stenosis on CCTA (11). AI analysis showed 99.7% accuracy in detecting >70% stenosis and 94.8% accuracy in detecting >50% stenosis. Among the vessels analyzed, the mean difference in maximal diameter stenosis between AI and L3 readers was minimal at −0.8 %. AI analysis to determine the Coronary Artery Disease Reporting and Data System (CAD-RADS) categorization compared to L3 readers was also examined.

AI generated a CAD-RADS score that was in agreement with the readers in 78% of scans, and generated a score that was in agreement within 1 category in 98% of the scans. A subsequent analysis by Griffin et al. evaluated a multi-center cohort of patients undergoing core-lab quantitative invasive angiography (QCA) and found that AI CCTA had high diagnostic accuracy when compared to QCA in detecting >50% stenosis (AUC 0.88) and >70% stenosis (AUC 0.92) . The analysis time was approximately 10 mins, which represents an improvement over the several hours that previous methods have required. The deep convolutional neural network based approach utilized in these studies has been cleared by the Food and Drug Administration (FDA), and is clinically available and are expected to enable widespread generalizability of the studied approaches.

Coronary Atherosclerosis Quantification

Beyond coronary stenosis or coronary artery calcium contemporary evidence has shown that the quantification of adverse atherosclerotic plaque characteristics enhances prognostication of patients at elevated risk for acute coronary syndrome (ACS) Rosendael et al. showed that calcium density (calculated from semi-automated software) can be associated with ACS risk. In thisstudy, patients with and without ACS had similar calcified plaque volume. However, those who experienced ACS had less highly dense plaque, termed by the authors as "1K plaque" (HU > 1,000) than ACS-free subjects, suggesting that 1K plaque has lower risk for acute plaque rupture. The SCOT-HEART trial showed that low-attenuation plaque (HU <30) was associated with three times the risk of coronary heart disease death or nonfatal MI (30). Other features of plaques which contribute to the prognosis of CAD were studied by Yang et al. The investigators used machine learning to analyze vessels in CCTA that had low fractional flow reserve (FFR) (≤ 0.80). In these vessels, adverse plaque features beyond lumen area which were found to be associated with low FFR vessels that included: percent atheroma volume, fibrofatty/necrotic core volume, plaque volume, proximal left anterior descending coronary artery involvement, and remodeling index. Al' Aref et al. trained a machine learning model to detect culprit lesions (which had been confirmed on invasive coronary angiography) by combining quantitative and qualitative plaque features on CCTA. The machine learning model yielded an area under the curve of 0.77 for identifying the culprit lesion, significantly outperforming other models that were based solely on diameter stenosis or high-risk plaque features.

Quantification of plaque and identifying high risk plaque features is time consuming, often taking several hours for a single study, and requires a high level of expertise in a dedicated research core lab limiting such application to real world practice.Machine learning offers tremendous potential to allow for interpretation of imaging matrices that encompass the millions of pixels required to fully quantify atherosclerotic plaque from CCTA data in the clinical world. The aforementioned CLARIFY study by Choi et al. and the subsequent evaluation by Griffin et al. has evaluated a broad range of atherosclerosis plaque features using AI analysis . Subsequent initial analysis has further shown that AI detected high risk features, such as lumen volume and low-attenuation, more often than experienced level 3 readers as well as accuracy when compared to fractional flow reserve. Furthermore, the analysis was performed as little as under 10 mins.There are a number of important ongoing applications of plaque quantification. Budoff et al. demonstrated that in CAD patients with elevated triglyceride levels and already taking a statin, icosapent ethyl significantly decreased the volume of low-attenuation plaque compared to placebo over an 18 month period. The application of well-validated AI guided approach to atherosclerosis quantification may enable important advances in assessing the response to preventive therapies.

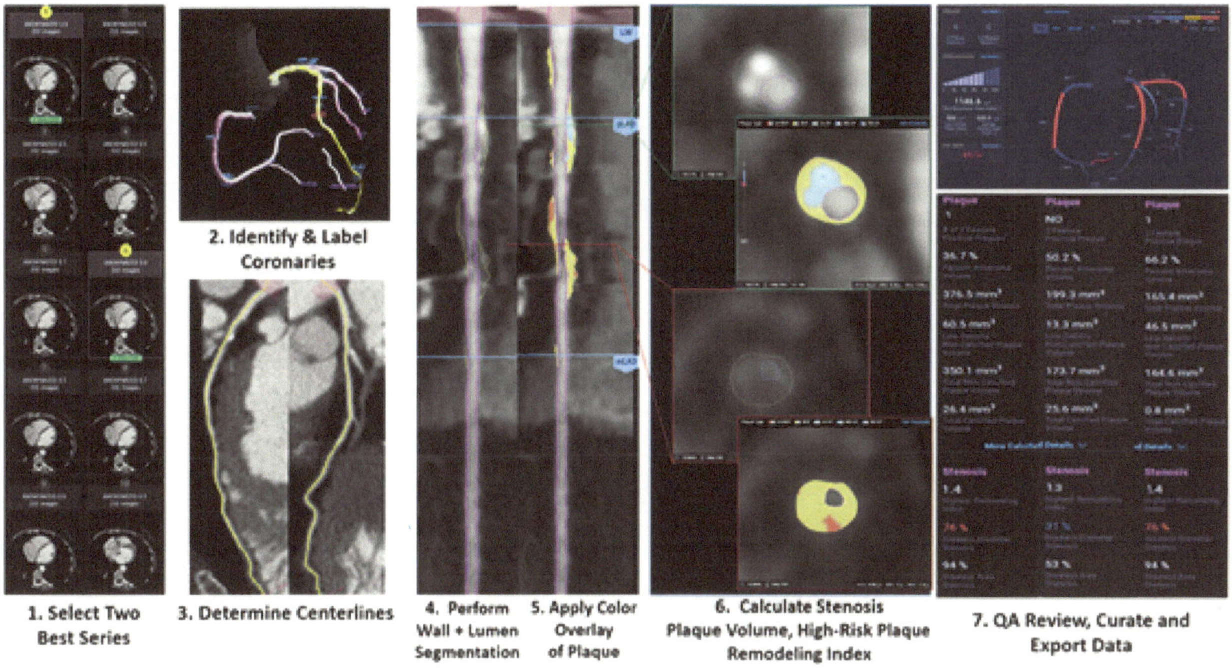

Fig.23.1 Case example of AI-guided coronary computed tomography angiography. Using a series of validated convolutional neural network models (including VGG19 network, 3D U-Net, and VGG Network variant) for image quality assessment, the machine learning algorithm (Cleerly, New York, NY) selects the best series, identifies and labels all of the major epicardial coronaries and their side branches, determines centerlines, performs coronary segmentation and labeling and then performs a rapid assessment of % stenosis, plaque volume and of adverse plaque characteristics. The data is then displayed in a graphical output to allow for clinical review.

Nuclear Myocardial Perfusion Imaging

AI has also been applied to the field of nuclear medicine. Its utility has been demonstrated in the evaluation of coronary artery disease via single photon emission computed tomography (SPECT). Hu et al. studied 1980 patients with suspected CAD . Those patients underwent SPECT imaging and later invasive coronary angiography. ML utilized multiple clinical, imaging, and stress test variables to predict the need for early coronary revascularization (ECR). On a per vessel basis, ML better predicted the need for ECR (AUC = 0.79) vs. Regional Stress Tissue perfusion deficit (TPD) (AUC = 0.71), combined view TPD (AUC = 0.71), or ischemic TPD (AUC = 0.72). This was also true on a per patient basis (AUC = 0.81). Interestingly, ML also outperformed expert nuclear readers on the need for ECR in a per patient basis. Arsanjani et al. showed that machine learning can improve the accuracy of SPECT in identifying significant CAD (≥70% stenosis).AI performed with similar, if not better, accuracy (87%) in detecting these lesions compared to two expert readers (86 and 82%). A similar study found that support vector machines algorithm was superior to two expert readers in detecting obstructive CAD (AUC 0.92 vs. 0.87 and 0.88) . Betancur et al. also showed that compared to current clinical method (total perfusion deficit), deep learning was able to predict obstructive CAD with more accuracy per patient (AUC 0.80 vs. 0.78) and also per vessel (AUC 0.76 vs. 0.73) . While identifying obstructive CAD is certainly important, what is of greater clinical value is predicting those patients who will go on to have adverse outcomes. In one study, machine learning demonstrated superiority to visual analysis by physicians in predicting 3-year major adverse cardiovascular events (MACE) (AUC 0.78 vs. 0.65). When incorporating clinical information (age, gender, risk factors, family history) into the algorithm, machine learning performed with even greater accuracy in predicting MACE (AUC 0.81) Furthermore, Alonso et al. showed that by analyzing SPECT data, a machine learning model outperformed logistic regression in predicting cardiac death (AUC 0.83 vs. 0.76) . In analyzing patients with obstructive CAD, AI has also proven its ability to predict those that may require intervention in the future. Arsanjani et al. explored the utility of AI in predicting the need for revascularization. The researchers discovered that by incorporating clinical parameters such as age, smoking history, hypertension, diabetes, and family history, machine learning algorithm could predict the need for revascularization with similar or better accuracy compared to two expert readers (AUC 0.81 vs. 0.81 and 0.72). As AI interpretion of nuclear imaging continues to improve, its clinical value may increase the automated identification of ischemia beyond currently available perfusion mapping.

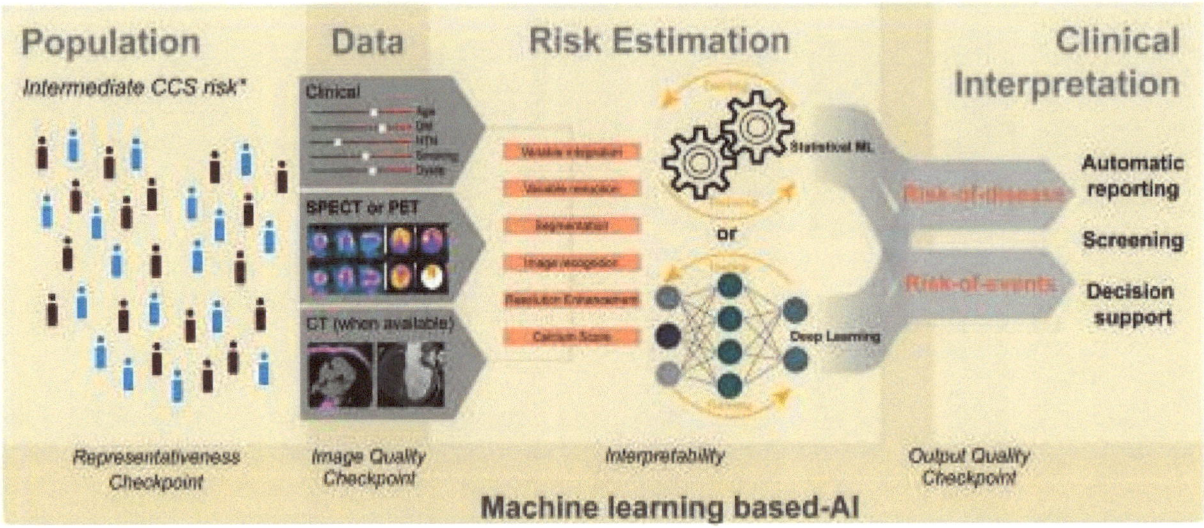

Fig.23.2 As machine learning-based artificial intelligence (AI) continues to revolutionize the way in which we analyze data, the field of nuclear cardiology provides fertile ground for the implementation of these complex analytics in the continuous search for optimizing the evaluation of known or suspected cardiovascular disease, mainly in the form of coronary artery disease (CAD)

Coronary Flow

In 2011, the non-invasive evaluation of fractional flow reserve by computed tomography (FFRCT) was introduced into the field of cardiac imaging by the DISCOVER-FLOW trial . Machine learning has been subsequently applied to the analysis of non-invasive coronary flow. The MACHINE registry was the first study comparing CT FFR from machine learning algorithm vs. CT FFR from computational fluid dynamics (CFD) algorithm . The study demonstrated that machine learning CT FFR algorithm distinguished functionally significant obstructive CAD equally well as FFR derived from a hybrid CFD approach. Tesche et al. found that machine learning CT FFR had a per-lesion sensitivity of 79% and specificity of 94% in detecting lesion-specific ischemia. The area under the curve for detecting lesion-specific ischemia was 0.89 for machine learning CT FFR, equal to CFD CT FFR (AUC 0.89) and significantly higher than CCTA (AUC 0.61) and quantitative coronary angiography (AUC 0.69). The diagnostic value of machine learning CT FFR was also studied by Dugua et al. who retrospectively investigated patients with symptoms of ACS who were worked up with CCTA followed by invasive coronary angiography. The investigators identified non-culprit lesions (≥ 25% stenosis, not intervened on during invasive coronary angiography). In an average of 19.5 month follow-up period, 14 patients (29%) suffered a MACE due to these non-culprit lesions. The mean FFR CT for these non-culprit lesions was 0.78, therefore showing that FFR CT ≤ 80% in patients with symptoms consistent with ACS can be a predictor of future MACE. These studies show the clinical utility of machine learning FFR CT, which also has the potential to be more efficient. Calculating FFR CT using computational flow dynamics is technologically demanding and can take up to 10 mins .

On the other hand Itu et al. demonstrated how machine learning models could generate FFR CT in as little as 2.4 s. Mannil et al. conducted a proof-of-concept study showing that machine learning and texture analysis of low-dose cardiac CT was able to detect myocardial infarction that was not visible to radiologists.

Perivascular Adipose Inflammation by CT

Vascular inflammation is a significant contributor to atherosclerosis and plaque destabilization. Perivascular Adipose Tissue (PVAT) can be monitored by CT fat attenuation to predict coronary artery disease due to the inflammatory effects from the vessels to the PVAT . Higher fat attenuation index (FAI) is associated with increased cardiovascular mortality . One study found that there is higher FAI in culprit lesions compared to non-culprit lesions in ACS . Oikonomou et al. studied the use of ML in PVAT in three different studies/methodologies for enhanced cardiac risk prediction beyond looking at the coronary vessel anatomy and risk factors. The first study analyzed 167 patients undergoing cardiac surgery. PVAT was biopsied for transcriptional factors and CT scan to image the PVAT was performed. This demonstrated a non-invasive method of detecting and adipose tissue microvacuolar remodeling by correlation with increased levels of Collagen Type 1 Alpha 1 Chain. Study 2 analyzed the Fat Radiomic Profile (FRP) of 1,575 patients from the SCOT-HART trial and concluded that high FRP (designated as ≥ 0.63) was associated with a 10.8 fold increase of MACE after adjustment for risk factors . Lastly in study 3,44 patients with acute myocardial infarctions (AMI) underwent CT scans on admission and 6 months later. The authors found that there were higher FRP values consistent with adverse PVAT remodeling with persistence at 6 months compared to perivascular Fat attenuation index (FAI) which was present at only with initial presentation of AMI.

Epicardial Fat Quantification

In multiple studies, the location of the epicardial fat, particularly in the left atrioventricular groove has been a modest predictor of obstructive CAD. In a study by Commanduer et al. (56), deep learning to quantify epicardial adipose tissue (EAT) was compared to quantification from two expert readers. 70 patients underwent non-contrast calcium scans and correlation of EAT volumes with deep learning quantification highly correlated with expert readers R = 0.973 and R = 0.979; p <0.001. Deep learning quantification was also associated with increased non-calcified plaque on subsequent CCTA (5.7 vs. 1.8%, p = 0.026). Deep learning quantification was performed with a mean of 1.57 s ± 0.49 s compared to 15 mins for expert readers.

Coronary Artery Calcium

Increased coronary artery calcium has demonstrated to have important prognostic significance across age and diverse ethnic group. In addition, CAC now has an importanguideline-level role in risk-stratification and treatment decisions of CAD for patients at intermediate risk. For example, in non-diabetic adults aged 40–75 with LDL-C between 70 and 189 mg/dl and a 10-year ASCVD risk between 7.5 and 19.9%, current guidelines encourage the use of CAC score to guide clinicians on de-risking patients or initiating intensive lipid lowering therapy (60). Typically, calcium scores are obtained from regular dose, ECG-gated chest CT's and require some degree of manual input (the provider selecting/confirming areas of calcification and the software subsequently generating a calcium score).

There has been recent interest in using artificial intelligence/ machine learning to allow for the automated quantification of coronary artery calcium as well as incorporating a calculated coronary artery calcium score to improve current risk prediction models. Isgum et al. demonstrated that coronary artery calcium score can also be obtained from low-dose chest CT performed for lung cancer screening in the smoking population. Investigators identified CAC with a statistical pattern recognition system, and then utilized support vector machines to correctly classify cardiovascular risk category in 82% of the subjects based on Agatston score. The accuracy of fully automated calcium scores from low-dose CT has also been evaluated in other studies.Takx et al. , examined automatic calcium scores derived from low-dose CT. There was good reliability between fully automated calcium scores and reference scores set by human readers (kappa 0.85). Most of the discordance was due to the automated method failing to detect calcifications in the right coronary artery. Isgum et al. , also yielded similar results. The study showed agreement of CVD risk category (based on Agatston score) not only between fully automatic and manual calcium scores derived from low dose CT (kappa 0.89), but also between fully automatic calcium score from low dose CT and calcium score from dedicated calcium scoring CT (kappa 0.74).). Winkel et al. used deep-learning software to calculate vessel-specific CAC sub-scores (right coronary artery, left main, left main, left anterior descending, and circumflex). The risk class assignment determined by AI showed agreement with that of human readers (kappa = 0.91). Given the association of smoking history with cardiovascular disease, and the abundance of lung cancer screening CT scans, the ability to automatically estimate calcium scores from such scans could provide the added benefit of identifying patients at increased cardiovascular risk.

Ethics, Limitations and Standards of Artificial Intelligence in CAD Imaging

The ease in which ML can acquire data can present ethical dilemmas. Big data can be analyzed in minutes (11) raising issues such as proper consent and safe storage of protected health information (PHI). The “black box” nature of AI may lead to uncertainty for physicians seeking to apply these approaches to practice. Clinicians must be aware of the specific validation of AI and the limitations to avoid unintended extrapolation and biased results. As automated analysis improves to better address gaps in expert level care, the field of cardiovascular imaging training may be inadvertently depleted of the “Human Neural Network” when there is overreliance on AI to create the foundations of analyzing images. The use of AI in cardiovascular medicine needs to be tailored to specific patient-centered goals to avoid unintended or false discoveries .

In the imaging of coronary artery disease, it is important to establish appropriate ground truth standards such as quantitative coronary angiography, fractional flow reserve and invasive ultrasound.In addition, new artificial intelligence and machine learning based approaches should be validated in randomized controlled trials (RCT). An RCT in which one arm receives usual care and the other arm receives AI assisted care can be extremely influential and may be a novel trial approach to further create an evidence base for the use AI in clinical practice. It is important that these tools are vetted by the Food and Drug Administration and similar regulatory bodies, through peer-reviewed studies as well as through the professional societies. The field will also need to further develop models for integration into clinical practice, its use as a clinical decision support tool as well as addressing scenarios in which the AI/ML tool disagrees with clinical readers. It is also expected there may be clinical scenarios in which the AI/ML has not been fully trained. For example, in an acute coronary syndrome, the AI/ ML may be able to identify severity of stenosis and adverse plaque characteristics, but not recognize a coronary artery dissection. With its various application to cardiovascular medicine, there will be a continued and ongoing need to apply ethnical and scientific standards in AI/ML in coronary imaging.

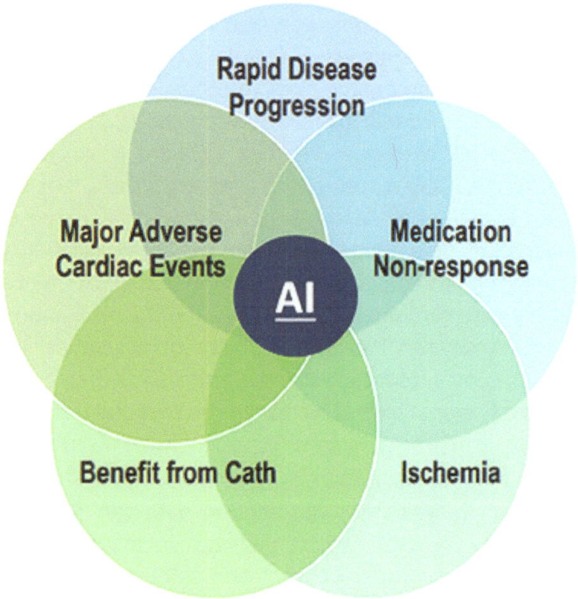

Fig.23.3 New paradigm of AI guided coronary artery disease imaging. An artificial intelligence (AI) guided approach to coronary artery disease in CAD imaging opens several new frontiers in the evaluation and treatment of atherosclerosis. These include the evaluation of rapid disease progressors, accessing response or non-response to statin and other lipid lowering therapies, improved prediction of ischemia, enhanced selection for guideline based invasive angiography and prognostication of major adverse cardiovascular events.

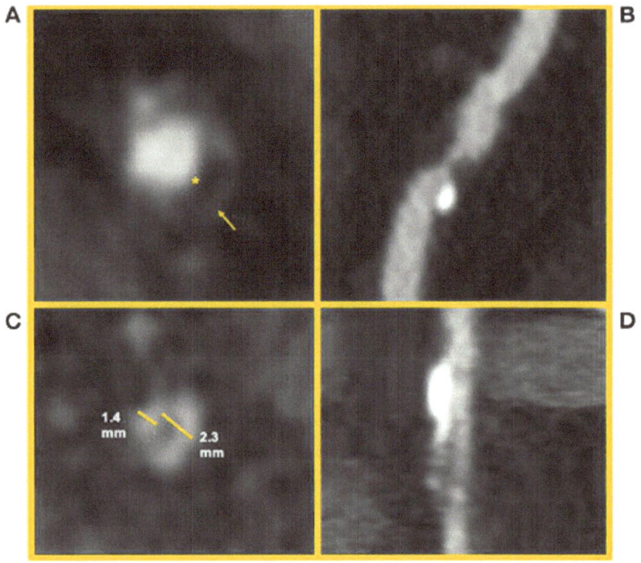

Fig.23.4 High risk features of coronary artery plaques. The figure shows clinical examples of high-risk plaque feature. (A) Depicts an example of a Napkin-ring sign. The asterisk identifies the hypodense necrotic core; the arrow identifies the hyperdense ring-like thin cap. (B) Depicts a high-risk coronary plaque with spotty calcifications and low attenuation (i.e., attenuation <30 HU). (C,D) Depict a coronary artery plaque with positive remodeling (i.e., a positive ratio between diameter of the vessel outside the plaque and its internal diameter) in short and long axis, respectively.

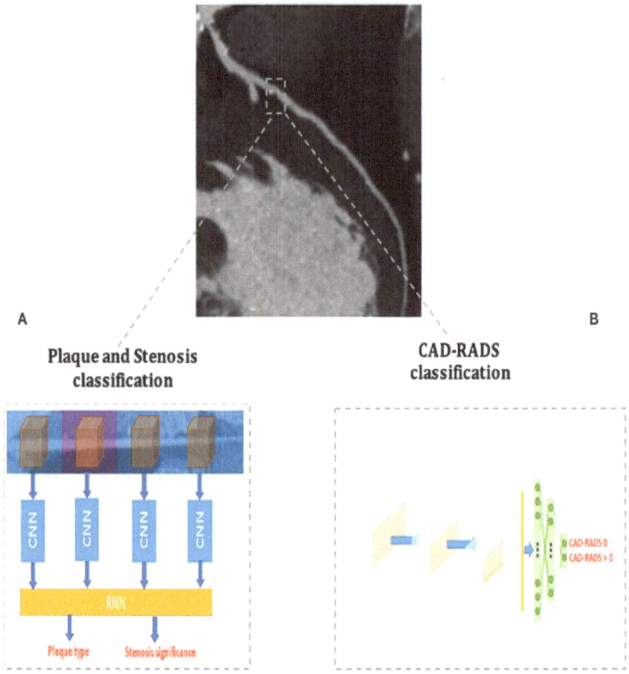

Fig.23.5 AI applications to cardiac CT. The figure depicts two examples of AI workflow applied to the automatic analysis of coronary artery stenoses by Coronary Computed Tomography Angiography (CCTA). (A) Schematizes the algorithm proposed by Zreik et al. (72) and composed of a 3D convolutional neural network (CNN) used for coronary artery features extraction and a subsequent recurrent neural network for a two-task classification of plaque phenotype and stenosis degree. (B) Schematizes the algorithm applied by Muscogiuri et al. (68) for the fully automatic CAD-RADS classification of CCTA scans with a CNN.

The promise of artificial intelligence lies in leveraging modern algorithms to improve decision making and risk prediction beyond current models that are patient-centered (. In the opinion of this author group, the recently validated stenosis and atherosclerosis quantification methods discussed in this paper, with their FDA approval and clinical availabilityrepresent a practice ready approach. Application of an AI/ML guided CCTA approach opens several new frontiers in the assessment and treatment of atherosclerosis. Specific examples include the opportunity to evaluate rapid disease progressors and those that do not respond to lipid lowering therapies. AI/ML may also allow for non-invasive evaluation of those that demonstrate plaque regression after intensified, personalized medical therapies. AI/ML guided atherosclerosis evaluation may better predict ischemia as well as those patients that will require invasive angiographyA future paradigm includes utilization of AI so that the cardiologist may use the AI/ML guided information to make improved clinical decisions and enhance patient-centered outcomes. With continued research in the field and promising outcomes it is expected that the next decade will see AI applied broadly in clinical practice to allow improved outcomes while care remains led by the cardiovascular clinician.

Bibliography and Acknowledgement

- Al'Aref SJ, Maliakal G, Singh G, van Rosendael AR, Ma X, Xu Z, et al. Machine learning of clinical variables and coronary artery calcium scoring for the prediction of obstructive coronary artery disease on coronary computed tomography angiography: analysis from the CONFIRM registry. Eur Heart J. (2020) 41:359–67. doi: 10.1093/eurheartj/ehz565
- Antonopoulos AS, Sanna F, Sabharwal N, Thomas S, Oikonomou EK, Herdman L, et al. Detecting human coronary inflammation by imaging perivascular fat. Sci Transl Med. (2017) 9:398. doi: 10.1126/scitranslmed.aal2658
- Arnett DK, Blumenthal RS, Albert MA, Buroker AB, Goldberger ZD, Hahn EJ, et al. 2019 ACC/AHA guideline on the primary prevention of cardiovascular disease: a report of the American College of Cardiology/American Heart Association Task Force on clinical practice guidelines. J Am Coll Cardiol. (2019) 74:e177–232. doi: 10.1161/CIR.0000000000000678
- Arsanjani R, Dey D, Khachatryan T, Shalev A, Hayes SW, Fish M, et al. Prediction of revascularization after myocardial perfusion SPECT by machine learning in a large population. J Nucl Cardiol. (2015) 22:877–84. doi: 10.1007/s12350-014-0027-x
- Arsanjani R, Xu Y, Dey D, Fish M, Dorbala S, Hayes S, et al. Improved accuracy of myocardial perfusion SPECT for the detection of coronary artery disease using a support vector machine algorithm. J Nucl Med. (2013) 54:549–55. doi: 10.2967/jnumed.112.111542
- Betancur J, Commandeur F, Motlagh M, Sharir T, Einstein AJ, Bokhari S, et al. Deep learning for prediction of obstructive disease from fast myocardial perfusion SPECT: a multicenter study. JACC Cardiovasc Imaging. (2018) 11:1654–63. doi: 10.1016/j.jcmg.2018.01.020
- Betancur J, Otaki Y, Motwani M, Fish MB, Lemley M, Dey D, et al. Prognostic value of combined clinical and myocardial perfusion imaging data using machine learning. JACC Cardiovasc Imaging. (2018) 11:1000–9. doi: 10.1016/j.jcmg.2017.07.024
- Bizopoulos P, Koutsouris D. Deep learning in cardiology. IEEE Rev Choi AD, Blankstein R. Becoming an expert practitioner: the lifelong journey of education in cardiovascular imaging. JACC Cardiovasc Imaging. (2021) 14:1594–7. doi: 10.1016/j.jcmg.2021.03.006
- Choi AD, Marques H, Kumar V, Griffin WF, Rahban H, Karlsberg RP, et al. CT EvaLuation by ARtificial Intelligence For Atherosclerosis, Stenosis and Vascular MorphologY (CLARIFY): a multi-center, international study. J Cardiovasc Comput Tomogr. (2021) 15:470–6. doi: 10.1016/j.jcct.2021.05.004
- Coenen A, Kim YH, Kruk M, Tesche C, De Geer J, Kurata A, et al. Diagnostic accuracy of a machine-learning approach to coronary computed tomographic angiography-based fractional flow reserve: result from the MACHINE Consortium. Circ Cardiovasc Imaging. (2018) 11:e007217. doi: 10.1161/CIRCIMAGING.117.007217
- Commandeur F, Goeller M, Razipour A, Cadet S, Hell MM, Kwiecinski J, et al. Fully automated CT quantification of epicardial adipose tissue by deep learning: a multicenter study. Radiol Artif Intell. (2019) 1:e190045. doi: 10.1148/ryai.2019190045
- Criqui MH, Denenberg JO, Ix JH, McClelland RL, Wassel CL, Rifkin DE, et al. Calcium density of coronary artery plaque and risk of incident cardiovascular events. JAMA. (2014) 311:271–8. doi: 10.1001/jama.2013.282535
- Currie G, Rohren E. Intelligent imaging in nuclear medicine: the principles of artificial intelligence, machine learning and deep learning. Semin Nucl Med. (2021) 51:102–11.
- DeFilippis AP, Young R, McEvoy JW, Michos ED, Sandfort V, Kronmal RA, et al. Risk score overestimation: the impact of individual cardiovascular risk factors and preventive therapies on the performance of the American Heart Association-American College of Cardiology-Atherosclerotic Cardiovascular Disease risk score in a modern multi-ethnic cohort. Eur Heart J. (2017) 38:598–608. doi: 10.1093/eurheartj/ehw301
- Dey D, Slomka PJ, Leeson P, Comaniciu D, Shrestha S, Sengupta PP, et al. Artificial intelligence in cardiovascular imaging: JACC state-of-the-art review. J Am Coll Cardiol. (2019) 73:1317–35. doi: 10.1016/j.jacc.2018.12.054
- Duguay TM, Tesche C, Vliegenthart R, De Cecco CN, Lin H, Albrecht MH, et al. Coronary computed tomographic angiography-derived fractional flow reserve based on machine learning for risk stratification of non-culprit coronary narrowings in patients with acute coronary syndrome. Am J Cardiol. (2017) 120:1260–6. doi: 10.1016/j.amjcard.2017.07.008
- Freiman M, Manjeshwar R, Goshen L. Unsupervised abnormality detection through mixed structure regularization (MSR) in deep sparse autoencoders. Med Phys. (2019) 46:2223–31. doi: 10.1002/mp.13464
- Goeller M, Achenbach S, Cadet S, Kwan AC, Commandeur F, Slomka PJ, et al. Pericoronary adipose tissue computed tomography attenuation and high-risk plaque characteristics in acute coronary syndrome compared with stable coronary artery disease. JAMA Cardiol. (2018) 3:858–63. doi: 10.1001/jamacardio.2018.1997 Google Scholar
- Griffin W, Choi A, Earls J, Marques H, Barkovich E, Riess J, et al. Evaluation of coronary stenosis on CT coronary angiography, comparison with quantitative coronary angiography and fractional flow reserve; A CREDENCE trial sub-study. JACC: Cardiovasc Imaging. (2022) S1936-878X(22)00001-8. doi: 10.1016/j.jcmg.2021.10.020
- Gulati M, Levy PD, Mukherjee D, Amsterdam E, Bhatt DL, Birtcher KK, et al. 2021 AHA/ACC/ASE/CHEST/SAEM/SCCT/SCMR guideline for the evaluation and diagnosis of chest pain: a report of the
- American College of Cardiology/American Heart Association Joint Committee on clinical practice guidelines. J Am Coll Cardiol. (2021) 78:e187–285. doi: 10.1016/j.jacc.2021.07.053
- Haro Alonso D, Wernick MN, Yang Y, Germano G, Berman DS, Slomka P. Prediction of cardiac death after adenosine myocardial perfusion SPECT based on machine learning. J Nucl Cardiol. (2019) 26:1746–54. doi: 10.1007/s12350-018-1250-7
- Išgum I, de Vos BD, Wolterink JM, Dey D, Berman DS, Rubeaux M, et al. Automatic determination of cardiovascular risk by CT attenuation correction maps in Rb-82 PET/CT. J Nucl Cardiol. (2018) 25:2133–42. doi: 10.1007/s12350-017-0866-3
- Isgum I, Prokop M, Niemeijer M, Viergever MA, van Ginneken B. Automatic coronary calcium scoring in low-dose chest computed tomography. IEEE Trans Med Imaging. (2012) 31:2322–34. doi: 10.1109/TMI.2012.2216889
- Kang D, Dey D, Slomka PJ, Arsanjani R, Nakazato R, Ko H, et al. Structured learning algorithm for detection of nonobstructive and obstructive coronary plaque lesions from computed tomography angiography. J Med Imaging. (2015) 2:014003.
- Koo BK, Erglis A, Doh JH, Daniels DV, Jegere S, Kim HS, et al. Diagnosis of ischemia-causing coronary stenoses by noninvasive fractional flow reserve computed from coronary computed tomographic angiograms. Results from the prospective multicenter DISCOVER-FLOW (Diagnosis of ischemia-causing stenoses obtained via noninvasive fractional flow reserve) study. J Am Coll Cardiol. (2011) 58:1989–97. doi: 10.1016/j.jacc.2011.06.066

- Lu MT, Meyersohn NM, Mayrhofer T, Bittner DO, Emami H, Puchner SB, et al. Central core laboratory versus site interpretation of coronary ct angiography: agreement and association with cardiovascular events in the PROMISE Trial. Radiology. (2018) 287:87–95. doi: 10.1148/radiol.2017172181
- Mannil M, von Spiczak J, Manka R, Alkadhi H. Texture analysis and machine learning for detecting myocardial infarction in noncontrast low-dose computed tomography: unveiling the invisible. Invest Radiol. (2018) 53:338–43. doi: 10.1097/RLI.0000000000000448
- Motwani M, Dey D, Berman DS, Germano G, Achenbach S, Al-Mallah MH, et al. Machine learning for prediction of all-cause mortality in patients with suspected coronary artery disease: a 5-year multicentre prospective registry analysis. Eur Heart J. (2017) 38:500–7. doi: 10.1093/eurheartj/ehw188
- Nakanishi R, Slomka PJ, Rios R, Betancur J, Blaha MJ, Nasir K, et al. Machine learning adds to clinical and CAC assessments in predicting 10-year CHD and CVD deaths. JACC Cardiovasc Imaging. (2021) 14:615–25. doi: 10.1016/j.jcmg.2020.08.024
- Oikonomou EK, Marwan M, Desai MY, Mancio J, Alashi A, Hutt Centeno E, et al. Non-invasive detection of coronary inflammation using computed tomography and prediction of residual cardiovascular risk (the CRISP CT study): a post-hoc analysis of prospective outcome data. Lancet. (2018) 392:929–39. doi: 10.1016/S0140-6736(18)31114-0
- Peper J, Suchá D, Swaans M, Leiner T. Functional cardiac CT-going beyond anatomical evaluation of coronary artery disease with Cine CT, CT-FFR, CT perfusion and machine learning. Br J Radiol. (2020) 93:20200349. doi: 10.1259/bjr.20200349
- Quer G, Arnaout R, Henne M. Machine learning and the future of cardiovascular care: JACC state-of-the-art review. J Am Coll Cardiol. (2021) 77:300–13. doi: 10.1016/j.jacc.2020.11.030
- Rana JS, Tabada GH, Solomon MD, Lo JC, Jaffe MG, Sung SH, et al. Accuracy of the atherosclerotic cardiovascular risk equation in a large contemporary, multiethnic population. J Am Coll Cardiol. (2016) 67:2118–30. doi: 10.1016/j.jacc.2016.02.055
- Ridker PM, Libby P, MacFadyen JG, Thuren T, Ballantyne C, Fonseca F, et al. Modulation of the interleukin-6 signalling pathway and incidence rates of atherosclerotic events and all-cause mortality: analyses from the Canakinumab Anti-Inflammatory Thrombosis Outcomes Study (CANTOS). Eur Heart J. (2018) 39:3499–507. doi: 10.1093/eurheartj/ehy310
- Seetharam K, Brito D, Farjo PD, Sengupta PP. The role of artificial intelligence in cardiovascular imaging: state of the art review. Front Cardiovasc Med. (2020) 7:618849. doi: 10.3389/fcvm.2020.618849
- Seetharam K, Shrestha S, Sengupta PP. Artificial intelligence in cardiovascular medicine. Curr Treat Options Cardiovasc Med. (2019) 21:25.doi:10.1007/s11936-019-0728-1
- Sengupta PP, Shrestha S, Berthon B, Messas E, Donal E, Tison GH, et al. Proposed requirements for cardiovascular imaging-related machine learning evaluation (PRIME): a checklist: reviewed by the American College of Cardiology Healthcare Innovation Council. JACC CardiovascImaging.(2020)13:2017–35.
- Sengupta PP, Shrestha S. Machine learning for data-driven discovery: the rise and relevance. JACC Cardiovasc Imaging. (2019) 12:690–2. doi:10.1016/j.jcmg.2018.06.030
- Shameer K, Johnson KW, Glicksberg BS, Dudley JT, Sengupta PP. Machine learning in cardiovascular medicine: are we there yet? Heart. (2018)104:1156–64.doi:10.1136/heartjnl-2017-311198
- Shaw LJ, Blankstein R, Bax JJ, Ferencik M, Bittencourt MS, Min JK, et al. Society of Cardiovascular Computed Tomography/North American Society of cardiovascular imaging—expert consensus document on coronary CT imaging of atherosclerotic plaque. J Cardiovasc Comput Tomogr. (2021) 15:93–109. doi: 10.1016/j.jcct.2020.11.002
- Shen YW, Wu YJ, Hung YC, Hsiao CC, Chan SH, Mar GY, et al. Natural course of coronary artery calcium progression in Asian population with an initial score of zero. BMC Cardiovasc Disord. (2020) 20:212. doi: 10.1186/s12872-020-01498-x
- Singh G. Al'Aref SJ, Van Assen M, Kim TS, van Rosendael A, Kolli KK, et al. Machine learning in cardiac CT: basic concepts and contemporary data. J Cardiovasc Comput Tomogr. (2018) 12:192–201. doi: 10.1016/j.jcct.2018.04.010
- Takx RA, de Jong PA, Leiner T, Oudkerk M, de Koning HJ, Mol CP, et al. Automated coronary artery calcification scoring in non-gated chest CT: agreement and reliability. PLoS ONE. (2014) 9:e91239. doi: 10.1371/journal.pone.0091239
- Tesche C, De Cecco CN, Baumann S, Renker M, McLaurin TW, Duguay TM, et al. Coronary CT angiography-derived fractional flow reserve: machine learning algorithm versus computational fluid dynamics modeling. Radiology. (2018) 288:64–72. doi: 10.1148/radiol.2018171291
- van Rosendael AR, Narula J, Lin FY, van den Hoogen IJ, Gianni U, Al Hussein Alawamlh O, et al. Association of high-density calcified 1K plaque with risk of acute coronary syndrome. JAMA Cardiol. (2020) 5:282–90. doi: 10.1001/jamacardio.2019.5315
- Williams MC, Kwiecinski J, Doris M, McElhinney P, D'Souza MS, Cadet S, et al. Sex-specific computed tomography coronary plaque characterization and risk of myocardial infarction. JACC Cardiovasc Imag. (2021) 14:1804–14. doi: 10.1016/j.jcmg.2021.03.004
- Williams MC, Newby DE. Understanding quantitative computed tomography coronary artery plaque assessment using machine learning. JACC Cardiovasc Imaging. (2020) 13:2174–6. doi: 10.1016/j.jcmg.2020.04.027
- Winkel DJ, Suryanarayana VR, Ali AM, Görich J, Buß SJ, Mendoza A, et al. Deep learning for vessel-specific coronary artery calcium scoring: validation on a multi-centre dataset. Eur Heart J Cardiovasc Imaging. (2021) jeab119. doi: 10.1093/ehjci/jeab119
- Wu FZ, Chou KJ, Huang YL, Wu MT. The relation of location-specific epicardial adipose tissue thickness and obstructive coronary artery disease: systemic review and meta-analysis of observational studies. BMC Cardiovasc Disord. (2014) 14:62. doi: 10.1186/1471-2261-14-62
- Wu FZ, Huang YL, Wang YC, Lin HS, Chen CS, Ju YJ, et al. Impact of location of epicardial adipose tissue, measured by coronary artery calcium-scoring computed tomography on obstructive coronary artery disease. Am J Cardiol. (2013) 112:943–9. doi: 10.1016/j.amjcard.2013.05.022
- Wu YJ, Mar GY, Wu MT, Wu FZ. A LASSO-derived risk model for subclinical CAC progression in Asian population with an initial score of zero. Front Cardiovasc Med. (2020) 7:619798. doi: 10.3389/fcvm.2020.619798
- Yang S, Koo BK, Hoshino M, Lee JM, Murai T, Park J, et al. CT Angiographic and plaque predictors of functionally significant coronary disease and outcome using machine learning. JACC Cardiovasc Imaging. (2021) 14:629–41. doi: 10.1016/j.jcmg.2020.08.025
- Yu M, Dai X, Deng J, Lu Z, Shen C, Zhang J. Diagnostic performance of perivascular fat attenuation index to predict hemodynamic significance of coronary stenosis: a preliminary coronary computed tomography angiography study. Eur Radiol. (2020) 30:673–81. doi: 10.1007/s00330-019-06400-8

CHAPTER

24

Artificial Intelligence-(AI) Empowered Echocardiography Interpretation : A Review

Echocardiography (Echo), also known as cardiac ultrasound (CUS), is currently the most widely used noninvasive imaging modality for assessing patients with various cardiovascular disorders. It plays a vital role in evaluation of patients with symptoms of heart disease by identifying structural as well as functional abnormalities and assessing intracardiac hemodynamics. However, accurate echo measurements can be hampered by variability between interpreters, patients, and operators and image quality. Therefore, there is a clinical need for standardized methods of echo measurements and interpretation to reduce these variabilities. Artificial-intelligence-empowered echo (AI-Echo) can potentially reduce inter-interpreter variability and indeterminate assessment and improve the detection of unique conditions as well as the management of various cardiac disorders.

In this review chapter , a brief background on transthoracic echocardiography (TTE) and artificial intelligence (AI) followed by a summary of the advances in echo interpretation using deep learning (DL) with its self-learning ability would be provided. Since DL approaches have shown superior performance compared to machine-learning (ML) approaches based on hand-crafted features, we ,therefore try to focus on DL progress in this review The AI advances could potentially allow objective evaluation of echocardiography, improving clinical workflow, and reducing healthcare costs. Subsequently, we will present currently available AI-Echo applications, delve into challenges of current AI applications using DL, and share our view on future trends in AI-Echo.

Transthoracic Echocardiogram

Transthoracic echocardiogram transmits and receives sound waves with frequencies higher than human hearing using an ultrasound transducer. It generates ultrasound waves and transmits to the tissue and listens to receive the reflected sound wave (echo). The reflected echo signal is recorded to construct an image of the interrogated region. The sound waves travel through soft tissue medium with a speed of approximately 1540 m/s. The time of flight between the transmitted and received sound waves is used to locate objects and construct an image of the probed area. The recorded echo data can be either a single still image or a movie/cine clip over multiple cardiac cycles. CUS has several advantages compared to cardiac magnetic resonance, cardiac computed tomography, and cardiac positron emission tomography imaging modalities. CUS does not use ionizing radiation, is less expensive, portable for point-of-care (POCUS) applications, and provides actual real-time imaging. It can be carried to a patient's bedside for examining patients and monitoring changes over time. Disadvantages of TTE include its dependence on operator and interpreter skill, with variability in data acquisition and interpretation. In addition to operator variability, it includes patient specific variability (e.g., signal-to-noise ratio and limited acoustic window due to anatomical or body mass differences) and machine specific variability (e.g., electronic noise and post-processing filters applied to acquired images). Image quality plays an important factor for accurate measurements. Suboptimal image quality can affect all measurements and can result in misdiagnosis.Diverse image types are formed by using cardiac ultrasound . The most common types used in clinics are:

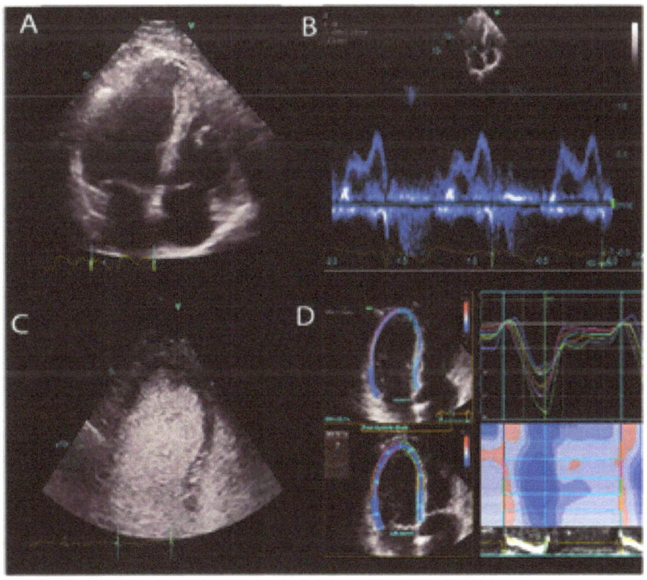

Fig.24.1 Sample US images showing different US modes. (A) B-mode image of the apical 4 chamber view of a heart. (B) Doppler image of mitral inflow. (C) Contrast enhanced ultrasound image of left ventricle. (D) Strain imaging of the left ventricle.

B-mode: It is also called brightness mode (B-mode), which is the most well-known US image type. An ultrasound beam is scanned across the tissue to construct a 2D cross section image of the tissue.

M-mode: Motion mode (M-mode) is used to examine motion over time. For example, it provides a single scan line of the heart, and all of the reflectors along this line are shown along the time axis to measure temporal resolution of the cardiac structures.

Doppler ultrasound: A change in the frequency of a wave occurs when the source and observer are moving relative to each other, this is called the Doppler effect. An US wave is transmitted with a specific frequency through an ultrasound probe (the observer). The US waves that are reflected from moving objects (e.g., red blood cells in vessels) return to the probe with a frequency shift. This frequency shift is used to estimate the velocity of the moving object. In blood flow, the velocity of red blood cells moving towards and away from the probe is recorded to construct Doppler signals. The velocity of information overlaid on top of a B-mode anatomical image to show color Doppler images of blood flow.

Contrast enhanced ultrasound (CEUS): CEUS is a functional imaging that suppresses anatomical details but visualizes blood pool information. It exploits the non-linear response of ultrasound contrast agents (lipid coated gas bubbles). Generally, two consecutive US signals are propagated through the same medium, and their echo response is subtracted to obtain contrast signal. Since the tissue generates linear echo response, the subtraction cancels out the tissue signal, and only the difference signal from non-linear responses of bubbles remains. This imaging technique is used to enhance cardiac chamber cavities when B-mode US provides poor quality images. It is useful to detect perfusion abnormalities in tissues and enhance the visibility of tissue boundaries.

Strain imaging: This technique detects myocardial deformation patterns such as longitudinal, radial, and circumferential deformations, and early functional abnormalities before they become noticeable as regional wall motion abnormalities or reduced ejection fraction on B-mode cardiac images.

Artificial Intelligence

Artificial intelligence (AI) is considered to be a computer-based system that can observe an environment and takes actions to maximize the success of achieving its goals. Some examples include a system that has the ability of sensing, reasoning, engaging, and learning, are computer vision for understanding digital images, natural language processing for interaction between human and computer languages, voice recognition

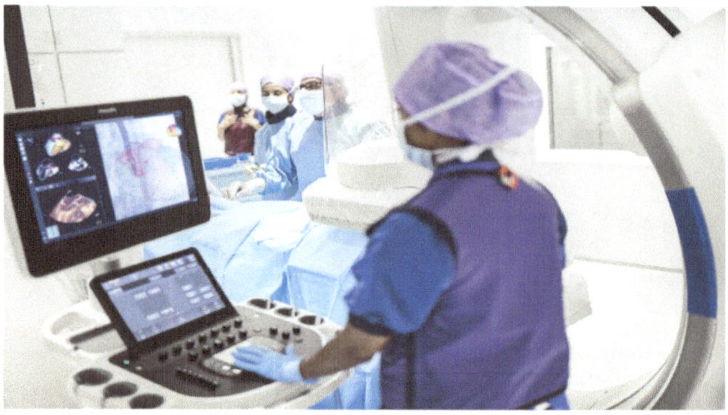

Fig.24.2 The Philips EPIQCVxi with Echonavigator streamlines communication between the interventional cardiologist and the echocardiographer.

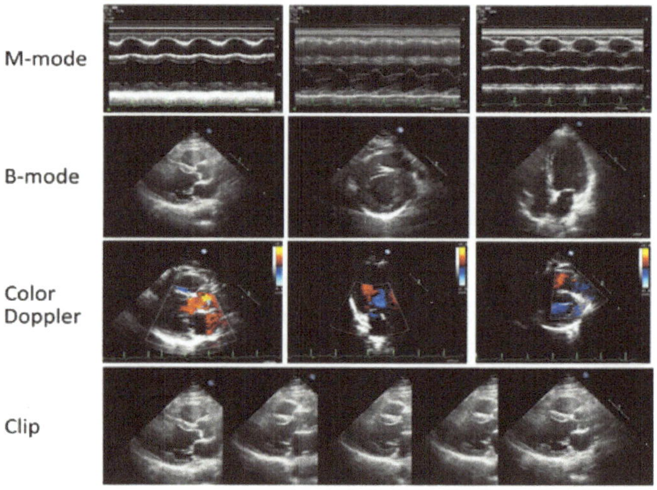

Fig.24.3 Variety of echocardiographic images needed to be recognized by artificial intelligence systems.

for detection and translation of spoken languages, robotics and motion, planning and organization, and knowledge capture. ML is a subsection of AI that covers the ability of a system to learn about data using supervised or unsupervised statistical and ML methods such as regression, support vector machines, decision trees, and neural networks. Deep learning (DL), which is a subclass of ML, learns a sequential chain of pivotal features from input data that maximizes the success of the learning process with its self-learning ability. This is different from statistical ML algorithms that require handcrafted feature selection.Artificial neural networks (ANN) are the first DL network design where all nodes are fully connected to each other. It mimics biological neurons for creating representation from an input signal, including many consecutive layers that learn a hierarchy of features from an input signal. ANN and the advance in graphics processing units (GPU) processing power have enabled the development of deep and complex DL models with simultaneous multitasking at the same time. DL models can be trained with thousands or millions of samples to gain robustness to variations in data. The representation power of

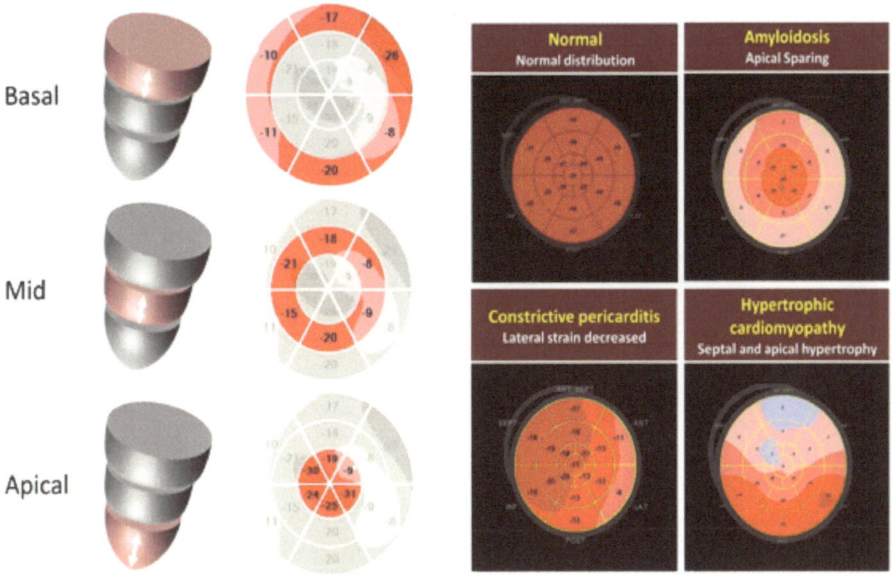

Fig.24.4 Examples of strain distribution in amyloidosis, constrictive pericarditis and hypertrophic cardiomyopathy.

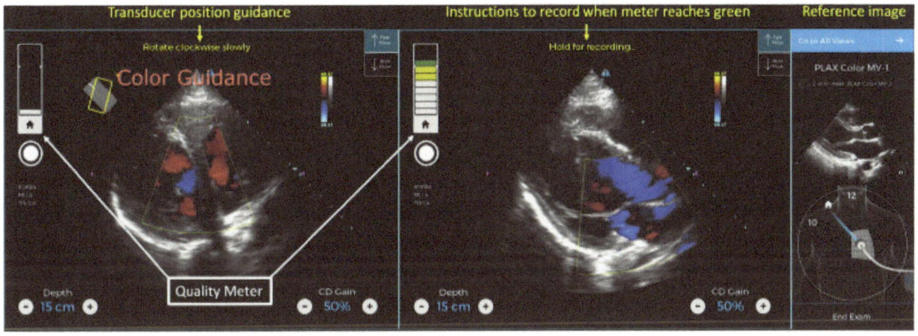

Fig.24.5 AI guidance user interface. Initial (left) and captured (center) PLAX color Doppler image of aortic outflow and mitral regurgitation using AI guidance. The reference image (right) instructs the novice where to place the transducer initially. Instructions on transducer movement result in an optimal image and increase in quality meter from white to yellow to green. While the color box position is optimized for PLAX mitral valve color Doppler, the scanner is required to use their own knowledge to optimally position the color box in the software version available during the study. Once the meter is in green, the scanner is instructed to manually acquire the image.

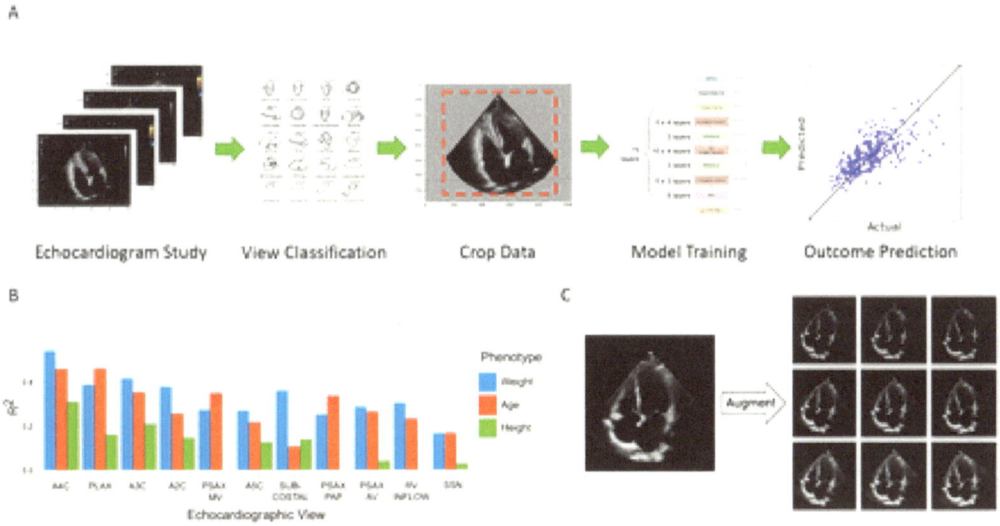

Fig.24.6 A. EchoNet workflow for image selection, cleaning, and model training. B. Comparison of model performance with different cardiac views as input. C. Examples of data augmentation. The original frame is rotated (left to right) and its intensity is increase (top to bottom) as augmentations.

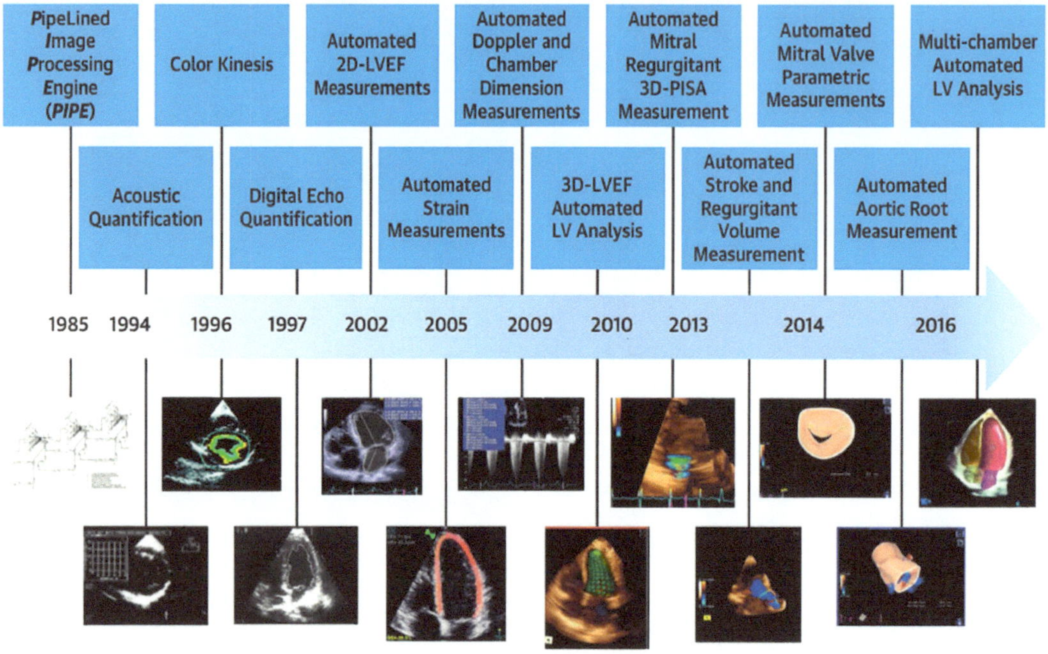

Fig.24.7 Temporal progression in automated quantification in echocardiography. Adapted from Nolan et al. (10). Permission obtained from the publisher.

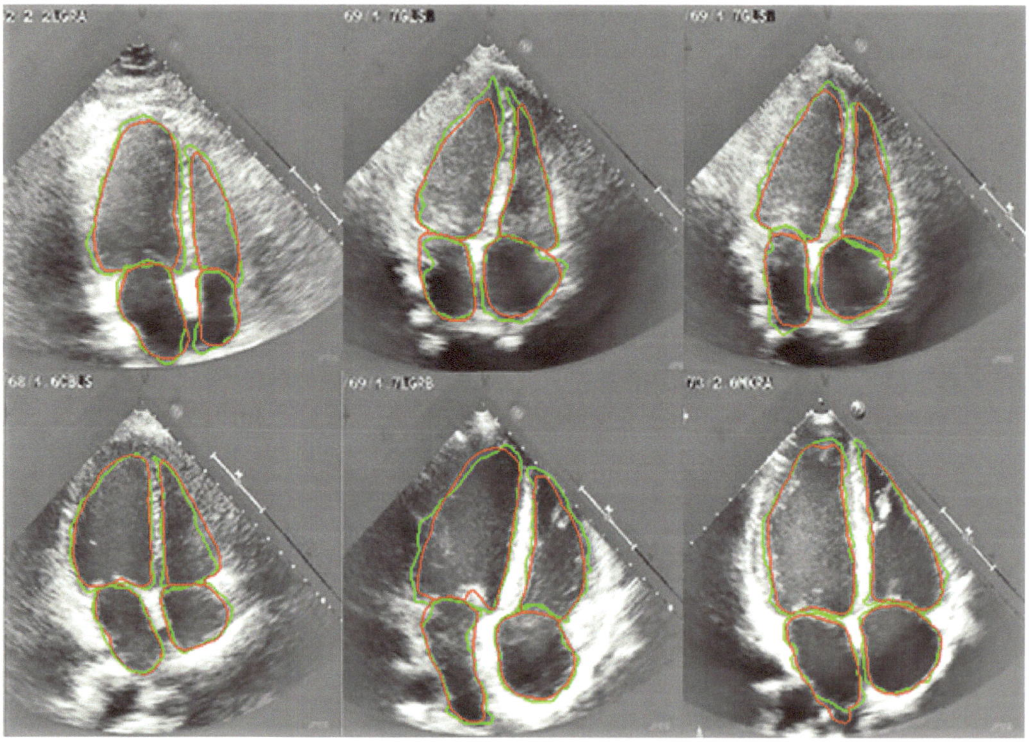

Fig.24.8 UCI Engineers Develop a New AI-based Method for Analyzing Echocardiograms UC Irvine engineers have developed a novel artificial intelligence method for assessing echocardiograms that could help cardiologistmore accurately determine heart function and disease. The machine learning platform will automatically segment the heart's four chambers and calculate their volumes, eliminating the variability in human assessment of cardiac function, using echocardiography data. The research, led by Samueli School professors Arash Kheradvar and Hamid Jafarkhani, was recently published in the Journal of the Royal Society Interface.

DL models is massive and can create representation for any given variation of a signal. Recent accomplishments of DL, especially in image classification and segmentation applications, made it very popular in the data science community. Traditional ML methods use hand-crafted features extracted from data and process them in decomposable pipelines.This makes them more comprehensible as each component is explainable. On the other hand, they tend to be less generalizable and robust to variations in data. With DL models, we give up interpretability in exchange for obtaining robustness and greater generalization ability, while generating complex and abstract features

State-of-the-art DL models have been developed for a variety of tasks such as object detection and segmentation in computer vision, voice recognition, and genotype/phenotype prediction. There are different types of models that include convolutional neural networks (CNNs), deep Boltzmann machines, stacked auto-encoders , and deep belief neural networks . The most commonly used DL method for processing images that are CNNs as fully connected ANN is computationally heavy for 2D/3D images and requires extensive GPU memory. CNNs share weights across each feature map or convolutional layers to mitigate this. CNN approaches have gained enormous awareness, achieving impressive results in the ImageNet competition in 2012 , which includes natural photographic images. They were utilized to classify a dataset of around a million images that comprise a thousand diverse classes, achieving half the error rates of the most popular traditional ML approaches . CNNs have been widely utilized for medical image classification and segmentation tasks with great success Since DL algorithms outperform ML algorithms in general and exploit the GPU processing power, it allows real-time processing of US images. We will only focus on DL applications of AI-powered US cardiology in this review.

To assess the performance of ML models, data are generally split into training, validation, and test sets. The training set is used for learning about the data. The validation set is employed to establish the reliability of learning results, and the test set is used to assess the generalizability of a trained model on the data that are never seen by the model. When training samples are limited, k-fold cross validation approaches (e.g., leave-one-out, five-fold, or ten-fold cross validation) are utilized. In cross-validation, the data are divided randomly into k equal sized pieces. One piece is reserved for assessing the performance of a model, and the remaining pieces (k-1) are utilized for training models. The training process is typically performed in a supervised way, which involves ground truth labels for each input data and minimizes a loss function over training samples iteratively,. Supervised learning is the most common training approach for ML, but it requires a laborious ground truth label generation In medical imaging, ground truth labels are generally obtained from clinical notes for diagnosis or quantification. Furthermore, manual outlining of structures by experts are used to train ML models for segmentation tasks.

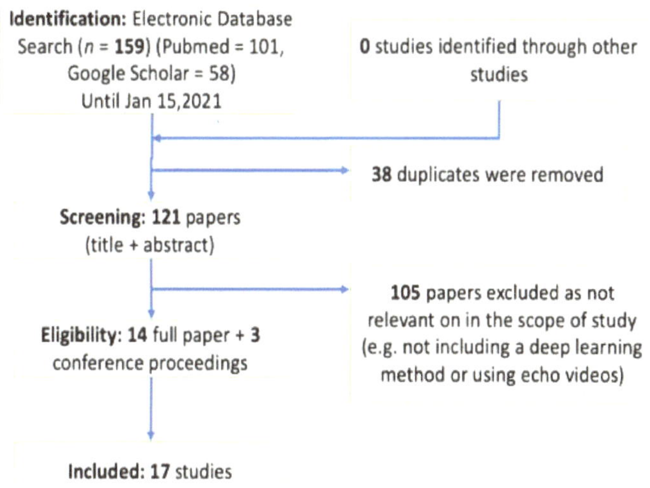

Fig.24.9 The flowchart of systematic review that includes identification, screening, eligibility, and inclusion.

Methods and Results: Automated Echo Interpretation

A thorough analysis of the literature using Google Scholar and PubMed search engines was carried out. This analysis also included ,a peer-reviewed journal publications and conference proceedings in this field (IEEE Transactions on Medical Imaging, IEEE Journal of Biomedical and Health Informatics, Circulation, Nature, and conference proceedings from SPIE, the Medical Image Computing and Computer Assisted Intervention Society, the Institute of Electrical and Electronics Engineers, and others) that describe the application of DL to cardiac ultrasound images .

Current Echo-AI applications require several successive processing steps such as view labelling and quality control, segmentation of cardiac structures, echo measurements, and disease diagnosis . AI-Echo can be used for low-cost, serial, and automated evaluation of cardiac structures and function by experts and non-experts in cardiology, primary care, and emergency clinics. This would also allow triaging incoming patients with chest pain in an emergency department by providing preliminary diagnosis and longitudinally monitoring patients with cardiovascular risk factors in a personalized mannerWith the advancing ultrasound technology, the current clinical cart-based ultrasound systems could be replaced with portable point-of-care ultrasound (POCUS) systems or could be used together. GE Vscan, Butterfly IQ, and Philips Lumify are popular POCUS devices. A single Butterfly IQ probe contains 9000 micro-machined semiconductor sensors and emulates linear, phased, and curved array probes. While the Butterfly IQ probe using ultrasound-on-chip technology ,could be used for imaging the whole body, Philips Lumify provides different probes for

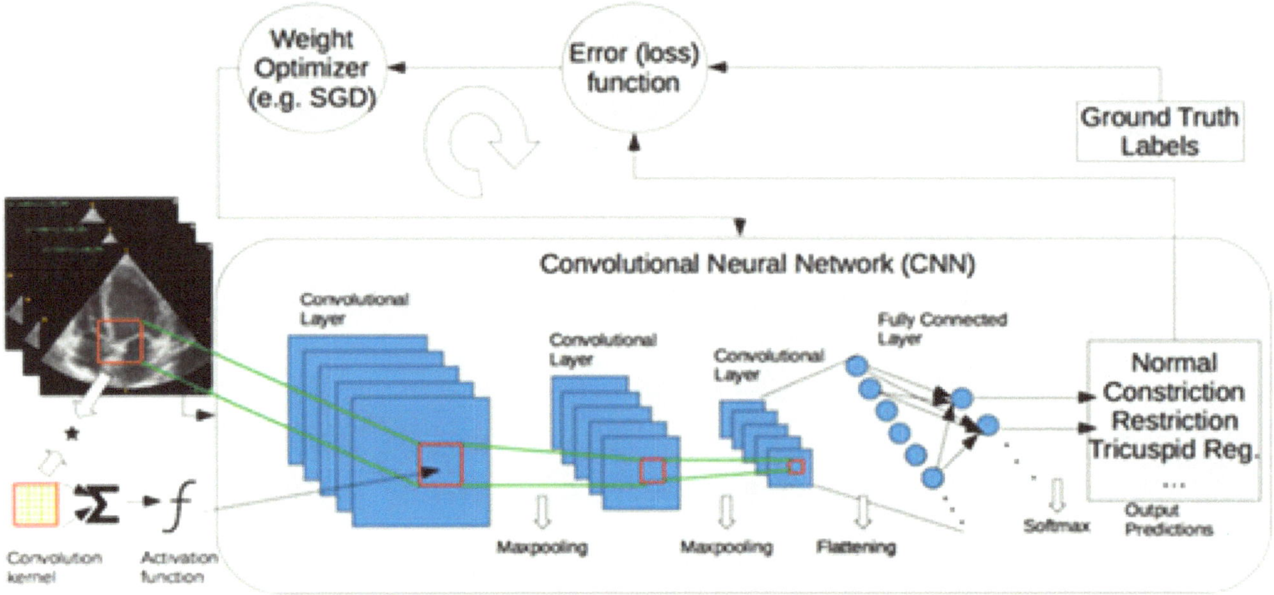

Fig 24.10 A framework of training a deep-learning model for classification of myocardial diseases. Operations between layers are shown with arrows. SGD: Stochastic Gradient Descent.

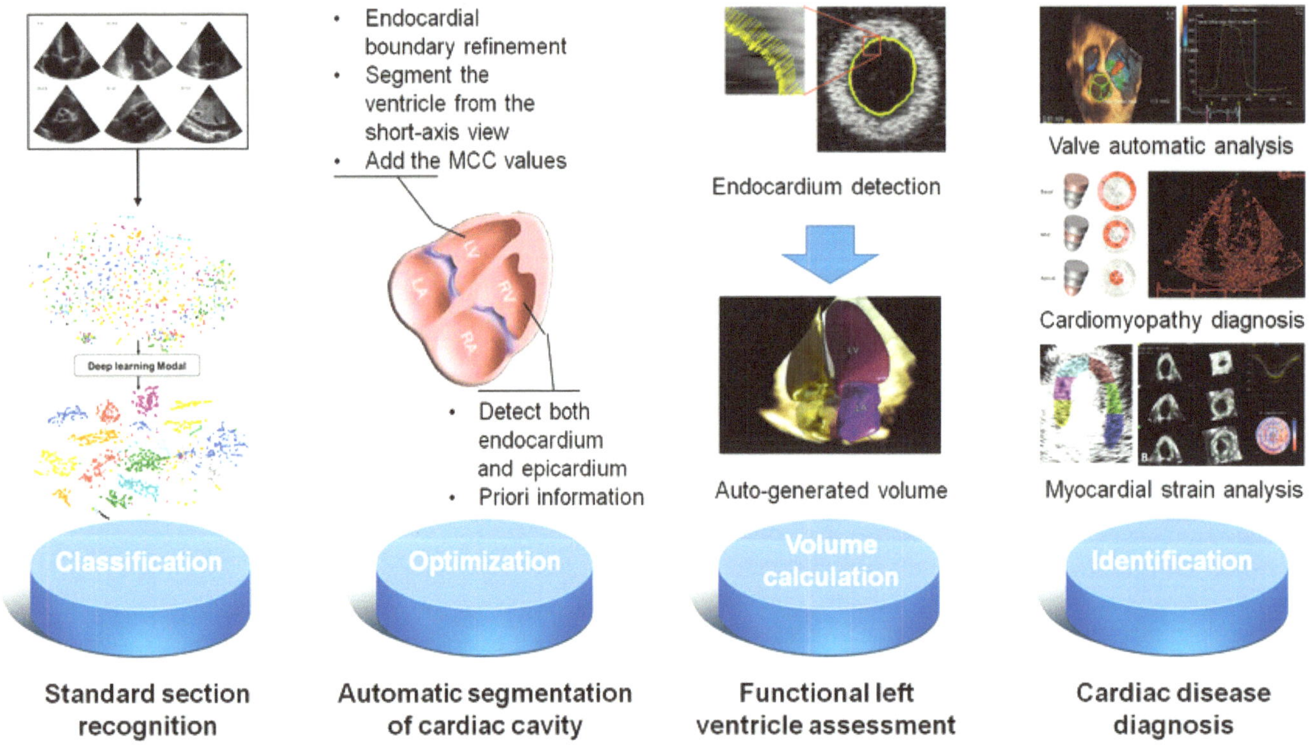

Fig 24.11 Artificial intelligence in echocardiography: detection, functional evaluation, and disease diagnosis

each organ (e.g., s4-1 phased array probe for cardiac applications). GE Vscan comes with two transducers placed in one probe and can be used for scanning deep and superficial structures. Using POCUS devices powered with cloud-based AI-Echo interpretation at point of care locations could significantly reduce the US cost and increase the utility of AI-Echo by non-experts in primary and emergency department A number of promising studies using DL approaches have been published for classification of standard echo views (e.g., apical and parasternal views), segmentation of heart structures (e.g., ventricle, atrium, septum, myocardium, and pericardium), and prediction of cardiac diseases (e.g., heart failure, hypertrophic cardiomyopathy, cardiac amyloidosis, and pulmonary hypertension) in recent years In addition, several companies such as TOMTEC IMAGING SYSTEMS GMBH, Munich, Germany and Ultromics, Oxford, United Kingdom have already obtained premarket FDA clearance on auto ejection fraction (EF) and echo strain packages using artificial intelligence.

View Identification and Quality Control

A typical TTE study includes the acquisition of multiple cine clips of the heart's chambers from five standardized windows that are left parasternal window (i.e., parasternal long and short axis views), apical window (i.e., two, three, four, five chamber views), subcostal window (i.e., four chamber view, long axis inferior vena cava view), and suprasternal notch window (i.e., aortic arch view), right parasternal window (i.e., ascending aorta view). In addition to these, the study includes several other cine clips of color Doppler, strain imaging, and 3D ultrasound and still images of valves, walls, and the blood vessels (e.g., aorta and pulmonary veins). View identification and quality control are essential prerequisite steps for a fully automated echo interpretation.

Zhang et al. presented a fully automated echo interpretation pipeline that includes 23 view classifications. They trained a 13-layer CNN model with 7168 labelled cine clips and used five-fold cross validation to assess the performance of their model. In evaluation, they selected 10 random frames per clip and averaged the resulting probabilities. The overall accuracy of their model was 84% at an individual image level. They also reported that distinguishing the various apical views was the greatest challenge in the setting of partially obscured left ventricles. They made their source code and model weights publicly available at. Mandani et al. presented the classification of 15 standard echo views using DL. They trained a VGG CNN network with 180,294 images of 213 studies and tested their model on 21,747 images of 27 studies. They obtained 91.7% overall accuracy on the test dataset at a single image level and 97.8% overall accuracy when considering the model's top two guesses. Akkus et al. [20] trained a CNN inception model with residual connections on 5544 images of 140 patients for predicting 24 Doppler image classes and automating Doppler mitral inflow analysis. They obtained overall accuracy of 97% on thetest set that included 1737 images of 40 patients.Abdi et al. trained a fully connected CNN with 6196 apical four chamber (A4C) images that were scored between 0 to 5 to assess the A4C quality of echo images. They used three-fold cross validation and reported an error comparable to intra-rater reliability (mean absolute error: 0.71 ± 0.58). Abdi et al. later extended their previous work and trained a CNN regression architecture that includes five regression models with the same weights in the first few layers for assessing the quality of cine loops across five standard view planes (i.e., apical 2, 3, and 4 chamber views and parasternal short axis views at papillary muscle and aortic valve levels). Their dataset included 2435 cine clips, and they achieved an average of 85% accuracy compared to gold standard scores assigned by experienced echo sonographers on 20% of the dataset. Zhang et al. calculated the averaged probability score of views classification across all videos in their study to define an image quality score for each view. They assumed that poor quality cine clips tended to have a more ambiguous view assignment, and the view classification probability could be used for quality assessment. Dong et al. presented a generic quality control framework for fetal ultrasound cardiac four chamber planes (CFPs). Their proposed framework consists of three networks that roughly classify four-chamber views from the raw data, determine the gain and zoom of images, and detect the key anatomical structures on a plane. The overall quantitative score of each CFP was achieved based on the output of the three networks. They used five-fold cross validation to assess their model across 2032 CFPs and 5000 non-CFPs and obtained a mean average precision of 93.52%. Labs et al. trained a hybrid model including CNN and LSTM layers to assess the quality of apical four-chamber view images for three proposed attributes (i.e., foreshortening, gain/contrast, and axial target). They split a dataset of 1039 unique apical four-chamber views into 60:20:20% ratio for training, validation, and testing, respectively, and achieved an average accuracy of 86% on the test set.View identification and quality assessment of cine clips are the most important pieces of a fully automated echo interpretation pipeline. There is an error range of 3–16% in the current studies for both view identification and quality control. The proposed models were generally trained with a dataset from a single or a few vendors or a single center. Apart from the study of Zhang et al., none of the studies shared their source code and model weights for comparisons. In some studies, customized CNN models were used, but not enough evidence or comparisons were shown to support that their choices perform better than the state-of-the-art CNN models such as Resnet, Inception, and Densenet.

Image Segmentation and Quantification

Partitioning of an identified view into the region of interests such as left/right ventricle or atrium, ventricular septum, and

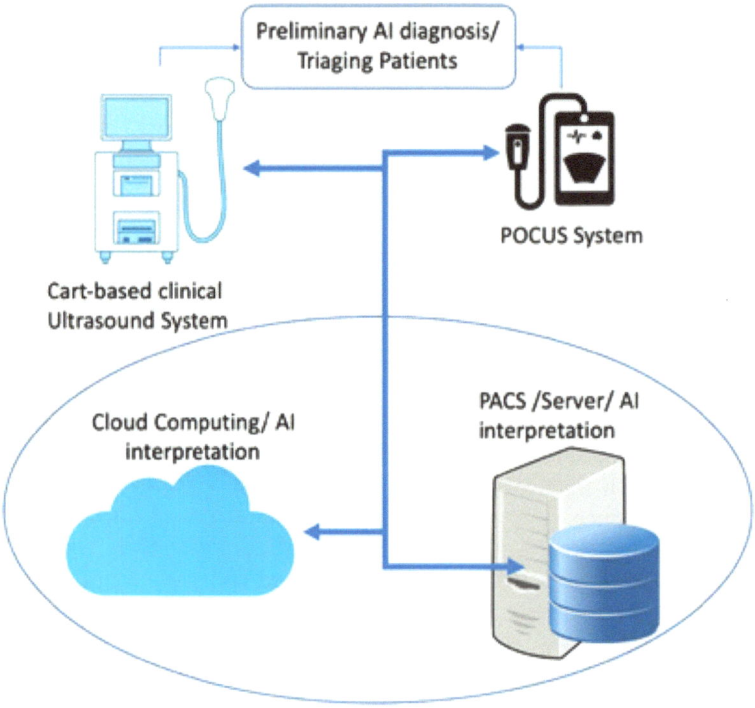

Fig 24.12 A schematic diagram of AI (artificial intelligence) interpretation of echocardiography images for preliminary diagnosis and triaging patients in emergency and primary care clinics. POCUS: point of care ultrasound.

Table 24.1 The list of commercial software packages that provides automated measurements or diagnosis.

Company	Software Package	AI-Empowered Tools
Siemens Medical Solutions Inc., USA	syngo Auto Left Heart, Acuson S2000 US system.	Auto EF, Auto LV and LA volumes, Auto Strain for manually selected views.
GE Healthcare, Inc., USA	Ultra Edition Package, Vivid Ultrasound Systems	Auto EF, Auto LV and LA volumes, Auto Strain for manually selected views
TOMTEC Imaging Systems GmbH, Germany	Tomtec-Arena/Tomtec-Zero	Auto EF, Auto LV and LA volumes, Auto Strain for manually selected views
Ultromics Ltd., United Kingdom	Echo Go/Echo Go Pro	Auto EF, Auto LV and LA volumes, Auto Strain, Auto identification of CHD (Fully automated)
Dia Imaging Analysis Ltd., Israel	DiaCardio'sLVivoEF Software/LVivo Seamless	Auto EF and Auto standard echo view identification (Fully automated)
Caption Health, Inc., USA	The Caption Guidance software	AI tool for assisting to capture images of a patient's heart

EF: ejection fraction. CHD: coronary heart disease.

mitral/tricuspid valves is necessary to quantify certain biomarkers such as ejection fraction, volume changes, and velocity of septal or distal annulus. Several studies have used DL methods to segment left ventricles from apical four and two chamber views.

Zhang et al. presented a fully automated echo interpretation pipeline that includes segmentation of cardiac chambers in five common views and quantification of structure and function. They used five-fold cross validation on 791 images that have manual segmentation of left ventricle and reported the intersection over union metric ranging from 0.72 to 0.90 for the performance of their U-Net-based segmentation model. In addition, they produced automated measurements such as LV ejection fraction (LVEF), LV volumes, LV mass, and global longitudinal strain from the resulting segmentations. Compared to manual measurements, median absolute deviation of 9.7% (n = 6407 studies) was achieved for LVEF; median absolute deviation of 15–17% was obtained for LV volume and mass measurements; median absolute deviation of 7.5% (n = 419) and 9.0% (n = 110) was obtained for strain. They concluded that they obtained cardiac structure measurements comparable with values in study reports. Leclerc et al. studied the state-of-art encoder–decoder type DL methods (e.g., U-Net for segmenting cardiac structures and made a large dataset (500 patients) publicly available with segmentation labels of end diastole and systole frames. They showed that their U-Net-based model outperformed the state-of-the-art non-deep-learning methods for measurements of end-diastolic and end-systolic left ventricular volumes and LVEF. They achieved a mean correlation of 0.95 and an absolute mean error of 9.5 mL for LV volumes and a mean correlation coefficient of 0.80 and an absolute mean error of 5.6% for LVEF. Jafari et al. [30] presented a recurrent CNN and optical flow for segmentation of the left ventricle in echo images. Jafari et al. also presented biplane ejection fraction estimation with POCUS using multi-task and learning and adversarial training. The performance of the proposed model for the segmentation of LV was an average Dice score of 0.92 and, for the automated ejection fraction, was shown to be around an absolute error of 6.2%. Chen et al. proposed an encoder–decoder type CNN with multi-view regularization to improve LV segmentation. The method was evaluated on 566 patients and achieved an average Dice score of 0.88. Oktay et al. incorporated anatomical prior knowledge in their CNN model that allows following the global anatomical properties of the underlying anatomy. Ghorbani et al. used a custom CNN model, named EchoNet, to predict left ventricular end systolic and diastolic volumes ($R2 = 0.74$ and $R2 = 0.70$), and ejection fraction ($R2 = 0.50$). Ouyang et al. trained a semantic segmentation model using atrous convolutions on echocardiogram videos. Their model obtained Dice similarity coefficient of 0.92 for left ventricle segmentation of apical four-chamber view and used a spatiotemporal 3D CNN model with residual connections and predicted ejection fraction with mean absolute errors of 4.1 and 6% for internal and external datasetsrespectively.Ouyanget al. de-identified 10,030 echocardiogram videos, resized them into 112 × 112 pixels, and made their dataset publicly available at .U-Net is the most common DL model used for echo image segmentation. The error range for LVEF is ranging between 4 and 10%, while it ranges between 10 and 20% for LV and LA volume measurements.

Disease Diagnosis

Several studies have shown that DL models can be used to assess cardiac diseases (see Table 4). Zhang et al.] presented a fully automated echo interpretation pipeline for disease detection. They trained a VGG network using three random images per video as an input and provided two prediction outputs (i.e., diseased or normal). The ROC curve performance of their model for prediction of hypertrophic cardiomyopathy, cardiac amyloidosis, and pulmonary hypertension were 0.93, 0.87, and 0.85, respectively. Ghorbani et al. trained a customized CNN model that includes inception connections, named EchoNet, on a dataset of more than 1.6 million echocardiogram images from 2850 patients to identify local cardiac structures, estimate cardiac function, and predict systemic risk factors. The proposed CNN model identified the presence of pacemaker leads with AUC = 0.89, enlarged left atrium with AUC = 0.86, and left ventricular hypertrophy with AUC = 0.75. Ouyang et al. trained a custom model that includes spatiotemporal 3D convolutions with a residual connection network together with semantic segmentation of the left ventricle to predict the presence of heart failure with reduced ejection fraction. The output of the spatiotemporal network and semantic segmentation were combined to classify heart failure with reduced ejection fraction. Their model achieved an area under the curve of 0.97 for predicting heart failure with reduced ejection fraction. Omar et al. trained a modified VGG-16 CNN model on a 3D Dobutamine stress echo dataset to detect wall motion abnormalities and compared its performance to hand-crafted approaches: support vector machines (SVM) and random forests (RF). They achieved slightly better accuracy with the CNN model: RF (72.1%), SVM (70.5%), and CNN (75.0%). In another study, Kusunose et al. [36] investigated whether a CNN model could provide improved detection of wall motion abnormalities.

They presented that the area under the AUC produced by the deep-learning algorithm was comparable to that produced by the cardiologists and sonographer readers (0.99 vs. 0.98, respectively) and significantly higher than the AUC result of the resident readers (0.99 vs. 0.90, respectively). Narula et al. trained SVM, RF, and artificial neural network (ANN) with hand-crafted echo measurements (i.e., LV wall thickness, end-diastolic volume, end-systolic volume, and ejection fraction, pulsed-wave Doppler-derived transmitral early diastolic velocity (E), the late diastolic atrial contraction wave velocity (A), and the ratio E/A to differentiate hypertrophic cardiomyopathy (HCM) from physiological hypertrophy seen in athletes (ATH). They reported overall sensitivity and specificity of 87 and 82%, respectively.Unlike other hand-crafted feature-based ML approaches, the DL approaches may extract features from data beyond human perception. DL-based AI approaches have the potential to support accurate diagnosis and discovering crucial features from echo images. In the near future, these tools may aid physicians in diagnosis and decision making and reduce the misdiagnosis rate.

Discussion and Outlook

Automated image interpretation that mimics human vision with traditional machine learning has existed for a long time. Recent advances in parallel processing with GPUs and deep-learning algorithms, which extract patterns in images with their self-learning ability, have changed the entire automated image interpretation practice with respect to computation speed, generalizability, and transferability of these algorithms. AI-empowered echocardiography has been advancing and moving closer to be used in routine clinical workflow in cardiology due to the increased demand for standardizing acquisition and interpretation of cardiac US images. Even though DL-based methods for echocardiography provide promising results in diagnosis and quantification of diseases, AI-Echo still needs to be validated with larger study populations including multi-center and multi-vendor datasets. High intra-/inter-variability in echocardiography makes standardization of image acquisition and interpretation challenging. However, AI-Echo will provide solutions to mitigate operator-dependent variability and interpretability. AI applications in cardiac US are more challenging than those in cardiac CT and MR imaging modalities due to patient-dependent factors (e.g., obesity, limited acoustic window, artifacts, and signal drops) and natural US speckle noise pattern. These factors that affect US image quality will remain as challenges with cardiac ultrasound.Applications of DL in echocardiography are rapidly advancing as evidenced by the growing number of studies recently. DL models have enormous representation power and are hungry for large amounts of data in order to obtain generalization ability and stability. Creating databases with large datasets that are curated and have good quality data and labels is the most challenging and time-consuming part of the whole AI model development process. Although it has been shown that AI-echo applications have superb performance compared to classical ML methods, most of the models were trained and evaluated on small datasets. It is important to train AI models on large multi-vendor and multi-center datasets to obtain generalization and validate on large multi-vendor datasets to increase reliability of a proposed model. An alternative way to overcome the limitation of having small training datasets would be augmenting the dataset with realistic transformations (e.g., scaling, horizontal flipping, translations, adding noise, tissue deformation, and adjusting image contrast) that could help improve generalizability of AI models. On the other hand, realistic transformations need to be used to genuinely simulate variations in cardiac ultrasound images, and transformations-applied images should not create artifacts. Alternatively, generative adversarial networks, which include a generator and a discriminator model, are trained until the model generates images that are not separable by the discriminator. This could be used to generate realistic cardiac ultrasound B-mode images of the heart. Introducing such transformations during the training process will make AI models more robust to small perturbations in input data space. Making predictions and measurements based on only 2D echo images could be considered as a limitation of AI-powered US systems. Two-dimensional cross section images include limited information and do not constitute the complete myocardium. Training AI models on 3D cardiac ultrasound data that include the entire heart or the structure of interest would potentially improve the diagnostic accuracy of an AI model . It is important to design AI models that are transparent for the prediction of any disease from medical images. The AI models developed for diagnosis of a disease must elucidate the reasons and motivations behind their predictions in order to build trust in them. Comprehension of the inner mechanism of an AI model necessitates interpreting the activity of feature maps in each layer . However, the extracted features are a combination of sequential layers and become complicated and conceptual with more layers. Therefore, the interpretation of these features become difficult compared to handcrafted imaging features in traditional ML methods. Traditional ML methods are designed for separable components that are more understandable, since each component of ML methods has an explanation but usually is not very accurate or robust. With DL-based AI models, the interpretability is given up for the robustness and complex imaging features with greater generalizability. Recently, a number of methods have been introduced about what DL models see and how to make their predictions. Several CNN architectures employed techniques such as deconvolutional networks gradient back-propagation , class activation maps (CAM) gradient-weighted CAM , and saliency maps to make CNN understandable. With these techniques, gradients of a model have been projected back to the input image space, which shows what parts in the input image contribute the most to the prediction outcome that maximizes the classification accuracy. Although making AI models understandable has been an active research topic in the DL community, there is still much further research needed in the area. Despite the fact that high prediction performances were achieved and reported in the studies discussed in this review, none of the studies have provided an insight on which heart regions play an important role in any disease prediction

Developing AI models that standardize image acquisition and interpretation with less variability is essential considering that echocardiography is an operator- and interpreter-dependent imaging modality. AI guidance during data acquisition for the optimal angle, view, and measurements would make echocardiography less operator-dependent and smarter, while standardizing data acquisition. Cost-effective and easy access of POCUS systems with AI capability would help clinicians and non-experts perform swift initial examinations on patients and progress with vital and urgent decisions in emergency and primary care clinics. In the near future, POCUS systems with AI capability could replace the stethoscopes that doctors use in their daily practice to listen to patients' hearts. Clinical cardiac ultrasound or POCUS systems empowered with AI, which can assess multi-mode data, steer sonographers during acquisition, and deliver objective qualifications, measurements, and diagnoses, will assist with decision making for diagnosis and treatments, improve echocardiography workflow in clinics, and lower healthcare cost.

Utilization of Artificial Intelligence in Echocardiography

In the modern era, artificial intelligence (AI) is spreading into all parts of daily life. AI is a program that has tasks based on algorithms in an intelligent manner. Machine learning is a subset of AI and focuses on the machine's ability to receive a set of data and learn for itself. The tasks in machine learning can be classified into supervised and unsupervised learning problems. In the former, the task of assigning data to one of the discrete categories is called classification, whereas the task of fitting the desired output consisting of ≥1 continuous variables is called regression. In the latter, the goal may be to discover some groups categorized with similar variables, or features, called "clustering". Deep learning is a subset of machine learning that can solve a problem by using multilayered neural networks (Figure 1). Deep learning has led to state-of-the art improvements in word recognition, visual object recognition, object detection, etc.1 Image recognition by machines trained through deep learning in some situations is superior to that of humans. Just a few years ago, we were surprised by a machine learning-based computer program ("AlphaGo") that defeated the world champion of Go.2 The AI algorithm continues to be enhanced every year. Medical imaging also seems to be changing and undergoing an important revolution because of AI methods such as deep learning based on neural networks.Data are an essential component of AI, and the quality and size of a dataset used to build a model will strongly influence the outcomes. When datasets are biased, the results are unusable in the clinical setting. Preprocessing is also important because echocardiographic data are nonstructural and there are differences in image properties in the dataset. Cardiologists need to make a labeled dataset to develop the model. After development of models, a clinical trial is key to this flow because developed models must be validated in different cohorts. A typical model development process is shown in Figure 2. AI researchers follow this process when developing a new model.Recently, there have been some reports on AI in the medical imaging modalities. For example, calcium scoring in low-dose chest computed tomography (CT), identification of functionally significant stenosis in CT angiography, and diagnosis of chronic myocardial infarction on cine magnetic resonance image (MRI) have been developed.3–5 Compared with CT and MRI, in echocardiography there is an issue of high observer variation in the interpretation of images. Thus, AI might be help to improve observer variation and provide accurate diagnosis in echocardiography. In this review, we focus on the current status and future directions of AI in the field of echocardiography.

Direction of AI in Echocardiography

Echocardiography has a central role in the diagnosis and management of cardiovascular disease.6 Precise and reliable echocardiographic assessment is required for clinical decision-making.7–10 Even in the development of new technologies (3-dimentional echocardiography, speckle-tracking, semi-automated analysis, etc.), the final analytical decision is strongly dependent on operator experience. For example, left ventricular ejection fraction (LVEF) is subjective, and variability could be influenced by observer experience. Several institutes have several readers with a wide range of experience levels.Until now, many interventions for reduction of variability in LVEF have been tested to overcome this issue. Our multicenter group suggested that a simple teaching intervention can reduce the variability in LVEF assessment, especially for readers with limited experience. However, there are several limitations, including a lack of ground truth, limited number of sample sizes, etc. Thus, diagnostic errors are a major unresolved problem. Moreover, not only can cardiologists differ from one another in image interpretations, but the same observer may come to different conclusion when a reading is repeated. Daily high workloads in clinical practice may lead to this error, and all cardiologists require precise perception in this field. AI will likely help to overcome these issues. The AI algorithms might provide an aid to diagnostics with fewer errors and provide hidden features for accurate diagnosis. One landmark echocardiographic paper was recently published. The authors used a deep learning model to build a fully automated echocardiogram interpretation program, including view identification, image segmentation, quantification of structure and function, and disease detection. Since then, many cardiologists can see a potential role for AI in the echocardiographic field. Our laboratory also investigated the building of models of automated diagnosis of myocardial infarction using a deep learning algorithm.

AI for View Classifications

Echocardiographic images consist of several video clips, still images (M-mode and B-mode) and Doppler recordings

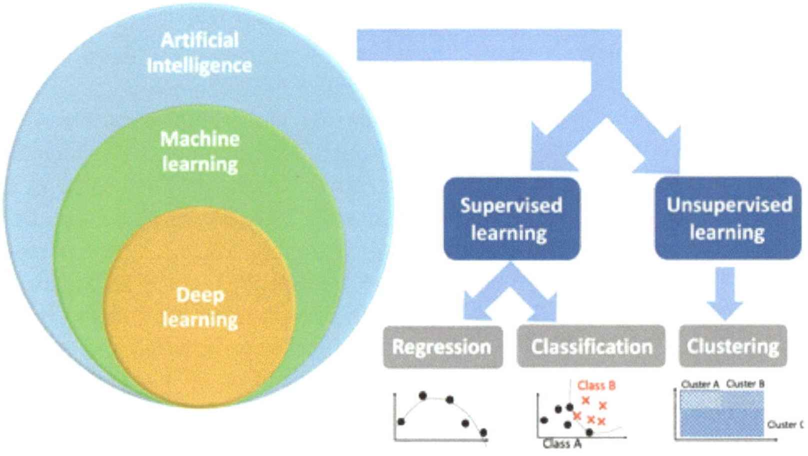

Fig 24.13 .Artificial intelligence, including machine learning and deep learning and their tasks.

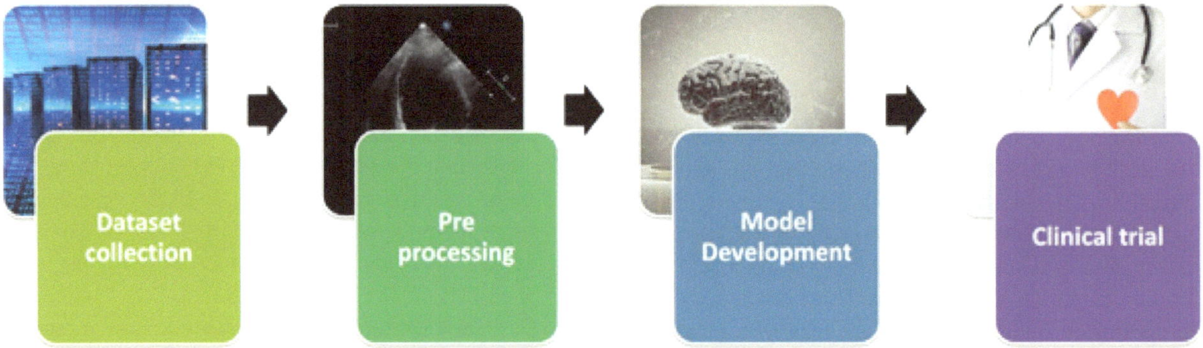

Fig 24.14 Development process for artificial intelligence models.

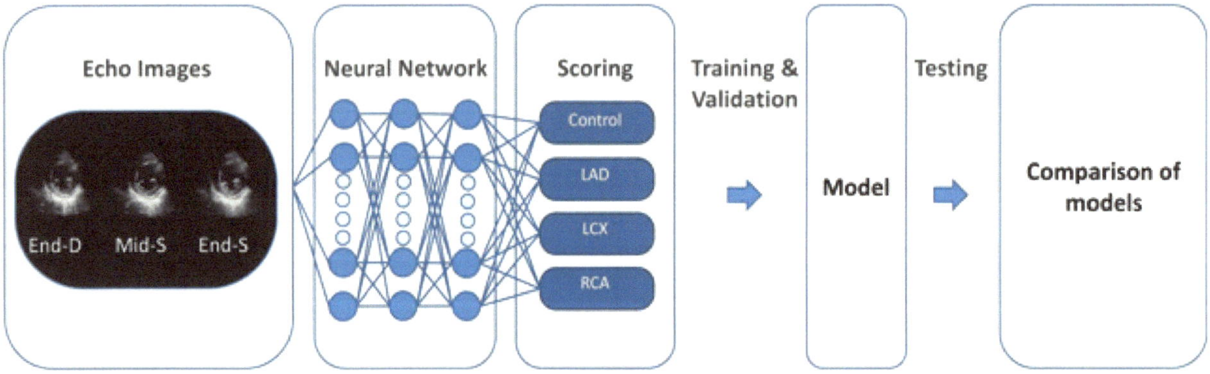

Fig 24.15 An example of a convolutional neural network model for detection of coronary artery disease. LAD, left anterior descending coronary artery; LCX, left circumflex coronary artery; RCA, right coronary artery.

because the heart's structure and function are complex and require many views to diagnose cardiovascular diseases Because of the nonstructural data in echocardiography, determination of the view is the essential first step in interpreting an echocardiogram. Recent studies applied deep learning with convolutional neural networks for view classification of echocardiograms.

They trained a convolutional neural network to simultaneously classify 15 standard views (12 video, 3 still), based on labeled still images and videos from 267 transthoracic echocardiograms with over 800,000 images that captured a range of real-world clinical variations. Their model classified among 12 video views with 97.8% overall test accuracy without overfitting. Another group reported that a model for view classification was successfully trained with more layers and a larger number of echocardiography view classes. Thus, this method may be reasonable for application to image classification. On the other hand, there are some limitations, including lack of explanation of the learning process and less than perfect classification. The utility is questionable in the current version of models. Moreover, they did not adequately resolve the problem of vendor differences and image qualities. A future enhanced model to classify the correct views would be required.

AI for Size and Function

Quantification of heart size and function is an essential part of echocardiography. Fully automated 3D echocardiographic analysis can obtain quantitative results without any observer interaction (e.g., selection of views, positioning markers and modifying borders). Commercially available software has been tested for accuracy and reproducibility. The algorithms are knowledge-based probabilistic contouring algorithms or adaptive analytics algorithms. The most frequently used software is the HeartModel algorithm in the Philips EPIQ series.This software shows automated tracings of the left ventricular and left atrial endocardial borders with 3D analysis. There are many studies comparing fully automated methods and either cardiac magnetic resonance or manual echocardiography,but there are some limitations from the clinical setting viewpoint. One is the dependency on image quality, which has an important role, because results obtained with poor but analyzable image quality provide inaccurate results. On the other hand, although measurement accuracy using this analysis still depends on image quality, its degree becomes obviously smaller than with current semi-automated software. The number of datasets for training also affects measurement accuracy. The current adaptive analytics algorithm does not work very well in patients with distorted LV shape, such as LV aneurysms and apical hypertrophic cardiomyopathy because of the limited number of datasets for machine learning.These limitations also exist for deep learning in echocardiography. Deep learning algorithms require a high-quality database to provide a sound estimation model with a small sample size. Zhang et al proposed a pipeline based on a deep learning approach for a fully automated analysis of echocardiographic data.They proposed to train a U-net deep learning model for automatic segmentation of the LV in the apical 4- and 2-chamber views. For LV segmentation, their model had a Dice score of approximately 85% in the apical 2-chamber view, and approximately 80% in the apical 4-chamber view, and a mean absolute percentage error of approximately 10% for EF from the apical 2-chamber view, and 20% for EF from the apical 4-chamber view. The correlation is good; however, their dataset did not include a wide range of LVEF. In addition, EF values were evaluated after segmentation of the LV, so may include segmentation errors. We believe that a direct evaluation of EF with larger training sets that include extremes of LV range will be needed for training and validation.

AI for Wall Motion Abnormality

One of the most important assessments in echocardiography is evaluating regional wall motion abnormalities (RWMAs) for the management of ischemic coronary artery disease (CAD). Assessment of RWMAs is a Class I recommendation in the guidelines by trained echocardiographic technicians for patients with chest pain in the emergency department. Conventional assessment of RWMAs, which is based on visual interpretation of endocardial excursion and myocardial thickening, is subjective and experience-dependent. A useful method for reducing the misreading of RWMAs is required.Machine-learning models have been evaluated to identify and quantify RWMAs. A convolutional neural network provided good models with high sensitivity for diagnosis of CAD. Recently, our laboratory investigated building models of automated diagnosis for myocardial infarction using a deep learning algorithm . For detection of the presence of RWMA, the area under the receiver-operating characteristic curve (AUC) by deep learning algorithm was similar to that for a reading by cardiologist/sonographer, and significantly higher than the AUC for resident readers. Interestingly, deep learning had relatively low ratios of misclassification of the right coronary artery, left circumflex coronary artery, and control groups except for the left anterior descending coronary artery (LAD). It seems to reflect the real-world assessment (e.g., overdiagnoses in ischemic groups by human observers or importance of LAD in the clinical setting). The results of a deep learning model in echocardiography might provide new insights in the medical field

AI for Diagnosis of Cardiovascular Diseases

Several techniques have been applied to identify clinical disease states. In the echocardiographic field, speckle-tracking imaging is widely used in cases of cardiomyopathy. Clinical reports on speckle-tracking imaging show significant differences in regional strain in several cardiomyopathies, even in the absence of ischemia. Knowledge of the characteristic LV strain distribution pattern might facilitate diagnosis of constrictive pericarditis, cardiac amyloidosis, hypertrophic cardiomyopathy, hypertensive heart disease, tachycardia-induced cardiomyopathy, and aortic stenosis. On the other hand, recent American and European consensus paper describe reginal longitudinal strain assessment by speckle-tracking

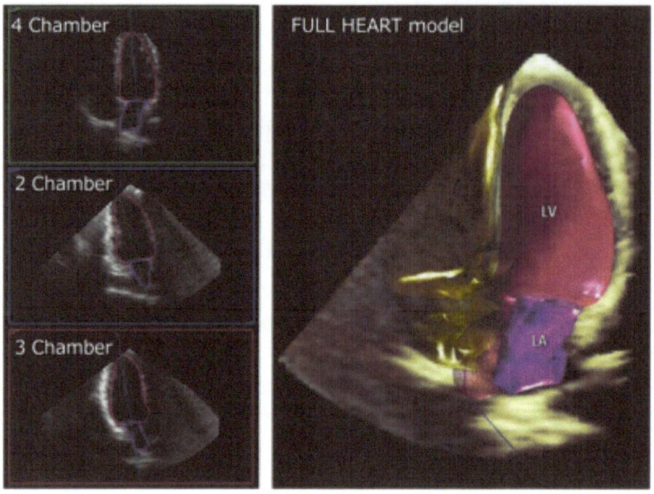

Fig 24.16 Representative fully automated analysis software, HeartModel

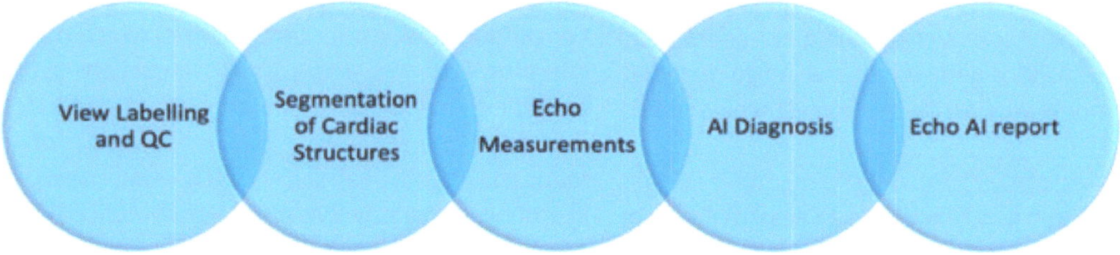

Fig 24.17 The flowchart of automated artificial-intelligence-empowered echo (AI-Echo) interpretation pipeline using a chain approach. QC: Quality Control.

analysis as still too immature to adopt in the clinical setting.The limitation should be overcome in the future. Recently, machine-learning algorithms have revealed clinical disease conditions and new futures. Sengupta et al applied a cognitive machine-learning algorithm to differentiate constrictive pericarditis from restrictive cardiomyopathy with multimodality imaging and pathology. The same group showed a machine-learning approach to assessing the potential role diagnosing hypertrophy in athletes and hypertrophic cardiomyopathy. Sanchez-Martinez et al and Tabassian et al showed that machine learning using echocardiographic data, including strain imaging at rest and during exercise, may improve diagnosis and understanding of heart failure with preserved EF. In this field, investigators try to not only assess the accuracy of diagnosis, but also discover new findings in cardiovascular disease. Zhang et al proposed a model based on a deep learning approach for differentiating cardiomyopathy and pulmonary hypertension from the parasternal long-axis views. Unlike other machine-learning approaches, the deep learning approach may automatically encode optimal features from data beyond human recognition. Big data have the potential to lead to precise diagnosis and discovering important features from the echocardiographic images. In the future, AI may aid physicians in accurate diagnosis without requiring pathologicalsamples.

Future of AI in Echocardiography

Cardiologists will determine the capability of AI in diagnosis, and they will be responsible for the final decisions. Thus, cardiologists will be required to have the capacity e to manage AI and advanced knowledge. Some recent studies have been concerned about adversarial examples in the medical imaging field.48 Adversarial examples are inputs to learning models that an attacker has intentionally designed to cause the model to make a mistake; they are like optical illusions for machines. In echocardiography, data are just pixel images, not structured data. Echocardiographic imaging systems may be vulnerable to adversarial attacks. For example, insurance companies will use a deep learning system that receives images as part of a claim to verify that heart surgery would be necessary in the future. An adversarial example may be used to deceive the insurance company's system. In these cases, cardiologists should have adequate and solid knowledge in this field. The era of AI is almost here.

Coronary Flow Assessment Using 3-Dimensional Ultrafast Ultrasound Localization Microscopy

Coronary microcirculation (ie, flow in vessels smaller than 300 µm) plays a key role in the control of cardiac perfusion.1 Patients with coronary microvascular disease (CMD) have poor prognoses with significantly higher rates of cardiovascular events, including hospitalization for heart failure, sudden cardiac death, and myocardial infarction (MI). Likewise, microvascular obstruction after reperfusion of a MI, a phenomenon called no-reflow, is the most relevant predictor of adverse outcome.Up to date, although the anatomy of large vessels can be easily assessed, only functional assessments of the coronary microcirculation are available either through imaging (positron emission tomography, cardiac magnetic resonance, and contrast echocardiography) or through invasive measurements.These examinations can provide hemodynamic information such as myocardial blood flow and coronary flow reserve (CFR) in response to the vasodilator adenosine. However, there is currently no available tool to image directly the entire coronary microcirculation in clinical or preclinical settings, which in turn has limited considerably the knowledge on the coronary microcirculation pathophysiology and the development of effective therapeutic strategies. Indeed, direct visualization of the full coronary architecture including complex microvascular network remains out of reach of current cardiac imaging modalities mainly because of the low spatial and temporal resolutions or sensitivity limitations.6 The association of anatomic and hemodynamic exploration at the microscopic scale could allow a better understanding of the adaptation of the coronary microcirculation to physiological conditions (aging, exercise) or to pathophysiological stresses (proximal artery stenosis, O2 consumption/perfusion imbalance). Moreover, besides contrast echocardiography, none of the examinations for the microcirculation evaluation can be easily repeated because of their availability, the risk of irradiation, and the risk of complications for invasive assessment. Consequently, we are currently lacking of a technique that would allow repeated anatomical and functional evaluation of the coronary microcirculation to determine the mechanisms of the functional alterations but also to address the effect of the different treatments.

Recently, ultrafast ultrasound broke the conventional resolution barrier via localization of single circulating microbubbles (MB) in the blood flow. Ultrafast ultrasound localization microscopy (ULM) allowed mapping microvascular flows at high spatial resolution (10 µm), an order of magnitude smaller than the ultrasound diffraction limit, and at depths much greater than the traditionally frequency-limited imaging depth.8 However, coronary network arrangement is complex and arbitrarily oriented in all 3 dimensions, which greatly limits 2- dimensional (2D) ULM assessed in cross-sections. Furthermore, deformation of the heart as well as large and rapid out-of-plane motion induced by physiological events, mostly cardiac and respiratory motions, create significant errors in localizationand cannot be efficiently corrected without 3-dimensional (3D) imaging.

Here, we overcome these issues and demonstrate coronary ultrasound localization microscopy (CorULM) for direct visualization and quantification of the microvascular flows in beating perfused rat hearts. Our approach relies on volumetric ultrafast imaging with a matrix transducer connected to a high channel–count ultrafast electronics.10 3D-ULM is used to track the individual MB and quantify the flow velocity in the entire vasculature. A multiscale 3D motion correction is applied on the localization center over a few tens of cardiac cycles, which enabled reconstructing the microvascular anatomy, flow velocity, and flow rate of beating hearts

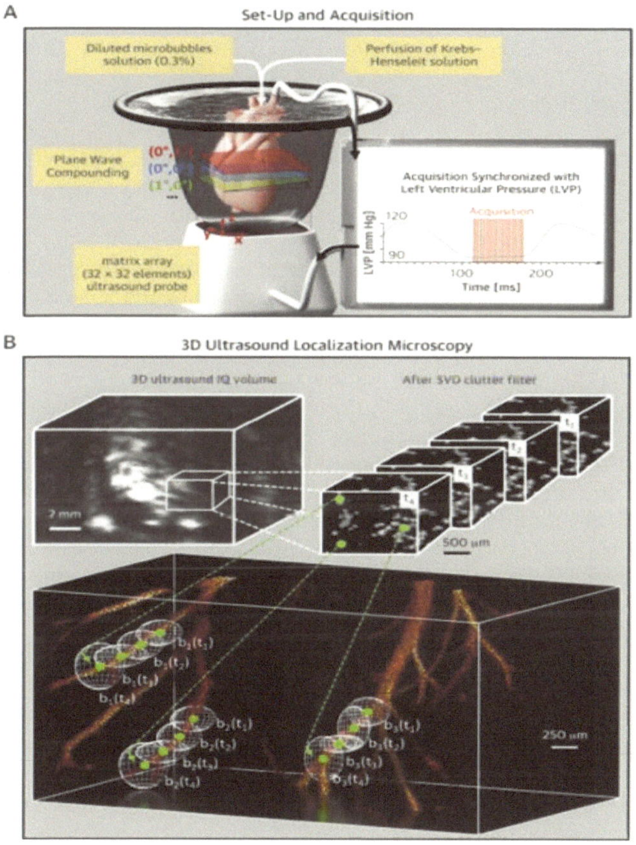

Fig 24.18 3D-CorULM Principles (A) Experimental set-up: plane waves are transmitted at high repetition rate at different angles during diastole in a perfused isolated beating rat heart. (B) 3D ULM processing: after SVD filtering, MBs are localized with a 3D paraboloid bn and are tracked over acquisition times ti to determine tracks. (C) 3D intensity-based rigid registration is computed to correct motion between diastolic phases. Then, a fine ICP correction is applied at a subwavelength scale. Corrected MB coordinates are eventually aggregated to create a 3D vascular volume. 3D = 3-dimensional; CorULM = coronary ultrasound localization microscopy; ICD = XXX; IQ = in-phase and quadrature; LVP = left ventricular pressure; MB = microbubble; SVD = XXX; ULM = ultrasound localization microscopy.

Bibliography and Acknowledgement

- Abdi A.H., Luong C., Tsang T., Allan G., Nouranian S., Jue J., Hawley D., Fleming S., Gin K., Swift J., et al. Proceedings of the Medical Imaging 2017: Image Processing; International Society for Optics and Photonics. Volume 10133. IEEE; Piscataway, NJ, USA: 2017. Automatic quality assessment of apical four-chamber echocardiograms using deep convolutional neural networks; p. 101330S. [Google Scholar]
- Abdi A.H., Luong C., Tsang T., Allan G., Nouranian S., Jue J., Hawley D., Fleming S., Gin K., Swift J., et al. Automatic Quality Assessment of Echocardiograms Using Convolutional Neural Networks: Feasibility on the Apical Four-Chamber View. IEEE Trans. Med. Imaging. 2017;36:1221–1230. doi: 10.1109/TMI.2017.2690836. [PubMed] [CrossRef] [Google Scholar]
- Abdi A.H., Luong C., Tsang T., Jue J., Gin K., Yeung D., Hawley D., Rohling R., Abolmaesumi P. Proceedings of the Medical Image Computing and Computer Assisted Intervention–MICCAI 2017. Springer International Publishing; Berlin/Heidelberg, Germany: 2017. Quality Assessment of Echocardiographic Cine Using Recurrent Neural Networks: Feasibility on Five Standard View Planes; pp. 302–310. [Google Scholar]
- Badrinarayanan V., Kendall A., Cipolla R. SegNet: A Deep Convolutional Encoder-Decoder Architecture for Image Segmentation. IEEE Trans. Pattern Anal. Mach. Intell. 2017;39:2481–2495. doi: 10.1109/TPAMI.2016.2644615. [PubMed] [CrossRef] [Google Scholar]
- Cai J.C., Akkus Z., Philbrick K.A., Boonrod A., Hoodeshenas S., Weston A.D., Rouzrokh P., Conte G.M., Zeinoddini A., Vogelsang D.C., et al. Fully Automated Segmentation of Head CT Neuroanatomy Using Deep Learning. Radiol. Artif. Intell. 2020;2:e190183. doi: 10.1148/ryai.2020190183. [CrossRef] [Google Scholar]
- Chattopadhay A., Sarkar A., Howlader P., Balasubramanian V.N. Grad-CAM++: Generalized Gradient-Based Visual Explanations for Deep Convolutional Networks; Proceedings of the 2018 IEEE Winter Conference on Applications of Computer Vision (WACV); Lake Tahoe, NV, USA. 12–15 March 2018; pp. 839–847. [Google Scholar]
- Chen H., Zheng Y., Park J.-H., Heng P.-A., Zhou S.K. Iterative Multi-domain Regularized Deep Learning for Anatomical Structure Detection and Segmentation from Ultrasound Images; Proceedings of the Medical Image Computing and Computer-Assisted Intervention–MICCAI 2016; Athens, Greece. 17–21 October 2016; pp. 487–495. [Google Scholar]
- Deng J., Dong W., Socher R., Li L.-J., Li K., Li F.-F. Proceedings of the 2009 IEEE Conference on Computer Vision and Pattern Recognition. IEEE; Piscataway, NJ, USA: 2009. ImageNet: A large-scale hierarchical image database. [Google Scholar]
- Dong J., Liu S., Liao Y., Wen H., Lei B., Li S., Wang T. A Generic Quality Control Framework for Fetal Ultrasound Cardiac Four-Chamber Planes. IEEE J. Biomed. Health Inform. 2020;24:931–942. doi: 10.1109/JBHI.2019.2948316. [PubMed] [CrossRef] [Google Scholar]
- E.A., Zou J.Y. Deep learning interpretation of echocardiograms. NPJ Digit. Med. 2020;3:10. doi: 10.1038/s41746-019-0216-8. [PMC free article] [PubMed] [CrossRef] [Google Scholar]
- He K., Zhang X., Ren S., Sun J. Deep Residual Learning for Image Recognition. arXiv. 20151512.03385 [Google Scholar]
- Hinton G.E., Osindero S., Teh Y.-W. A Fast Learning Algorithm for Deep Belief Nets. Neural Comput. 2006;18:1527–1554. doi: 10.1162/neco.2006.18.7.1527. [PubMed] [CrossRef] [Google Scholar]
- Jafari M.H., Girgis H., Liao Z., Behnami D., Abdi A., Vaseli H., Luong C., Rohling R., Gin K., Tsang T., et al. Proceedings of the Deep Learning in Medical Image Analysis and Multimodal Learning for Clinical Decision Support. Springer International Publishing; Granada, Spain: 2018. A Unified Framework Integrating Recurrent Fully-Convolutional Networks and Optical Flow for Segmentation of the Left Ventricle in Echocardiography Data; pp. 29–37. [Google Scholar]
- Kusunose K., Abe T., Haga A., Fukuda D., Yamada H., Harada M., Sata M. A Deep Learning Approach for Assessment of Regional Wall Motion Abnormality from Echocardiographic Images. JACC Cardiovasc. Imaging. 2020;13:374–381. doi: 10.1016/j.jcmg.2019.02.024. [PubMed] [CrossRef] [Google Scholar]
- Labs R.B., Vrettos A., Azarmehr N., Howard J.P., Shun-shin M.J., Cole G.D., Francis D.P., Zolgharni M. Automated Assessment of Image Quality in 2D Echocardiography Using Deep Learning; Proceedings of the International Conference on Radiology, Medical Imaging and Radiation Oncology; Paris, France. 25–26 June 2020. [Google Scholar]
- Leclerc S., Smistad E., Pedrosa J., Ostvik A. Cardiac Acquisitions for Multi-Structure Ultrasound Segmentation. [(accessed on 26 March 2021)]; Available online: https://camus.creatis.insa-lyon.fr/challenge/
- Li G., Yu Y. Visual Saliency Detection Based on Multiscale Deep CNN Features. IEEE Trans. Image Process. 2016;25:5012–5024. doi: 10.1109/TIP.2016.2602079. [PubMed] [CrossRef] [Google Scholar]
- Madani A., Arnaout R., Mofrad M., Arnaout R. Fast and accurate view classification of echocardiograms using deep learning. NPJ Digit. Med. 2018;1 doi: 10.1038/s41746-017-0013-1. [PMC free article] [PubMed] [CrossRef] [Google Scholar]
- Narula S., Shameer K., Salem Omar A.M., Dudley J.T., Sengupta P.P. Machine-Learning Algorithms to Automate Morphological and Functional Assessments in 2D Echocardiography. J. Am. Coll. Cardiol. 2016;68:2287–2295. doi: 10.1016/j.jacc.2016.08.062. [PubMed] [CrossRef] [Google Scholar]
- Ouyang D. EchoNet-Dynamic. [(accessed on 26 March 2021)]; Available online: https://echonet.github.io/dynamic/
- Ouyang D., He B., Ghorbani A., Yuan N., Ebinger J., Langlotz C.P., Heidenreich P.A., Harrington R.A., Liang D.H., Ashley E.A., et al. Video-based AI for beat-to-beat assessment of cardiac function. Nature. 2020;580:252–256. doi: 10.1038/s41586-020-2145-8. [PMC free article]
- Philbrick K.A., Yoshida K., Inoue D., Akkus Z., Kline T.L., Weston A.D., Korfiatis P., Takahashi N., Erickson B.J. What Does Deep Learning See? Insights from a Classifier Trained to Predict Contrast Enhancement Phase from CT Images. AJR Am. J. Roentgenol. 2018;211:1184–1193. doi: 10.2214/AJR.18.20331. [PubMed] [CrossRef] [Google Scholar]
- Ronneberger O., Fischer P., Brox T. U-Net: Convolutional Networks for Biomedical Image Segmentation. In: Navab N., Hornegger J., Wells W.M., Frangi A.F., editors. Medical Image Computing and Computer-Assisted Intervention–MICCAI 2015. Volume 9351. Springer International Publishing; Munich, Germany: 2015. pp. 234–241. Lecture Notes in Computer Science. [Google Scholar]
- Simonyan K., Zisserman A. Very Deep Convolutional Networks for Large-Scale Image Recognition. arXiv. 20141409.1556 [Google Scholar]
- Springenberg J.T., Dosovitskiy A., Brox T., Riedmiller M. Striving for Simplicity: The All Convolutional Net. arXiv. 20141412.6806
- Szegedy C., Ioffe S., Vanhoucke V., Alemi A.A. Inception-v4, inception-resnet and the impact of residual connections on learning; Proceedings of the Thirty-First AAAI Conference on Artificial Intelligence; San Francisco, CA, USA. 4–6 February 2017. [Google Scholar]
- Szegedy C., Vanhoucke V., Ioffe S., Shlens J., Wojna Z. Rethinking the inception architecture for computer vision; Proceedings of the IEEE Conference on Computer Vision and Pattern Recognition; Las Vegas, NV, USA. 27–30 June 2016; pp. 2818–2826. [Google Scholar]
- Vincent P., Larochelle H., Lajoie I., Bengio Y., Manzagol P.-A. Stacked Denoising Autoencoders: Learning Useful Representations in a Deep Network with a Local Denoising Criterion. J. Mach. Learn. Res. 2010;11:3371–3408. [Google Scholar]
- Zamzmi G., Hsu L.-Y., Li W., Sachdev V., Antani S. Harnessing Machine Intelligence in Automatic Echocardiogram Analysis: Current Status, Limitations, and Future Directions. IEEE Rev. Biomed. Eng. 2020 doi: 10.1109/RBME.2020.2988295. [PMC free article] [PubMed] [CrossRef]

CHAPTER 25

AI Empowered Diagnosis Of Epicardial ,Pericardial Fat And Pericardial effusion. A- Review

The compartments of adipose tissue surrounding the heart are metabolically active organs. In recent years, a relationship has been demonstrated between epicardial adipose tissue (EAT) and heart diseases including coronary artery disease, heart failure with preserved ejection fraction, and atrial fibrillation Obesity could cause unbalanced adipogenesis in EAT resulting in secretion of proinflammatory cytokines. Furthermore, the paracrine activity of the adipose tissue seems to be affected by other changes of hormonal status such as diabetes mellitus or menopause

The metabolic syndrome (MetS) comprised of obesity, hyperglycemia, hypertension and atherogenic dyslipidemia, can lead to proinflammatory state and is a risk factor for cardiovascular diseases. Moreover, the accumulation of visceral adipose tissue associated with MetS, non-alcoholic fatty liver disease (NAFLD) and EAT has been advocated as biomarker of cardiometabolic risk.

Computed tomography (CT) and magnetic resonance imaging (MRI) allow for non-invasive quantification of adipose tissue depots, including pericardial fat. However, quantification of pericardial adipose tissue depots is rarely performed outside research setting. Indeed, while CT is in the literature the most validated and reproducible technique for fat quantification, given the higher spatial resolution compared to MRI, many practical challenges remain.When quantification is performed, manual segmentation of epicardial fat volume (EFV) quantification is today the method of choice. Nevertheless, this approach requires a laborious stepwise manual segmentation of relevant anatomical structures, being therefore operator-dependent and time-consuming, not suitable for routine clinical practice .Therefore, development of computer-assisted tools aimed at tissue segmentation and quantification is of paramount importance to improve consistency of results and reduce processing times .

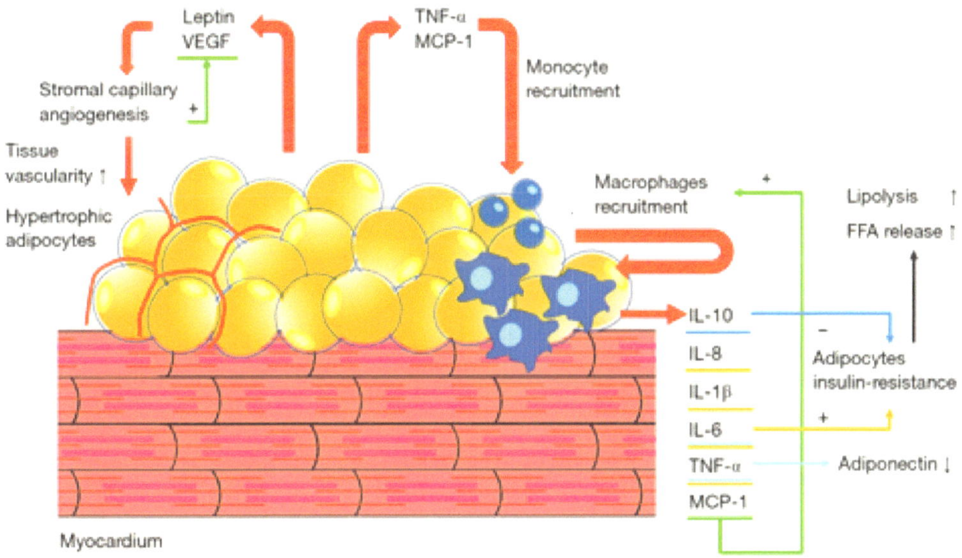

Fig.25.1 Pathophysiology of hypertrophic epicardial adipocytes. In obese subjects, triglycerides accumulation in adipocytes makes them hypertrophic. This result in a cellular and molecular inflammatory cascade with both positive and negative feedbacks involving VEGF and MCP-1. The mechanism determines macrophages accumulation with release of cytokines and relative local insulin-resistance with acceleration of lipolysis and release of FFA and reduction of adiponectin levels, and the increase in vascularization due to the increase in leptin and VEGF. VEGF, vascular endothelial growth factor; TNF-α, tumor necrosis factor α; MCP-1, monocyte chemoattractant protein-1; IL-10, interleukin-10; IL-8, interleukin-8; IL-1β, interleukin-1β; IL-6, interleukin-6; FFA, free fatty acids.

In this context, artificial intelligence (AI) solutions, including machine learning and deep learning, has been recently proposed as solution to obtain fast, automatic, and reliable measures of abdominal adipose tissue on CT and MRI.

Machine learning is a group of techniques allowing to extrapolate or classify models through computer learning. These algorithms have the potential to offer robust and feasible solutions to quantify adipose tissue compartments of the human body, including epicardial and pericardial fat, possibly enhancing, in an opportunistic fashion, the value of images acquired for other purposes.

The present literature review will be focused on AI supervised methods for epicardial and pericardial fat analysis using CT Images. Neither other imaging modalities (such as ultrasound or MRI) nor other adipose tissue compartments (such as paracardial adipose tissue) will be addressed in detail.

The aim of this chapter is to provide an overview of the available evidence on AI algorithms proposed for the segmentation and quantification of epicardial and pericardial adipose tissues on CT images.

Anatomy and physiology

The adipose tissue surrounding the heart is divided into several compartments. EAT is the adipose tissue localized between the myocardium and the visceral layer of the pericardium. The contiguity between epicardial fat and myocardium is an important anatomical feature, given the epicardial tissue distinct properties. Within the EAT there is the pericoronary adipose tissue (PCAT), consisting of adipose tissue located in a radial distance to the external wall of the vessel equal to the diameter of the coronary vessel . PCAT is contiguous with the adventitial layer in large vessels, while adipocytes are present in vascular wall of small vessels and microvessels . The pericardial adipose tissue is located outside the EAT. It is lined internally by the visceral layer (located between the EAT and the pericardial adipose tissue) and externally by the parietal layer, located between the pericardial adipose tissue and the paracardial adipose tissue. Hence, from the inner to the outer layer this anatomy can be summarized with the following scheme: ((((((heart) perivascular adipose tissue) EAT) [pericardial adipose tissue = PCAT + EAT + pericardial adipose tissue] pericardial sac) paracardial adipose tissue) mediastinum).EAT covers 80% of cardiac surface, with a greater concentration in the atrioventricular sulci, interventricular sulci and around the epicardial coronary arteries . Epicardial adipocytes are smaller in size than adipocytes of the subcutaneous and visceral adipose tissue. EAT also contains immune, stromal, inflammatory, nodal, and nerve tissue cells. There are several known physiological functions of EAT related to cardiac physiology. It holds a protective function for the heart and a support for the coronary arteries against the torsion caused by the arterial pulse and cardiac contraction . Moreover, EAT derives from the same (splanchnopleuric) mesoderm as brown adipose tissue and omental fat cells.It is also a barrier against pathogens through immune activity, protects against

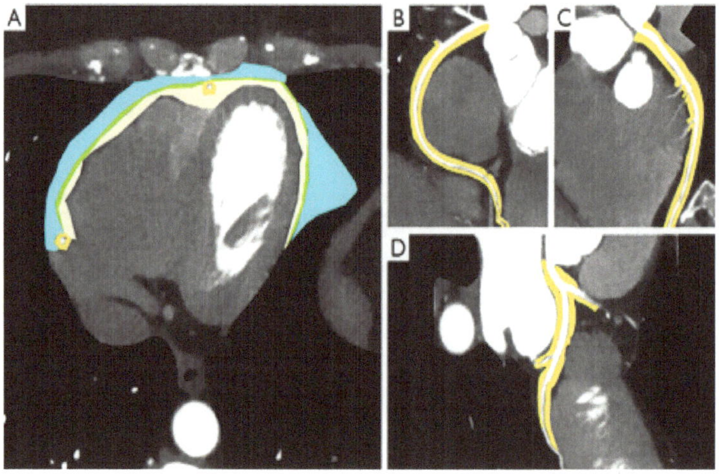

Fig.25.2 Coronary CT on axial plane (A) shows regions of interest (ROIs) of PCAT (light orange ROI), EAT (light yellow ROI), pericardial adipose tissue (green ROI) and paracardial adipose tissue (light blue ROI). Curved plane reconstructions of right coronary artery (B), left anterior descending artery (C) and circumflex artery (D), with highlighted perivascular adipose tissue (light orange ROI). CT, computed tomography; PCAT, pericoronary adipose tissue; EAT, epicardial adipose tissue

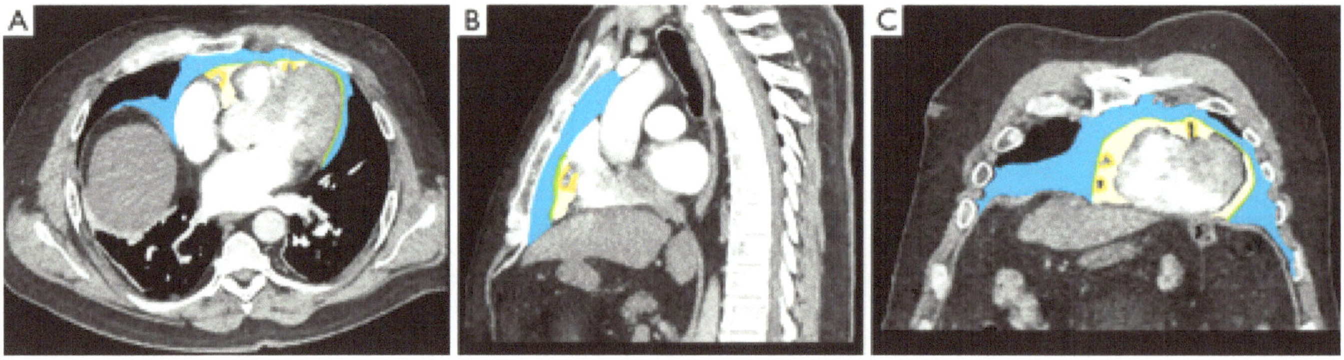

Fig.25.3 Thoracic CT on axial (A), sagittal (B) and coronal (C) planes. See regions of interest (ROIs) of PCAT (light orange ROI), EAT (light yellow ROI), pericardial adipose tissue (green ROI) and paracardial adipose tissue (light blue ROI). CT, computed tomography; PCAT, pericoronary adipose tissue; EAT, epicardial adipose tissue.

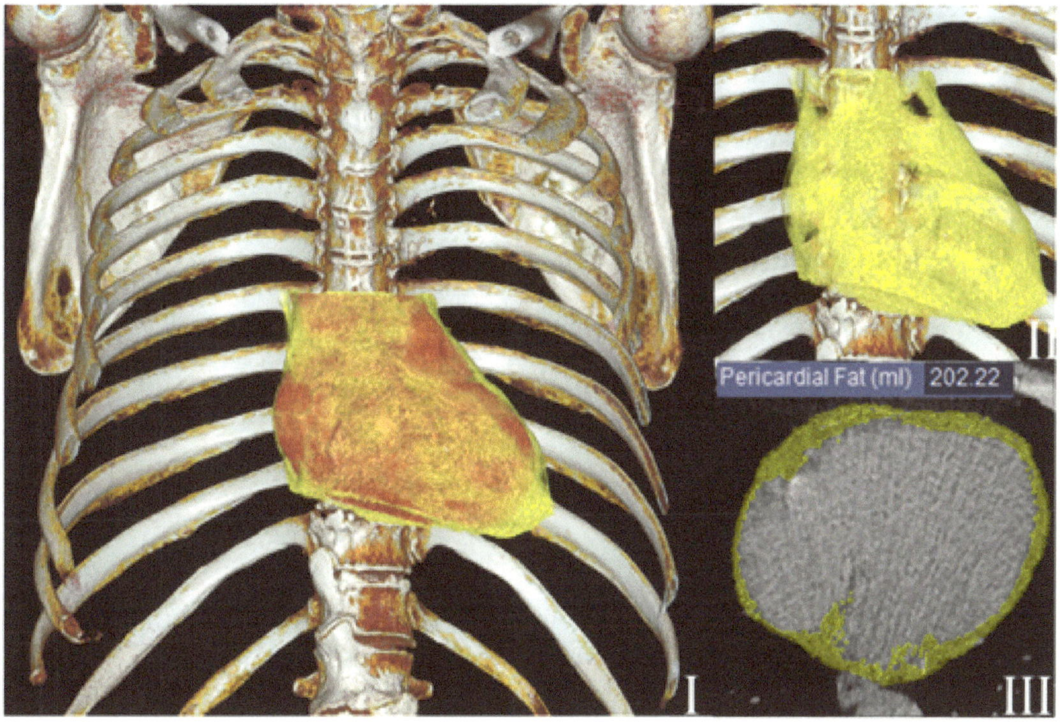

Fig.25.4 Schematic diagram of epicardial adipose tissue. Two 3D volume rendering images (I and II) and an axial CT image (III) show the heart (red color) and epicardial adipose tissue (yellow)

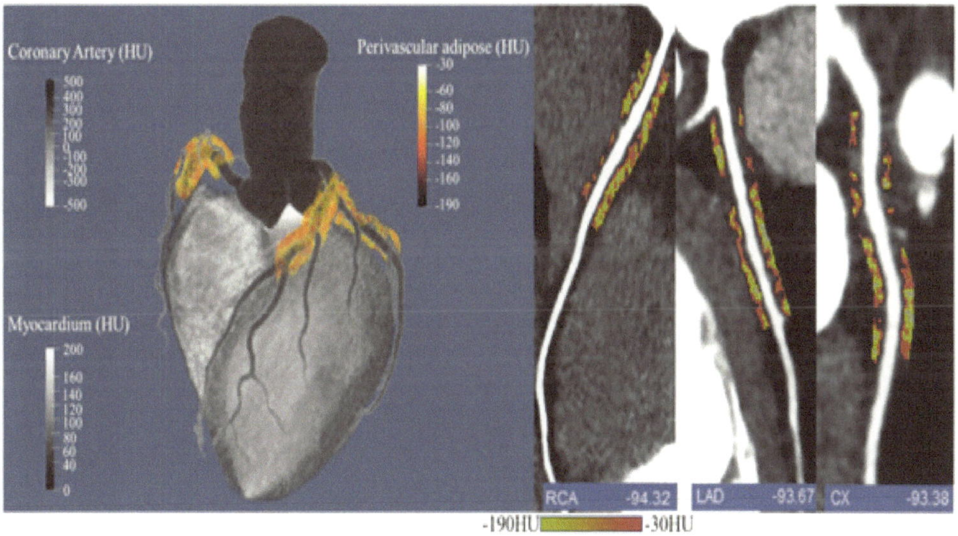

Fig.25.5 Schematic diagram of pericoronary adipose tissue and FAI. (left) 3D volume rendering image of pericoronary adipose tissue (orange color); (right) the numbers in the lower right corner represent the values of fat attenuation index. RCA = right coronary artery; LAD = left anterior descending artery; CX = circumflex artery; HU = Hounsfield unit

hypothermia thanks to the activity of adipocytes that have brown or beige characteristics, adipocytes typically involved in thermogenesis, and regulates the energy supply to the myocardium through lipolytic and lipogenic activities. Furthermore, it is now known that EAT is an endocrine organ having a unique secrotome. In fact, it exerts a paracrine and vasocrine activity on the myocardium and coronary arteries through the release of adipokines with vasodilator, antioxidant, antifibrotic and anti-inflammatory activities .Indeed, EAT and pericardial adipose tissue correlate with several markers of oxidative stress, inflammation, and vascular dysfunction, underlining the importance of pericardial adipose tissue segmentation in addition to the other compartments.Taken together, these arguments underline that adipose tissue surrounding the heart is of anatomical and physiological paramount importance.

Clinical applications of machine learning in EAT

EAT plays an important role in the development of CVD through pathophysiological mechanisms (Mazurek et al. 2003; Cheng et al. 2008). Evidence suggests that abundant EAT is a predictor of adverse cardiovascular events (Mahabadi et al. 2013; Goeller et al. 2018). Since machine learning algorithms can maximize the data mining of image features and clinical factors, researchers have used them to analyze EAT. In a prospective study, Commandeur et al. developed a machine learning-derived risk score based on the extreme gradient boosting (XGBoost) algorithm, which combined clinical risk factors with the coronary artery calcium (CAC) score and automatically quantified EAT to predict the long-term risk of myocardial infarction (MI) and cardiac death (Commandeur et al. 2020). The machine learning-derived risk score (AUC = 0.82) performed better than the risk factors for atherosclerotic CVD (AUC = 0.77) and CAC score (AUC = 0.77). Otaki et al. applied the same algorithm (XGBoost) and found that the epicardial fat volume was an independent predictor of impaired myocardial flow reserve (Otaki et al. 2015). Compared with the CAC score (AUC = 0.66) and epicardial fat volume (AUC = 0.67), the AUC of the combined risk score integrating the CAC score and epicardial fat volume was 0.73, which improved the prediction ability of impaired myocardial flow reserve. In general, the existing evidence suggests that EAT, with the support of machine learning, can improve the diagnosis and prognostic prediction of CVD.

Clinical applications of machine learning in PCAT

PCAT is the adipose tissue enveloping the coronary artery, which involves the evolution of atherosclerosis (Dey et al. 2010). The pericoronary fat attenuation index (FAI) is a novel imaging biomarker that maps the spatial changes in PCAT attenuation in CCTA images. The FAI has been used to identify subclinical coronary artery disease (Antonopoulos et al. 2017) and improve the risk prediction of all-cause cardiac mortality (Oikonomou et al. 2018). In addition to the FAI that simply represents the CT value, radiomics can mine the high-throughput quantitative information of the PCAT. Oikonomou et al. reported that the radiomics signature of the PCAT was associated with the fibrosis and vascularity of the PCAT, and the PCAT represented the adipose tissue remodelling caused by coronary inflammation (Oikonomou et al. 2019). In addition, they proposed a random forest method to analyze 1391 radiomic features of the PCAT extracted from 101 patients who had major adverse cardiac events (MACEs) within 5 years after undergoing CCTA and 101 matched controls. Their machine learning-based model performed better than the existing clinical risk factor model (Δ[C-statistic] = 0.126, $p < 0.001$) in predicting the outcome of MACEs. Lin et al. explored the ability of the radiomics signature of the PCAT in CCTA images to discriminate patients with MI from those with stable or no coronary artery disease (Lin et al. 2020). Using an XGBoost that combined clinical factors, PCAT attenuation, and radiomics features, their method significantly improved the discrimination ability of acute MI (AUC = 0.87) compared with a model with clinical factors and PCAT attenuation (AUC = 0.77) or clinical factors alone (AUC = 0.76). In brief, the implementation of machine learning can maximize the information extracted from PCAT and play an important role in the diagnosis and risk prediction of coronary artery disease.

Multi-modal imaging of cardiac adipose tissue

Multiple types of equipment can be used to evaluate EAT, including CT, CMR, and echocardiography. CT offers volumetric visualization and quantification of cardiac adipose tissue with high spatial resolution. However, CT has the disadvantage of unavoidable radiation exposure. CMR is considered to be the best imaging method for adipose tissue because of its superb fat signal display (Wong et al. 2017). According to the results of Mahajan et al., there was a significant correlation between CMR and autopsy for measuring the mass of adipose tissue with an intraclass correlation coefficient > 0.8 (Mahajan et al. 2013). The main disadvantages of CMR are its limited availability and high costs. Echocardiography is widely used, but the image quality is poor and not conducive to quantitative analysis. The quantification of EAT by echocardiography was limited to the thickness of adipose tissue on the right ventricular free wall (related to EAT thickness on CMR: R = 0.905) (Iacobellis et al. 2003; Gaborit et al. 2017).

Compared with the CT widely used in EAT analysis, research based on echocardiography and CMR is limited. In the included studies, only one used deep learning to segment EAT in CMR images with a low DSC of 0.56. More studies are expected to investigate EAT using AI and multi-modal imaging.

AI-derived epicardial fat measurements improve cardiovascular risk prediction from myocardial perfusion imaging

Epicardial adipose tissue (EAT) volume and attenuation are associated with cardiovascular risk, but manual annotation is time-consuming. We evaluated whether automated deep learning-based EAT measurements from ungated computed tomography (CT) are associated with death or myocardial infarction (MI). We included 8781 patients from 4 sites without known coronary artery disease who underwent hybrid myocardial perfusion imaging. Of those, 500 patients from one site were used for model training and validation, with the remaining patients held out for testing (n = 3511 internal testing, n = 4770 external testing).We modified an existing deep learning model to first identify the cardiac silhouette, then automatically segment EAT based on attenuation thresholds. Deep learning EAT measurements were obtained in <2 s compared to 15 min for expert annotations

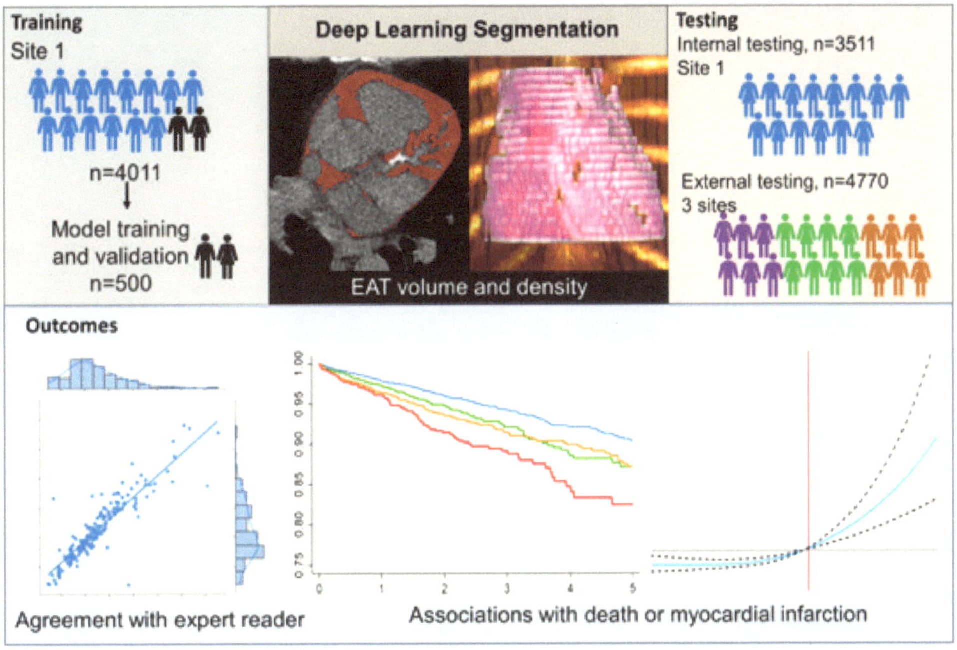

Fig.25.6: Overview of study design The deep learning model for epicardial adipose tissue (EAT) segmentation was trained and then tested in internal and external testing populations. Outcomes included agreement with expert reader segmentation and associations with death or myocardial infarction (MI).

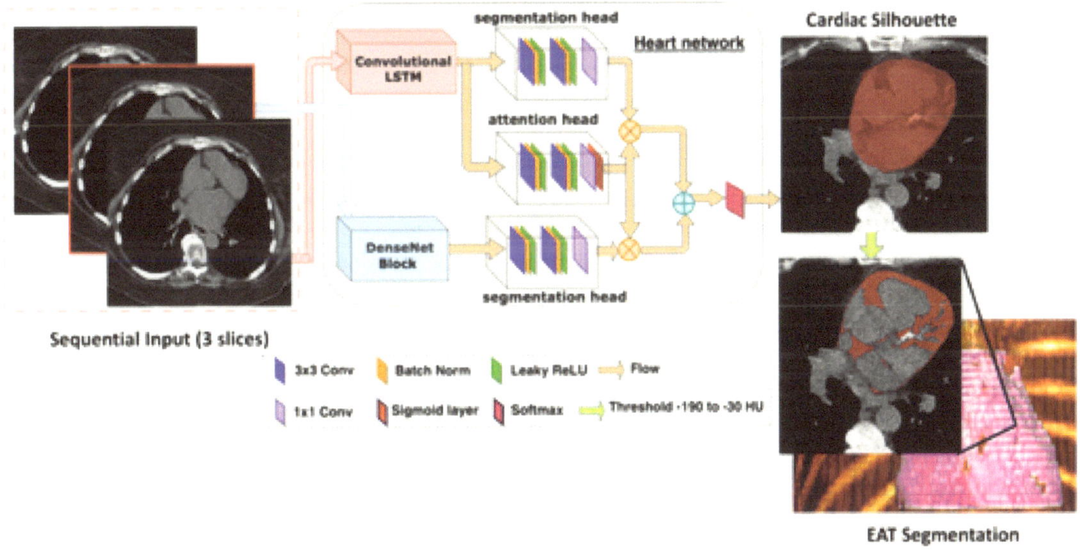

Fig.25.7: Overview of deep learning model architecture.A convolutional long short-term memory (LSTM) model is used to generate a cardiac silhouette mask. Attenuation thresholds are then applied to the mask to automatically segment epicardial adipose tissue (EAT).

There was excellent agreement between EAT attenuation (Spearman correlation 0.90 internal, 0.82 external) and volume (Spearman correlation 0.90 internal, 0.91 external) by deep learning and expert segmentation in all 3 sites (Spearman correlation 0.90–0.98). During median follow-up of 2.7 years (IQR 1.6–4.9), 565 patients experienced death or MI. Elevated EAT volume and attenuation were independently associated with an increased risk of death or MI after adjustment for relevant confounders. Deep learning can automatically measure EAT volume and attenuation from low-dose, ungated CT with excellent correlation with expert annotations, but in a fraction of the time. EAT measurements offer additional prognostic insights within the context of hybrid perfusion imaging.

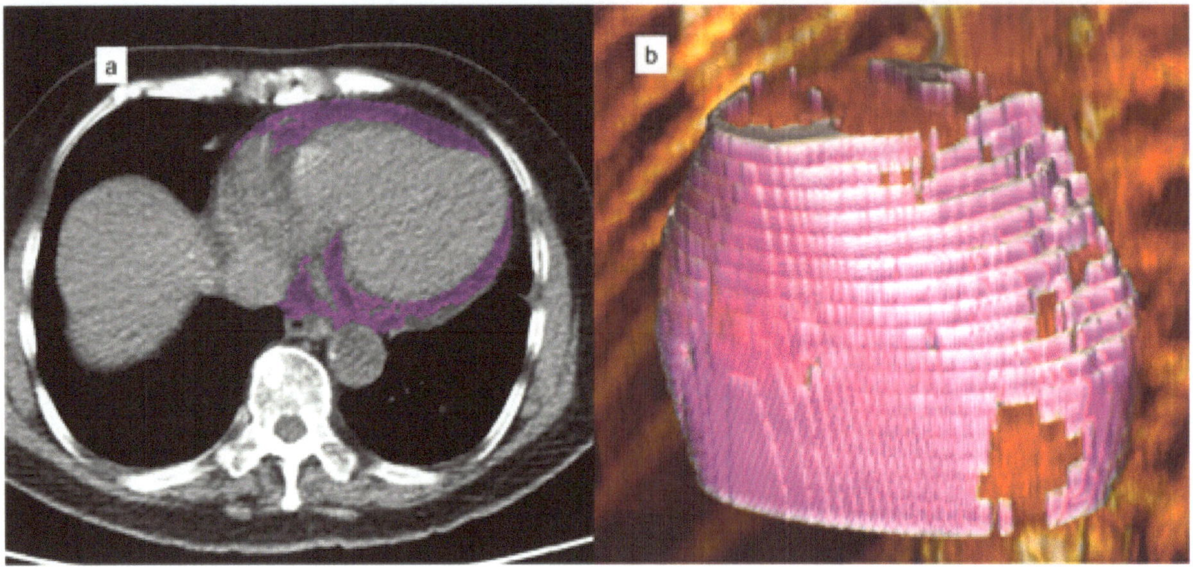

Fig.25.8 Example of EAT segmentation The deep learning model segments epicardial adipose tissue (EAT) for each slice, shown in purple (a). The combined three-dimensional volume is used to quantify EAT volume (b). The patient was a 70-year-old woman with body mass index of 21.5 kg/m2, but EAT volume was elevated at 209 mL. The patient died 425 days after the scan.

Comparison of manual and DL-based EAT measurements

Manual EAT measurements took a mean time of 15 min. DL EAT measurements took a mean time <2 s. The per-pixel EAT attenuation values for one patient are shown in Supplementary Fig. 1. A subset of patients from the testing population underwent both manual and DL-based EAT measurements in each site (internal n = 256, external n = 382). Figure 4 shows the correlation between median EAT attenuation measurements for internal (Spearman correlation 0.90) and external testing (Spearman correlation 0.82). Similarly, the correlation for EAT volume was excellent in internal (Spearman correlation 0.90) and external testing (Spearman correlation 0.91). Bland-Altman plots (Supplementary Fig. 1) demonstrate that the agreement between DL and an expert reader was comparable to the agreement between two expert readers. Two case examples of EAT annotation by DL .

Discussion

We evaluated a DL model which measures EAT attenuation and volume from low-dose, ungated CT. We showed that the DL model had an excellent correlation with expert segmentation, demonstrating similar agreement as was seen between two experts, but in a fraction of the time. We went on to demonstrate that patients with higher EAT volume or higher EAT attenuation were more likely to experience death or MI during follow-up. Importantly, we also demonstrated that the increase in risk was independent of other imaging findings including perfusion, LVEF and CAC in large internal and external testing populations.

EAT has primarily been quantified from ECG-gated cardiac CT. The gating minimizes cardiac motion, simplifying the task of segmenting EAT. EAT thickness (measured by echocardiography) varies through the cardiac cycle21, with some authors suggesting that measurements should be averaged across three points in the cardiac cycle22. Grodecki et al. demonstrated that DL could quantify EAT from ungated chest CT images in patients with COVID-19 infection.

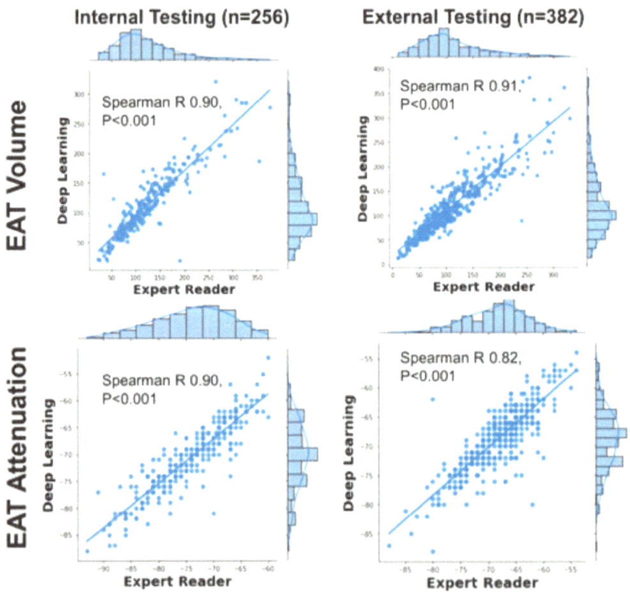

Fig.25.9 Correlation between experts and deep learning.Epicardial adipose tissue (EAT) attenuation and volume measurements are shown for deep learning and expert interpreters.

Similar to our results, they found that both higher EAT volume and attenuation were associated with increased risk. In the present work, we demonstrate that EAT can be automatically segmented by DL from ungated CT for hybrid MPI, which are acquired with lower radiation doses and subsequently lower image quality compared to standard ungated chest CT. The DL EAT measurements had an excellent correlation with expert EAT annotations for both volume and median attenuation. However, the DL annotations were automatically generated within a few seconds compared to approximately 15 minutes for expert annotations. This rapid and accurate quantification can facilitate routine evaluation within a typical clinical workflow. We also expand on existing studies by demonstrating that EAT volume and attenuation carry prognostic significance in patients undergoing MPI. Importantly, this allowed us to evaluate the independent association of EAT with death or MI after accounting for age, sex, and medical history as well as imaging parameters including myocardial perfusion, ventricular function, and CAC.

The independent prognostic utility of EAT attenuation was expected based on the hypothesized relationships between EAT and CAD. EAT interacts with the heart through local paracrine effects and inflammatory signaling3. Higher EAT attenuation values may be a marker of coronary inflammation24. In fact, peri-coronary adipose tissue (which is a component of EAT) attenuation is positively correlated with sodium fluoride uptake25, which is a measure of microcalcification that reflects atherosclerotic plaque activity26. Additionally, while CAD may lead to inflammatory changes within EAT, EAT inflammation also accelerates atherosclerosis in adjacent coronary arteries27. Therefore, measurement of EAT attenuation allows physicians to capture relevant information regarding cardiac inflammatory state which previously could not be evaluated with MPI.

We also anticipated that higher EAT volume would be associated with increased cardiovascular risk. Prior studies have shown that visceral fat is superior to BMI and waist circumference for predicting cardiovascular risk28. EAT volume is correlated with BMI and waist circumference;28 however, EAT volume is a direct measure of visceral adipose tissue. In fact, in an analysis of the multi-ethnic study of atherosclerosis, EAT volume, but not BMI, was predictive of future coronary atherosclerosis.. In our study, while patients with elevated BMI were more likely to have high EAT volume, we found that almost one-third of patients with elevated EAT volume had a BMI < 30 kg/m2. Lastly, it is worth noting that a small study have suggested that dapagliflozin may decrease EAT volum,, suggesting a possible therapeutic intervention for patients with elevated EAT volume. Therefore, the measurement of EAT volume potentially provides physicians with prognostic and therapeutic information to consider following MPI.

Our study has a few important limitations in addition to its retrospective nature. We only utilized ungated CT scans and therefore EAT values may differ from those obtained from gated chest CT. However, this is representative of

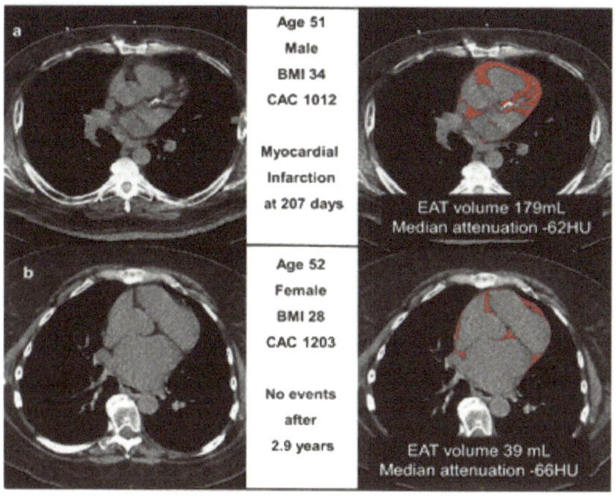

Fig. 25.10 (a) 51-year-old man with a body mass index (BMI) of 34, coronary artery calcium 1012, and normal perfusion. Epicardial adipose tissue (EAT) volume (red overlay) was 179 mL and median attenuation −62 (both high risk). He experienced a myocardial infarction 207 days after the scan. (b) 52-year-old woman with BMI 28, CAC 1203, and abnormal perfusion. Her EAT volume (red overlay) was 39 mL and median attenuation was -66 (both low risk). She was managed medically and did not experience death or myocardial infarction during 2.9 years of follow-up.

the CT scans typically used for attenuation correction. We used set thresholds for EAT segmentation. It is possible that the thresholds should vary according to acquisition protocol. Different thresholds would influence both EAT volume and median attenuation values. As a result, optimal cutoffs for EAT volume and attenuation may vary by protocol and may vary by sex. However, in our study the thresholds for abnormal cutoffs were established within the internal testing site, then applied to the external site which has a different acquisition protocol, suggesting that the thresholds are still generalizable. The model was trained in a random selection of patients with and without known CAD. However, patients with known CAD were excluded from the internal and external testing populations (since this can influence the association between MPI findings and outcomes). Future studies should evaluate the prognostic of EAT measurements in these patients. Additionally, cardiovascular mortality was not available in the registry, but existing methods for identifying cardiovascular mortality have limited accuracy30. However, we would expect even stronger associations if we were able to ascertain cardiovascular mortality since EAT is pathophysiologically related to cardiovascular outcomes. Similarly, we do not have information regarding inflammatory markers or use of anti-inflammatory medications, so we are not able to evaluate these potential pathophysiologic links. Lastly, we do not have information regarding race or ethnicity in our cohort.

Our study demonstrates that deep learning can automatically measure EAT volume and attenuation from low-dose, ungated CT with excellent correlation with expert annotations, but in a fraction of the time. EAT measurements provide independent prognostic information regarding inflammation and metabolism which complement the functional and anatomic information available through hybrid perfusion imaging.

Development and validation of a deep learning pipeline to measure pericardial effusion in echocardiography

Pericardial effusion (PE) is a condition characterized by the accumulation of fluid within the pericardial space, which is typically diagnosed using transthoracic echocardiography. The buildup of fluid increases pressure within the pericardial sac, potentially leading to cardiac tamponade and decreased cardiac output. PE is a serious condition that requires timely intervention, making early detection and accurate measurement of the width of the effusion critical.

Echocardiography is considered the gold standard for the detection of PE due to its accessibility, portability, and ability to provide a comprehensive assessment of both anatomy and function . However, the presence and severity of PE can be uncertain, with mild effusion sometimes indicating pericardial fat rather than true effusion .Additionally, image quality can be compromised by factors such as breast tissue or obscuration from bone or lung. These challenges highlight the need for an accurate and reliable method for measuring PE that is not dependent on operator experience.

Artificial intelligence (AI) has been applied in various clinical settings to aid in the diagnosis of conditions based on echocardiograms, with considerable effort devoted to areas such as left ventricular function assessment, regional wall motion abnormality, right ventricular function, valvular heart disease, cardiomyopathy, and intracardiac mass .In particular, a study conducted in 2020 employed a deep learning model to detect PE in echocardiography and achieved an accuracy of 0.87–0.9 . In clinical practice, information on PE width and severity is crucial for initiating appropriate interventions. To the best of our knowledge, no study has yet analyzed the grading of PE using machine learning. Therefore, our study aimed to develop a deep learning model using echocardiography for PE detection and PE width measurement. Additionally, to facilitate the deployment of the deep learning model, we proposed an end-to-end guideline that can output detection results from raw ultrasound files.

Data collection

During the data collection process, we utilized the keyword "pericardial effusion" to search the Hybrid Picture Report System in EDH in order to gather a list of examination records. We obtained raw data from transthoracic echocardiography examinations with a diagnosis of pericardial effusion, These data were divided into training and validation datasets based on the respective examination dates.

Echocardiography

Images were gathered in a normal manner, with patients lying in the left lateral decubitus position. The ultrasound system (IE33, Philips Healthcare; S70, GE Healthcare; or SC2000, Siemens Healthineers) was used to perform echocardiographic examinations in EDH Data from CGMH for external validation were acquired using EPIC7 (Philips Healthcare), Vivid E9 (GE Healthcare), or SC2000 (Siemens Healthineers).

All examinations were saved in picture archiving and communication systems in the Digital Imaging and Communications in Medicine (DICOM) format. After extracting the raw DICOM files, we processed the image from each patient to select the proper echocardiography views for developing a deep learning pipeline. The selected views were the parasternal long-axis (PLAX), parasternal short-axis (PSAX), apical four-chamber (A4C), and subcostal (SC) views. Two cardiologists manually measured the thickest point of pericardial effusion during each cardiac cycle as ground truth for width of PE. We employed ImageJ, an open-source software platform specifically designed for the scientific analysis and processing of images, to label and annotate the segmented masks corresponding to the echocardiography images. Upon completing the labeling process, the data was subsequently stored as CSV files on a secure, encrypted hard drive to ensure data integrity and confidentiality.

Deep learning model development

we developed an end-to-end pipeline for the automated measurement of PE based on the steps outlined below.The training subset of videos from EDH was used for the three main tasks of our pipeline

Step one: moving window view selection (MWVS)

We proposed a pipeline for managing echocardiography files directly from the workstation, similar to the work done by Zhang et al. and Huang et al., with some adjustments To distinguish the four primary views (PLAX, PSAX, A4C, and SC) from other views during each examination, we developed the first deep neural network model. This model was a ResNet-50-based two-dimensional model that aimed to classify each frame from the extracted DICOM files of echocardiography into the selected view types. To train this model, we randomly selected 6,434 images from the training dataset of EDH and labeled them according to the four primary views or other views, including low-quality views. We trained the model with a data split of 80% for the training set and 20% for the validation set. The model weight with the best detection performance in the validation set during the training process was preserved. The detection accuracy was assessed for each view class and weighted average result.In order to effectively manage the input video from patients during data collection, a 48-frame moving window was utilized to filter all videos. For each video, the best 48 frames with regard to specific view type and image quality were selected using a majority voting method .This process, known as MWVS concept, served not only as a view classifier but also as a quality control measure. Videos that did not contain at least 48 consecutive frames that met the image quality criteria of 50% or higher from one of the four primary views were excluded from further analysis. Additionally, the average view-classifying confidence levels for all images obtained from the selected 48-frame clip were used to evaluate the overall image quality and its correlation with performance. Videos with an average confidence level of less than 0.8 were also excluded from automated segmentation.

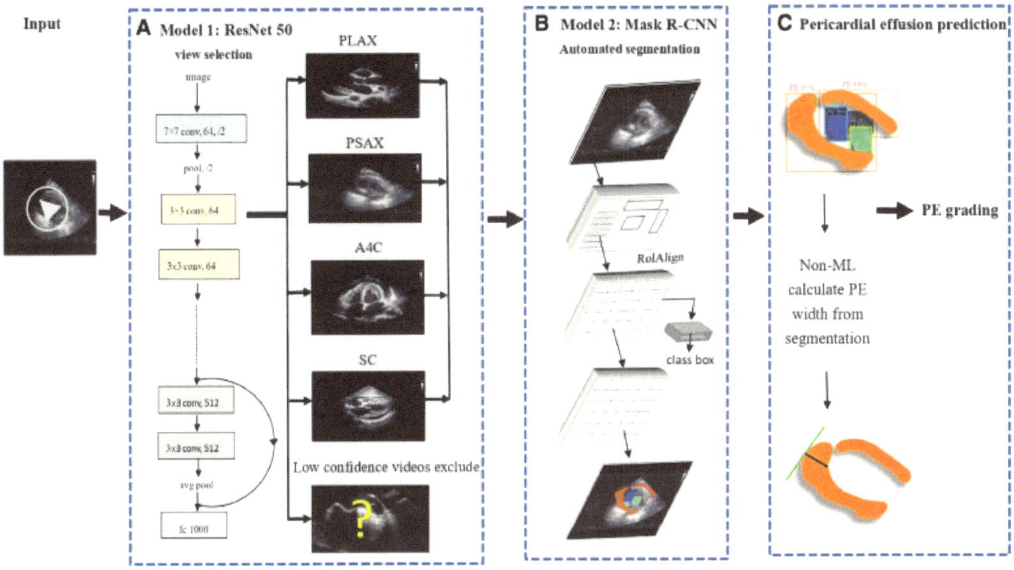

Fig. 25.11 End-to-end pipeline for the automated measurement of pericardial effusion.

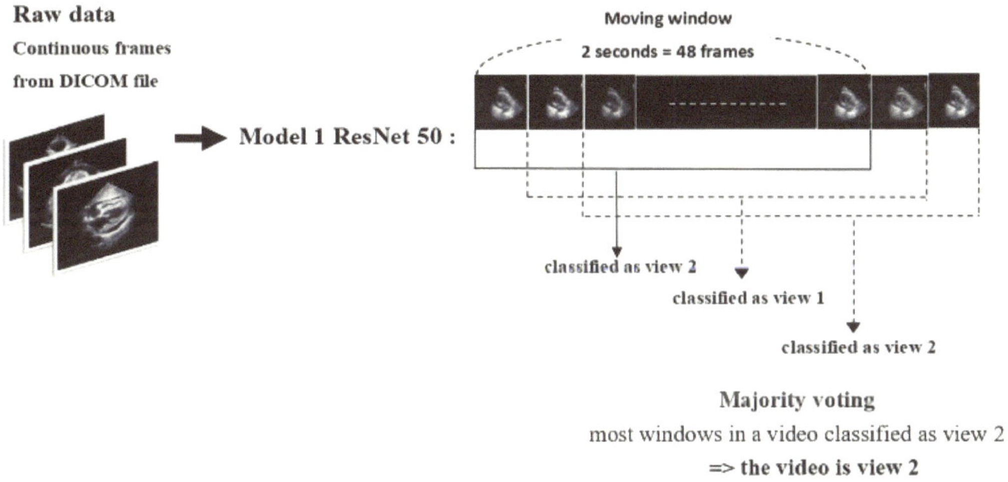

Fig. 25.12 Moving window view selection concept.

Step Two : Automated segmentation

From the dataset, we randomly selected and annotated 2,548 frames in the EDH training dataset, ensuring an even distribution across the four primary views. We manually labeled the segmented area for pericardial effusion (PE) at three different phases in the cardiac cycle: end-systolic, end-diastolic, and the middle phase between the two aforementioned phases. The differentiation between epicardial adipose tissue and pericardial fluid was established. During this labeling phase, experienced clinicians manually segmented the area of PE based on its characteristic appearances in ultrasound images, while explicitly excluding epicardial adipose tissue. Additionally, we labeled the segmented areas for the four cardiac chambers to enhance the model's performance in separating these fluid-containing areas.To train object instance segmentation based on the labeled ground truth, we utilized a Mask Region-Convolutional Neural Network (R-CNN) framework . The model was trained with a data split of 80% for the training set and 20% for the validation set. Mask R-CNN is commonly used in medical applications for instance segmentation tasks as it can simultaneously perform pixel-level segmentation and classification of multiple target lesions .The implemented model generates bounding boxes and targeting masks for each instance of an object in an image. The input comprised consecutive ultrasound frames, and the output was a segmented mask indicating the corresponding four cardiac chambers and PE. The accuracy of the segmentation model was assessed using the Dice coefficient metric.

Step Three : Measurement of pericardial effusion

After generating a segmented mask for pericardial effusion (PE), we proposed a computer vision technique, known as the maximal width calculator, to calculate the largest width of the PE in each ultrasound frame . To accomplish this, we iterated through the vertical axis in each frame and hypothetically drew a horizontal line to determine if there was an intersection between the segmented mask and the horizontal line. If an intersection existed, we obtained a normal line from the edge of the mask over the intersection point. The length of the normal line that passed through the segmented mask was counted as the width of the PE at that intersection point. The largest width of the PE obtained through the iteration over the vertical axis was regarded as the width of the PE of the frame. This technique was applied to all 48 frames in the ultrasound video to provide the optimal PE width

Discussion

In recent years, computer vision and deep learning techniques have been utilized to aid in the interpretation of echocardiography, estimate cardiac function, and identify local cardiac structures. Deep learning algorithms have also been applied to facilitate the diagnosis of PE. Nayak et al. developed a CNN that detected PE in the apical four-chamber (A4C) and short-axis (SC) views with accuracies of 91% and 87%, respectively..In this study, we propose a deep learning pipeline that can process raw DICOM files from ultrasound and predict the PE width in a clinical setting. This pipeline combines two deep learning models and one technical calculation algorithm to accurately predict PE width. There have been few efforts to predict PE existence, with some studies being based on computed tomography scans. To the best of our knowledge, this is the first video-based machine learning model to measure PE width using echocardiography. The correlation between the measurement of our model and human experts was high in both the internal and external validation datasets, with the best performance observed in the parasternal long-axis (PLAX) view. The inference speed of our model, using one graphics processing unit (NVIDIA RTX 3090), was approximately 30–40 s for one examination, which is usually faster than human assessment.The present study introduces two novel concepts for echocardiography analysis: the MWVS and the maximal width calculator of the segmented mask. These methods are particularly important for real-world applications, particularly when working with relatively smaller datasets

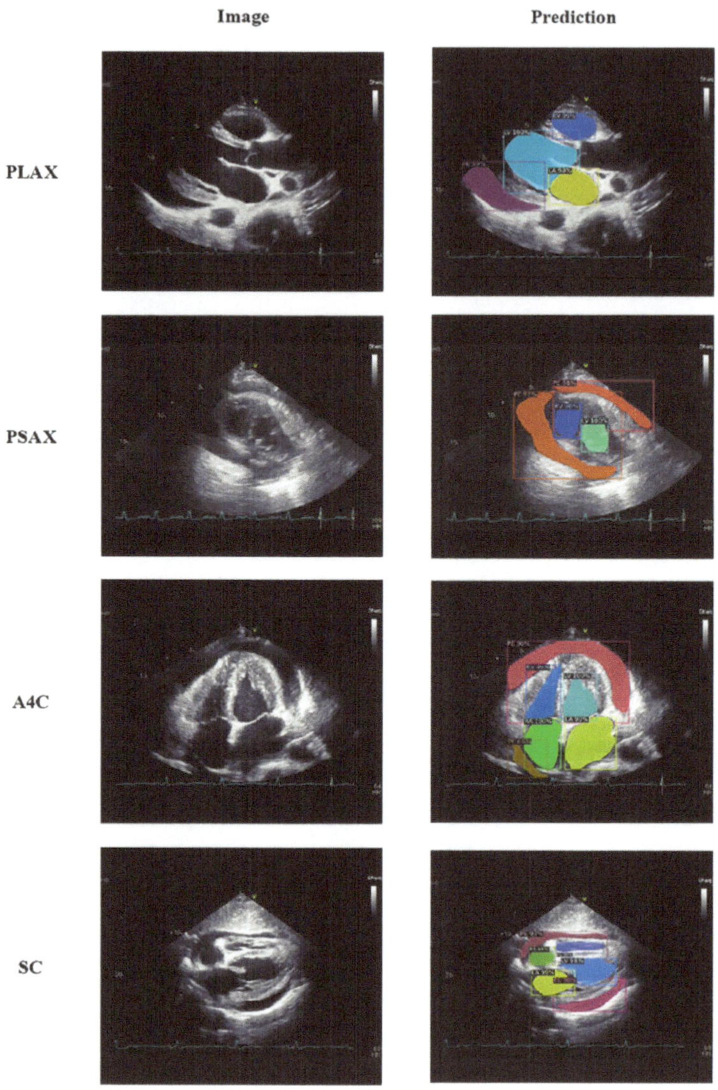

Fig. 25.13 Image segmentation over cardiac chambers and pericardial effusion.

Previous studies often rely on datasets manually selected by human experts during dataset cleaning, and use only "textbook-quality" images for training. In contrast, the present study proposes an analytical pipeline that can automatically analyze echocardiograms and be easily applied to personal devices or web applications, thus eliminating the need for expert sonographers or cardiologists. Madani et al. developed a CNN that simultaneously classified 15 standard echocardiogram views acquired under a range of real-world clinical variations, and the model demonstrated high accuracy for view classification. Similarly, this study used echocardiogram video clips obtained from the real world, taken for a variety of clinical purposes, including ejection fraction calculation, and detecting PE, valve disease, regional wall abnormality, cardiomyopathy, and pulmonary arterial hypertension.An initial screening model for view classification and quality control was developed.

All raw images from the medical image database were input into the screening model, leaving a specific view of sufficient quality for diagnosis. Additionally, the "moving window" concept was used to retrieve only clips with 48 consecutive frames that fulfilled the image quality criteria. By avoiding limited or idealized training datasets, it is believed that this model is broadly applicable to clinical practice.

The method of MWVS is a novel concept that has not yet been proposed in the field of echocardiography assisted by machine learning. MWVS serves as an image quality filter and plays a crucial role in ensuring that the images are of sufficient quality for the next step in the pipeline. In the EDH dataset, echocardiography is performed by well-trained technicians who adhere to a protocol established by the echocardiologist consensus committee. As such, the original images from EDH were of relatively homogeneous quality, and MWVS filtered out fewer patients. Conversely, at CGMH, echocardiography is performed by individual echocardiologists who may have varying techniques. As a result, the original images from CGMH were less homogeneous, and MWVS filtered out more patients. This finding highlights the significance of MWVS in maintaining image quality and highlights the importance of image homogeneity in the applicability of machine learning models.

After segmenting the PE area, we developed a novel computer vision-based technique to calculate the largest PE width in ultrasound video. The current categorization of PE size relies on linear measurements of the largest width of the effusion at end-diastole, and is graded as small (<1 cm), moderate (1–2 cm), or large (>2 cm. This semiquantitative classification method is prone to errors due to asymmetric, loculated effusions and shifts in fluid location during the cardiac cycle .Therefore, an automated calculation system could help identify the largest width of the PE in every ultrasound frame without any errors. In comparison to AI-based models, the computer vision technique is more similar to the method used by human experts. AI-based models not only consume more computing resources, but also require a large number of datasets for training and validation. To the best of our knowledge, our study is the first to not only detect but also classify the grade of PE.Our model's ability to automate the process of classifying PE severity, traditionally categorized as mild, moderate, or severe, signifies a meaningful advancement in this field. Although this may appear straightforward for experienced clinicians, automated segmentation and measurement can be invaluable, especially in contexts where echocardiography expertise may be limited or entirely absent. Importantly, even though our model does not currently provide prediction on hemodynamic instability such as cardiac tamponade, its ability to differentiate moderate to severe PE from none or mild is crucial.

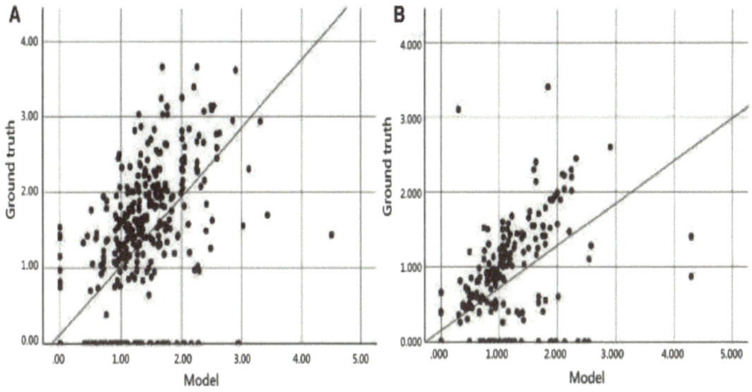

Fig. 25.14 Scatter plot of pericardial effusion width measurement between model and manual annotation.

This feature allows for early risk stratification in patients, prompting clinicians to initiate appropriate assessments and interventions as early as possible. Moreover, our work lays the groundwork for the future development of models designed to predict complex clinical scenarios, such as early hemodynamic instability. The integration of our model's segmentation and classification capabilities with other clinically relevant parameters may, in time, lead to major advancements in the prediction and management of such conditions.

This study had certain limitations that should be considered when interpreting the results. Firstly, the study was conducted retrospectively and the model was trained using data from only one hospital. This resulted in a limited sample size and a lack of ethnic diversity, which may impact the generalizability of the findings to other populations. To address this, future studies should utilize a multicenter design with greater heterogeneity in the dataset. However, it is important to note that the images used in this study were obtained using different ultrasonography machines and were interpreted by multiple echocardiographers, and the model achieved similar results during external validation. Secondly, while the proposed pipeline did grade the amount of PE, there was no information on whether there were signs of cardiac tamponade, as PE volume does not necessarily correlate with clinical symptoms (24). Additionally, due to the small sample size, we were unable to conduct subgroup analysis to distinguish the algorithm's performance on transudative vs. exudative effusions. To increase the clinical applicability of the findings, larger studies and validation cohorts are needed to reproduce the results of this study. Further research should also evaluate the collapsibility of the cardiac chambers and the presence of tamponade signs.

Conclusion

The machine-learning pipeline developed in this study can automatically calculate the width of PE from raw ultrasound clips. The novel concepts of moving window view selection for image quality control and computer vision techniques for maximal PE width calculation seem useful in the field of ultrasound. This pipeline could potentially provide a standardized and objective approach to the measurement of PE, reducing operator-dependency and improving accuracy.

Bibliography and Acknowledgement

- Aarthy D, Priya C, Sudha S (2019) Deep Learning for Quantification of Epicardial Fat from Non-Contrast CT. 2019 IEEE International Conference on Intelligent Techniques in Control, Optimization and Signal Processing (INCOS). https://doi.org/10.1109/INCOS45849.2019.8951387
- Abe I, Teshima Y, Kondo H, Kaku H, Kira S, Ikebe Y, Saito S, Fukui A, Shinohara T, Yufu K, Nakagawa M, Hijiya N, Moriyama M, Shimada T, Miyamoto S, Takahashi N (2018) Association of fibrotic remodeling and cytokines/chemokines content in epicardial adipose tissue with atrial myocardial fibrosis in patients with atrial fibrillation. Heart Rhythm 15(11):1717–1727. https://doi.org/10.1016/j.hrthm.2018.06.025
- Avanzo M, Wei L, Stancanello J, Vallières M, Rao A, Morin O, Mattonen SA, el Naqa I (2020) Machine and deep learning methods for radiomics. Med Phys 47(5):e185–e202. https://doi.org/10.1002/mp.13678
- Bambace C, Telesca M, Zoico E, Sepe A, Olioso D, Rossi A, Corzato F, Di Francesco V, Mazzucco A, Santini F, Zamboni M. Adiponectin gene expression and adipocyte diameter: a comparison between epicardial and subcutaneous adipose tissue in men. Cardiovasc Pathol 2011;20:e153-6. 10.1016/j.carpath.2010.07.005 [PubMed] [CrossRef] [Google Scholar]
- Ceriani E, Cogliati C. Update on bedside ultrasound diagnosis of pericardial effusion. Intern Emerg Med. (2016) 11:477–80. 10.1007/s11739-015-1372-8 [Abstract] [CrossRef] [Google Scholar]
- Chartrand G, Cheng PM, Vorontsov E, Drozdzal M, Turcotte S, Pal CJ, Kadoury S, Tang A (2017) Deep learning: a primer for radiologists. RadioGraphics37(7):2113–2131.https://doi.org/10.1148/rg.2017170077
- Chechi K, Richard D. Thermogenic potential and physiological relevance of human epicardial adipose tissue. Int J Obes Suppl 2015;5:S28-34. 10.1038/ijosup.2015.8 [PMC free article] [PubMed] [CrossRef] [Google Scholar]
- Cheng KH, Chu CS, Lee KT, Lin TH, Hsieh CC, Chiu CC, Voon WC, SheuSH,LaiWT(2008) Adipocytokines and proinflammatory mediators from abdominal and epicardial adipose tissue in patients with coronaryarterydisease.IntJObes32(2):268–274.https://doi.org/10.1038/sj.ijo.0803726
- Bengio Y. Learning deep architectures for AI. Foundations and Trends® in Machine Learning 2009;2:1-127.
- Betancur J, Commandeur F, Motlagh M, Sharir T, Einstein AJ, Bokhari S, Fish MB, Ruddy TD, Kaufmann P, Sinusas AJ, Miller EJ, Bateman TM, Dorbala S, di Carli M, Germano G, Otaki Y, Tamarappoo BK, Dey D, Berman DS, Slomka PJ (2018) Deep learning for prediction of obstructive disease from fast myocardial perfusion SPECT: a multicenter study. JACC Cardiovasc Imaging 11(11):1654–1663.
- Ceriani E, Cogliati C. Update on bedside ultrasound diagnosis of pericardial effusion. Intern Emerg Med. (2016) 11:477–80. 10.1007/s11739-015-1372-8 [Abstract] [CrossRef] [Google Scholar]
- Chartrand G, Cheng PM, Vorontsov E, Drozdzal M, Turcotte S, Pal CJ, Kadoury S, Tang A (2017) Deep learning: a primer for radiologists. RadioGraphics37(7):2113–2131. https://doi.org/10.1148/rg.2017170077
- Chechi K, Richard D. Thermogenic potential and physiological relevance of human epicardial adipose tissue. Int J Obes Suppl 2015;5:S28-34. 10.1038/ijosup.2015.8 [PMC free article] [PubMed]
- Cheng KH, Chu CS, Lee KT, Lin TH, Hsieh CC, Chiu CC, Voon WC, Sheu SH, Lai WT (2008) Adipocytokines and proinflammatory mediators from abdominal and epicardial adipose tissue in patients with coronary artery disease. Int J Obes 32(2):268–274. https://doi.org/10.1038/sj.ijo.0803726
- Choy G, Khalilzadeh O, Michalski M, Do S, Samir AE, Pianykh OS, Geis JR, Pandharipande PV, Brink JA, Dreyer KJ. Current Applications and Future Impact of Machine Learning in Radiology. Radiology 2018;288:318-28. 10.1148/radiol.2018171820 [PMC free article] [PubMed] [CrossRef] [Google Scholar]
- Commandeur F, Goeller M, Betancur J, Cadet S, Doris M, Chen X, Berman DS, Slomka PJ, Tamarappoo BK, Dey D. Deep Learning for Quantification of Epicardial and Thoracic Adipose Tissue From Non-Contrast CT. IEEE Trans Med Imaging 2018;37:1835-46. 10.1109/TMI.2018.2804799 [PMC free article] [PubMed] [CrossRef] [Google Scholar]
- Commandeur F, Goeller M, Betancur J, Cadet S, Doris M, Chen X, Berman DS, Slomka PJ, Tamarappoo BK, Dey D (2018) Deep learning for quantification of epicardial and thoracic adipose tissue from non-contrast CT. IEEE Trans Med Imaging 37(8):1835–1846. https://doi.org/10.1109/TMI.2018.2804799
- Commandeur F, Goeller M, Razipour A, Cadet S, Hell MM, Kwiecinski J, Chen X, Chang HJ, Marwan M, Achenbach S, Berman DS, Slomka PJ, Tamarappoo BK, Dey D. Fully Automated CT Quantification of Epicardial Adipose Tissue by Deep Learning: A Multicenter Study. Radiol Artif Intell 2019;1:e190045. 10.1148/ryai.2019190045 [PMC free article] [PubMed] [CrossRef] [Google Scholar]
- Commandeur F, Goeller M, Razipour A, Cadet S, Hell MM, Kwiecinski J, Chen X, Chang HJ, Marwan M, Achenbach S, Berman DS, Slomka PJ, Tamarappoo BK, Dey D (2019) Fully Automated CT Quantification of Epicardial Adipose Tissue by Deep Learning: A Multicenter Study. Radiol Artif Intell 1(6):e190045. https://doi.org/10.1148/ryai.2019190045
- Commandeur F, Slomka PJ, Goeller M, Chen X, Cadet S, Razipour A, McElhinney P, Gransar H, Cantu S, Miller RJH, Rozanski A, Achenbach S, Tamarappoo BK, Berman DS, Dey D (2020) Machine learning to predict the long-term risk of myocardial infarction and cardiac death based on clinical risk, coronary calcium, and epicardial adipose tissue: a prospective study. Cardiovasc Res 116(14):2216–2225. https://doi.org/10.1093/cvr/cvz321
- Dey D, Wong ND, Tamarappoo B, Nakazato R, Gransar H, Cheng VY, Ramesh A, Kakadiaris I, Germano G, Slomka PJ, Berman DS (2010) Computer-aided non-contrast CT-based quantification of pericardial and thoracic fat and their associations with coronary calcium and metabolic syndrome. Atherosclerosis 209(1):136–141. https://doi.org/10.1016/j.atherosclerosis.2009.08.032
- Eckel RH, Grundy SM, Zimmet PZ. The metabolic syndrome. Lancet 2005;365:1415-28. 10.1016/S0140-6736(05)66378-7 [PubMed] [CrossRef] [Google Scholar]
- Eisenberg E, McElhinney PA, Commandeur F, Chen X, Cadet S, Goeller M, Razipour A, Gransar H, Cantu S, Miller RJH, Slomka PJ, Wong ND, Rozanski A, Achenbach S, Tamarappoo BK, Berman DS, Dey D. Deep Learning-Based Quantification of Epicardial Adipose Tissue Volume and Attenuation Predicts Major Adverse Cardiovascular Events in Asymptomatic Subjects. Circ Cardiovasc Imaging 2020;13:e009829. 10.1161/CIRCIMAGING.119.009829 [
- El Khoudary SR, Shields KJ, Janssen I, Budoff MJ, Everson-Rose SA, Powell LH, Matthews KA. Postmenopausal Women With Greater Paracardial Fat Have More Coronary Artery Calcification Than Premenopausal Women: The Study of Women's Health Across the Nation (SWAN) Cardiovascular Fat Ancillary Study. J Am Heart Assoc 2017;6:004545. 10.1161/JAHA.116.004545 [PMC free article]
- Fulton MR, Givan AH, Fernandez-del-Valle M, Klingensmith JD (2020) Segmentation of epicardial adipose tissue in cardiac MRI using deep learning. Proceedings of the SPIE - Progress in Biomed Opt Imaging 11317:113170Q(113177 pp.). https://doi.org/10.1117/12.2550013

- Goeller M, Achenbach S, Marwan M, Doris MK, Cadet S, Commandeur F, Chen X, Slomka PJ, Gransar H, Cao JJ, Wong ND, Albrecht MH, Rozanski A, Tamarappoo BK, Berman DS, Dey D (2018) Epicardial adipose tissue density and volume are related to subclinical atherosclerosis, inflammation and major adverse cardiac events in asymptomatic subjects. J Cardiovasc Comput Tomogr 12(1):67–73. https://doi.org/10.1016/j.jcct.2017.11.007
- Gohmann RF, Temiz B, Seitz P, Gottschling S, Lücke C, Krieghoff C, Blume C, Horn M, Gutberlet M. Segmentation and characterization of visceral and abdominal subcutaneous adipose tissue on CT with and without contrast medium: influence of 2D- and 3D-segmentation. Quant Imaging Med Surg 2021;11:4258-68. 10.21037/qims-21-178
- Hasebe H, Yoshida K, Nogami A, Ieda M (2020) Difference in epicardial adipose tissue distribution between paroxysmal atrial fibrillation and coronary artery disease. Heart Vessels 35(8):1070–1078.
- He X, Guo BJ, Lei Y, Wang T, Curran WJ, Liu T, Zhang LJ, Yang X (2020b) Automatic quantification of myocardium and pericardial fat from coronary computed tomography angiography: a multicenter study. Eur Radiol 31(6):3826–3836. https://doi.org/10.1007/s00330-020-07482-5
- Huber FA, Del Grande F, Rizzo S, Guglielmi G, Guggenberger R. MRI in the assessment of adipose tissues and muscle composition: how to use it. Quant Imaging Med Surg 2020;10:1636-49. 10.21037/qims.2020.02.06 [PMC free article] [PubMed] [CrossRef] [Google Scholar]
- Iacobellis G, Assael F, Ribaudo MC, Zappaterreno A, Alessi G, Di Mario U et al (2003) Epicardial fat from echocardiography: a new method for visceral adipose tissue prediction. Obes Res 11(2):304–310. https://doi.org/10.1038/oby.2003.45
- Iacobellis G, Corradi D, Sharma AM (2005) Epicardial adipose tissue: anatomic, biomolecular and clinical relationships with the heart. Nat Clin Pract Cardiovasc Med 2(10):536–543. https://doi.org/10.1038/ncpcardio0319
- Iacobellis G. Epicardial adipose tissue in endocrine and metabolic diseases. Endocrine 2014;46:8-15. 10.1007/s12020-013-0099-4

  Koitka S, Kroll L, Malamutmann E, Oezcelik A, Nensa F. Fully automated body composition analysis in routine CT imaging using 3D semantic segmentation convolutional neural networks. Eur Radiol 2021;31:1795-804. 10.1007/s00330-020-07147-3 [PMC free article] [PubMed] [CrossRef] [Google Scholar
- Lambin P, Rios-Velazquez E, Leijenaar R, Carvalho S, van Stiphout RGPM, Granton P, Zegers CML, Gillies R, Boellard R, Dekker A, Aerts HJWL (2012) Radiomics: Extracting more information from medical images using advanced feature analysis. Eur J Cancer 48(4):441–446. https://doi.org/10.1016/j.ejca.2011.11.036
- Lin A, Dey D, Wong DTL, Nerlekar N. Perivascular Adipose Tissue and Coronary Atherosclerosis: from Biology to Imaging Phenotyping. Curr Atheroscler Rep 2019;21:47. 10.1007/s11883-019-0817-3
- Lin A, Wong ND, Razipour A, McElhinney PA, Commandeur F, Cadet SJ, Gransar H, Chen X, Cantu S, Miller RJH, Nerlekar N, Wong DTL, Slomka PJ, Rozanski A, Tamarappoo BK, Berman DS, Dey D. Metabolic syndrome, fatty liver, and artificial intelligence-based epicardial adipose tissue measures predict long-term risk of cardiac events: a prospective study. Cardiovasc Diabetol 2021;20:27. 10.1186/s12933-021-01220-x [PMC free article] [PubMed] [CrossRef] [Google Scholar]
- Litjens G, Ciompi F, Wolterink JM, de Vos BD, Leiner T, Teuwen J et al (2019) State-of-the-art deep learning in cardiovascular image analysis. JACC Cardiovasc Imaging 12(8, Part 1):1549–1565
- Mahabadi AA, Berg MH, Lehmann N, Kälsch H, Bauer M, Kara K, Dragano N, Moebus S, Jöckel KH, Erbel R, Möhlenkamp S (2013) Association of epicardial fat with cardiovascular risk factors and incident myocardial infarction in the general population: the Heinz Nixdorf Recall Study. J Am Coll Cardiol 61(13):1388–1395. https://doi.org/10.1016/j.jacc.2012.11.062
- Mahabadi AA, Lehmann N, Kälsch H, Bauer M, Dykun I, Kara K, Moebus S, Jöckel KH, Erbel R, Möhlenkamp S. Association of epicardial adipose tissue and left atrial size on non-contrast CT with atrial fibrillation: the Heinz Nixdorf Recall Study. Eur Heart J Cardiovasc Imaging 2014;15:863-9. 10.1093/ehjci/jeu006 [PubMed] [CrossRef] [Google Scholar]
- Mahajan R, Kuklik P, Grover S, Brooks AG, Wong CX, Sanders P, Selvanayagam JB (2013) Cardiovascular magnetic resonance of total and atrial pericardial adipose tissue: a validation study and development of a 3 dimensional pericardial adipose tissue model. J Cardiovasc Magn Reson 15(1):73. https://doi.org/10.1186/1532-429X-15-73
- Malik SB, Chen N, Parker RA, III, Hsu JY. Transthoracic echocardiography: pitfalls and limitations as delineated at cardiac CT and MR imaging. Radiographics. 2017;37:383–406. 10.1148/rg.2017160105 [Abstract] [CrossRef] [Google Scholar]
- Norlén A, Alvén J, Molnar D, Enqvist O, Norrlund RR, Brandberg J, Bergström G, Kahl F (2016) Automatic pericardium segmentation and quantification of epicardial fat from computed tomography angiography. J Med Imaging (Bellingham) 3(3):034003. https://doi.org/10.1117/1.JMI.3.3.034003
- Ouyang D, He B, Ghorbani A, Yuan N, Ebinger J, Langlotz CP, et al. Video-based AI for beat-to-beat assessment of cardiac function. Nature. (2020) 580:252–6. 10.1038/s41586-020-2145-8 [Europe PMC free article] [Abstract] [CrossRef] [Google Scholar]
- Packer M. Epicardial Adipose Tissue May Mediate Deleterious Effects of Obesity and Inflammation on the Myocardium. J Am Coll Cardiol 2018;71:2360-72. 10.1016/j.jacc.2018.03.509 [PubMed] [CrossRef] [Google Scholar]
- Quattrocchi CC, Mallio CA, Presti G, Beomonte Zobel B, Cardinale J, Iozzino M, Della Sala SW. The challenge of COVID-19 low disease prevalence for artificial intelligence models: report of 1,610 patients.

  Renganathan V. Overview of artificial neural network models in the biomedical domain. Bratisl Lek Listy 2019;120:536-40. 10.4149/BLL_2019_087 [PubMed] [CrossRef] [Google Scholar]
- Sun J, Lv H, Li M, Zhao L, Liu Y, Zeng N, Wei X, Chen Q, Ren P, Liu Y, Zhang P, Yang Z, Zhang Z, Wang Z. How much abdominal fat do obese patients lose short term after laparoscopic sleeve gastrectomy? A quantitative study evaluated with MRI. Quant Imaging Med Surg 2021;11:4569-82. 10.21037/qims-20-1380 [PMC free article] [PubMed]
- Tadros TM, Massaro JM, Rosito GA, Hoffmann U, Vasan RS, Larson MG, Keaney JF, Jr, Lipinska I, Meigs JB, Kathiresan S, O'Donnell CJ, Fox CS, Benjamin EJ. Pericardial fat volume correlates with inflammatory markers: the Framingham Heart Study. Obesity (Silver Spring) 2010;18:1039-45. 10.1038/oby.2009.343 [PMC free article] [PubMed] [CrossRef] [Google Scholar]
- Vakamudi S, Ho N, Cremer PC. Pericardial effusions: causes, diagnosis, and management. Prog Cardiovasc Dis. (2017) 59:380–8. 10.1016/j.pcad.2016.12.009 [Abstract] [CrossRef] [Google Scholar]
- Villasante Fricke AC, Iacobellis G. Epicardial Adipose Tissue: Clinical Biomarker of Cardio-Metabolic Risk. Int J Mol Sci 2019;20:5989. 10.3390/ijms20235989 [PMC free article] [PubMed] [CrossRef] [Google Scholar]

  Wang J, Wang LJ, Peng YP, Zhang LJ, Jiang SS, Gong JB (2013) Association of pericardial adipose tissue volume with presence and severity of coronary atherosclerosis. Clin Invest Med 36(3):E143–E150. https://doi.org/10.25011/cim.v36i3.19725
- Zhou J, Du M, Chang S, Chen Z. Artificial intelligence in echocardiography: detection, functional evaluation, and disease diagnosis. Cardiovasc Ultrasound. (2021) 19:1–11. 10.1136/heartjnl-2021-319725 [Europe PMC free article] [Abstract] [CrossRef] [Google Scholar]
- Zlokolica V, Krstanović L, Velicki L, Popović B, Janev M, Obradović R, Ralević NM, Jovanov L, Babin D (2017) Semiautomatic epicardial fat segmentation based on fuzzy c-means clustering and geometric ellipse fitting. J Healthc Eng 2017:5817970. https://doi.org/10.1155/2017/5817970

CHAPTER

26

Implantable Cardiac Pacemakers Embedded with Artificial Intelligence

A cardiac pacemaker is a medical equipment that generates impulses within the heart in case of an abnormal heart rhythm and coordinates the electrical signaling between the heart's chambers. Since the development of the first cardiac pacemaker in 1958, this therapeutic device has undergone several modifications. Every year, thousands of surgeries are performed in cardiac patients for pacemaker placement or revision. Although a pacemaker is commonly indicated in patients over 60 years old, it is placed in infants and children if indicated.

There are two types of pacemakers- permanent and temporary. While temporary pacemakers are used in situations where arrhythmias are anticipated to be temporary, permanent pacemakers are often recommended for patients with bradyarrhythmia or tachyarrhythmia. Advancements in implantable pacemakers have resulted in several modifications, such as reducing the size of the device, remote monitoring using the internet, and a considerable increase in battery longevity.

France based **Implicity** is a startup that can monitor implanted cardiac-connected devices remotely with artificial intelligence. Their product connects with pacemakers and implanted defibrillators to facilitate heartbeat at a regular pace and also treat in cases of emergency such as heart attack. All devices being connected also enables to transmit the data back to the server and the physician. The technology at **Implicity** examines the patients' data from the implanted pacemaker and from the patient's medical record to identify high-risk patients that would require modifications in medication or change in the treatment plan.

A research team at **Bios** leverages machine learning to identify patterns of neural biomarkers and then synchronize them based on other organ functions to develop an algorithm. Towards this, they record raw neural data through neural interfaces. They compare with the recordings of physiological signals such as heart rate, blood pressure, glucose levels, body temperature, and physical activity levels.

France based Implicity is a startup that can monitor implanted cardiac-connected devices remotely with artificial intelligence. Their product connects with pacemakers and implanted defibrillators to facilitate heartbeat at a regular pace and also treat in cases of emergency such as heart attack. All devices being connected also enables to transmit the data back to the server and the physician. The technology at Implicity examines the patients' data from the implanted pacemaker and from the patient's medical record to identify high-risk patients that would require modifications in medication or change in the treatment plan.

A research team at Bios leverages machine learning to identify patterns of neural biomarkers and then synchronize them based on other organ functions to develop an algorithm. Towards this, they record raw neural data through neural interfaces. They compare with the recordings of physiological signals such as heart rate, blood pressure, glucose levels, body temperature, and physical activity levels.

Usually, patients with pacemakers have certain contraindications while undergoing medical and dental treatments. One such contraindication is undergoing MRI imaging. But the recent FDA-approved MRI pacemakers have revolutionized the way cardiac patients undergo imaging examinations without adverse effects, and **Biotronik** is one such example.

Shallow Blue is a startup that deals with pacemaker predictive analytics. Their system can predict the onset of cardiac arrest in a person with a pacemaker or ICD so that appropriate intervention can be administered in advance.

Furthermore, scientists at Rice University and the Texas Heart Institute (THI) are working on machine learning algorithms that could improve the current pacemaker algorithm's overall sensitivity. It aims to identify an algorithm that can distribute the pacemaker's effect across several areas in the heart in a synchronized and accurate manner with the help of machine learning algorithms and validate the machine learning algorithm to classify different pathophysiology.Another application of implantable pacemaker is the detection of an electrical storm (ES) that is a dangerous arhythmic condition with increased mortality and morbidity. There is ongoing research to construct and validate machine learning models to predict ES based on an intracardiac device's remote monitoring possibility (ICD). A recent study by Professor Saeed Shakibfar from the University of Copenhagen showed that in patients with ICD, the occurrence of ES could be predicted one day in advance based on the data stored in ICD summaries with good diagnostic accuracies.

Professor Truong and the team at the Linder Research Centre, Ohio, investigated the feasibility of predicting pacemaker risk following transcatheter aortic valve replacement using ECG data and comparing the traditional logistic regression with machine learning approaches. It was found that machine learning methodology is significantly more robust than conventional logistic regression in predicting permanent pacemaker implantation risk following transcatheter aortic valve replacement with good diagnostic accuracy.

Future

Bioelectronic devices are revolutionizing the pacemaker industry primarily by replicating neural signals. These control the activity of abnormal neural circuits that possibly cause the disease. But there is a need for a better understanding of neural biomarkers to receive signals and deliver appropriate treatment autonomously. There is a need to develop a more efficient implantable device for improved interpretation of neural data. But it may not be as easy as it sounds because the human heart does not function alone in conjunction with other organs. Impulses from different organs and activities heavily affect the functioning of the heart. What's more, machine learning can also utilize medical data to support patients' personalized clinical decisions after running validated models.

A. Next-generation pacemakers: from small devices to biological pacemakers

Cardiac conduction system

1.Normal cardiac conduction system

A healthy heart beats >3 billion times in a typical lifetime owing to the remarkable capacity of the endogenous pacemaker to produce rhythmic, spontaneous electrical impulses. The cardiac conduction system then spreads the impulse throughout the heart, exciting the upper (atrial) and lower (ventricular) cardiac pumping chambers in a coordinated manner, appropriately responsive to modulation by the autonomic nervous system.

The main pacemaker of the heart resides in the sinus node, also known as the sinoatrial node (SAN), located at the junction of the superior vena cava and right atrium,. Electrical impulses originate in the SAN, travel rapidly across the right and left atrial muscle to initiate atrial contraction, and then slow when encountering the atrioventricular (AV) node.The AV node delay allows the atria to contract and prime the ventricles with blood for their subsequent contraction. The AV node is also a secondary pacemaker that can serve as a backup (albeit at a much slower rate) in the event of primary SAN failure. After the AV node, the electrical impulse proceeds along the His bundle, the only electrical connection between the atria andthe ventricles and then rapidly spreads throughout the ventricles via a network of specialized Purkinje fibres, which make contact with the working cardiomyocytes. Cells from the different areas of the conduction system have characteristic complements of ion channels and gap junctions that generate different action potential profiles , allowing each tissue to function in a specific manner.

During embryonic development, as early as embryonic day 7.5 (E7.5) in mice, the cells of the primitive heart tube beat spontaneously, with most of the automaticity originating in cells from the precardiac mesoderm located in the inflow tract region8. In mice, these cells reside in the sinus venosus and express potassium/ sodium hyperpolarization-activated cyclic nucleotidegated channel 4 (HCN4) and the transcription factor homeobox protein NKX2.5 . A series of transcription factors including insulin gene enhancer protein ISL1, short stature homeobox protein 2 (SHOX2), and the T-box transcription factors TBX3 and TBX5 activate the SAN gene programme in the sinus venosus whereas NKX2.5, TBX3, and TBX18 repress the chamber myocyte gene programme in the sinus venosus, the AV canal, and the inner curvature, thereby allowing pacemaking cells to dominate in these regions9. Re-expression of transcription factors such as SHOX2 and TBX18 in postnatal mouse ventricular cardiomyocytes has been used to transform chamber cardiomyocytes into pacemaker cells that possess all the main characteristics of SAN cells; this finding is the basis for a strategy to create biological pacemakers, as discussed below. By the time looping occurs at E9 the conduction system activation pattern in the heart tube follows that of the adult heart.SAN cells have dual oscillators to provide stable rhythmic diastolic depolarization for triggering pacemaker action potentials. These two oscillators are referred to as the 'membrane clock' and the 'calcium clock' . The membrane clock oscillator is in the plasma membrane and relies on the pacemaker current — or funny current (If) which is generated through HCN4. The generated inward current causes diastolic depolarization and subsequent activation of T-type and L-type calcium channel currents (ICaL; which in the SAN is generated predominantly by the Cav calcium channe. Depolarization mediated by the inward calcium current (ICa) provides the characteristic slow depolarization of the SAN action potential compared with chamber cardiomyocytes, which rely on the inward sodium current — generated by the sodium channel Nav1.5 — for the action potential rapid upstroke phase. The membrane clock works in concert with the internally driven calcium clock In this second oscillator, diastolic depolarization is facilitated by rhythmic release of calcium from the sarcoplasmic reticulum and consequent depolarization by the electrogenic sodium-calcium exchanger (NCX)The inward current carried by If and NCX acting synergistically suffices to depolarize the surface membrane to the threshold of activation of ICa. Although sodium currents do not have a major role in SAN pacemaker activity, these currents do facilitate conduction out of the SAN and into the surrounding atrial tissue.

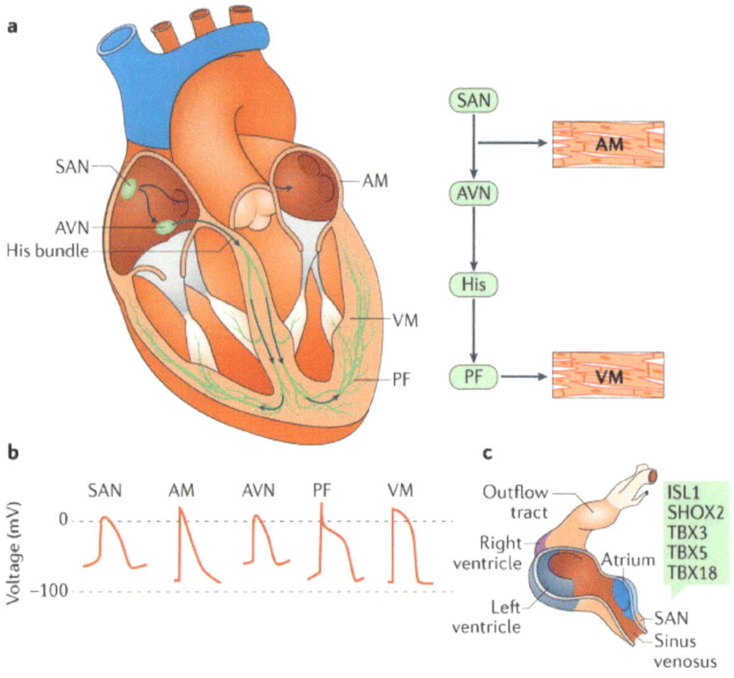

Fig. 26.1 Cardiac conduction system.

a| Schematic representation of the anatomy and cellular electrophysiology of the cardiac conduction system. The cardiac impulse (arrows) originates in the sinoatrial node (SAN), travels across the atrial myocardium (AM), and moves through the atrioventricular node (AVN), the His bundle, and left and right bundle branches. The simultaneous activation of both bundle branches and their terminal Purkinje fibres (PF) provides antegrade activation of the ventricular myocardium (VM) in a synchronized fashion. b | Distinct action potential morphologies at different levels of the conduction system impose specialized electrical behaviours. c | Development of the SAN in mice. The SAN forms in the sinus venosus; during early embryonic development of the heart, transcription factors (green box) activate the SAN gene programme in the sinus venosus, while repressing the chamber myocyte gene programme. Chamber myocardium is depicted in purple, grey, and blue; non-chamber myocardium in dark pink; and non-myocardial tissue in light pink. ISL1, insulin gene enhancer protein ISL1; SHOX2, short stature homeobox protein 2; TBX, T-box transcription factor. Part c adapted from REF 9. http://creativecommons.org/licenses/by/3.0/.

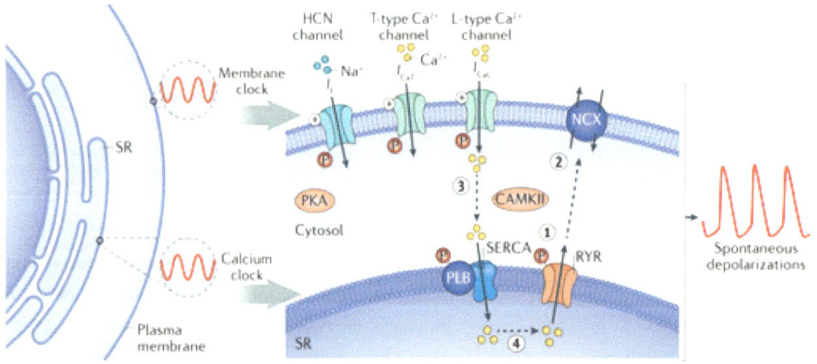

Fig. 26.2 Mechanisms of sinoatrial node automaticity.

A dual oscillator system consisting of a membrane clock and a calcium clock provides stable rhythmic depolarizations. The membrane clock relies on the pacemaker current (via hyperpolarization-activated cyclic nucleotide-gated (HCN) channels), L-type calcium channels, and T-type calcium channels for diastolic depolarization. The calcium clock works in synchrony with the membrane clock by releasing calcium from the sarcoplasmic reticulum (SR) through ryanodine receptors (RYRs) (step 1), thereby depolarizing the cell in diastole by activating the sodium-calcium exchanger (NCX) (step 2). The sarcoplasmic/endoplasmic reticulum calcium ATPase (SERCA), modulated by cardiac phospholamban (PLB), moves the calcium entering through the calcium channels in the plasma membrane back into the SR (step 3) to prime the calcium for the next cycle (step 4). Both the membrane clock and the calcium clock act in synchrony to create spontaneous depolarizations and are regulated by the autonomic nervous system through β-adrenergic and muscarinic stimulation, which modulates the activity of protein kinases (cAMP-dependent protein kinase (PKA) and calcium/calmodulin-dependent protein kinase type II (CAMKII)) that phosphorylate multiple proteins in the system. The calcium cycle is represented by the dashed grey arrows. ICaL, L-type calcium channel current; ICaT, T-type calcium channel current; If, funny current.

If can be modulated by the autonomic nervous system through adrenergic and muscarinic stimulation, as well as by drugs such as ivabradine that alter the pacemaker rate by influencing the slope of diastolic depolarization. Autonomic receptor stimulation modulates the activity of cAMP-dependent protein kinase (PKA) and calcium/ calmodulin-dependent protein kinase type II (CAMKII), which in turn influence both the membrane clock and calcium clock by regulating the phosphorylation of hyperpolarization-activated cyclic nucleotide-gated (HCN) channels, calcium channels, ryanodine receptors, and other proteins that regulate sarcoplasmic reticulum refilling and release of calcium. Elevations in intracellular calcium increase calcium-dependent phosphorylation, whereas phosphodiesterases, when active, counteract the effects of phosphorylation.

Although other parts of the conduction system (AV node, His bundle, bundle branches, and Purkinje fibres) can fire spontaneously, they do so at a slower rate than that of the SAN and usually at rates insufficient to support the circulation. Therefore, the SAN sets the heart rate by overriding the slower pacemakers below it. If spontaneous pacing below the SAN were faster, such ectopic pacemakers would compete with the SAN and could potentially cause arrhythmias.

2.Conduction system Dysfunctions

Pacemaker and/or conduction system disturbances can result from a failure in impulse generation by the SAN or from a block of impulse propagation at any point in the conduction system. Other causes of conduction failure, which we do not describe here, include abnormal pathways of conduction owing to developmental accidents.

The most common identifiable causes of conduction block arise from physical destruction of part of the conduction system; for example, valvular infections owing to endocarditis can form abscesses that compress or erode the AV node. Likewise, implantation of a prosthetic valve can impinge the adjacent conduction system, leading to reversible or irreversible heart block. In rare cases, congenital, complete heart block develops in response to circulating factors (possibly antibodies that impede AV conduction) transferred from the mother to the fetus. Nevertheless, the most common cause of conduction disturbance is progressive cardiac conduction disease (or Lev-Lenegre disease), an idiopathic, age-related condition characterized by fibrosis of the conduction system. Regardless of the aetiology, treatment of these irreversible conditions is determined primarily by the presence of associated symptoms (such as fatigue, dizziness, or fainting) and the degree of heart-rate slowing

B. Electronic pacemakers

Evolution of device technology

Electronic pacemakers are the mainstay of therapy for slow heart rhythms (bradycardia) owing to cardiac conduction system disease. Every year, >200,000 patients undergo permanent pacemaker implantation to treat these conditions in the USA alone.The first successful applications of electrotherapy in patients with bradycardia involved external pulse generators connected to the chest wall or directly to the heart via wires. For obvious reasons, mobility was limited, and the devices were uncomfortable. In 1958, the first fully implantable pacemaker was placed by open thoracotomy at the Karolinska Institute, Sweden . The device, designed by Rune Elmqvist and Ake Senning, had epicardial electrodes that connected directly to the heart, the pacemaker supported the patient's heart rhythm for 3 h and then had to be replaced by a new device. This patient required a total of 26 pacemaker changes throughout his lifetime, dying aged 86 years from an unrelated cause32. In the USA, implantable electronic pacemakers designed and built by Wilson Greatbatch using mercury-based battery technology were introduced for human use in the 1960s. The first patient implanted with the Greatbatch pacemaker lived for 18 months.

Since the first implantable electronic pacemakers were developed 6 decades ago, we have witnessed continuous improvements in device technology, with advances in lead design, generator size, battery longevity, and software algorithms that have resulted in smaller devices with improved functionality . One of the main limitations of early electronic devices was the extremely short battery lifespan. In an attempt to solve this issue, multiple companies developed nuclear-powered pacemakers. The first isotope-based pacemaker (238Pu) was implanted in April 1970 in France. Such isotope-based devices were capable of producing stable pacing for >30 years to provide fixed or asynchronous pacing. Later generations of isotope-based pacemakers had synchronous pacing capabilities, which allowed for sensing of the intrinsic patient rhythm and then pacing only on demand when no underlying intrinsic rhythm was present. Despite their extraordinary battery longevity, these devices were replaced by next-generation devices with lithium-based battery technology and improved software algorithms. Given the obvious safety concerns of isotope-powered devices, lithium-based batteries quickly became the standard source of power for modern electronic pacemakers

Modern device technologies

Implantable electronic pacemaker technology has continued to evolve, and we now have a variety of technologically advanced devices capable of providing reliable pacing for different patient populations Today's modern devices can sense the intrinsic rhythm in both the atrium and ventricle and can pace either chamber on demand at a programmable baseline heart rate.

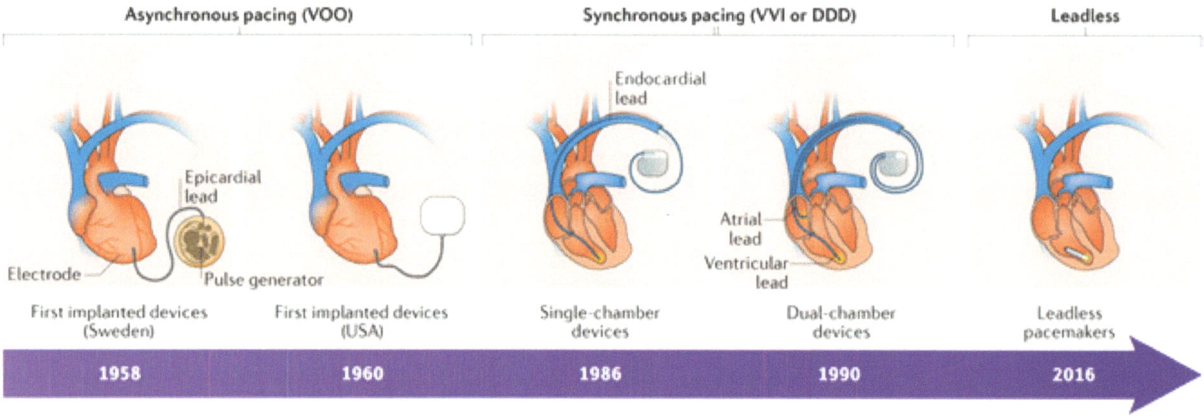

Fig. 26.3| Timeline of the evolution of electronic pacemakers. Early electronic pacemaker devices were big, had epicardial leads, and were implanted by open thoracotomy. Modern devices (single-chamber devices and dual-chamber devices) are much smaller, use endocardial leads, and can be implanted with minimally invasive techniques. First-generation devices provided only asynchronous (VOO) pacing, whereas modern devices are capable of synchronous and/or on-demand (VVI/DDD) pacing. Leadless pacemakers have a self-contained capsule that includes the battery, generator, and pacing electrodes, and are implanted percutaneously through the femoral vein.

Although current lithium-based battery technologies can provide stable pacing for >0 years, battery longevity can be extended further by software algorithms. Algorithms that iteratively test the minimum output required (pacing threshold) to capture the myocardium (autocapture) can automatically adjust the output, increasing the longevity of the pacemaker to >10 years. Additionally, modern software algorithms can monitor for the presence of AV nodal conduction and minimize right ventricular (RV) pacing in those patients with intermittent AV nodal block. The goal is to avoid (when possible) the potential deleterious effects of chronic RV pacing, such as electrical and mechanical dyssynchrony and RV pacing-induced cardiomyopathy. An additional pacing modality to treat RV pacing-induced cardiomyopathy, which also revolutionized the management of heart failure (HF), is cardiac resynchronization therapy (CRT), also known as biventricular pacing Biventricular pacing, achieved by placing a left ventricular (LV) lead through a coronary venous branch in addition to a conventional RV lead, has been proven to prolong survival and improve symptoms and LV ejection fraction (EF) in patients with HF with widened QRS complexes (corresponding to ventricular depolarization) on the electrocardiogram (ECG)Given that approximately one-third of patients do not show improvements in functional capacity or EF with CRT, novel, multipoint pacing modalities have been developed47 to pace the left ventricle at multiple points48. Randomized clinical trials to compare the effects of bipolar versus quadripolar leads in patients with CRT are ongoingThe capacity to capture the His-Purkinje network by placing a pacing electrode in the His bundle region has given rise to an additional pacing modality, His bundle pacing . This modality creates fast antegrade (forward) activation of the ventricles, with the consequent narrow QRS complex on surface ECG. Interestingly, His-Purkinje recruitment by His bundle pacing occurs not only in patients with AV block at the level of the AV node, but also in patients with AV block below the AV node (infranodal block). Although larger studies are needed to understand better the long-term benefits of this modality, His-bundle pacing might be a superior alternative to apical RV pacing.

Electronic pacemakers with a subcutaneous generator connected to endovascular pacing lead(s) can provide different pacing modalities: single-chamber, dual-chamber, biventricular, and His-bundle pacing. Additionally, some modern devices have software algorithms that detect and treat atrial tachyarrhythmias by overdrive-pacing the atria and interrupting the arrhythmia circuit.

Although effective, these devices do entail substantial risks; complications are often related to either lead insertion or malfunction or to infections of the leads and/or generators. Such infections can be life-threatening and generally require removal of all hardware, during which time temporary pacing strategies are required.Additionally, leads can be thrombogenic, creating upper extremity deep venous thrombosis. Leads can also affect tricuspid valve leaflet motion, causing clinically significant tricuspid regurgitation .Given the potential of lead-related complications, leadless pacemakers have been developed In such devices, the pulse generator, the battery, and the sensing and pacing electrodes are self-contained in a small capsule designed to be delivered into the right ventricle through a steerable sheath inserted through the femoral vein.The major limitations of current leadless pacemakers are the need for a large-bore (18–24 French) venous delivery system, the uncertainty about infectious and thrombogenic risks, and their capacity to provide only single-chamber RV pacing. Single-chamber pacing prevents the use of leadless pacemakers for common indications for cardiac pacing such as sick sinus syndrome, where atrial pacing is preferred, or in conditions where AV synchrony is desired, such as sinus rhythm with chronic AV block.

Next-generation devices

As discussed above, current-generation pacemakers have limitations related to lead(s) or generator malfunction, thrombosis, infections, and lack of a physiological autonomic response. Additionally, pacemaker implantation in children has additional challenges owing to the smaller body size, rapid growth, and long life-expectancy of children and the anatomical variations associated with congenital heart defects In general, epicardial pacing (with leads placed via thoracotomy) is recommended for patients with <15 kg of body weight and/or unfavourable anatomy (for example, presence of an intracardiac shunt or a single ventricle). However, epicardial pacing leads are more prone to fracture and often need to be replaced by either a new epicardial lead or an endocardial system when possible With contemporary battery technologies, generators need to be replaced every >10 years (depending on pacemaker utilization), requiring multiple generator changes, with the associated cumulative risk of procedure-related complications. Alternative energy sources, such as conformal piezoelectric energy harvesting and solar-powered pacemakers66, are currently being studied at preclinical stages. Conformal piezoelectric energy harvesting technology, long-used in wristwatches, uses the movements of internal organs such as heart, lung, and diaphragm to enable mechanical-to-electrical energy conversion. By contrast, solar-powered devices utilize a subcutaneous solar module to convert transcutaneous light into the electrical energy required for self-sustainable cardiac pacing. Additional preclinical testing is required to assess the reliability and duration of these self-sustained power technologies.To solve lead-related complications as well as infections associated with subcutaneous (extravascular) generators, leadless pacemakers have some promise

Although leadless pacemakers have been used in patients with device-related infections, the risk of bacteraemic 'seeding' of the leadless device remains to be studied in the long term. Additionally, current-generation leadless pacemakers can provide only single-chamber RV pacing44. With advances in wireless communication technologies, we foresee the development of next-generation, dual leadless pacemakers capable of sensing and/or pacing in both cardiac chambers, resulting in sequential AV pacing

Although device manufacturers have developed different sensing systems and software algorithms to provide rate adaptation, current-generation pacemakers do not have true autonomic responsiveness to satisfy physiological needs. Impedance measurements from the pacing electrode have been used to estimate myocardial contractile performance (as a surrogate of sympathetic activation)69. More commonly, most electronic pacemakers have a programmable accelerometer to detect patient activity and adjust pacing rate in response to exercise..Although these systems are designed to satisfy physiological demands, given the complexity of the autonomic innervation of the cardiac conduction system5, it is difficult to conceive that device-based technologies will be able accurately to reproduce physiological rate responses. Nevertheless, with ongoing advancements in sensors and wearable technologies, next-generation pacemakers are likely to combine different sensing systems (that is, accelerometer, impedance, cardiac output, and blood pressure) and complex software algorithms to support more accurately the physiological needs.

Biological pacemakers

Despite continuous improvements in device technologies, electronic pacemakers still have limitations and complications.Several situations warrant non-device options. Patients with hardware-related infections who require a pacemaker have a contraindication to re-implantation before effective antibiosis is established. In at least one instance (congenital heart block), life-threatening bradycardia cannot be treated by electronic pacemakers. This condition results in fetal death or stillbirth in >80% of cases and would necessitate in utero pacing, which is not yet feasible. Consequently, biological pacemakers are being developed to provide a therapeutic alternative to electronic devices.

Proof-of-concept studies

Different biological approaches to enhance cardiac automaticity have been investigated over the years .The common goal is to generate an ectopic region of automaticity in the heart that can function as a surrogate for the SAN. Various gene-based and cell-based approaches to generate biological pacemakers have been described .

Gene-based approaches

The earliest 'genes-only' approach to increase automaticity involved overexpression of the genes encoding the human ß2-adrenergic receptors in mouse. and porcine atria. Although this approach did not generate a biological pacemaker, endogenous SAN rate was accelerated by increasing the number of β2-adrenergic

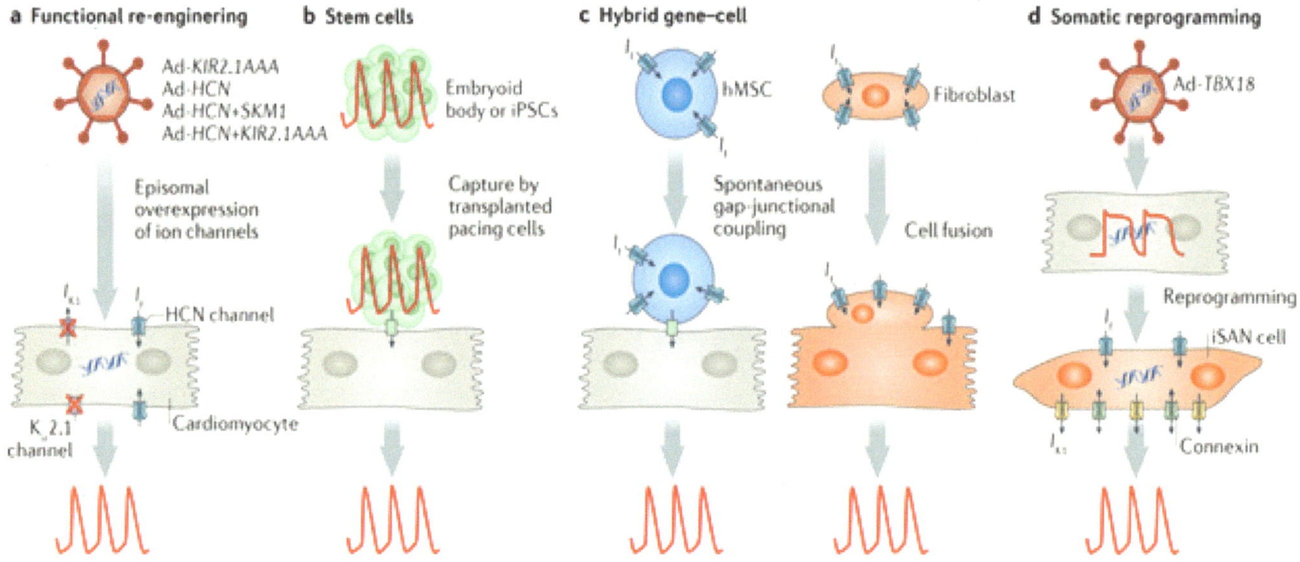

Fig. 26.4 **Biological pacemaker approaches.** a | In a functional re-engineering approach, adenoviral (Ad) vectors are used to overexpress genes encoding ion channels (single channel or a combination of channels) in cardiomyocytes to create automaticity, for example, to increase the number of hyperpolarization-activated cyclic nucleotidegated (HCN) channels and to reduce the number of functional inward-rectifier potassium channels (Kir2.1) by overexpressing a dominant negative construct (KIR2.1AAA). b | With a stem cell approach, a cluster of beating cells derived from human embryonic stem cells (called an embryoid body) or induced pluripotent stem cells (iPSCs) are transplanted into a specific location in the heart to capture surrounding myocardium, thereby creating biological pacing. c | In a hybrid approach, cells (human mesenchymal stem cells (hMSCs) or fibroblasts) are used to deliver ion channel genes (for example, genes encoding components of HCN channels) to produce cardiac automaticity. Delivery by hMSCs requires gap-junctional coupling between the cardiomyocyte and the hMSC, whereas delivery by fibroblasts involves cell fusion. d | In somatic reprogramming, overexpression of the T-box transcription factor TBX18 by use of Ad vectors reprogrammes adult cardiac chamber cardiomyocytes into induced sinoatrial node (iSAN) cells, recapitulating the features of the SAN and therefore creating pacemaker activity. If, funny current; IK1, inward rectifier current.

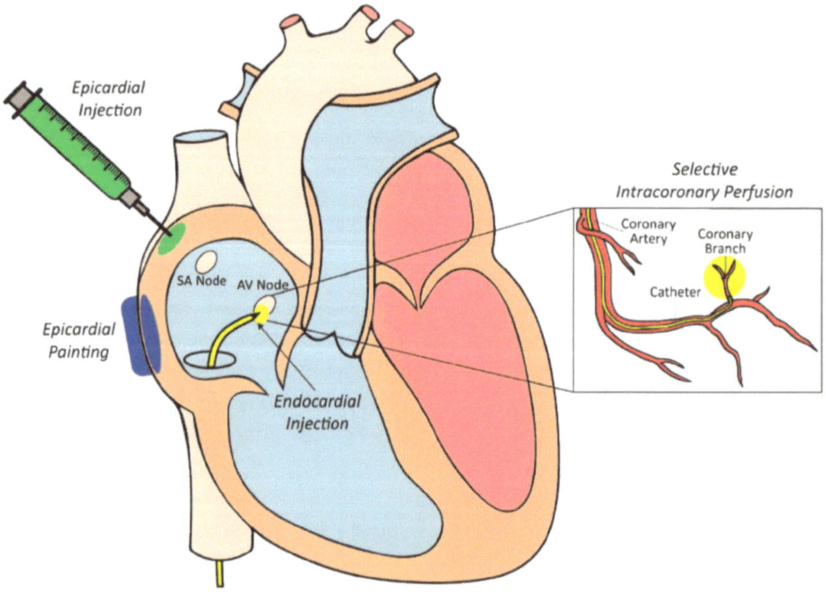

Fig. 26.5 Showing Researchers successfully used gene therapy to create a "biological pacemaker" that could replace electronic pacemakers currently used to treat human heart conditions.

receptors available for binding to endogenous catecholamines The first de novo biological pacemaker was created by gene therapy and reported in 2002 . The strategy was to release the 'electrical brake' that suppresses automaticity in ventricular cardiomyocytes by inhibiting the endogenous inward rectifier potassium current (7K1). Miake et al. reduced the number of functional inward rectifier potassium ion channels (encoded by the KIR2 gene family; also known as KCNJ2) in the myocardium by overexpressing a KIR2.1 -dominant-negative construct (KIR2.1AAA) in guinea pig hearts This suppression of IK1 released the intrinsic capacity of ventricular cardiomyocytes to depolarize spontaneously, thereby generating biological pacemaker activity Notably, the strategy was not designed to create a genuine phenocopy of the SAN; instead, this technique was a 'functional engineering' approach whereby manipulation of a single ionic current unleashed biological pacemaker activity in ventricular cardio-myocytes that otherwise remained structurally and genetically unaltered. Follow-up studies demonstrated that KIR2.1AAA overexpression not only affected the resting membrane potential (generating spontaneous depolarizations), but also led to prolongation of action potential duration when KIR2.1AAA was less-intensely expressed in the heart81. Although diffuse suppression of IK1 in ventricular myocardium can predispose to arrhythmias, as seen clinically in familial long QT syndrome type 7 , the potential pro-arrhythmic effects of focal suppression of IK1 (as required for generating biological pacemaker activity) were not characterized in these proof-of-concept, small-animal studies. Given this important consideration, every biological therapy that has the potential to increase cardiac automaticity (regardless of changes in action potential duration) should be carefully characterized in several preclinical models (including large animals with slow heart rates, like that of humans) to rule out potential pro-arrhythmic effects (see next section).

In the SAN, If has an important role in cardiac pacemaking83. An additional functional re-engineering (gene-based) approach, first reported by Qu et al. in a canine model, involved the overexpression of Hcn2 to elicit biological pacemaker activity84. Adenoviral constructs with mouse Hcn2 were delivered by open thoracotomy to the root of the left atrial appendage; 4 days after the injection, the anaesthetized dogs had spontaneous rhythms that originated from the left atria after suppressing sinus rhythm by vagal stimulation84. Follow-up studies from the same group demonstrated that injection of Hcn2-expressing adenovirus into the left bundle branch resulted in spontaneous ventricular rhythms after vagal stimulation85. Taken together, these independent, proof-of-concept studies demonstrated the capacity to create biological pacemaker activity by functional re-engineering by either suppressing IK1 (releasing the intrinsic beating capacity of cardiomyocytes) or by expressing If channels in normal working cardiomyocytes.

Cell-based approaches.

In cell-based approaches, a cluster of spontaneously beating cells is transplanted into the heart to elicit ectopic biological pacemaker activity. The earliest attempt utilized fetal cardiomyocytes injected in the hearts of two dogs with iatrogenic AV block with a resultant ventricular escape rhythm not observed in two control dogs. The cell transplantation approach has been sporadically mimicked since then with various spontaneously beating cell types.

Human embryonic stem cells (hESCs) readily differentiate into spontaneously beating cardiomyocytes. In vivo transplantation of hESC-derived cardiomyocytes into guinea pigs resulted in biological pacemaker activity confirmed by ex vivo optical mapping89. After AV nodal ablation, those animals that had previously been injected with hESC-derived cardiomyocytes exhibited spontaneous biological pacemaker activity originating at the injection site (demonstrated by optical mapping). Given the human origin of these cells, immunosuppression was required to prevent rejection.

SAN-like cardiomyocytes derived from human induced pluripotent stem cells (iPSCs) have been used to create biological pacemaker activity in vitro and in vivo . In another study from an independent group, iPSC-derived cardiomyocytes were delivered into dog hearts by open thoracotomy. Biological pacemaker activity was seen in only 50% of the animals, with beating rates of 40–50 bpm . Although attractive, iPSC-derived biological pacemakers face substantial hurdles for clinical translation: current iPSC technologies produce a mixed population of cells with various phenotypes. This issue not only affects the function of iPSC-derived biological pacemakers (as previously reported, but is also a safety concern given the potential of immature cells to migrate or to differentiate into different cell types (such as teratomas). Moreover, generating iPSCs requires weeks to months; any given patient would have to defer implantation until their autologous cardiomyocytes became available, which limits the potential patient candidates to those not requiring urgent chronotropic support.

Hybrid gene-cell approaches.

One combined or hybrid approach has been the delivery of cells carrying pacemaker genes (for example, genes encoding HCN channels) into the heart to generate biological pacemaker activity (FIG. 4c). Human mesenchymal stem cells (hMSCs) engineered to express the pacemaker channel HCN2 were delivered by open thoracotomy in dogs with complete AV block93. Animals injected with engineered HCN2-expressing hMSCs showed biological pacemaker activity with ventricular rates of 50–60 bpm and no evidence of cellular or humoral rejection93. Potential advantages of this approach include avoiding a viral vector (used in most gene therapy approaches) and immunosuppression (given the low immunogenicity of hMSCs). Although the absence of rejection without immunosuppression is an important advantage of this approach, the fairly low heart rates achieved and concerns about potential migration and further differentiation of hMSCs are important limitations of this strategy.

Another hybrid approach used engineered syngeneic fibroblasts expressing HCN1 injected into guinea pig hearts in a vehicle designed to induce cell fusion with surrounding endogenous ventricular cells95. The study documented the formation of fibroblast-myocyte heterokaryons and biological pacemaker activity originating at the injection site. Although this alternative represents a non-viral, non-stem-cell approach to biological pacemakers, additional preclinical studies with optimized, minimally invasive delivery systems are needed if translational efforts for cell-fusion biological pacemakers are to proceed.

Somatic reprogramming approaches.

Starting in 2013, a conceptually different alternative has been developed with a view to clinical translation. Unlike functional re-engineering approaches, which transferred either mutant80 or wild-type ion channel genes to generate biological pacemaker activity, transfer of genes encoding transcription factors has the potential to create faithful replicas of genuine pacemaker cells. This 'somatic reprogramming' approach has been applied in practice by overexpressing the gene coding for the human embryonic transcription factor TBX18 in ventricular cardiomyocytes. Transfer of TBX18 induced the conversion of cardiomyocytes into induced SAN (iSAN) cells that resembled endogenous SAN pacemaker cells. With this approach, no single determinant of excitability is selectively overexpressed; instead, the entire geneexpression programme is altered, with resultant changes in fundamental cell physiology and morphology.Initial studies demonstrated that TBX18-induced reprogramming created electrical automaticity by both voltage clock and calcium clock mechanisms). Interestingly, iSAN cells had many of the phenotypic and functional characteristics of native SAN cells. Moreover, in vivo somatic reprogramming by TBX18 created a biological pacemaker rhythm in guinea pig hearts that not only originated from the injection site, but also responded to catecholamines.As described below, this somatic reprogramming technology has been advanced into a large-animal model of complete heart block

Large-animal studies

To develop a biological pacemaker candidate ready for clinical testing, addressing the following considerations is important: delivery system, preferred biological agent, and target patient population. The most notable large-animal studies differ in the choice of animal model (swine versus canine), the duration of follow-up, and, most importantly, the assessment of efficacy and safety. Most studies used repeated ECGs and/or serial Holter recordings to assess biological pacemaker activity and potential pro-arrhythmic effects,but only one study used real-time, continuous ECG telemetry to characterize biological pacemaker activity and cardiac safety (check for arrhythmias) Although short-term biological pacemakers have been successfully generated in large-animal models by gene-based, cell-based, and reprogramming-based therapies, the delivery methods have been extremely invasive (open-chest or transarterial approaches limiting the potential for human translation. Gene-based biological pacemakers have been successfully delivered by catheter-based techniques, but cell-based biological pacemakers have yet to be delivered by minimally invasive (catheter) techniques. As described in the previous section, cell-based biological pacemakers rely on successful transplantation and engraftment of a cluster of spontaneously beating cells capable of electrically entraining the surrounding myocardium. A critical mass of clustered beating cells (derived from hESCs or iPSCs) is required to capture the heart successfully and create biological pacemaker activity. Given the limitations of open-chest and transarterial approaches, we have developed a right-sided (venous) delivery approach in a swine model of complete heart block whereby biological pacemaker vectors can be delivered percutaneously through a catheter placed in the femoral vein.

To date, studies on ion channel-based (functional re-engineering) biological pacemakers have used recombinant adenovirus as the gene delivery vector. Adenoviral vectors have been used in >40 human clinical trials (completed) as an alternative to standard therapies in different disease conditions. Additionally, various clinical trials of adenoviral gene therapy in patients with different cardiac diseases are currently in the recruitment phase. One limitation of the use of adenoviral vectors is their temporary nature: transduced cells express the transgene robustly for several weeks, but the cells are then cleared by the immune system. However, given the generally favourable safety profile in human clinical trials, the lack of genomic integration, and the proven safety and efficacy in preclinical studies, adenoviral vectors remain a viable option for certain clinical applications After the initial proof-of-concept studies showing somatic reprogramming by TBX18 both in vitro and in vivo Hu et al. delivered TBX18 by a minimally invasive technique in a swine model of complete heart block. Adenovirus carrying TBX18 was delivered to the His-bundle region by a single venous catheter (introduced through an 8 French venous sheath) without the need for thoracotomy or arterial access. Animals were monitored by implanted, continuous ECG telemetry, and activity was measured by a built-in accelerometer. TBX18-treated animals had stable biological pacemaker activity originating at the injection site (as demonstrated by in vivo electroanatomical mapping) and improved exercise capacity. Moreover, no signs of local (proarrhythmic) or systemic adverse effects occurred during follow-up98. The reprogramming-based strategy, by transforming adult cardiac cells into iSAN cells, might be a more physiologically-based biological pacemaker than previously described, ion channel-based strategies.

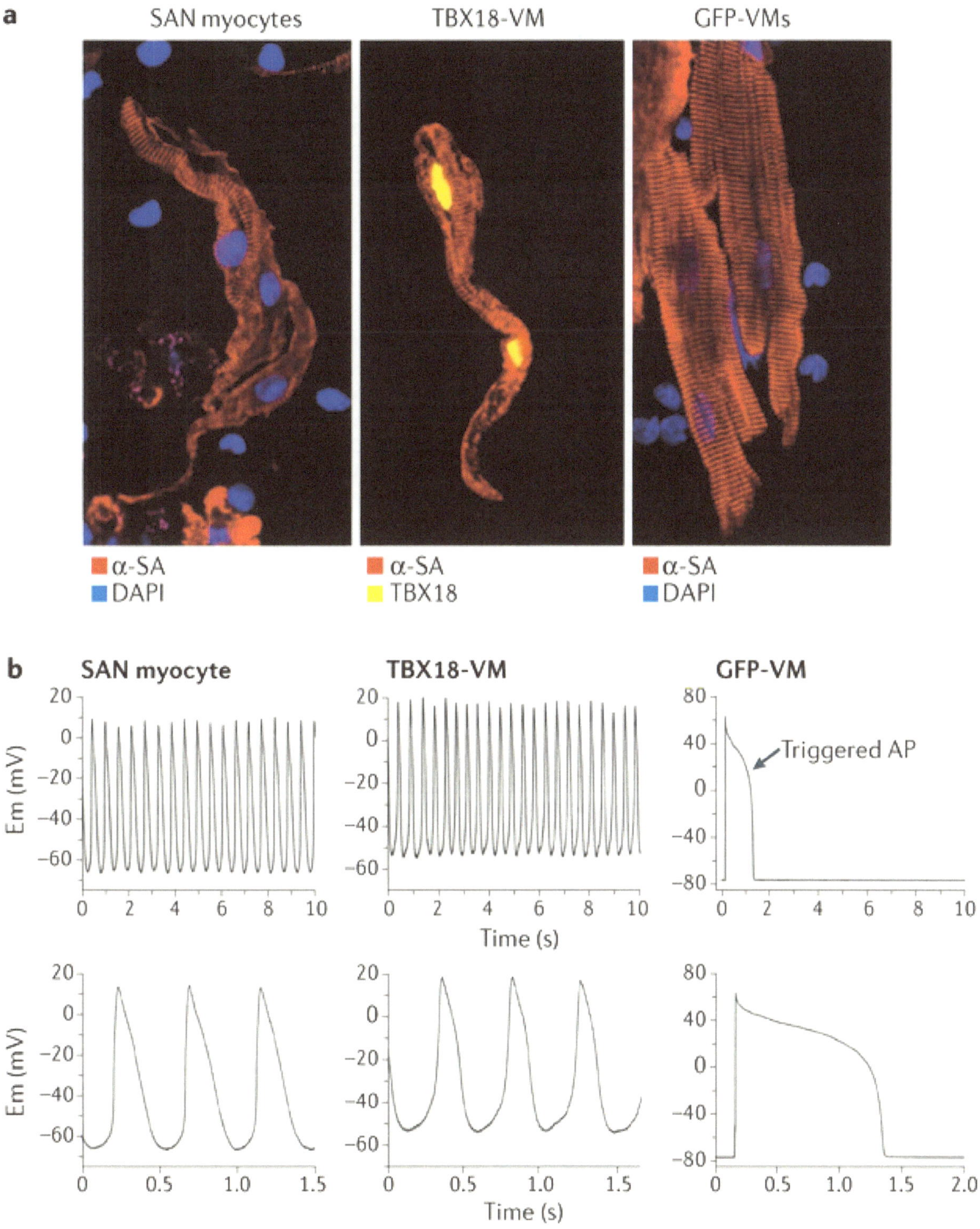

Fig. 26.6 Somatic reprogramming by TBX18.

In summary, large-animal studies performed in two clinically relevant models (swine and canine) using either open thoracotomy or catheter-based delivery systems have shown the feasibility and safety of biological pacing. The most robust preclinical data come from gene-based and reprogramming-based approaches.

Ideal population for first-in-human-trial

Although biological pacemakers might supplant electronic pacemakers in the future, we should be realistic about potential first-in-human applications. If effective and safe, a biological pacemaker can be extremely valuable in the following conditions: device-related infections, chronic atrial fibrillation (AF) with slow ventricular response, and congenital (intrauterine) AV block.

Device-related infections.

Device-related infections have been increasing in the past decade as a result of not only the increase in pacemaker implantations but also the higher incidence of bacterial infections worldwide and the substantial associated morbidity and mortality. The presence of an indwelling foreign body such as a pacemaker device predisposes a patient to life-threatening infections of the leads and/or the generator. Patients with device-related infections generally require complete removal of all hardware until they become infection-free on systemic antibiotics For those patients who depend on the pacemaker, a temporary transvenous pacing device needs to be utilized during the antibiotic treatment, which typically requires >2 weeks. Moreover, the presence of an indwelling catheter can potentially undermine the capacity of systemic antibiotics to clear the infection. Device-related infections are independent markers of long-term mortality and are costly. A hardware-free, temporary pacing alternative would be desirable in such patients to support the circulation in the interval after removal of the infected hardware and before implantation of a new, definitive permanent electronic pacemaker. An effective biological pace-maker could potentially provide temporary pacing, eliminating the need for indwelling hardware during antibiotic therapy and improving the outcomes and effectiveness of such therapy by removing any possible nidus of infection associated with temporary, transvenous leads.

Chronic atrial fibrillation.

Chronic AF associated with AV nodal disease can present with slow ventricular response and symptoms such as fatigue, dizziness, and syncope. These patients do not require AV synchrony (like in persistent AF); therefore, these patients are often treated with either single-chamber pacemakers or, more recently, leadless pacemakers. Biological pacemakers delivered by a minimally invasive delivery system could, in principle, be a viable, hardware-free alternative to single-chamber pacing or could decrease battery utilization (by diminishing pacemaker utilization) in those patients with a previously implanted pacemaker.

Congenital AV block.

Congenital AV block, when severe, can result in hydrops fetalis, stillbirth, and postpartum circulatory collapse. This disease is more common in mothers with systemic lupus erythematosus, and severe forms of this disorder do not respond to conventional therapies (systemic steroids). Moreover, electronic devices cannot be implanted in utero or in newborn babies. If safely delivered, a biological pacemaker could (in principle) be the only available therapy for congenital AV block.

Before the first-in-human biological pacemaker clinical trial, performing long-term efficacy and safety studies using a clinically realistic animal model with the proposed biological candidate is critical. Being able to deliver the biological pacemaker product through a minimally invasive delivery system is an obvious advantage. Additionally, efficacy and safety studies need to be replicated with the use of vectors (or cells) generated under good manufacturing practice conditions. Formal toxicology and biodistribution studies need to be performed according to the standards of regulatory agencies, such as the FDA.

The first clinical application of the ICD was reported 10 years later. Patient selection was restricted to those with recurrent cardiac arrest episodes despite receiving conventional therapy, and implantation was performed by open thoracotomy110. The device turned out to be highly efficacious. Over the next 3 decades, implantation of the ICD became entirely percutaneous, and the ICD is now part of routine care for those patients at general risk of fatal arrhythmias; indeed, ICDs are implanted prophylactically in hundreds of thousands of patients annually. With the biological pacemaker, we remain at the preclinical stage. As with the ICD, the technology has been ridiculed by an establishment cardiologist. Only time will tell whether the biological pacemaker will succeed in clinical translation and, if so, how major the effect will be in clinical practice.

Conclusions

Conduction system disorders are currently treated with electronic pacemakers. Electronic pacemaker technologies continue to evolve, and latest-generation devices are smaller, have longer battery duration, and improved functionality compared with previous devices. In the future, we will probably see further improvements in electronic devices: progressive miniaturization; dual-chamber, leadless pacing; and improved sensor technologies to better adjust to metabolic and physiological needs. Different electronic pacemakers are currently available to treat specific patient populations (such as single-chamber or leadless devices in chronic AF or biventricular pacemakers in HF with wide QRS complex), and device technologies will probably have further improvements tailored to specialized patient needs. If successfully tested in niche populations (for example, patients with device-related infections), biological pacemakers might provide a therapeutic alternative to devices in the future management of patients with conduction system disorders.

Cardiac Pacemakers – The Route To Implantable Artificial Intelligence

Since the dawn of the 20th century, the field of medical science has undergone remarkable advancements, largely driven by the integration of technology. Notably, the utilization of embedded technology to restore malfunctioning organs to a state closer to their natural functionality has found its pinnacle in the realm of permanent transvenous pacemaker therapy, emerging as an indispensable therapeutic approach for patients afflicted by symptomatic bradyarrhythmia.

The evolution of cardiac pacemakers has unfolded in parallel with the evolution of microelectronics and its profound role in information technology. As silicon-based microcontrollers and microprocessors have advanced, they have ushered in a digital revolution that has left an indelible mark on pacemaker technology. Contemporary pacemaker hardware is endowed with the remarkable ability to be programmed and reprogrammed without the need for invasive procedures. This capability, coupled with its diverse feature set, is enabled or disabled, and seamlessly synchronized with specialized external devices through wireless connectivity. Starting in the 1980s, manufacturers of cardiac pacemakers, themselves pioneers of cutting-edge technology, began harnessing the potential of expert systems and early artificial intelligence techniques to optimize therapy selection and analyze complex electrocardiogram results.

Today, the rapid progress in artificial intelligence, amplified by exponential growth in computational power and the proliferation of correlated devices, is ushering in a transformative era. AI-powered applications and the vast landscape of Big Data analytics are revolutionizing the quality of life for patients and their caregivers through enhanced atrial fibrillation detection. This transformation is facilitated by the ubiquitous expansion of the Internet of Things and breakthroughs in telecommunication technologies.

This research embarks on a journey through the realm of AI-aided innovations in cardiac health. It explores the frontiers of 3D imaging, the creation of virtual hearts, the simulation of cardiac arrhythmias, robotics, non-invasive ablation therapies, and the integration of augmented reality. These advancements are driving the realization of a future where pacemakers evolve into genuine implantable Artificial Intelligence entities, revolutionizing the landscape of cardiac arrhythmia care.

1. Artificial intelligence in cardiac pacemakers – Current advances and future horizons

The field of cardiac pacemakers has evolved significantly over the years, and the integration of artificial intelligence (AI) has played a pivotal role in these advancements. This section provides an overview of the current status of AI applications in cardiac pacemakers, exploring the convergence of technology, medicine, and AI, and their implications for the future of cardiac arrhythmia care.

Since the dawn of the 20th century, cardiac pacemakers have been an essential therapeutic approach for patients suffering from symptomatic bradyarrhythmia (Bachtiger, et al., 2020). These devices have undergone a remarkable transformation in parallel with the growth of microelectronics and information technology (Dassen, Den Dulk, & Wellens, 1988). Modern pacemakers are equipped with silicon-based microcontrollers and microprocessors, allowing for non-invasive programming and reprogramming, as well as seamless synchronization with external devices through wireless connectivity (Dassen, Den Dulk, & Wellens, 1988). In the 1980s, manufacturers of cardiac pacemakers began harnessing the potential of expert systems and early AI techniques to optimize therapy selection and analyze electrocardiogram results (Dassen, Den Dulk, & Wellens, 1988). This marked the initial steps toward the integration of AI in cardiac pacemakers.

Today, the rapid progress in AI, coupled with the exponential growth in computational power and the proliferation of connected devices, is ushering in a transformative era in cardiac health (Kim, et al., 2022). AI-powered applications and Big Data analytics are revolutionizing atrial fibrillation detection, improving the quality of life for patients and caregivers (Isaksen, Baumert, Hermans, Maleckar, & Linz, 2022). These advancements are facilitated by the expansion of the Internet of Things and breakthroughs in telecommunication technologies (Nakamura & Sasano, 2022).

This research embarks on a journey through the realm of AI-aided innovations in cardiac health, delving into 3D imaging, the creation of virtual hearts, the simulation of cardiac arrhythmias, robotics, non-invasive ablation therapies, and the integration of augmented reality (Nakamura & Sasano, 2022). These advancements are driving the realization of a future where pacemakers evolve into genuine implantable Artificial Intelligence entities, revolutionizing the landscape of cardiac arrhythmia care (Kim, et al., 2022).

The integration of AI in cardiac pacemakers is a dynamic field that has evolved significantly over the years. Current advancements in AI technology offer the potential to revolutionize the landscape of cardiac arrhythmia care, and this section will explore the latest developments and future prospects.

1.1 The evolution of cardiac pacemakers

The history of cardiac pacemakers is marked by remarkable technological and medical advancements. This section delves into the evolution of cardiac pacemakers, tracing their development from the early days to the present while highlighting key milestones along the way.

The concept of artificial pacing of the heart dates back to the early 20th century. The first breakthrough in this field can be traced to the pioneering work of Dr. Albert Hyman in the 1930s. Dr. Hyman's invention of the "artificial pacemaker" paved the way for the development of modern cardiac pacemakers (Dassen, Den Dulk, & Wellens, 1988).

In the 1950s, Dr. Paul Zoll introduced the external cardiac pacemaker, which was a major advancement in cardiac pacing technology. This device allowed for temporary pacing of the heart and proved to be life-saving in critical situations (Dassen, Den Dulk, & Wellens, 1988).

However, it was in the 1960s that the first implantable pacemaker was developed by Dr. Rune Elmqvist and Dr. Åke Senning. This implantable device significantly improved patient outcomes and quality of life. Over the subsequent decades, various iterations and improvements were made to implantable pacemakers, incorporating advancements in microelectronics and materials (Dassen, Den Dulk, & Wellens, 1988).

The evolution of cardiac pacemakers unfolded in parallel with the advancement of microelectronics and information technology (Dassen, Den Dulk, & Wellens, 1988). Silicon-based microcontrollers and microprocessors became integral components of modern pacemakers, allowing for programmability and non-invasive adjustments, a pivotal milestone in their evolution.

With the integration of artificial intelligence and Big Data analytics in recent years, pacemakers have continued to progress. These devices are now capable of providing advanced diagnostics and personalized therapy options, further enhancing patient care (Isaksen, Baumert, Hermans, Maleckar, & Linz, 2022).

The history of cardiac pacemakers is a testament to the relentless pursuit of innovation in medical technology. The development from early external devices to sophisticated implantable AI-enhanced systems has transformed cardiac arrhythmia care, and this evolution forms the foundation for the future discussed in this article.

1.2 The role of artificial intelligence in modern cardiac pacemakers

Modern cardiac pacemakers have transcended their original purpose as simple rhythm-keeping devices to become sophisticated AI-powered systems that offer personalized therapy and enhanced diagnostics. In this section, we explore the integral role of artificial intelligence (AI) in contemporary cardiac pacemakers, including the key AI techniques and technologies utilized.

1.2.1 AI Integration in Cardiac Pacemakers. Modern cardiac pacemakers have evolved to include AI-driven components (Isaksen, Baumert, Hermans, Maleckar, & Linz, 2022). These AI systems leverage complex algorithms and data analysis techniques to enhance their functionality and adapt to the unique needs of individual patients (Isaksen, Baumert, Hermans, Maleckar, & Linz, 2022).

1.2.2 AI-Enhanced Diagnostics. AI algorithms are employed to analyse electrocardiogram (ECG) data, enabling pacemakers to detect and diagnose cardiac arrhythmias with a high degree of accuracy (Isaksen, B aumert, Hermans, Maleckar, & Linz, 2022). These AI-enhanced diagnostics ensure timely and precise identification of irregular heart rhythms.

1.2.3 Personalized Therapy. AI in pacemakers allows for the customization of therapy based on the patient's specific cardiac needs (Isaksen, Baumert, Hermans, Maleckar, & Linz, 2022). This personalization includes adjusting pacing rates and configurations to optimize heart function, all in real time.

1.2.4 Data Sensors and Interconnectivity. Data sensors embedded within pacemakers collect information on various physiological parameters. These sensors, in conjunction with AI, provide insights into a patient's heart health, which can be transmitted to healthcare providers for remote monitoring and timely interventions (Bachtiger, et al., 2020).

1.2.5 Expert Systems. Expert systems, a subset of AI, are employed to assist in the selection of optimal pacing settings and to aid in the interpretation of ECG results (Dassen, Den Dulk, & Wellens, 1988). These systems have contributed to the increased precision and efficiency of pacemaker therapies.

1.2.6 Machine Learning and Predictive Modelling. Machine learning algorithms are used to predict and manage atrial fibrillation episodes and other cardiac arrhythmias (Kim, et al., 2022). These predictive models enable timely intervention and tailored treatments.

Artificial intelligence is seamlessly integrated into modern cardiac pacemakers, enabling advanced diagnostics, personalized therapy, and real-time adaptability. These AI-driven systems represent a significant advancement in the field of cardiac arrhythmia care, offering improved patient outcomes and quality of life. This section sets the stage for a deeper exploration of the impact of AI on the future of cardiac pacemakers in the subsequent sections.

1.3 Benefits of ai in cardiac pacemakers

The integration of artificial intelligence (AI) into cardiac pacemakers offers a multitude of benefits, revolutionizing the landscape of cardiac arrhythmia care. This section highlights the advantages that AI brings to cardiac pacemakers, including improved diagnostic accuracy, personalized therapy, and remote monitoring.

1.3.1 Improved Diagnostic Accuracy. AI algorithms in cardiac pacemakers enhance diagnostic accuracy by effectively identifying and differentiating various cardiac arrhythmias (Isaksen, Baumert, Hermans, Maleckar, & Linz, 2022). The precision of AI-driven diagnostics leads to timely and accurate treatment decisions.

1.3.2 Personalized Therapy. AI enables the tailoring of therapy to each patient's specific needs, adjusting pacing rates and configurations in real-time (Isaksen, Baumert, Hermans, Maleckar, & Linz, 2022). This personalized approach optimizes the patient's heart function, resulting in improved quality of life.

1.3.3 Remote Monitoring. AI-powered pacemakers, equipped with data sensors, facilitate remote monitoring of patients' heart health (Bachtiger, et al., 2020). Physicians and healthcare providers can access real-time data, allowing for proactive interventions and reducing the need for frequent in-person visits.

1.3.4 Early Detection of Atrial Fibrillation. AI algorithms can detect and predict atrial fibrillation episodes with high sensitivity (Kim, et al., 2022). Early detection of atrial fibrillation is crucial for timely intervention and the prevention of potentially life-threatening complications.

1.3.5 Efficient Treatment Selection. AI-assisted expert systems aid in selecting optimal pacing settings and interpreting ECG results, improving the efficiency of treatment decisions (Dassen, Den Dulk, & Wellens, 1988). This ensures that patients receive the most effective therapies.

1.3.6 Data-Driven Insights. AI analyses data collected by pacemakers, providing valuable insights into a patient's heart health (Bachtiger, et al., 2020). These insights inform clinical decisions, allowing for a more comprehensive understanding of a patient's condition.

AI integration in cardiac pacemakers results in enhanced diagnostic accuracy, personalized therapy, and the ability for remote monitoring. These advantages collectively contribute to improved patient outcomes, increased quality of life, and more efficient healthcare delivery. The benefits of AI in cardiac pacemakers set the stage for the transformative impact of AI on the future of cardiac arrhythmia care, which will be further explored in this chapter.

1.4 Challenges and ethical considerations

The integration of artificial intelligence (AI) into cardiac pacemakers brings about numerous advantages, but it also presents challenges and ethical dilemmas that must be addressed. This section discusses the complexities associated with AI-powered cardiac pacemakers, including concerns related to data privacy, cybersecurity, and the potential for bias in AI algorithms.

1.4.1 Data Privacy. The use of AI in cardiac pacemakers involves the collection and analysis of sensitive patient data. Ensuring the privacy and security of this data is paramount (Bachtiger et al., 2020). Striking a balance between utilizing patient data for improved care and safeguarding individual privacy remains a significant challenge.

1.4.2 Cybersecurity. The interconnected nature of AI-powered pacemakers exposes them to potential cybersecurity threats (Bachtiger, et al., 2020). Protecting these devices from hacking and unauthorized access is essential to prevent harm to patients and their health data.

1.4.3 Bias in AI Algorithms. AI algorithms used in cardiac pacemakers must be carefully designed and tested to mitigate biases and ensure equitable care (Siontis & Friedman, The role of artificial intelligence in arrhythmia monitoring.). Bias in algorithms could lead to disparities in diagnosis and treatment, impacting patient outcomes.

1.4.4 Informed Consent. Ethical considerations extend to informed consent, as patients must be aware of the AI-driven functionalities and the potential consequences of using such technology (Sanchez de la Nava, Atienza, Bermejo, & Fernandez-Aviles, 2021). Providing comprehensive information and obtaining informed consent can be challenging.

1.4.5 Regulatory Oversight. Effective regulatory oversight is crucial to ensure the safety and effectiveness of AI-powered pacemakers (Nakamura & Sasano, 2022).

Regulatory bodies face the challenge of keeping pace with rapidly evolving technology and its applications in healthcare.

1.4.6 Long-Term Reliability. AI systems in pacemakers must demonstrate long-term reliability and resilience, as these devices are intended to operate over extended periods (Dassen, Den Dulk, & Wellens, 1988). Ensuring their continued functionality and safety is a substantial challenge.

In summary, the integration of AI into cardiac pacemakers offers numerous benefits, but it also raises ethical and practical challenges, such as data privacy, cybersecurity, and algorithmic bias. Addressing these challenges is essential to harness the full potential of AI while ensuring the safety, privacy, and equity of cardiac arrhythmia care. These considerations underscore the importance of striking a delicate balance between technological innovation and ethical responsibility.

1.5 Future directions and potential impacts

The integration of artificial intelligence (AI) into cardiac pacemakers offers promising avenues for future developments and broader implications for patient care, healthcare systems, and research. This section explores the potential future directions and impacts of AI-enhanced cardiac pacemakers.

1.5.1 *Enhanced Patient Care.* Future AI-enhanced cardiac pacemakers are expected to introduce advanced predictive algorithms that can anticipate and respond to the patient's cardiac needs in real-time (Kim, et al., 2022). This level of personalization is anticipated to optimize therapy, improve patient outcomes, and enhance the quality of life.

1.5.2 Data-Driven Research. AI-powered pacemakers are poised to generate vast datasets, providing a wealth of information for cardiovascular research and the development of novel therapies (Nakamura & Sasano, 2022). These datasets will serve as valuable resources for understanding cardiac arrhythmias and exploring innovative treatment strategies.

1.5.3 *Healthcare System Efficiency*. The remote monitoring capabilities of AI-enhanced pacemakers will contribute to the efficiency of healthcare systems by enabling proactive care, reducing the burden on hospitals, and decreasing the need for frequent in-person visits (Bachtiger, et al., 2020). This transformation is expected to lead to more streamlined healthcare delivery and resource allocation.

1.5.4 *Early Detection and Prevention*. Advancements in AI algorithms will continue to improve the early detection of cardiac arrhythmias, including atrial fibrillation (Kim, et al., 2022). Timely detection and intervention have the potential to prevent life-threatening complications and reduce healthcare costs.

1.5.5 *Regulatory Framework Development*. The evolving landscape of AI in pacemakers will necessitate the development of comprehensive regulatory frameworks to ensure patient safety, data privacy, and the quality of AI algorithms (Nakamura & Sasano, 2022). Regulatory bodies will play a pivotal role in shaping the future of this technology.

1.5.6 *Collaboration and Interconnectivity*. Future AI-enhanced pacemakers will become integral components of a broader interconnected ecosystem of medical devices (Bachtiger et al., 2020). This interconnected healthcare environment will promote collaboration among healthcare professionals and deliver a more holistic approach to patient care.

AI-enhanced cardiac pacemakers hold the potential to transform the landscape of patient care, research, and healthcare systems. These developments are expected to be characterized by increased personalization, improved patient outcomes, and enhanced healthcare efficiency. The integration of AI in cardiac pacemakers marks a significant leap toward the future of cardiology, shaped by advanced technology and its implications for better cardiac arrhythmia care.

1.6 Case studies and clinical applications

AI-powered cardiac pacemakers have found meaningful applications in clinical scenarios, offering tangible benefits to patients with cardiac arrhythmias. This section highlights specific case studies and examples that demonstrate how AI has been successfully applied to improve patient care, with reference to relevant literature.

1.6.1 *Atrial Fibrillation Detection*. Researchers have implemented AI algorithms for atrial fibrillation (AF) detection using data from cardiac implantable electronic devices (CIEDs) (Kim et al., 2022). In a case study, AI accurately predicted clinically relevant atrial high-rate episodes, enabling timely intervention and improved patient outcomes (Kim et al., 2022).

1.6.2 *Personalized Therapy*. AI-driven pacemakers have been employed to provide personalized therapy by continuously adapting pacing settings to the patient's unique cardiac needs (Nakamura & Sasano, 2022). Case studies have shown that this personalization leads to optimized heart function, enhancing the quality of life for patients (Nakamura & Sasano, 2022).

1.6.3 *Remote Monitoring and Early Intervention*. AI-enhanced pacemakers enable remote monitoring of patients' heart health. In clinical applications, these devices have facilitated early intervention in cases of cardiac arrhythmias, reducing the need for hospital visits (Bachtiger, et al., 2020). Patients benefit from improved care and reduced healthcare burdens.

1.6.4 *Predictive Analytics*. AI algorithms have been used for predictive analytics in cardiac pacemakers, forecasting atrial fibrillation episodes and other arrhythmias (Kim, et al., 2022). By identifying potential issues in advance, these applications help prevent complications and provide more effective treatments.

1.6.5 *Real-World Data Insights*. Real-world data collected by AI-powered pacemakers offer insights into patients' heart health and treatment outcomes (Nakamura & Sasano, 2022). These insights can guide clinical decisions and advance our understanding of cardiac arrhythmias in real-world settings.

These case studies and clinical applications underscore the practical impact of AI in cardiac pacemakers. They demonstrate how AI technology is enhancing patient care, enabling early detection and intervention, and contributing to a more personalized and efficient approach to managing cardiac arrhythmias. These real-world examples serve as compelling evidence of the potential benefits that AI offers to patients and healthcare providers in the field of cardiology.

1.7 Regulatory and policy considerations

The integration of artificial intelligence (AI) in cardiac pacemakers raises critical regulatory and policy considerations. This section addresses the regulatory framework and the challenges of approving and monitoring AI-powered medical devices, including pacemakers, with reference to relevant literature.

1.7.1 *Regulatory Oversight*. Ensuring the safety and effectiveness of AI-enhanced pacemakers necessitates robust regulatory oversight (Nakamura & Sasano, 2022). Regulatory bodies, such as the Food and Drug Administration (FDA) and their international counterparts, must develop and update regulatory frameworks to keep pace with rapidly evolving AI technologies.

1.7.2 *Data Privacy and Security*. Regulatory policies need to address data privacy and security in AI-powered pacemakers (Bachtiger, et al., 2020). Stringent guidelines are essential to protect patient's health data and ensure the security of interconnected devices.

1.7.3 *Informed Consent*. Policies related to informed consent are critical as patients must be fully aware of the functionalities and potential implications of AI-enhanced pacemakers (Sanchez de la Nava, Atienza, Bermejo, &

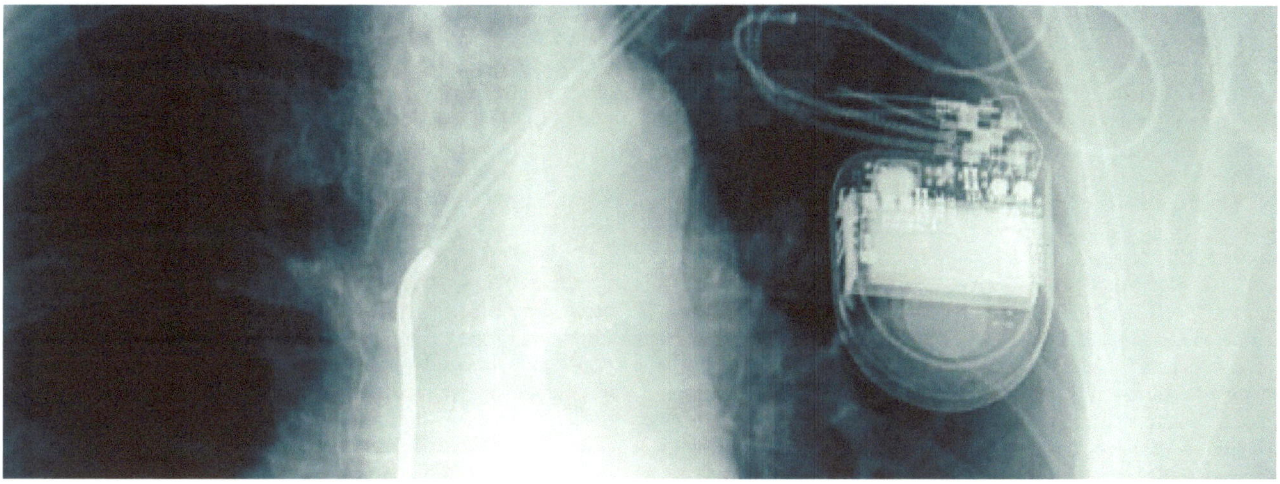

Fig. 26.7 A new pacemaker equipped with artificial intelligence will combat cardiac insufficiency The new pacemaker starts by using a neural network to analyze electrical activity in this muscle, and then it stimulates the left ventricle to synchronize it with the patient's breathing. The device has a built-in neural network that will improve heart function by 20%.

Fernandez-Aviles, 2021). Clear guidelines for informed consent will ensure that patients make informed decisions regarding their treatment.

1.7.4 *Pre-market Approval.* *AI-powered medical devices, including pacemakers, require thorough pre-market approval processes to assess their safety and efficacy (Nakamura & Sasano, 2022). Regulatory agencies should establish rigorous evaluation criteria to evaluate these devices before they enter the market.*

1.7.5 Post-market Surveillance. *Post-market surveillance is crucial for continuously monitoring the performance and safety of AI-enhanced pacemakers (Nakamura & Sasano, 2022). Regulatory bodies must establish mechanisms for ongoing device monitoring and reporting of adverse events.*

1.7.6 *International Harmonization.* Collaboration among regulatory agencies on an international scale is essential to harmonize standards for AI-powered medical devices (Nakamura & Sasano, 2022). Standardization and coordination across borders are necessary to facilitate global adoption and patient safety. The integration of AI into cardiac pacemakers presents regulatory and policy challenges related to safety, data privacy, and informed consent. Regulatory bodies must adapt to the evolving landscape of AI in healthcare to ensure that AI-powered medical devices are safe, effective, and comply with ethical standards. Addressing these considerations is critical to realizing the potential of AI-enhanced pacemakers and ensuring the well-being of patients.

Pacemaker neurons and neuronal networks

Rhythmically active neuronal networks give rise to rhythmic motor activities but also to seemingly non-rhythmic behaviors such as sleep, arousal, addiction, memory and cognition. Many of these networks contain pacemaker neurons. The ability of these neurons to generate bursts of activity intrinsically lies in voltage- and time-dependent ion fluxes resulting from a dynamic interplay among ion channels, second messenger pathways and intracellular Ca2+ concentrations, and is influenced by neuromodulators and synaptic inputs. This complex intrinsic and extrinsic modulation of pacemaker activity exerts a dynamic effect on network activity. The nonlinearity of bursting activity might enable pacemaker neurons to facilitate the onset of excitatory states or to synchronize neuronal ensembles — an interactive process that is intimately regulated by synaptic and modulatory processes. Pacemaker neurons are defined by their intrinsic ability to generate rhythmic bursting activity. The rhythmicity that emerges through voltage- and time-dependent ion fluxes in single neurons could be central to understanding how neuronal networks generate many rhythmic activities 1.••, 2.. This is an intriguing possibility, because many mammalian neuronal networks generate rhythmic activity 1.••, 2., 3.••, including networks in the neocortex, basal ganglia, thalamus, locus coeruleus, hypothalamus, ventral tegmentum area, hippocampus and amygdala.

These structures are associated with sleep, wakefulness, arousal, motivation, addiction, memory consolidation, cognition and fear. All of these neuronal networks contain rhythmically active neurons that possess ion channels crucial for generating pacemaker activity. For example, hippocampal neurons and dopaminergic ventral tegmentum area neurons possess a hyperpolarization-activated current (Ih), the 'pacemaker current' that also produces the heart beat.

Bibliography and Acknowledgement

- Ahmed FZ et al. One-month global longitudinal strain identifies patients who will develop pacing-induced left ventricular dysfunction over time: the Pacing and Ventricular Dysfunction (PAVD) Study. PloS ONE 12, e0162072 (2017). [PMC free article] [PubMed] [Google Scholar]
- Aquilina O A brief history of cardiac pacing. Images Paediatr. Cardiol. 8, 17–81 (2006). [PMC free article] [PubMed] [Google Scholar]
Athan E et al. Clinical characteristics and outcome of infective endocarditis involving implantable cardiac devices. JAMA 307, 1727–1735 (2012). [PubMed] [Google Scholar]
- Baddour LM et al. Update on cardiovascular implantable electronic device infections and their management: a scientific statement from the American Heart Association. Circulation 121, 458–477 (2010).
- Baruscotti M, Bucchi A & Difrancesco D Physiology and pharmacology of the cardiac pacemaker ("funny") current. Pharmacol. Ther. 107, 59–79 (2005). [PubMed] [Google Scholar]
- Biffi M et al. Actual pacemaker longevity: the benefit of stimulation by automatic capture verification. Pacing Clin. Electrophysiol. 33, 873–881 (2010). [PubMed] [Google Scholar]
- Bleiziffer S et al. Predictors for new-onset complete heart block after transcatheter aortic valve implantation. JACC Cardiovasc. Interv. 3, 524–530 (2010). [PubMed] [Google Scholar]
- Bogdanov KY, Vinogradova TM & Lakatta EG Sinoatrial nodal cell ryanodine receptor and Na+-Ca2 + exchanger: molecular partners in pacemaker regulation. Circul. Res 88, 1254–1258 (2001). [PubMed] [Google Scholar]
- Boriani G & Padeletti L Management of atrial fibrillation in bradyarrhythmias. Nat. Rev. Cardiol. 12, 337–349 (2015).
- Boriani G et al. Role of ventricular Autocapture function in increasing longevity of DDDR pacemakers: a prospective study. Europace 8, 216–220 (2006). [PubMed] [Google Scholar]
- Bornzin GA et al. Dual-chamber leadless intracardiac medical device with intra-cardiac extension. U.S. Patent 8634912 (2014).
- Bristow MR et al. Cardiac-resynchronization therapy with or without an implantable defibrillator in advanced chronic heart failure. N. Engl. J. Med. 350, 2140–2150 (2004).
- Cabell CH et al. Increasing rates of cardiac device infections among Medicare beneficiaries: 1990–1999. Am. Hear: J. 147, 582–586 (2004).
- Chardack WM, Gage AA & Greatbatch W A transistorized, self-contained, implantable pacemaker for the long-term correction of complete heart block. Surgery 48, 643–654 (1960). [
- Chauveau S et al. Induced pluripotent stem cell-derived cardiomyocytes provide in vivo biological pacemaker function. Circul. Arrhythmia Electrophysiol. 10, e004508 (2017). [PMC free article]
- Christoffels VM & Moorman A F Development of the cardiac conduction system: why are some regions of the heart more arrhythmogenic than others? Circul. Arrhythmia Electrophysiol 2, 195–207 (2009).
- Chua JD et al. Diagnosis and management of infections involving implantable electrophysiologic cardiac devices. Ann. Intern. Med 133, 604–608 (2000). [PubMed] [Google Scholar]
- Cingolani E & Marbán E Recreating the sinus node by somatic reprogramming: a dream come true? Rev. Esp. Cardiol. 68, 743–745 (2015). [PubMed] [Google Scholar]
- Crick SJ et al. Innervation of the human cardiac conduction system. A quantitative immunohistochemical and histochemical study. Circulation 89, 1697–1708 (1994). [PubMed] [Google Scholar]
- Dagdeviren C et al. Conformal piezoelectric energy harvesting and storage from motions of the heart, lung, and diaphragm. Proc. Natl Acad. Sci. USA 111, 1927–1932 (2014). [PMC free article]
- Dagdeviren C et al. Conformal piezoelectric systems for clinical and experimental characterization of soft tissue biomechanics. Nat. Mater. 14, 728–736 (2015). [PubMed] [Google Scholar]
- Dassen, W. R., Den Dulk, K., & Wellens, H. J. (1988). Modern pacemakers: Implantable artificial intelligence? Pacing and Clinical Electrophysiology, 11, 2114-2120.
- Edelberg JM, Aird WC & Rosenberg RD Enhancement of murine cardiac chronotropy by the molecular transfer of the human β2 adrenergic receptor cDNA. J. Clin. Invest. 101, 337–343 (1998). [PMC free article] [PubMed] [Google Scholar]
- Edelberg JM, Huang DT, Josephson ME & Rosenberg RD Molecular enhancement of porcine cardiac chronotropy. Heart 86, 559–562 (2001). [PMC free article] [PubMed] [Google Scholar]
- Eisner DA & Cerbai E Beating to time: calcium clocks, voltage clocks, and cardiac pacemaker activity. Am. J. Physiol. Heart Circ. Physiol. 296, H561–H562 (2009). [PubMed] [Google Scholar]
- Fortescue EB et al. Patient, procedural, and hardware factors associated with pacemaker lead failures in pediatrics and congenital heart disease. Hear: Rhythm 1, 150–159 (2004). [PubMed] [Google Scholar]
- Friedman D, Duncanson L, Glickstein J & Buyon J A review of congenital heart block. Images Paediatr. Cardiol. 5, 36–48 (2003). [PMC free article] [PubMed] [Google Scholar]
- Gillis AM et al. Reducing unnecessary right ventricular pacing with the managed ventricular pacing mode in patients with sinus node disease and AV block. Pacing Clin. Electrophysiol. 29, 697–705 (2006). [PubMed] [Google Scholar]
- Greenspon AJ et al. Trends in permanent pacemaker implantation in the United States from 1993 to 2009: increasing complexity of patients and procedures. J. Am. Coll. Cardiol. 60, 1540–1545 (2012). [PubMed] [Google Scholar]
- Haeberlin A et al. The first batteryless, solar-powered cardiac pacemaker. Heart Rhythm 12, 1317–1323 (2015). [PubMed] [Google Scholar]
- Harmon, D. M., Sehrawat, O., Maanja, M., Wight, J., & Noseworthy, P. A. (n.d.). Artificial intelligence for the detection and treatment of atrial fibrillation. Arrhythmia & Electrophysiology Review., 12.
- Hauser RG et al. Clinical experience with pacemaker pulse generators and transvenous leads: an 8-year prospective multicenter study. Heart Rhythm 4, 154–160 (2007). [PubMed] [Google Scholar]
- Ionta V et al. SHOX2 overexpression favors differentiation of embryonic stem cells into cardiac pacemaker cells, improving biological pacing ability. Stem Cell Rep. 4, 129–142 (2015). [PMC free article] [PubMed]
- Isaksen, J. L., Baumert, M., Hermans, A. N., Maleckar, M., & Linz, D. (2022). Artificial intelligence for the detection, prediction, and management of atrial fibrillation. Herzschrittmachertherapie+ Elektrophysiologie., 33(1), 34-41.
- Izmirly PM. et al. Clinical and pathologic implications of extending the spectrum of maternal autoantibodies reactive with ribonucleoproteins associated with cutaneous and now cardiac neonatal lupus from SSA/Ro and SSB/La to U1RNP. Autoimmun. Rev 16, 980–983 (2017). [PubMed] [Google Scholar]
- Kapoor N, Liang W, Marban E & Cho HC Direct conversion of quiescent cardiomyocytes to pacemaker cells by expression of Tbxl8. Nat. Biotechnol. 31, 54–62 (2013). [PMC free article] [PubMed] [Google Scholar]
- Karar, M. E. (2018). Robust RBF neural network–based backstepping controller for implantable cardiac pacemakers. International Journal of Adaptive Control and Signal Processing., 32(7), 1040-1051.
- Kehat I et al. Electromechanical integration of cardiomyocytes derived from human embryonic stem cells. Nat. Biotechnol. 22, 1282–1289 (2004). [PubMed] [Google Scholar]
- Larsson B, Elmqvist H, Rydén L & Schüller H Lessons from the first patient with an implanted pacemaker: 1958–2001. Pacing Clin. Electrophysiol. 26, 114–124 (2003). [PubMed] [Google Scholar]
- Leclercq C et al. A randomized comparison of triplesite versus dual-site ventricular stimulation in patients with congestive heart failure. J. Am. Coll. Cardiol. 51, 1455–1462 (2008). [PubMed] [Google Scholar]
- Leocadio, P. H. (2022). Cardiac Pacemakers: A Closer Look at Technological Innovations. Medhealth Outlook(Biotech). doi:10.6084/M9.FIGSHARE.21096010
- Liang W, Cho HC & Marban E Wnt signalling suppresses voltage-dependent Na+ channel expression in postnatal rat cardiomyocytes. J. Physiol. 593, 1147–1157 (2015). [PMC free article] [PubMed] [Google Scholar]

- Lloyd M et al. Rate adaptive pacing in an intracardiac pacemaker. Heart Rhythm 14, 200–205 (2017). [PubMed] [Google Scholar]
- Lown B & Axelrod P Implanted standby defibrillators. Circuíation 46, 637–639 (1972). [PubMed] [Google Scholar]
- Madhavan M, Mulpuru SK, McLeod CJ, Cha YM & Friedman PA Advances and future directions in cardiac pacemakers: part 2 of a 2-part series. J. Am. Coll. Cardiol. 69, 211–235 (2017).
- Mangoni ME et al. Functional role of L-type Cav1.3 Ca2+ channels in cardiac pacemaker activity. Proc. Natl Acad. Sci. USA 100, 5543–5548 (2003). [PMC free article] [PubMed] [Google Scholar]
- Marban E & Cingolani E Direct reprogramming: bypassing stem cells for therapeutics. JAMA 314, 19–20 (2015). [PubMed] [Google Scholar]
- Marban E Cardiac channelopathies. Nature 415, 213–218 (2002).
- Miake J, Marban E & Nuss HB Biological pacemaker created by gene transfer. Nature 419, 132–133 (2002). [PubMed] [Google Scholar]
- Miake J, Marban E & Nuss HB Functional role of inward rectifier current in heart probed by Kir2.1 overexpression and dominant-negative suppression. J. Clin. Invest. 111, 1529–1536 (2003). [PMC free article] [PubMed] [Google Scholar]
- Milasinovic G et al. Percent ventricular pacing with managed ventricular pacing mode in standard pacemaker population. Europace 10, 151–155 (2008). [PubMed] [Google Scholar]
- Miller MA, Neuzil P, Dukkipati SR & Reddy VY Leadless cardiac pacemakers: back to the future. J. Am. Coll. Cardiol. 66, 1179–1189 (2015). [PubMed] [Google Scholar]
- Miranda JO, Ramalho C, Henriques-Coelho T & Areias JC Fetal programming as a predictor of adult health or disease: the need to reevaluate fetal heart function. Heart Fail. Rev. 22, 861–877 (2017). [PubMed] [Google Scholar]
- Mirowski M et al. Termination of malignant ventricular arrhythmias with an implanted automatic defibrillator in human beings. N. Engí. J. Med 303, 322–324 (1980). [PubMed] [Google Scholar]
- Mirowski M, Mower MM, Staewen WS, Tabatznik B & Mendeloff AI Standby automatic defibrillator. An approach to prevention of sudden coronary death. Arch. Intern. Med 126, 158–161 (1970).
- Mond HG & Freitag G The cardiac implantable electronic device power source: evolution and revolution. Pacing Clin. Electrophysiol. 37, 1728–1745 (2014). [PubMed] [Google Scholar]
- Mond HG & Proclemer A The 11th world survey of cardiac pacing and implantable cardioverter-defibrillators: calendar year 2009 — a World Society of Arrhythmia's project. Pacing Ciin. Eiectrophysioí 34, 1013–1027 (2011). [PubMed] [Google Scholar]
- Monfredi O, Maltsev VA & Lakatta EG Modern concepts concerning the origin of the heartbeat. Physiology 28, 74–92 (2013). [PMC free article] [PubMed] [Google Scholar]
- Moss AJ et al. Cardiac-resynchronization therapy for the prevention of heart-failure events. N. Engl. J. Med. 361, 1329–1338 (2009).
- Mulpuru SK, Cha YM & Asirvatham SJ Synchronous ventricular pacing with direct capture of the atrioventricular conduction system: functional anatomy, terminology, and challenges. Heart Rhythm 13, 2237–2246 (2016). [PubMed] [Google Scholar]
- Mulpuru SK, Madhavan M, McLeod CJ, Cha YM & Friedman PA Cardiac pacemakers: function, troubleshooting, and management: part 1 of a 2-part series. J. Am. Coll. Cardiol. 69, 189–210 (2017).
- Muruve DA The innate immune response to adenovirus vectors. Hum. Gene Ther 15, 1157–1166 (2004). [PubMed] [Google Scholar]
- Nakamura, T., & Sasano, T. (2022). Artificial intelligence and cardiology: Current status and perspective. Journal of Cardiology., 79(3), 326-333.
- Parsonnet V, Driller J, Cook D & Rizvi SA Thirty-one years of clinical experience with "nuclear-powered" pacemakers. Pacing Clin. Electrophysiol. 29, 195–200 (2006). [PubMed] [Google Scholar]
- Piccini JP et al. Long-term outcomes in leadless Micra transcatheter pacemakers with elevated thresholds at implantation: results from the Micra Transcatheter Pacing System Global Clinical Trial. Hear: Rhythm 14, 685–691 (2017). [PubMed] [Google Scholar]
- Plotnikov AN et al. Biological pacemaker implanted in canine left bundle branch provides ventricular escape rhythms that have physiologically acceptable rates. Circulation 109, 506–512 (2004). [PubMed] [Google Scholar]
- Plotnikov AN et al. HCN212-channel biological pacemakers manifesting ventricular tachyarrhythmias are responsive to treatment with If blockade. Hear:Rhythm 2, 282–288 (2008). [PMC free article] [PubMed] [Google Scholar]
- Potapova I et al. Human mesenchymal stem cells as a gene delivery system to create cardiac pacemakers. Circuí. Res 94, 952–959 (2004). [PubMed] [Google Scholar]
- Protze SI et al. Sinoatrial node cardiomyocytes derived from human pluripotent cells function as a biological pacemaker. Nat. Biotechnol. 35, 56–68 (2017). [PubMed] [Google Scholar]
- Qu J et al. Expression and function of a biological pacemaker in canine heart. Circulation 107, 1106–1109 (2003). [PubMed] [Google Scholar]
- Ramos S, Matturri L, Rossi L & Rossi M Scleroatrophy of the atrioventricular junctional specialized tissue (Lenegre-Lev Disease) in chronic chagas' heart disease. Acta Cardiol. 50, 483–487 (1995). [PubMed] [Google Scholar]
- Reddy VY et al. Permanent leadless cardiac pacing: results of the LEADLESS trial. Circulation 129, 1466–1471 (2014). [PubMed] [Google Scholar]
- Ruhparwar A et al. Transplanted fetal cardiomyocytes as cardiac pacemaker. Eur. J. Cardiothorac. Surg. 21, 853–857 (2002). [PubMed] [Google Scholar]
- Saito M et al. Effect of right ventricular pacing on right ventricular mechanics and tricuspid regurgitation in patients with high-grade atrioventricular block and sinus rhythm (from the protection of left ventricular function during right ventricular pacing study). Am. J. Cardiol. 116, 1875–1882 (2015). [PubMed] [Google Scholar]
- Sanchez de la Nava, A. M., Atienza, F., Bermejo, J., & Fernandez-Aviles, F. (2021). Artificial intelligence for a personalized diagnosis and treatment of atrial fibrillation. American Journal of Physiology-Heart and Circulatory Physiology., 320(4), H1347-H1347.
- Schaldach M & Hutten H Intracardiac impedance to determine sympathetic activity in rate responsive pacing. Pacing Clin. Electrophysiol. 15, 1778–1786 (1992). [PubMed] [Google Scholar]
- Scott JS & Taylor PV Congenital AV-block: role of anti-Ro and anti-La antibodies. Springer Semin. Immunopathol. 11, 397–408 (1989).
- Shlapakova IN et al. Biological pacemakers in canines exhibit positive chronotropic response to emotional arousal. Heart Rhythm 12, 1835–1840 (2010). [PubMed] [Google Scholar]
- Singh HR, Batra AS & Balaji S Pacing in children. Ann. Pediatr. Cardiol. 6, 46–51 (2013). [PMC free article] [PubMed] [Google Scholar]
- Siontis, K. C., & Friedman, P. A. (n.d.). The role of artificial intelligence in arrhythmia monitoring. Cardiac Electrophysiology Clinics., 13(3), 543-554.
- Siontis, K. C., Noseworthy, P. A., Attia, Z. I., & Friedman, P. A. (2021). Artificial intelligence-enhanced electrocardiography in cardiovascular disease management. Nature Reviews Cardiology., 18(7), 465-478
- Sohail MR, Henrikson CA, Braid-Forbes MJ, Forbes KF & Lerner DJ Mortality and cost associated with cardiovascular implantable electronic device infections. Arch. Intern. Med 171, 1821–1828 (2011). [PubMed] [Google Scholar]
- Torrente AG et al. Burst pacemaker activity of the sinoatrial node in sodium-calcium exchanger knockout mice. Proc. Natl Acad. Sci. USA 112, 9769–9774 (2015). [PMC free article] [PubMed] [Google Scholar]
- Turakhia MP et al. Reduced mortality associated with quadripolar compared to bipolar left ventricular leads in cardiac resynchronization therapy. JACC Clin. Electrophysiol. 2, 426–433 (2016). [PubMed] [Google Scholar]
- van Hemel NM & van der Wall EE 8 October 1958, D Day for the implantable pacemaker. Neth. Heart J 16 (Suppl. 1), S3–S4 (2008).
- Vijayaraman P, Dandamudi G, Worsnick S & Ellenbogen KA Acute His-bundle injury current during permanent His-bundle pacing predicts excellent pacing outcomes. Pacing Clin. Electrophysiol. 38, 540–546 (2015).
- Walsh KB & Kass RS Regulation of a heart potassium channel by protein kinase A and C. Science 242, 67–69 (1988). [PubMed] [Google Scholar]
- Xu C, Police S, Rao N & Carpenter MK Characterization and enrichment of cardiomyocytes derived from human embryonic stem cells. Circul. Res 91, 501–508 (2002). [PubMed] [Google Scholar]

Artificial Intelligence,Wearables &Remote Monitoring for Heart Failure.Current & Future Applications

CHAPTER

27

Despite progress in understanding the pathophysiology of heart failure (HF), it remains a significant contributor to global morbidity and mortality. While continuous efforts to improve the understanding of HF over the past two decades have translated into a reduction in mortality, HF-related hospitalizations have increased over time. Moreover, with increasing complexity of HF patients and an increasing proportion of these patients receiving implantable devices, the consequent costs incurred by the United States healthcare system was $43 billion in 2020 alone and are projected to increase to $78 billion by 2030. Inpatient hospitalizations, contributing around 80 percent of the total medical costs for HF, have critical prognostic implications. HF hospitalizations are also associated with a high readmission rate, with nearly 1 in 5 patients getting readmitted within 30 days and every other patient getting rehospitalized by 6 months .Therefore, there is a pressing need for novel approaches to reduce the incidence of HF-related hospitalizations .While guideline-directed medical therapy coupled with close follow-up can reduce the incidence of HF hospitalizations, the paucity of widely available medical resources and workforce limits the ability to tackle the issue of HF hospitalizations and readmissions.

The use of wearable device technology and implantable cardiac devices have ushered in a new approach in the field of cardiovascular diagnostics in recent years, offering healthcare providers with an opportunity to monitor disease dynamics remotely and creating a window of opportunity to intervene in a timely and more effective manner—thereby potentially avoiding hospitalizations secondary to hemodynamic decompensations and adverse cardiac events .This can translate into increased healthcare system productivity in two ways (i) a higher proportion of individuals can be intervened upon remotely, leading to better outcomes, and (ii) medical resources can be judiciously diverted to individuals with advanced HF who are prone to frequent decompensations, thereby improving overall outcomes.

While the current state of wearables aims to reduce adverse cardiac events, it can be potentially utilized in a multitude of ways owing to the unique nature of the remotely collected data. Clinical variables are transmitted longitudinally over time, and the massive chunks of timestamped data can be analyzed to study disease trajectories and identify impending cardiac events.

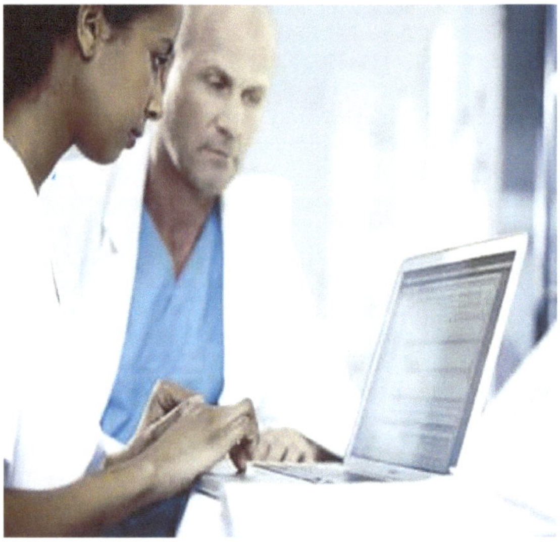

Fig.27.1 Remote monitoring Can reduce the rate of hospitalisation for patients with heart diseases

Moreover, when assembled from multiple patients, these variables can be used to phenogroup similar individuals, identify high-risk patients, develop risk and survival models, and discover new variables imparting worse prognoses. The current statistical models are limited by their ability to include finite datasets and the scientific assumptions inherent to the statistical model used. Conversely, artificial intelligence and machine learning (AI/ML) approaches require minimal assumptions, can illustrate complex, non-linear relationships as often observed in biologically derived data, and incorporate multiple variables for data modeling.

Given the above advantages, AI/ML models have been tested widely and have shown promising results when studied in conjunction with their statistical counterparts in the field of cardiovascular medicine [11]. With the evolution of AI/ML and the dawn of digital health in HF, AI/ML can be envisioned to play a significant role in improving the current understanding and monitoring of HF. In this review, we sought to introduce the concepts of AI/ML algorithms and time series analysis, the current state of wearable devices in HF, and the potential applications of AI/ML in wearable technology. Finally, we describe the limitations at present in adopting AI/ML technology, the challenges with digital data sharing and integration in healthcare, and discuss potential solutions.

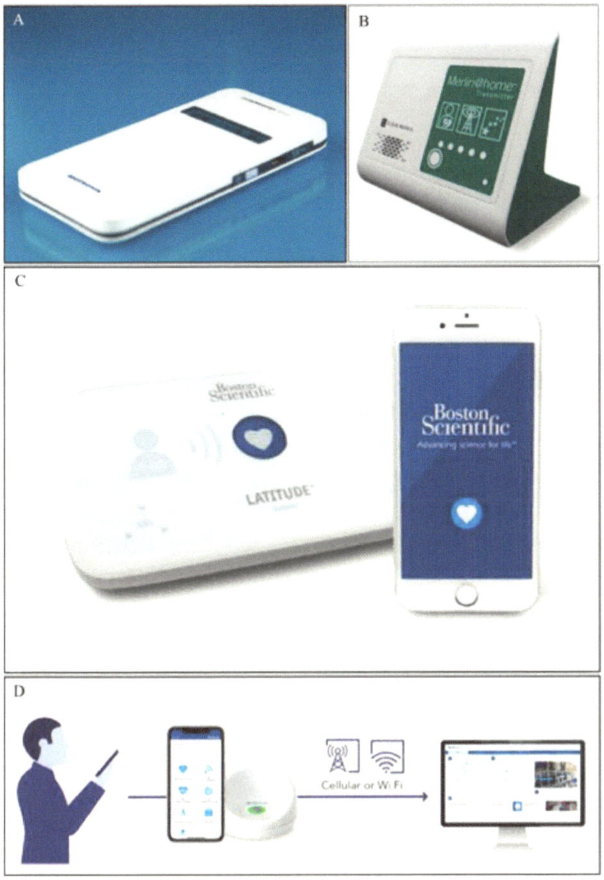

Fig.27.2 1Examples of currently available remote monitoring systems (A CardioMessenger Smart Homemonitoring system, BIOTRONIK SE & Co. KG., Berlin, Germany; B St. Jude Medical, Abbot Merlin@Home™ Transmitter;© 2022 Abbbott; C LATITUDE™ Home Monitoring System; Boston Scientific. Image provided courtesy of Boston Scientific. ©2022 Boston Scientific Corporation or its affiliates. All rights reserved D Medtronic CareLink™ System, Medtronic

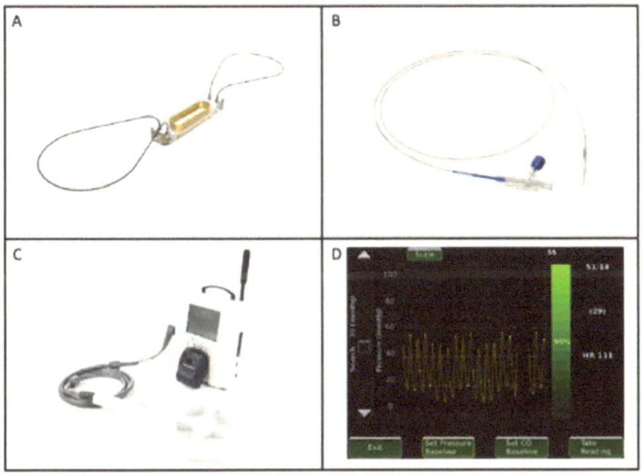

Fign 27.3 CardioMEMS™ HF system (A CardioMEMS™ PAP sensor; B CardioMEMS™ delivery catheter; C, D Hospital Electronics System CardioMEMS™ HF System Model CM3000; Micro-Electro-Mechanical HF System, Abbott Medical, Inc., Abbott Park, Illinois, USA,

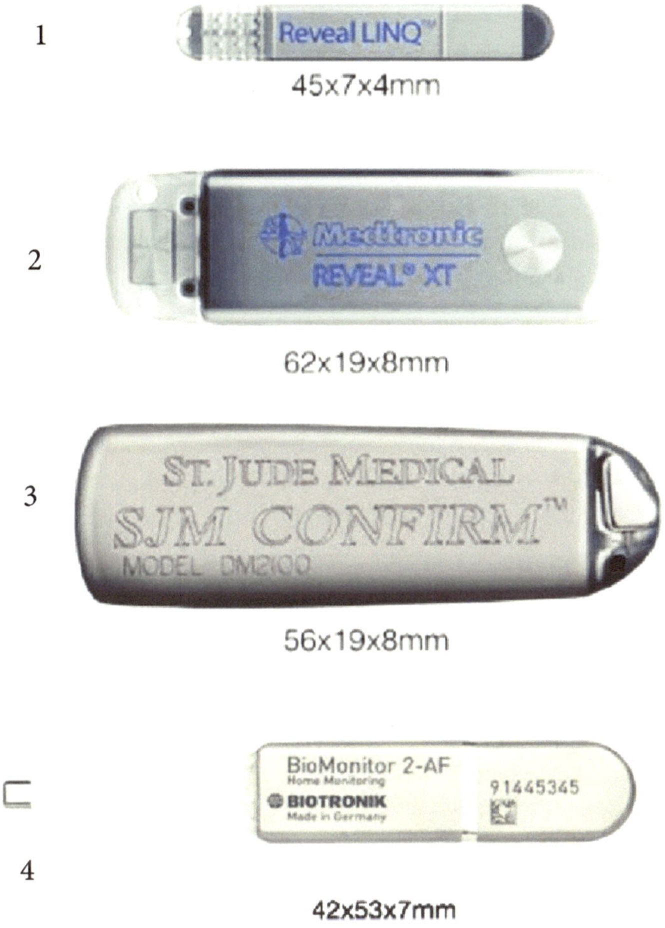

Fig.27.4 Examples of currently available insertable loop recorders 1.The Reveal LINQt ICM (Medtronic, Inc., Minneapolis, MN, USA) is much smaller than its predecessor,2. the Reveal XTt (Medtronic, Inc., Minneapolis, MN, USA), 3 .the Confirmt (Abbott Laboratories, Chicago, IL, USA) (third), and the 4. BioMonitor 2 (Biotronik, Berlin, Germany) (bottom).

Experts suggest that remote heart monitoring is one way to help people suffering from heart problems. Read on to know all the benefits of remote monitoring.

We live in a fast-paced world where digital advancements have helped in the availability of health services without having to meet the patient face to face. The current pandemic has further increased the scope and the importance of telemedicine. Experts have suggested that the efficient use of technology in heart care can help in enhancing patient safety and treatment. These technologies include telehealth, remote monitoring, wearables, cardiac imaging, etc, as well as leadless pacemakers and complex ablation (a medical procedure used to treat arrhythmia).

Teleconsultation is being widely used by patients with heart rhythm disorders (cardiac arrhythmia) who need regular medical intervention. Similarly, remote monitoring has become critical as it helps in timely intervention without visiting a hospital. This is because monitoring the heart rhythm for detecting any abnormality plays a crucial role in treating and managing arrhythmias. Cardiac arrhythmia patients who have undergone device implantations such as pacemakers especially require constant monitoring both from the doctor and patient's end. It is in such situations that technologies like remote monitoring enable heart patients with implants to monitor their heart rhythm within the comfort of their homes or anywhere in remote areas. Remote monitoring also makes it possible for the patient to transfer medical information about their condition to the doctor without meeting them in person

Role Of Remote Monitoring In Heart Patients

Remote cardiac monitoring, or remote heart monitoring, is a method by which information from a patient's implantable rhythm management device (pacemaker) can be communicated directly to the cardiac electrophysiologist (doctor) to review a patient's heart activity. It is a technological advancement for monitoring the heart rate and rhythm of patients suffering from heart conditions such as abnormal heart rhythms and heart failure. Such patients often undergo device implantation like ICD (implantable cardioverter-defibrillator) or CRT-D (cardiac resynchronization therapy defibrillator) for managing their condition. Remote monitoring involves syncing a transmitter with the implanted device to collect data on the heart's rate and rhythm. The transmitter then transfers this information through a secured website and server to the doctor. This helps the doctor, who already has access to the patient's medical history, offer the best medical advice remotely.

The newer generation devices use a technology that is inbuilt to send the device data to the patient's smartphone via Bluetooth. The phone then automatically transfers the data to the doctor enabling advanced remote monitoring capability. Thus, the patient does not need to carry the transmitter while travelling and is always connected with the doctor through his device and smartphone. This technology has been a boon to the patients, especially in situations like the current pandemic, where in-person consultations come with certain challenges.

Benefits Of Remote Monitoring

- Automatic checks for regular monitoring of the device
- Opportunity for an enhanced quality of life
- Option to reach out to the doctor directly at any time from anywhere
- Convenience and flexibility of securely communicating critical information to the doctor
- Immediately alerts the doctors via email or SMS in case of any life-threatening rhythm or any functioning abnormality in the device
- Patients with remote monitoring devices have been shown to have higher survival than those without it

Digitally empowered healthcare is the need of the hour, and remote care platforms provide patients with the convenience and comfort of accessing qualitative and quantitative healthcare from their homes. New-age technologies like remote monitoring can go a long way in ensuring patients are on top of their heart health and that their doctor is up to date on their condition at any given time.

Introduction to AI/ML and Time-Series Forecasting

As described by Arthur Samuel, ML is a field of study that provides learning capability to computers without being explicitly programmed. Learning happens when computers are fed with large amounts of data and a known output (i.e., training data). It often requires high computational power but can unravel non-linear, implicit relationships between the fed variables and the outcome of interest. Once trained, these computational algorithms can process unseen data to predict meaningful outcomes. ML has been applied widely in cardiovascular medicine in the last few years and can broadly be classified into unsupervised and supervised.

Unsupervised ML is a branch of ML whereby structured data, without any data labels, is fed into an algorithm to understand hidden relationships within data points. Data mining can be done to cluster similar data points into various groups, which can be used for phenogrouping (clustering algorithms such as k-means, hierarchical, etc.). Alternatively, association algorithms can be employed to help find relationships between data points themselves (Apriori and Equivalence Class Clustering and bottom-up Lattice Traversal (ECLAT) algorithms). Association algorithms have been applied vastly in market basket analysis to analyze customer purchasing patterns and have been recently employed in medicine. Moreover, unsupervised ML can also condense multiple data points into fewer dimensions (dimensionality reduction) via approaches such as principal component analysis. Supervised ML, on the other hand, requires an initial data labeling of the structured data, which is then fed through training algorithms to compute relationships between variables and an outcome of choice. The algorithms can be trained to either classify an output to predefined discrete categories (classification algorithms) or quantify relationships between variables (regression algorithms) The above-mentioned techniques have been applied in the field of HF for initial diagnosis, modeling disease prognoses, goal-directed medical therapy (GDMT) optimization, predicting outcomes for device therapy interventions, etc. Deep learning (DL) is a branch of AI/ML that can process large complex data, such as those derived from medical images or videos.. DL usually takes the form of neural networks consisting of multiple nodes (i.e., neurons) arranged into an input, multiple hidden layers, as well as an output layer. When a trained neural network is fed with data, specific neurons in the input layer are activated, which pass the command to a chain of neurons in the hidden layers and then the output layer; the command becomes increasingly complex as the information is passed along successive layers. Training of DL algorithms can be done in both unsupervised and supervised fashion and has been used widely in cardiovascular medicine to automate medical images interpretation, create multimodal prognostic models, as well as uncover unknown and undiscovered associations between phenotypes and a particular condition/outcome. For example, a DL algorithm has also been shown to be superior to sonographers for assessing left ventricular ejection fraction on 2-D echocardiography in the recently concluded EchoNet randomized controlled trial .

While these AI/ML techniques have been applied in the field of cardiovascular medicine, traditionally, data analysis via AI/ML usually has not taken into account the dimension of time. Continuously transmitted data via remote monitoring at regular intervals gives the opportunity to plot variables as a function of time and forecast future variables based on the prior trends, referred to as time series forecasting The concept of time series forecasting is not new and has been applied in fields outside of medicine. Modeling can be done to forecast the value of one variable independently (univariate) or as a function of multiple dependent variables (multivariate) with time. Statistical models developed for time-series analysis posit multiple assumptions about the data. Stationarity is a vital conceptin time-series analysis, which implies that the data's statistical properties (e.g., mean, variance, etc.) do not change with time. Real-world data is usually non-stationary, exhibiting trends, seasonality, or cyclical patterns when plotted chronologically.While traditional statistical models such as Autoregressive moving average (ARMA) necessitate the time-series data to beconverted to stationary data before model construction via approaches such as differencing and detrending, newer statistical and AI/ML models can be employed with non-stationary time series . Moreover, recurrent neural network (RNN)-based approaches that can handle large amounts of non-linear data have been described, which could prove ideal for the terabytes of data transmitted via remote monitoring. In contrast to traditional neural networks, which are strictly feed-forward neural networks, the output of the hidden layers of neurons can be fed back into neurons in RNNs, which is used in time-series forecasting . This hidden state output is then successfully combined with new input to generate the final output.During the training phase, the predicted output is then compared with the ground truth to calculate the error. Backpropagation is then done to calculate the gradients and adjust the weights of the layers for accurate prediction. RNNs might suffer from the 'vanishing' or 'exploding' gradient problem due to an exponential decrease or increase during backpropagation, respectively, leading to decreased performance of the model. Hence, RNNs can function well with a limited set of sequential data, with decreasing accuracy with increasing data. To solve this problem, Long short-term memory (LSTM) and gated recurrent units (GRU) models have been described, which can retain longer sequential data by the virtue of 'gates'

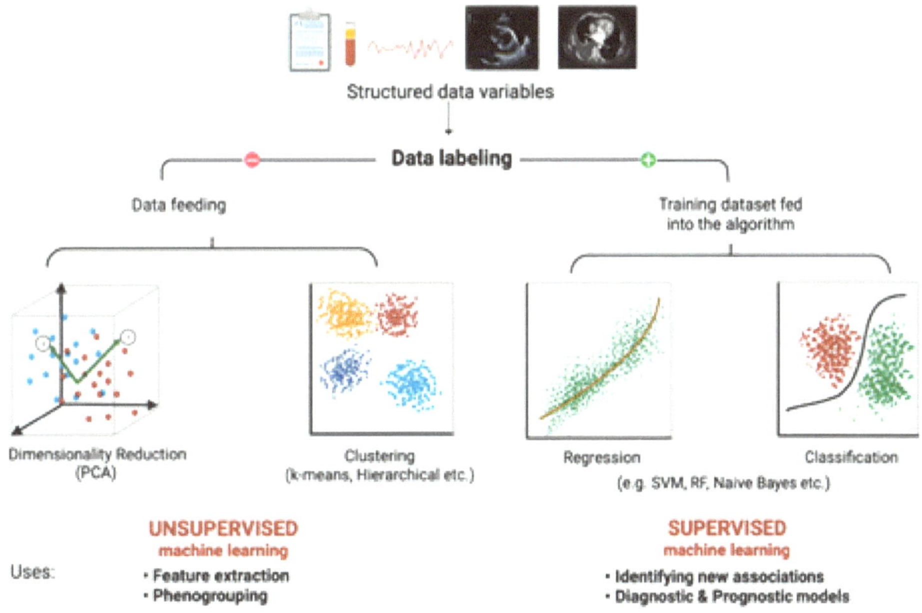

Fig. 27.5 An overview of unsupervised and supervised machine learning. Labeled data can be processed in an unsupervised fashion (i.e., without training data) to understand relationships between variables, clustering, etc. Supervised machine learning, on the other hand, requires a training dataset, which can be used to either infer quantitative relationships (regression models) or classify data into training outcomes (classification). Abbreviations: SVM: Support Vector machines; RF: Random Forest. Adapted from Gautam et al

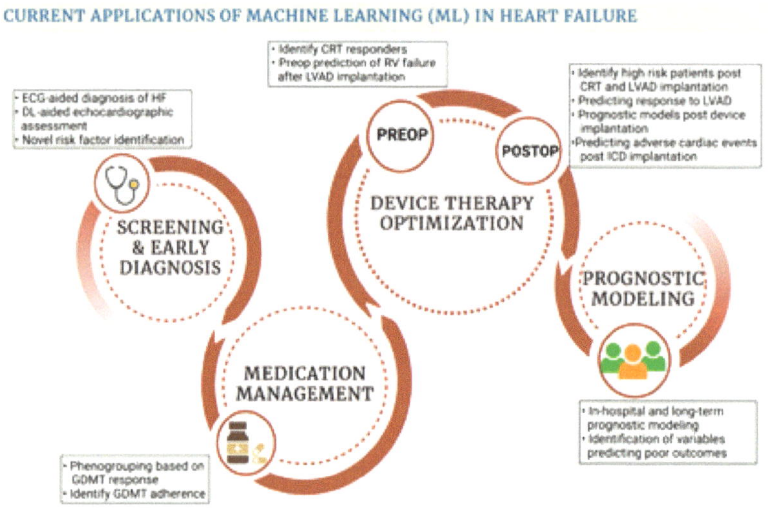

Fig. 27.6 Current applications of machine learning in Heart Failure. Abbreviations: CRT: Cardiac resynchronization therapy; DL: Deep learning; ECG: Electrocardiogram; GDMT: Guideline-directed medical therapy; ICD: Implantable cardiac defibrillator; LVAD: Left Ventricular Assist Device; RV: Right Ventricle.

Table 27.1 AI algorithms used in time-series forecasting.

Algorithms	Description
Support Vector Regression	Supervised ML algorithm based on support vector machines, whereby creation of hyperplane is done in order to minimize the error and maximizes the margin.
k-Nearest Neighbors	Supervised classifier or regression ML algorithm whereby the test variable is classified based on its proximity to k number of data points.
Recurrent Neuralnetwork (RNN)	DL algorithm whereby data is passed via multiple layers of neurons (consisting of input, hidden and output layers), with the output from one layer being looped back into the hidden layer, in order to predict sequential data. Associated with the vanishing and exploding gradient problem due to exponential decrease or increase of the gradient during backpropagation, leading to minimal change in adjusted weights in the earlier layers, thereby translating into a short-term memory which can limit its role in larger datasets.
Long short-term memory	Special form of RNN's (DL algorithms) useful for larger datasets, consisting of a memory unit, comprised of three gates. The forget gate is responsible for screening out irrelevant data, and the output gate is responsible for generation of the new cell state and the hidden state, and the process is repeated over again to yield the final model. Complex model, requiring higher computational power.
Gated recurrent units	Another form of RNN's (DL algorithms) consisting of two gates-update and the reset gate. The update gate decides the information to be omitted and added and the reset gate is to decide on how much past information can be omitted. Simpler model than LSTM, requiring lesser computational power, while retaining the long-term memory.

Abbreviations: DL: Deep learning; LSTM: Long short-term memory; ML: Machine learning; RNN: Recurrent Neural Network.

The Current State of Telemonitoring, Wearable, and Implantable Device Technology in HF

Trials aimed at monitoring patients via telephonic interventions and wearables have been attempted in the last decade, albeit with limited success. The Telemedical Interventional Management in Heart Failure (TIM-HF) trial enrolled 710 patients with a left ventricular ejection fraction (LVEF) of ≤35%, NYHA class II-III symptoms, and a 2-year history of HF decompensation and found no differences between telemonitoring (weight, blood pressure, and heart rhythm data transmission) and standard care in cardiovascular and all-cause mortality or hospitalizations at a median follow-up of 26 months .More recently, the TIM-HF2 trial showed superior results for web-based remote patient management than routine care in reducing HF hospitalizations and associated mortality . In contrast to TIM-HF, the TIM-HF2 study excluded patients with depression and recruited patients who had been hospitalized in the last 12 months. Of note, the investigators also broadened their selection criteria to include patients with LVEF ≤ 45% or LVEF ≥ 45% on diuretics. Their structured remote intervention was associated with a smaller proportion of days lost from unplanned HF-related hospital admissions (HR 0.80, 95% CI 0.65–1.00; p = 0.0460) and had lower all-cause mortality (HR 0.70 [95% CI 0.50–0.96], p = 0.28) compared to usual care . Furthermore, the Better Effectiveness After Transition- Heart Failure (BEAT-HF) trial, utilizing predischarge HF education coupled with regular telephone visits and telemonitoring, did not show any statistical difference in reducing 180-day readmission rates in patients with HF (HR: 1.03 [95% CI, 0.88–1.20]; p = 0.74) . Although telemonitoring was the backbone of the above trials, the recent emergence of wearables and novel sensor devices that can accurately detect intrinsic hemodynamic changes have demonstrated the potential to change the remote monitoring landscape.Most representative studies of wearables in HF patients have involved pedometers and actigraphy devices which, by analyzing the pattern of physical activity, can enable patients and physicians to engage in lifestyle modification and therapy modulation . Moreover, several emerging technologies have been tested in monitoring HF readmissions. While thoracic impedance monitoring via implantable cardioverter defibrillators (ICDs) has been shown to be a better predictor than daily weight monitoring for assessing pulmonary fluid status, studies of impedance-derived fluid index (Optivol index) for predicting HF hospitalizations in the ambulatory setting have yielded conflicting results . Remote dialectic sensing (RedS) has been recently proposed for monitoring pulmonary congestion in HF.

In a recent analysis, patients were provided with a vest, which they wore for a period of 90 s every day. Electromagnetic analysis of tissue dielectric properties, reflecting the degree of pulmonary congestion, was used to guide clinical management. ReDS-guided management decreased 90-day readmissions by 87% (HR: 0.07 [95% CI: 0.01–0.54], p < 0.01). Notably, discontinuation of ReDS increased readmissions by 79% (HR: 0.11 [95% CI: 0.012–0.88], p < 0.05) .

Similar to wearables, implantable devices, such as pacemakers, ICDs, and intracardiac pressure sensors, also generate an enormous amount of data that can be used to create algorithm-based risk prediction models aimed at early diagnosis treatment selection. For example, the MultiSENSE (Multisensor Chronic Evaluation in Ambulatory Heart Failure Patients) study tested the HeartLogic multisensor index and alert algorithm for predicting HF exacerbation . In 900 patients receiving cardiac resynchronization therapy, the HeartLogix algorithmic analysis of sensor data (the first and third heart sounds, thoracic impedance, respiration rate, ratio of respiration rate to tidal volume, heart rate, and patient activity) yielded a sensitivity of 70% (95% CI: 55.4–82.1%) for early detection of HF exacerbation with an unexplained alert rate of 1.47 (95% CI: 1.32 to 1.65) per patient-year, the median time from alert onset to a HF exacerbation being 34 days (interquartile range: 19.0 to 66.3 days). In addition, the algorithm's performance was assessed across a range of thresholds, providing an opportunity to customize its use for the individual patient.

The latest addition to the family of remote monitoring devices has been the implantable pulmonary artery and the left atrial pressure sensors, with the benefits of remote monitoring of pulmonary artery pressures (PAPs) in patients with HF being confirmed in multiple trials. More recently, with the VECTOR-HF trial showing positive results on the safety and usability of a digital, leadless intra-atrial pressure sensor (V-LAP system) in HF patients, the field is bound to grow . Moreover, with data being transmitted via multiple digital devices, parameters can be clubbed together via AI/ML techniques to tailor to better outcomes. Although remote PAP, LAP, and other monitoring devices have high costs and technical limitations, this can also be amenable to an AI/ML solution by developing algorithms from previous PAP-monitored patient data to 'learn' who benefits most, thus enabling targeting the intervention to a specific population.

Current Applications of AI/ML in Remote Monitoring via Wearables and Implantable Cardiac Devices

While AI/ML has increasingly been used for detecting and diagnosing a variety of cardiac diseases, its application to remote monitoring data is relatively new. While remote monitoring has been utilized for the detection of cardiac arrhythmias and for coronary vascular events, cutting-edge clinical applications in the realm of HF include the use of artificial neural networks trained with cardiac function parameters (QT interval, heart rate variability, seismocardiogram signals) from wearables to accurately identify early decompensation of HF, identify patients at higher risk of sudden cardiac death (SCD), etc. Accurate identification of pathophysiological dynamics may be helpful as it allows for the institution and optimization of medical therapies before the onset and progression of symptoms, thereby reducing the risk of HF hospitalizations and readmissions. Additionally, early identification of patients at high risk of SCD may allow for earlier intervention, translating into reduced morbidity and mortality.

Novel wearable devices have been integrated with AI/ML, with the goal of investigating surrogates for pulmonary vascular congestion, thereby leading to earlier detection of clinical decompensation. A pilot study on 45 patients by Inan et al. investigated the feasibility of wearable seismocardiogram patches to proactively assess and manage patients with HF . The researchers used wearable seismocardiogram patches to measure vibrations of the chest wall in response to each heartbeat. At-home hemodynamic changes were estimated with the 6-min walk test. The authors used an analytic graph mining–based approach to then quantify and compare the similarity of the structure of seismocardiogram signals before and after the 6-min walk test (graph similarity score). Since the decompensated (hospitalized) HF patients were unable to meet the increased cardiac requirement from the walking test, the changes in the graph similarity score (GSS) for decompensated HF patients were significantly lower than for compensated (outpatient) HF patients. This study showed that a small, wearable device could be used to identify HF states and preemptively treat patients before they required hospitalizations.

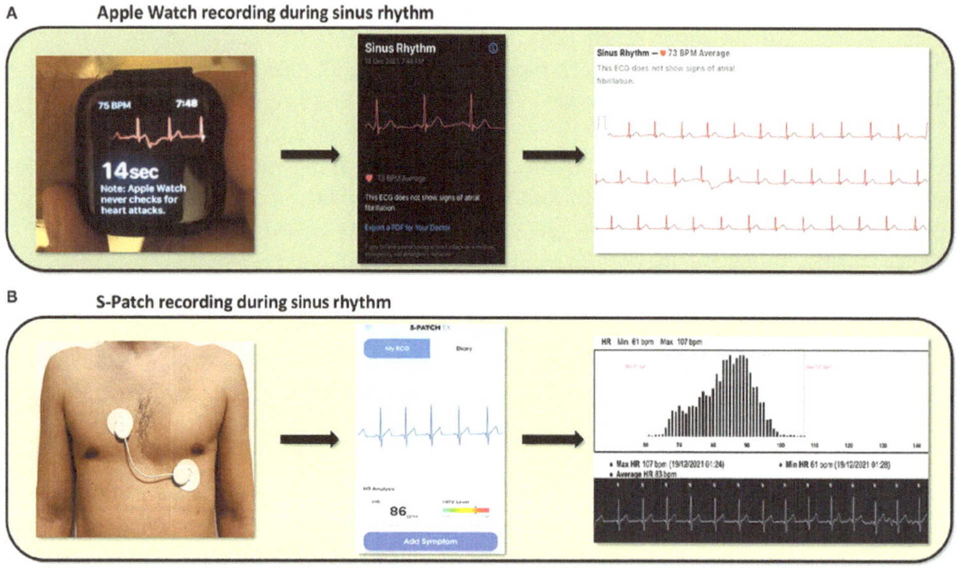

Fig. 27.7 Cardiac rhythm recordings derived from a smartwatch (Apple Watch) and a patch (S-Patch), (A) From left to right, the images show the process of data collection from an Apple Watch, the ECG presentation in the respective smartphone application and the final report, featuring a possible diagnosis, (B) From left to right, the images show the same process captured by the wearable S-Patch.

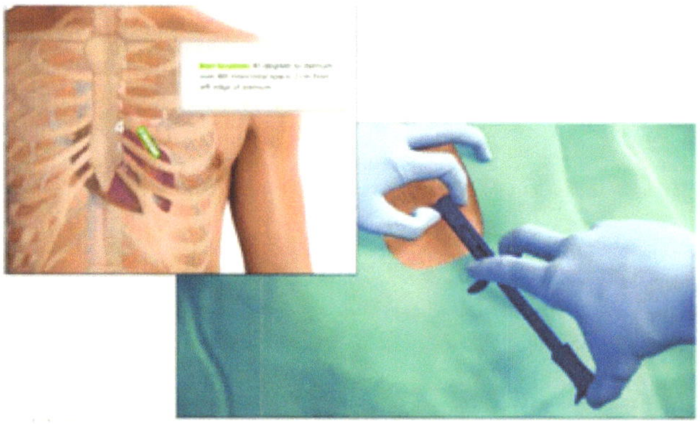

Fig. 27.8 The Reveal LINQt(Medtronic, Inc., Minneapolis, MN, USA) device may be implanted within minutes. During theprocedure, the skin is prepped/draped in a sterile fashion. A scalpel tool makes an incision at the fourth intercostal space, andthe ICM device is inserted into the subcutaneous space. The incision may be sealed with skin glue, staples, or suture material

More recently, using seismocardiogram-derived signals in 20 patients, good accuracies were reported for vasodilator-induced acute changes in mean pulmonary artery pressure (mPAP) and pulmonary capillary wedge pressure (PCWP) by the same group (root mean squared error of 2.5 mmHg and 1.9 mmHg for changes in mPAP and PCWP in the training dataset and 2.7 mmHg and 2.9 mmHg in the validation data sets, respectively), thus paving the way for easier tracking of monitoring of intracardiac hemodynamics . Moreover, a recent hierarchical clustering algorithm developed by Burton et al. aiming to identify phenogroups with elevated left ventricular end-diastolic volume (LVEDV) used electromechanical data collected via photoplethysmography and CorVista phase space analysis, thereby providing insights into the characteristics leading towards phenotypes of myocardial dysfunction .

Furthermore, Stehlik et al. investigated the accuracy and applications of noninvasive wearable monitoring in detecting HF exacerbations [39]. A total of 100 subjects (74 with HF with reduced ejection fraction and 26 with HF with preserved ejection fraction) were fitted with a wearable sensor that collected continuous ECG waveform, skin impedance, temperature, and patient activity data. Cloud-based analytic platforms used similarity-based modeling to evaluate the cumulated study subject data. The personalized AI/ML platform and wearable sensor predicted hospitalization secondary to HF exacerbation within a 10-day positive window with a sensitivity of 76% and a specificity of 85%, thus demonstrating the viability of timely detection and early intervention of HF with the use of AI/ML and wearables.

Apart from predicting HF decompensation, research has also focused on predicting sudden cardiac death (SCD) events in patients with HF . Acharya et al. developed a sudden cardiac death index (SCDI) utilizing discrete wavelet transform (DWT) and nonlinear AI/ML analysis of ECG signals four minutes before SCD onset . The ECG signals were retrospectively obtained from Holter monitor data and the normal sinus rhythm database. At one-minute intervals, nonlinear features were isolated from DWT decomposed ECG signals. Support Vector Machines, Decision Trees, and k-Nearest Neighbors were used to differentiate between normal variant ECG signals and ECG signals associated with SCD subjects. The most distinguishing features were then combined to form a single integrated index (i.e., SCDI), which was able to predict impending SCD with an accuracy of 92.1%, 98.7%, 93.4%, and 92.1% at one, two, three, and four minutes, respectively. More recently, using a prospective multicenter registry, Kim et al. used pacemaker-collected data to predict clinically relevant atrial high-rate episodes (AHREs). With data from 721 patients without a history of atrial fibrillation or flutter, AI/ML-based models were able to outperform logistic regression-based models in predicting clinically relevant AHREs (AUC for logistic regression and XgBoost 0.669 and 0.745, respectively) .

Additionally, DeMazumder et al. used ML algorithms (EntropyX) at the signal processing level to adapt to the signal noise and extract physiological dynamics with very highaccuracy and precision. In a prospective multicenter observational study of 852 HF patients in sinus rhythm, the EntropyX of cardiac repolarization (EntropyXQT) strongly predicted appropriate ICD shock as well as all-cause mortality, above and beyond a comprehensive set of conventional predictors and risk scores .Unlike conventional measures of variability, EntropyX analysis of a time series does not require equally sampled time intervals or preprocessing of data and is less sensitive to the presence of outlying points such as ectopic beats or noise. EntropyX analysis of physiological dynamics provides unique insight into subclinical physiological deterioration such as early changes in metabolic and redox properties that cannot be detected by contemporary clinical measures . This new paradigm has also proven important for highly accurate rhythm discrimination, including a ROC area under the curve of 98% for identifying very brief paroxysms of atrial fibrillation and outperforming ICD rhythm discrimination algorithms in a prospective multicenter study.

More recently, the DeepEntropy algorithm was developed for ML analysis of sinus rhythm during sleep to identify ostensibly healthy adults who will and will not develop new-onset atrial fibrillation over the next ten years. In a multicenter derivation study of 2807 community adults, the incorporation of DeepEntropy into a multivariate prediction model added major independent prognostic value to conventional risk factors and scores for predicting the incidence of new-onset AF . Whereas the performance of conventional risk predictors are limited in diverse populations, a subsequent validation study in the Multi-Ethnic Study of Atherosclerosis demonstrated that DeepEntropy performs well regardless of age, sex, race/ethnicity, etc., and has potential for broad application . Ultimately, randomized controlled trials are needed to definitively establish the clinical utility of AI/ML analysis of physiological time series for improving outcomes. With the initial success of wearable technology and the incorporation of AI/ML in pilot studies, multiple trials are underway employing AI/ML to further widen the scope of wearables in HF management, such as GDMT optimization, medication adherence, etc.. Moreover, innovative AI/ML algorithms are currently being designed utilizing ECG and acoustic recordings recorded by electronic stethoscopes, which can accurately detect changes in pulmonary artery pressures in patients with an implanted CardioMEMS device . If successful, such an approach allowing for accurate monitoring of HF dynamics via wearables can help alleviate the burden on outpatient healthcare providers while enabling the creation of 'personal' patient profiles. Analysis of troves of remotely monitored individual patient data can allow for delineation of daily patterns in activity, medication adherence, cardiac hemodynamics, etc., which will help patients by allowing for the creation of personalized health management plans, and simultaneously physicians by providing zettabytes of reliably collected real-world data, which can be used to further HF research.

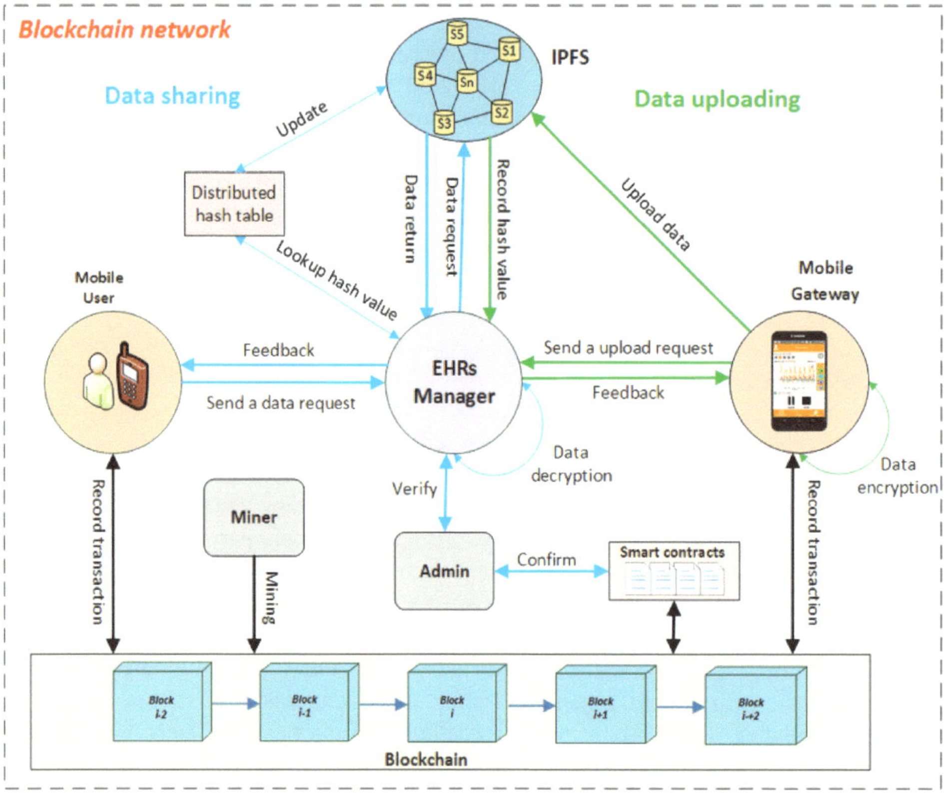

Fig. 27.9 Remote monitoring data, along with data from EHRs and medical images stored on local computers, can be transferred to a cloud computing network, allowing for data integration. Blockchain technology (a) can allow for secure data transfers between systems and allow for data decentralization. Such pools of data, once established, can be used to train powerful ML algorithms, which can be used to guide remote interventions and identify patients needing loser follow-ups. Abbreviations: EHRs: Electronic health records; GDMT: Guidelines directed medical therapy; ML: Machine learning.

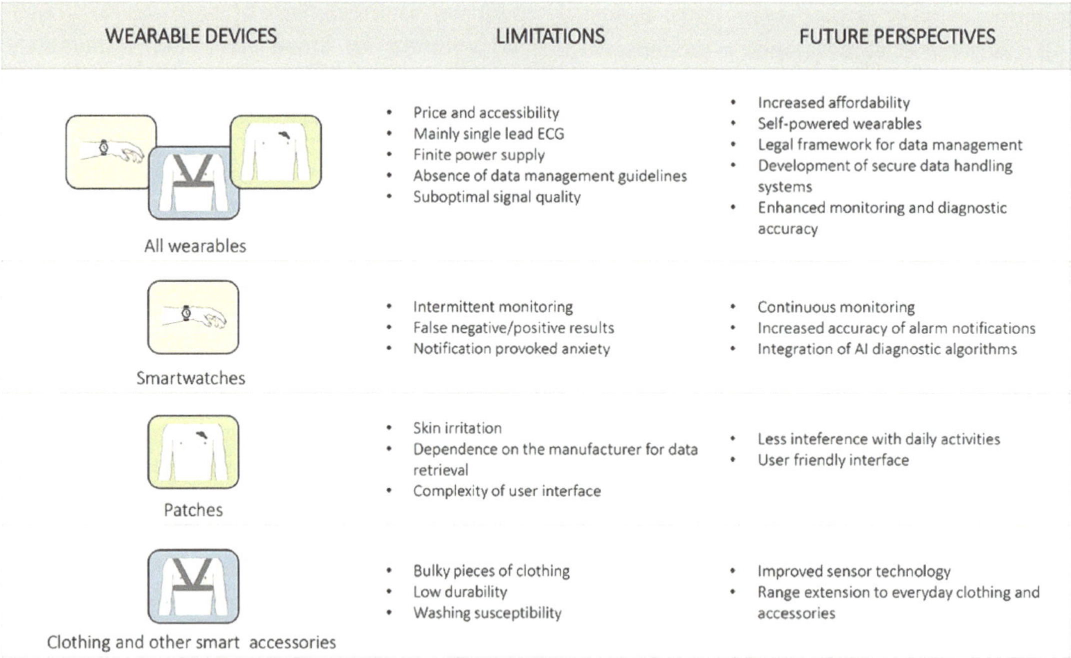

Fig.27.10 Main limitations and future perspectives of wearable devices for heart rhythm monitoring are presented. Specific information for each category of wearable devices is presented separately.

Table 27.2 Ongoing clinical trials investigating the application of digital devices and machine learning in HF cohorts.

Clinical Trial	Wearable/Implantable	Description	Current Stage
Activity-Aware Prompting to Improve Medication Adherence in Heart Failure Patients	Smartphone	Designing ML-based software algorithms aimed at analyzing daily behavior and to utilize it to improve medication compliance among patients with HF	Recruitment complete
AIM-POWER study	BiovitalsHF	To study the effectiveness of a cloud-based platform (BiovitalsHF) collecting data using remote wearable sensors in improving GDMT adoption among patients with HF.	Recruiting
ASE-INNOVATE study	Multiple digital health devices	To study the effectiveness of technology-based visitations (outpatient visit supplemented by focused echocardiography, ECG, and vitals collected by digital devices) on long term cardiovascular outcomes.	Unclear
Heart Failure Monitoring With Eko Electronic Stethoscopes (CardioMEMS)	Eko electronic stethoscopes (AI based)	Designing a ML-based algorithm which can correlate Eko stethoscope acoustic and ECG recordings with the pulmonary artery pressure measurements taken via the CardioMEMS device	Recruiting
Interactive Patient's Assistant-LUCY	Implanted CRT and ICD devices	Designing a ML-based algorithm based on remotely monitored data to determine the parameters in CRT/ICD requiring an ambulatory device clinic visit, overall	Unclear
LINK-HF2 study	Continuous remote monitoring via wearable sensors	To study the impact of remote monitoring on 90-day HF hospitalizations rate in patients with HF.	Recruiting
Validation of Ejection Fraction and Cardiac Output Using Biostrap Wristband	Wristband with photoplethysmgraphy sensor	Correlation of ejection fraction and cardiac output measured via AI-powered translation of wristband PPG recordings with echocardiogram and pulmonary artery catheter measurements.	Recruiting
VESTA study	Wearable sensor data	Validation of ML algorithm for early detection of HF events via multi-parametric sensor data.	Not yet recruiting

Abbreviations: AI: Artificial Intelligence; ECG: Electrocardiogram; CRT: Cardiac resynchronization therapy; GDMT: Guideline directed medical therapy; HF: Heart Failure; ICD: Implantable cardiac defibrillator; PPG: Photoplethysmography.

Data Extraction and Storage

Currently, medical information is stored in local data centers with a fixed computational capacity which requires extensive resources for storage expansion, data transmission, and integration across platforms. With remote monitoring likely to play a significant role in guiding cardiovascular care in the future, cloud computing solutions can bridge the unmet need for data storage and integration solutions for such large amounts of data. Cloud computing can accommodate terabytes of data while allowing for quick data retrieval from multiple sources (remote monitoring data, EHRs, medical images, etc.) .Apart from integration at the patient level, 'data decentralization' can help medical researchers by potentially creating more extensive repositories of data for improved disease modeling and forecasting. Moreover, while tons of data are stored in electronic health records, such troves of data are not readily employable and often need to be converted and restricted before being fed into an ML algorithm. More recently, Aslan et al. devised a convolutional neural network (CNN) based approach to convert numerical data into images, which can then be accurately classified for the purpose of diagnosing HF . Such an approach, along with data extraction methods that use natural language processing algorithms, can help expand the current data pool and thereby lead to improved performance of the current diagnostic and prognostic models.

Data Quality Challenges

Data privacy, sometimes also referred to as information privacy, is an area of data protection that concerns the proper handling of sensitive data, including personal data or other confidential data. Researchers are confronted with the issue of privacy when transmitting data over the internet. Data transmission over the internet is susceptible to cyber-attacks, misuse, tampering, etc., and technologies ensuring data encryption and safe data transmission need to be established. Blockchain technology, though initially introduced in cryptocurrency, can facilitate data decentralization, interoperability, and data integrity across institutions . Electronic computer code-based agreements (i.e., smart contracts) can help improve data transparency and allow for easier data sharing between parties while ensuring data integrity, owing to the blockchain-based timestamped nature of the data .

There is also a lack of regulations on using patient health information generated via consumer-owned wearables by third-party companies. Confidentiality is paramount regarding data transmission and sharing, with data sharing being protected by the Health Insurance Portability and Accountability Act (HIPAA) regulations . The HIPAA regulations currently cover physicians and associated business entities, but concrete guidelines are necessary to direct data handling by third-party companies .

Challenges to Digital Technology Adoption

There is a potential for a 'digital divide' with the dawn of wearable sensors in HF. Apart from the clinical heterogeneity observed in patients with HF, socioeconomic status (SES) plays a paramount role, with studies showing more than a 50% increase in HF risk with lower SES . While wearable technology has the potential to transform cardiovascular care, it can increase health inequity, owing to the need for adequate digital affordability and literacy associated with wearable technology. For instance, in a survey of 4551 adults in the United States, individuals with a higher annual household income (defined as \$75,000 or more per year) were more likely to use wearables than individuals with a household income of less than \$20,000 per year (OR 2.6; 95% CI [1.39–4.86], $p < 0.001$) . Incorporating device-related costs into healthcare insurance benefit packages is crucial for narrowing the digital divide based on economic disparities. Moreover, loaner digital wearables can help mitigate the financial implications on healthcare, provided checks are in place to ensure the return of the digital devices. The novel iShare program utilizing loaner iPhones and smartwatches in 200 patients demonstrated augmented participation of patients without access to smartphones in remote monitoring following an acute myocardial infarction. However, with a modest return percentage of 72% at the end of the 30-day follow-up period, a system of checks and incentives is needed for its widespread implementation . Nevertheless, the cost-effectiveness of wearable devices coupled with AI modalities needs to be studied in HF, with such devices being previously proven to be cost-effective in the screening of other cardiac pathologies, such as atrial fibrillation .

With pulmonary arterial pressure monitoring being shown to be cost-effective in multiple studies, complementing remote monitoring with AI is likely to improve the cost–benefit ratio, although it yet needs to be proven across a spectrum of population cohorts.

A lack of digital literacy can not only impede the adoption of digital technology but can also impact patient compliance with data transmission. Not surprisingly, individuals possessing college degrees or greater have been shown to be more receptive to the adoption of digital technology when compared to people with a lesser educational background .Moreover, elderly individuals are less likely to adopt the usage of digital technology and also to comply with regular data transmission . While it is essential to devise ways to improve the usage of wearables in this at-risk population, how these measures can be implemented in patients with neurocognitive disorders and visual/hearing impairment remains challenging.

Challenges Inherent to AI/ML Model Development and Processing

Apart from intensive computational power, model training requires diversely represented data and well-thought-of model assumptions. If overlooked, the above factors risk introducing implicit selection bias in terms of gender, race, socioeconomic status, etc. .

For instance, Obermeyer et al. described their observations on a healthcare algorithm aimed at recognizing the medical needs to be preferentially skewed towards white patients. By using healthcare spending as a proxy for the severity of medical illness, the algorithm underestimated the number of sicker black patients by more than half . Careful data curation and representation in the model pre-processing stage can help mitigate some of the inherent bias.

While AI/ML models have the advantage of incorporating more horizontal data, the model's predictive power starts decreasing with increasing dimensional complexity, often referred to as the 'Hughes phenomenon' . Multi-dimensional data, when fed, leads to a lower degree of bias but a high variability. This leads to higher accuracy when tested internally but a dismal external performance. Smaller retrospective databases are especially susceptible to overfitting, given the higher rate of data missingness and irregularities, leading to additional noise being incorporated into the model. Moreover, data mining approaches on national database registries face the unique challenge of a high degree of dimensional heterogeneity, predisposing to overfitting. While solutions such as k-fold cross-validation and regularization have been proposed to tackle this challenge, feature extraction techniques such as principal component analysis can be undertaken to condense high-dimensional data into fewer dimensions responsible for maximum variance in the dataset, thereby allowing for better generalizability. Furthermore, feature selection can be undertaken to eliminate noise and incorporate only the features accounting for the variance in output. While these techniques have been used in studies variably to overcome overfitting, external validation has been done only infrequently. A recent systematic review reported that >90% of studies not performing an external validation of their AI/ML algorithms, thereby indicating an urgent need to test for generalizability, albeit in prospectively trials, before its implementation in the clinical practice .

Despite the abundance of clinical trials on a yearly basis, inadequate infrastructure, lack of physician training, and incentives are significant hurdles to the process. Moreover, industry-based sponsorship for clinical trials might complicate matters further, as data withholding and the creation of proprietary algorithms might be undertaken for industrial purposes . With a push from the International Committee of Medical Journal Editors (ICMJE) and the National Institute of Health to encourage data sharing and the formulation of repositories such as BigData@Heart, and SWEDEHEART in recent years, the unification of data resources leading to more impactful clinical research might be attainable in the near future .Furthermore, some AI/ML models suffer from the black box problem, which refers to the limited interpretability of the AI/ML models, with the models becoming increasingly uninterpretable with the increasing complexity of AI/ML algorithms.

This becomes a problem in healthcare, as physicians and patients are interested in knowing the result and why the algorithm arrived at a specific result. Not surprisingly, much research has been focused in the past years on making the models more explainable, whereby intelligible approximations of how the model functions (e.g., variable importance plots) are made, helping unzip the black box nature of complex AI/ML models .

Apart from the above challenges of model overfitting and lack of interpretability, additional limitations exist specifically to AI/ML models employed for time-series forecasting. Data, once collected, might need to be carefully pre-processed to prevent the model from becoming unstable Moreover, training AI/ML models for time series forecasting is labor intensive, with neural network-based models requiring substantial computational power. Furthermore, while AI/ML models have been increasingly applied for time series forecasting, there have been few studies directly comparing statistical and AI/ML models, with some showing statistical models to be better than the current AI/ML models . Moreover, besides knowledge of the forecasted variable, researchers are also interested in knowing about the uncertainty surrounding the forecast, which is imperative to making decisions based on forecasts .This becomes especially useful in the clinical setting, whereby creating a parameter of uncertainty (analogous to confidence intervals) can help clinicians decide the significance of a forecasted variable and thereby make insightful medical decisions.

With the demonstrable success of artificial intelligence and the steps taken by the scientific community to address the aforementioned issues, the next decade is set to witness artificial intelligence techniques being employed and tested in randomized controlled trials against standard-of-care modeling, paving the way toward incorporation into clinical practice. Significant strides have already been made with the guidelines being made for the appropriate conduct of trials employing artificial intelligence Moreover, multiple trials are already underway aimed at testing the role of wearables and AI/ML in improving patient outcomes in HF . With AI/ML bound to advance further, future trials could see the unification of structured clinical variables and unstructured medical images to produce robust algorithms, hoping to further our knowledge in understanding disease characteristics and phenogroups within the domain of HF.

Conclusions

AI/ML and wearable technology, when used together, have the potential to induce a paradigm change in HF management. With few pilot studies showing the effectiveness of AI/ML approaches in conjunction with wearable technology and multiple trials currently underway, the field is only bound to expand. Notable limitations exist at present, which need to be addressed before digitization can be used to its fullest potential. While the scientific community is devising ways at present to address these limitations, the next few years could witness an expansion of the medical armamentarium physicians currently possess, with AI/ML complementing our current tools.

Bibliography and Acknowledgement

- Akintola AA, van de Pol V, Bimmel D, Maan AC, van Heemst D. Comparative analysis of the equivital EQ02 lifemonitor with holter ambulatory ECG device for continuous measurement of ECG, heart rate, and heart rate variability: A validation study for precision and accuracy. Front Physiol. (2016) 7:391. doi: 10.3389/fphys.2016.00391
- Al-Kaisey AM, Koshy AN, Ha FJ, Spencer R, Toner L, Sajeev JK, et al. Accuracy of wrist-worn heart rate monitors for rate control assessment in atrial fibrillation. Int J Cardiol. (2020) 300:161–4. doi: 10.1016/j.ijcard.2019.11.120
- Allen J. Photoplethysmography and its application in clinical physiological measurement. Physiol Meas. (2007) 28:R1–39. doi: 10.1088/0967-3334/28/3/R01
- Ballaji HK, Correia R, Korposh S, Hayes-Gill BR, Hernandez FU, Salisbury B, et al. A textile sleeve for monitoring oxygen saturation using multichannel optical fibre photoplethysmography. Sensors (Basel). (2020) 20:6568. doi: 10.3390/s20226568
- Barrett PM, Komatireddy R, Haaser S, Topol S, Sheard J, Encinas J, et al. Comparison of 24-hour Holter monitoring with 14-day novel adhesive patch electrocardiographic monitoring. Am J Med. (2014) 127:95.e11–17.doi:10.1016/j.amjmed.2013.10.003
- Bayoumy K, Gaber M, Elshafeey A, Mhaimeed O, Dineen EH, Marvel FA, et al. Smart wearable devices in cardiovascular care: where we are and how to move forward. Nat Rev Cardiol. (2021) 18:581–99.doi:10.1038/s41569-021-00522-7
- Bioelectron. (2018) 4:195–202. doi: 10.15406/ijbsbe.2018.04.00125 Boudreaux BD, Hebert EP, Hollander DB, Williams BM, Cormier CL, Naquin MR, et al. Validity of Wearable Activity Monitors during Cycling and Resistance Exercise. Med Sci Sports Exerc. (2018) 50:624–33.doi:10.1249/MSS.0000000000001471
- Bumgarner JM, Lambert CT, Hussein AA, Cantillon DJ, Baranowski B, Wolski K, et al. Smartwatch algorithm for automated detection of atrial fibrillation. J Am Coll Cardiol. (2018) 71:2381–8. doi: 10.1016/j.jacc.2018.03.003
- Caillol T, Strik M, Ramirez FD, Abu-Alrub S, Marchand H, Buliard S, et al. Accuracy of a smartwatch-derived ECG for diagnosing bradyarrhythmias, tachyarrhythmias, and cardiac ischemia. Circ Arrhythmia Electrophysiol. (2021) 14:e009260. doi: 10.1161/CIRCEP.120.009260
- Castaneda D, Esparza A, Ghamari M, Soltanpur C, Nazeran H. A review on wearable Castelletti S, Dagradi F, Goulene K, Danza AI, Baldi E, Stramba-Badiale M, et al. A wearable remote monitoring system for the identification of subjects with a prolonged QT interval or at risk for drug-induced long QT syndrome. Int J Cardiol. (2018) 266:89–94.doi:10.1016/j.ijcard.2018.03.097
- Dagher L, Shi H, Zhao Y, Marrouche NF. Wearables in cardiology: Here to stay. Hear Rhythm. (2020) 17:889–95. doi: 10.1016/j.hrthm.2020.02.023
- Derkac WM, Finkelmeier JR, Horgan DJ, Hutchinson MD. Diagnostic yield of asymptomatic arrhythmias detected by mobile cardiac outpatient telemetry and autotrigger looping event cardiac monitors. J Cardiovasc Electrophysiol. (2017) 28:1475–8. doi: 10.1111/jce.13342
- Ding EY, Han D, Whitcomb C, Bashar SK, Adaramola O, Soni A, et al. Accuracy and usability of a novel algorithm for detection of irregular pulse using a smartwatch among older adults: Observational study. JMIR Cardio. (2019) 3:e13850. doi: 10.2196/13850
- Engel JM, Mehta V, Fogoros R, Chavan A. Study of arrhythmia prevalence in NUVANT mobile cardiac telemetry system patients. Proc Annu Int Conf IEEE Eng Med Biol Soc EMBS. (2012) (4):2440–3. doi: 10.1109/EMBC.2012.6346457
- Fan YY, Li YG, Li J, Cheng WK, Shan ZL, Wang YT, et al. Diagnostic performance of a smart device with photoplethysmography technology for atrial fibrillation detection: Pilot study (pre-mafa II registry). JMIR mHealth uHealth. (2019) 7:e11437. doi: 10.2196/11437
- Guo Y, Lane DA, Wang L, Chen Y, Lip GYH, Eckstein J, et al. Mobile Health (mHealth) technology for improved screening, patient involvement and optimising integrated care in atrial fibrillation: The mAFA (mAF-App) II randomised trial. Int J Clin Pract. (2019) 73:e13352.doi:10.1111/ijcp.13352
- Guo Y, Lip GYH. Mobile health for cardiovascular disease: The new frontier for AF management: Observations from the huawei heart study and mAFA-II randomised trial. Arrhythmia Electrophysiol Rev. (2020) 9:5–7. doi: 10.15420/aer.2020.12
- Ha ACT, Verma S, Mazer CD, Quan A, Yanagawa B, Latter DA, et al. Effect of continuous electrocardiogram monitoring on detection of undiagnosed atrial fibrillation after hospitalization for cardiac surgery: a randomized clinical trial. JAMA Netw Open. (2021) 4:e2121867. doi: 10.1001/jamanetworkopen.2021.21867
- Hindricks G, Potpara T, Dagres N, Bax JJ, Boriani G, Dan GA, et al. 2020 ESC Guidelines for the diagnosis and management of atrial fibrillation developed in collaboration with the European Association for Cardio-Thoracic Surgery (EACTS). Eur Heart J. (2021) 42:373–498. doi:10.1093/eurheartj/ehaa612
- Honarbakhsh S, Sporton S, Monkhouse C, Lowe M, Earley MJ, Hunter RJ. Remote clinics and investigations in arrhythmia services: What have we learnt during Coronavirus disease 2019? Arrhythmia Electrophysiol Rev. (2021) 10:120–4. doi: 10.15420/aer.2020.37
- nui T, Kohno H, Kawasaki Y, Matsuura K, Ueda H, Tamura Y, et al. Use of a Smart watch for early detection of paroxysmal atrial fibrillation: validation study. JMIR Cardio. (2020) 4:e14857. doi:
- 10.2196/14857 Isakadze N, Martin SS. How useful is the smartwatch ECG? Trends Cardiovasc Med. (2020) 30:442–8. doi: 10.1016/j.tcm.2019.10.010
- Johnstone JA, Ford PA, Hughes G, Watson T, Garrett AT. BioharnessTM multivariable monitoring device. Part I: Validity. J Sport Sci Med. (2012) 11:400–8.
- Johnstone JA, Ford PA, Hughes G, Watson T, Garrett AT. BioharnessTM Multivariable Monitoring Device: Part. II: Reliability. J SportsSciMed.(2012)11:409–17.
- Johnstone JA, Ford PA, Hughes G, Watson T, Mitchell ACS, Garrett AT. Field based reliability and validity of the bioharnessTM multivariable monitoring device. J Sport Sci Med. (2012) 11:643–52.
- Joshi AK, Kowey PR, Prystowsky EN, Benditt DG, Cannom DS, Pratt CM, et al. First experience with a Mobile Cardiac Outpatient Telemetry (MCOT) system for the diagnosis and management of cardiac arrhythmia. Am J Cardiol. (2005) 95:878–81. doi: 10.1016/j.amjcard.2004.12.015
- Karunadas CP, Mathew C. Comparison of arrhythmia detection by conventional Holter and a novel ambulatory ECG system using patch and Android App, over 24 h period. Indian Pacing Electrophysiol J. (2020) 20:49–53.doi:10.1016/j.ipej.2019.12.013
- Khurshid S, Choi SH, Weng LC, Wang EY, Trinquart L, Benjamin EJ, et al. Frequency of cardiac rhythm abnormalities in a half million adults. Circ Arrhythmia Electrophysiol. (2018) 11. doi: 10.1161/CIRCEP.118.006273
- Khushhal A, Nichols S, Evans W, Gleadall-Siddall D, Page R, O'Doherty A, et al. Validity and reliability of the apple watch for measuring heart rate during exercise. Sport Med Int Open. (2017) 1:E206–E211. doi: 10.1055/s-0043-120195
- Kim JH, Roberge R, Powell JB, Shafer AB, Jon Williams W. Measurement accuracy of heart rate and respiratory rate during graded exercise and sustained exercise in the heat using the zephyr BioHarness TM. Int J Sports Med. (2013) 34:497–501. doi: 10.1055/s-0032-1327661

- Krittanawong C, Johnson KW, Rosenson RS, Wang Z, Aydar M, Baber U, et al. Deep learning for cardiovascular medicine: A practical primer. Eur Heart J. (2019) 40:2058–73. doi: 10.1093/eurheartj/ehz056
- Lindberg T, Wimo A, Elmståhl S, Qiu C, Bohman DM, Sanmartin Berglund J. Prevalence and incidence of atrial fibrillation and other arrhythmias in the general older population: findings from the swedish national study on aging and care. Gerontol Geriatr Med. (2019) 5:233372141985968.doi:10.1177/2333721419859687
- Liu Y, Zhu SH, Wang GH, Ye F, Li PZ. Validity and reliability of multiparameter physiological measurements recorded by the equivital lifemonitor during activities of various intensities. J Occup Environ Hyg. (2013) 10:78–85. doi: 10.1080/15459624.2012.747404
- Lobodzinski SS. ECG patch monitors for assessment of cardiac rhythm abnormalities. Prog Cardiovasc Dis. (2013) 56:224–9.
- Lown M, Yue AM, Shah BN, Corbett SJ, Lewith G, Stuart B, et al. Screening for atrial fibrillation using economical and accurate technology (From the SAFETY Study). Am J Cardiol. (2018) 122:1339–44.
- Lubitz SA, Faranesh AZ, Atlas SJ, McManus DD, Singer DE, Pagoto S, et al. Rationale and design of a large population study to validate software for the assessment of atrial fibrillation from data acquired by a consumer tracker or smartwatch: The Fitbit heart study. Am Heart J. (2021) 238:16–26. doi: 10.1016/j.ahj.2021.04.003
- Maines M, Zorzi A, Tomasi G, Angheben C, Catanzariti D, Piffer L, et al. Clinical impact, safety, and accuracy of the remotely monitored implantable loop recorder Medtronic Reveal LINQ TM. Europace. (2018) 20:1050–7. doi: 10.1093/europace/eux187
- Nault I, André P, Plourde B, Leclerc F, Sarrazin JF, Philippon F, et al. Validation of a novel single lead ambulatory ECG monitor – CardiostatTM – Compared to a standard ECG Holter monitoring. J Electrocardiol.(2019)53:57–63.doi:10.1016/j.jelectrocard.2018.12.01187
- Navalta JW, Montes J, Bodell NG, Salatto RW, Manning JW, DeBeliso
- Pagola J, Juega J, Francisco-Pascual J, Moya A, Sanchis M, Bustamante A, et al. Yield of atrial fibrillation detection with Textile Wearable Holter from the acute phase of stroke: Pilot study of Crypto-AF registry. Int J Cardiol. (2018) 251:45–50. doi: 10.1016/j.ijcard.2017.10.063
- Olhede SC, Wolfe PJ. The growing ubiquity of algorithms in society: Implications, impacts and innovations. Philos Trans R Soc A Math Phys Eng Sci. (2018) 376:2128. doi: 10.1098/rsta.2017.0364
- Olmos C, Franco E, Suárez-Barrientos A, Fortuny E, Martín-García A, Viliani D, et al. Wearable wireless remote monitoring system: An alternative for prolonged electrocardiographic monitoring. Int J Cardiol. (2014) 172:e43–4. doi: 10.1016/j.ijcard.2013.12.068
- Perez MV, Mahaffey KW, Hedlin H, Rumsfeld JS, Garcia A, Ferris T, et al. Large-scale assessment of a smartwatch to identify atrial fibrillation. N Engl J Med. (2019) 381:1909–17. doi: 10.1056/NEJMoa1901183
- Rajakariar K, Koshy AN, Sajeev JK, Nair S, Roberts L, Teh AW. Accuracy of a smartwatch based single-lead electrocardiogram device in detection of atrial fibrillation. Heart. (2020) 106:665–70. doi: 10.1136/heartjnl-2019-316004
- Rho R, Vossler M, Blancher S, Poole JE. Comparison of 2 ambulatory patch ECG monitors: The benefit of the P-wave and signal clarity. Am Heart J. (2018) 203:109–17. doi: 10.1016/j.ahj.2018.03.022
- Rosenberg MA, Samuel M, Thosani A, Zimetbaum PJ. Use of a noninvasive continuous monitoring device in the management of atrial fibrillation: A pilot study. PACE - Pacing Clin Electrophysiol. (2013) 36:328–33.doi:10.1111/pace.12053
- Selvaraj N, Nallathambi G, Moghadam R, Aga A. Fully disposable wireless patch sensor for continuous remote patient monitoring. Annu Int Conf IEEE Eng Med Biol Soc. (2018). p.1632-1635. doi: 10.1109/EMBC.2018.8512569
- Shcherbina A, Mikael Mattsson C, Waggott D, Salisbury H, Christle JW, Hastie T, et al. Accuracy in wrist-worn, sensor-based measurements of heart rate and energy expenditure in a diverse cohort. J PersMed.(2017)7:1–12.doi:10.3390/jpm7020003
- Steinhubl SR, Mehta RR, Ebner GS, Ballesteros MM, Waalen J, Steinberg G, et al. Rationale and design of a home-based trial using wearable sensors to detect asymptomatic atrial fibrillation in a targeted population: The mHealth Screening to Prevent Strokes (mSToPS) trial. Am Heart J. (2016) 175:77–85. doi: 10.1016/j.ahj.2016.02.011
- Steinhubl SR, Waalen J, Edwards AM, Ariniello LM, Mehta RR, Ebner GS, et al. Effect of a home-Based wearable continuous ECG monitoring patch on detection of undiagnosed atrial fibrillation the mSToPS randomized clinical trial. JAMA - J Am Med Assoc. (2018) 320:146–55.doi:10.1001/jama.2018.810283
- Svennberg E, Friberg L, Frykman V, Al-Khalili F, Engdahl J, Rosenqvist M. Clinical outcomes in systematic screening for atrial fibrillation (STROKESTOP): a multicentre, parallel group, unmasked, randomised controlled trial. Lancet. (2021) 398:1498–506. doi: 10.1016/S0140-6736(21)01637-8
- Tayal AH, Tian M, Kelly KM, Jones SC, Wright DG, Singh D, et al. Atrial fibrillation detected by mobile cardiac outpatient telemetry in cryptogenic TIA or stroke. Neurology. (2008) 71:1696–70. doi: 10.1212/01.wnl.0000325059.86313.31
- Teplitzky BA, McRoberts M, Ghanbari H. Deep learning for comprehensive ECG annotation. Hear Rhythm. (2020) 17:881–8. doi: 10.1016/j.hrthm.2020.02.015
- Thomson EA, Nuss K, Comstock A, Reinwald S, Blake S, Pimentel RE, et al. Heart rate measures from the Apple Watch, Fitbit Charge HR 2, and electrocardiogram across different exercise intensities electrocardiogram across different exercise intensities. J Sports Sci. (2019) 37:1–9. doi: 10.1080/02640414.2018.1560644
- Ummel JD, Hoilett OS, Walters BD, Bluhm NDP, Pickering AS, Wilson DA, et al. A multi-sensor ring capturing respiration, electrocardiogram, oxygen saturation, and skin temperature1. Annu Int Conf IEEE Eng Med Biol Soc. (2020) 4394–7. doi: 10.1109/EMBC44109.2020.9176654
- Van Gelder IC, Healey JS, Crijns HJGM, Wang J, Hohnloser SH, Gold MR, et al. Duration of device-detected subclinical atrial fibrillation and occurrence of stroke in ASSERT. Eur Heart J. (2017) 38:1339–44. doi: 10.1093/eurheartj/ehx042
- Wolf PA, Abbott RD, Kannel WB. Atrial fibrillation as an independent risk factor for stroke: The framingham study. Stroke. (1991) 22:983–8. doi: 10.1161/01.STR.22.8.983 worn device. Physiol Meas. (2019) 40:025003.doi:10.1088/1361-6579/ab029c
- Xie J, Wen D, Liang L, Jia Y, Gao L, Lei J. Evaluating the validity of current mainstream wearable devices in fitness tracking under various physical activities: Comparative study. JMIR mHealth uHealth. (2018) 6.doi:10.2196/mhealth.9754
- Yao X, Rushlow DR, Inselman JW, McCoy RG, Thacher TD, Behnken EM, et al. Artificial intelligence-enabled electrocardiograms for identification of patients with low ejection fraction: a pragmatic, randomized clinical trial. Nat Med. (2021) 27:815–9. doi: 10.1038/s41591-021-01335-4
- Zhang MJ, Roetker NS, Folsom AR, Alonso A, Heckbert SR, Chen LY. Feasibility of using a leadless patch monitor in community cohort studies: The Multi-ethnic Study of Atherosclerosis. PACE - Pacing Clin Electrophysiol. (2018) 41:1389–90. doi: 10.1111/pace.13507
- Zheng Q, Tang Q, Wang ZL, Li Z. Self-powered cardiovascular electronic devices and systems. Nat Rev Cardiol. (2021) 18:7–21. doi: 10.1038/s41569-020-0426-4

The Role Of Artificial Intelligence(AI) In Clinical Practice

CHAPTER

28

Artificial Intelligence (AI) is a rapidly evolving field of computer science that aims to create machines that can perform tasks that typically require human intelligence. AI includes various techniques such as machine learning (ML), deep learning (DL), and natural language processing (NLP). Large Language Models (LLMs) are a type of AI algorithm that uses deep learning techniques and massively large data sets to understand, summarize, generate, and predict new text-based content . LLMs have been architected to generate text-based content and possess broad applicability for various NLP tasks, including text generation, translation, content summary, rewriting, classification, categorization, and sentiment analysis. NLP is a subfield of AI that focuses on the interaction between computers and humans through natural language, including understanding, interpreting, and generating human language. NLP involves various techniques such as text mining, sentiment analysis, speech recognition, and machine translation. Over the years, AI has undergone significant transformations, from the early days of rule-based systems to the current era of ML and deep learning algorithms.

AI has evolved since the first AI program was developed in 1951 by Christopher Strachey. At that time, AI was in its infancy and was primarily an academic research topic. In 1956, John McCarthy organized the Dartmouth Conference, where he coined the term "Artificial Intelligence." This event marked the beginning of the modern AI era. In the 1960 and 1970 s, AI research focused on rule-based and expert systems. However, this approach was limited by the need for more computing power and data .

In the 1980 and 1990 s, AI research shifted to ML and neural networks, which allowed machines to learn from data and improve their performance over time. This period saw the development of systems such as IBM's Deep Blue, which defeated world chess champion Garry Kasparov in 1997. In the 2000s, AI research continued to evolve, focusing on NLP and computer vision, which led to the development of virtual assistants, such as Apple's Siri and Amazon's Alexa, which could understand natural language and respond to user requests

.Today, AI is transforming healthcare, finance, and and transportation, among other fields, and its impact is only set to grow. In academia, AI has been used to develop intelligent tutoring systems, which are computer programs that can adapt to the needs of individual students. These systems have improved student learning outcomes in various subjects, including math and science. In research, AI has been used to analyze large datasets and identify patterns that would be difficult for humans to detect; this has led to breakthroughs in fields such as genomics and drug discovery. AI has been used in healthcare settings to develop diagnostic tools and personalized treatment plans. As AI continues to evolve, it is crucial to ensure that it is developed responsibly and for the benefit of all .

The rapid progression of AI technology presents an opportunity for its application in clinical practice, potentially revolutionizing healthcare services. It is imperative to document and disseminate information regarding AI's role in clinical practice, to equip healthcare providers with the knowledge and tools necessary for effective implementation in patient care. This review article aims to explore the current state of AI in healthcare, its potential benefits, limitations, and challenges, and to provide insights into its future development. By doing so, this review aims to contribute to a better understanding of AI's role in healthcare and facilitate its integration into clinical practice.

AI Assistance In Diagnostics

Diagnosis accuracy

With all the advances in medicine, effective disease diagnosis is still considered a challenge on a global scale. The development of early diagnostic tools is an ongoing challenge due to the complexity of the various disease mechanisms and the underlying symptoms. AI can revolutionize different aspects of health care, including diagnosis. ML is an area of AI that uses data as an input resource in which the accuracy is highly dependent on the quantity as well as the quality of the input data that can combat some of the challenges and complexity of diagnosis .ML, in short, can assist in decision-making, manage workflow, and automate tasks in a timely and cost-effective manner. Also, deep learning added layers utilizing Convolutional Neural Networks (CNN) and data mining techniques that help identify data patterns. These are highly applicable in identifying key disease detection patterns among big datasets. These tools are highly applicable in healthcare systems for diagnosing, predicting, or classifying diseases .

AI is still in its early stages of being fully utilized for medical diagnosis. However, more data are emerging for the application of AI in diagnosing different diseases, such as cancer. A study was published in the UK where authors input a large dataset of mammograms into an AI system for breast cancer diagnosis. This study showed that utilizing an AI system to interpret mammograms had an absolute reduction in false positives and false negatives by 5.7% and 9.4%, respectively . Another study was conducted in South Korea, where authors compared AI diagnoses of breast cancer versus radiologists. The AI-utilized diagnosis was more sensitive to diagnose breast cancer with mass compared to radiologists, 90% vs. 78%, respectively. Also, AI was better at detecting early breast cancer (91%) than radiologists 74% .

Furthermore, a study utilized deep learning to detect skin cancer which showed that an AI using CNN accurately diagnosed melanoma cases compared to dermatologists and recommended treatment options . Researchers utilized AI technology in many other disease states, such as detecting diabetic retinopathy . and EKG abnormality and predicting risk factors for cardiovascular diseases . Furthermore, deep learning algorithms are used to detect pneumonia from chest radiography with sensitivity and specificity of 96% and 64% compared to radiologists 50% and 73%, respectively .Also, a study was done on a dataset of 625 cases to diagnose acute appendicitis early to predict the need for appendix surgery using various ML techniques; the results showed that the random forest algorithm achieved the highest performance, accurately predicting appendicitis in 83.75% of cases, with a precision of 84.11%, sensitivity of 81.08%, and specificity of 81.01%. The improved method aids healthcare specialists in making informed decisions for appendicitis diagnoses and treatment. Furthermore, the authors suggest that similar techniques can be utilized to analyze images of patients with appendicitis or even to detect infections such as COVID-19 using blood specimens or images .

AI tools can improve accuracy, reduce costs, and save time compared to traditional diagnostic methods. Additionally, AI can reduce the risk of human errors and provide more accurate results in less time. In the future, AI technology could be used to support medical decisions by providing clinicians with real-time assistance and insights. Researchers continue exploring ways to use AI in medical diagnosis and treatment, such as analyzing medical images, X-rays, CT scans, and MRIs. By leveraging ML techniques, AI can also help identify abnormalities, detect fractures, tumors, or other conditions, and provide quantitative measurements for faster and more accurate medical diagnosis.

Clinical laboratory testing provides critical information for diagnosing, treating, and monitoring diseases. It is an essential part of modern healthcare which continuously incorporates new technology to support clinical decision-making and patient safety . AI has the potential to transform clinical laboratory testing by improving the accuracy, speed, and efficiency of laboratory processes. The role of AI in clinical microbiology is currently progressing and expanding. Several ML systems were developed to detect, identify, and quantify microorganisms, diagnose and classify diseases, and predict clinical outcomes. These ML systems used data from various sources to build the AI diagnosis such as genomic data of microorganisms, gene sequencing, metagenomic sequencing results of the original specimen, and microscopic imaging [. Moreover, gram stain classification to gram positives/negatives and cocci/rods is another essential application of using deep convolutional neural networks that reveal high sensitivity and specificity . A published systematic review showed that numerous MLs were evaluated for microorganism identification and antibiotic susceptibility testing; however, several limitations are associated with the current models that must be addressed before incorporating them into clinical practice . For malaria, Taesik et al. found that using ML algorithms combined with digital in-line holographic microscopy (DIHM) effectively detected malaria-infected red blood cells without staining. This AI technology is rapid, sensitive, and cost-effective in diagnosing malaria .

The projected benefits of using AI in clinical laboratories include but are not limited to, increased efficacy and precision. Automated techniques in blood cultures, susceptibility testing, and molecular platforms have become standard in numerous laboratories globally, contributing significantly to laboratory efficiency . Automation and AI have substantially improved laboratory efficiency in areas like blood cultures, susceptibility testing, and molecular platforms. This allows for a result within the first 24 to 48 h, facilitating the selection of suitable antibiotic treatment for patients with positive blood cultures . Consequently, incorporating AI in clinical microbiology laboratories can assist in choosing appropriate antibiotic treatment regimens, a critical factor in achieving high cure rates for various infectious diseases .

ML research in medicine has rapidly expanded, which could greatly help the healthcare providers in the emergency department (ED) as they face challenging difficulties from the rising burden of diseases, greater demand for time and health services, higher societal expectations, and increasing health expenditures . Emergency department providers understand that integrating AI into their work processes is necessary for solving these problems by enhancing efficiency, and accuracy, and improving patient outcomes .Additionally, there may be a chance for algorithm support and automated decision-making to optimize ED flow measurements and resource allocation . algorithms can analyze patient data to assist with triaging patients based on urgency; this helps prioritize high-risk cases, reducing waiting times and improving patient flow . Introducing a reliable symptom assessment tool can rule out other causes of illness to reducethe number of unnecessary visits to the ED. A series of AI-enabled machines can directly question the patient, and a sufficient explanation is provided at the end to ensure appropriate assessment and plan.Moreover, AI-powered decision support systems can provide real-time suggestions to healthcare providers, aiding diagnosis, and treatment decisions. Patients are evaluated in the ED with little information, and physicians frequently must weigh probabilities when risk stratifying and making decisions. Faster clinical data interpretation is crucial in ED to classify the seriousness of the situation and the need for immediate intervention. The risk of misdiagnosing patients is one of the most critical problems affecting medical practitioners and healthcare systems. Diagnostic mistakes in the healthcare sector can be expensive and fatal. A study found that diagnostic errors, particularly in patients who visit the ED, directly contribute to a greater mortality rate and a more extended hospital stay.Fortunately, AI can assist in the early detection of patients with life-threatening diseases and promptly alert clinicians so the patients can receive immediate attention. Lastly, AI can help optimize health care sources in the ED by predicting patient demand, optimizing therapy selection (medication, dose, route of administration, and urgency of intervention), and suggesting emergency department length of stay. By analyzing patient-specific data, AI systems can offer insights into optimal therapy selection, improving efficiency and reducing overcrowding.

AI in genomic medicine

The fusion of AI and genotype analysis holds immense promise in the realms of disease surveillance, prediction, and personalized medicine . When applied to large populations, AI can effectively monitor for emerging disease threats (such as COVID-19), while genomic data can provide valuable insights into genetic markers associated with increased susceptibility to specific diseases . By training ML algorithms to identify these markers in real-time data, we can facilitate the early detection of potential outbreaks. Moreover, the use of genotype data can aid in refining disease risk predictions, as ML algorithms can recognize complex patterns of genetic variations linked with disease susceptibility that might elude traditional statistical methods .The prediction of phenotypes, or observable characteristics shaped by genes and environmental factors, also becomes possible with this combination.ML algorithms make it feasible to predict a spectrum of phenotypes ranging from simple traits like eye color to more intricate ones like the response to certain medications or disease susceptibility. A specific area where AI and ML have demonstrated significant efficacy is the identification of genetic variants associated with distinctive traits or pathologies. Examining extensive genomic datasets allows these techniques to detect intricate patterns often elusive to manual analysis. For instance, a groundbreaking study employed a deep neural network to identify genetic variants associated with autism spectrum disorder (ASD), successfully

predicting ASD status by relying solely on genomic data .In the field of oncology, categorizing cancers into clinically relevant molecular subtypes can be accomplished using transcriptomic profiling. Such molecular classifications, first developed for breast cancer and later extended to other cancers like colorectal, ovarian, and sarcomas, hold substantial implications for diagnosis, prognosis, and treatment selection . Traditional computational methods for subtyping cancers, such as support vector machines (SVMs) or k-nearest neighbors, are susceptible to errors due to batch effects and may only focus on a small set of signature genes, thus neglecting vital biological information

The advent of high-throughput genomic sequencing technologies, combined with advancements in AI and ML, has laid a strong foundation for accelerating personalized medicine and drug discovery . Despite being a treasure trove of valuable insights, the complex nature of extensive genomic data presents substantial obstacles to its interpretation. The field of drug discovery has dramatically benefited from the application of AI and ML. The simultaneous analysis of extensive genomic data and other clinical parameters, such as drug efficacy or adverse effects, facilitates the identification of novel therapeutic targets or the repurposing of existing drugs for new applications .One of the prevalent challenges in drug development is non-clinical toxicity, which leads to a significant percentage of drug failures during clinical trials. However, the rise of computational modeling is opening up the feasibility of predicting drug toxicity, which can be instrumental in improving the drug development process . This capability is particularly vital for addressing common types of drug toxicity, such as cardiotoxicity and hepatotoxicity, which often lead to post-market withdrawal of drugs.

AI Assistance In Treatment

Precision medicine and clinical decision support

Personalized treatment, also known as precision medicine or personalized medicine, is an approach that tailors medical care to individual patients based on their unique characteristics, such as genetics, environment, lifestyle, and biomarkers . This individualized approach aims to improve patient outcomes by providing targeted interventions that are more effective, efficient, and safe. AI has emerged as a valuable tool in advancing personalized treatment, offering the potential to analyze complex datasets, predict outcomes, and optimize treatment strategies . Personalized treatment represents a pioneering field that demonstrates the potential of precision medicine on a large scale Nevertheless, the ability to provide real-time recommendations relies on the advancement of ML algorithms capable of predicting patients who may require specific medications based on genomic

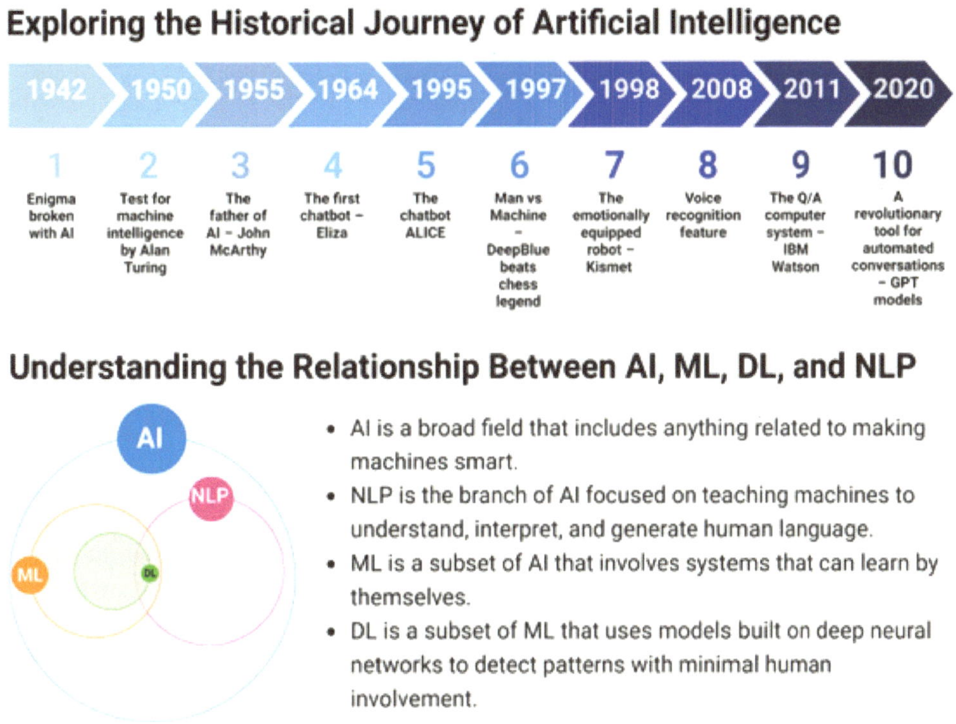

Fig.28.1 Tracing the Evolution of AI with a Better Understanding of the Relationship Between AI, ML, DL, and NLP

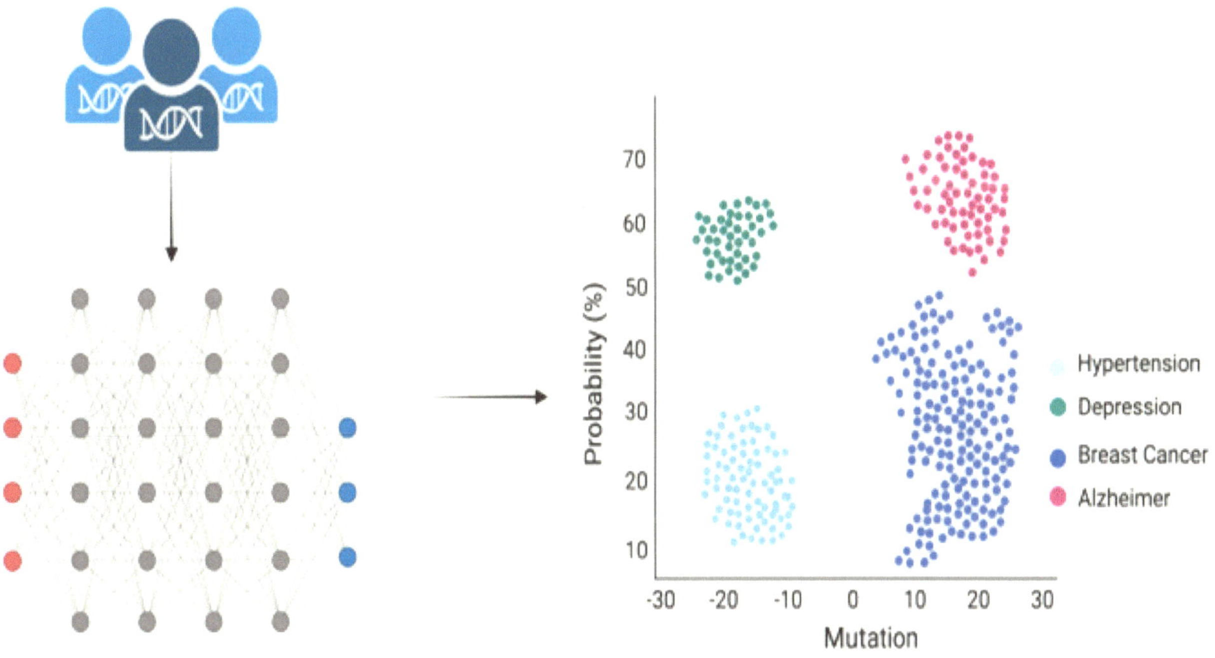

Fig.28.2 Schematic representation of the process starting with the extraction of DNA/RNA, followed by sequencing. The subsequent genotypic alignment is performed using neural networks and deep learning. Probability calculations are achieved through applying statistical methods and M: The graph's Y-axis denotes the probability (expressed in percentage) of a particular type of disease (hypertension, depression, breast cancer, and Alzheimer's disease), while the X-axis signifies the count of gene mutations. Negative numbers indicate gene deletions, whereas positive values represent gene additions or nucleic acid mutations

formation. The key to tailoring medications and dosages to patients lies in the pre-emptive genotyping of patients prior to the actual need for such information .

The potential applications of AI in assisting clinicians with treatment decisions, particularly in predicting therapy response, have gained recognition . A study conducted by Huang et al. where authors utilized patients' gene expression data for training a support ML, successfully predicted the response to chemotherapy . In this study, the authors included 175 cancer patients incorporating their gene-expression profiles to predict the patients' responses to various standard-of-care chemotherapies. Notably, the research showed encouraging outcomes, achieving a prediction accuracy of over 80% across multiple drugs. These findings demonstrate the promising role of AI in treatment response prediction. In another study performed by Sheu et al., the authors aimed to predict the response to different classes of antidepressants using electronic health records (EHR) of 17,556 patients and AI .The AI models considered features predictive of treatment selection to minimize confounding factors and showed good prediction performance. The study demonstrated that antidepressant response could be accurately predicted using real-world EHR data with AI modeling, suggesting the potential for developing clinical decision support systems for more effective treatment selection. While considerable progress has been made in leveraging AI techniques and genomics to forecast treatment outcomes, it is essential to conduct further prospective and retrospective clinical research and studies . These endeavors are necessary for generating the comprehensive data required to train the algorithms effectively, ensure their reliability in real-world settings, and further develop AI-based clinical decision tools.

Dose optimization and therapeutic drug monitoring

AI plays a crucial role in dose optimization and adverse drug event prediction, offering significant benefits in enhancing patient safety and improving treatment outcomes . By leveraging AI algorithms, healthcare providers can optimize medication dosages tailored to individual patients and predict potential adverse drug events, thereby reducing risks and improving patient care. In a study that aimed to develop an AI-based prediction model for prothrombin time international normalized ratio (PT/INR) and a decision support system for warfarin maintenance dose optimization . The authors analyzed data from 19,719 inpatients across three institutions, and the algorithm outperformed expert physicians with significant differences in predicting future PT/INRs and the generated individualized warfarin dose was reliable.

On the contrary, a novel dose optimization system—CURATE.AI—is an AI-derived platform for dynamically optimizing chemotherapy doses based on individual patient data.

A study was conducted to validate this system as an open-label, prospective trial in patients with advanced solid tumors treated with three different chemotherapy regimens. CURATE.AI generated personalized doses for subsequent cycles based on the correlation between chemotherapy dose variation and tumor marker readouts. The integration of CURATE.AI into the clinical workflow showed successful incorporation and potential benefits in terms of reducing chemotherapy dose and improving patient response rates and durations compared to the standard of care. These findings support the need for prospective validation through randomized clinical trials and indicate the potential of AI in optimizing chemotherapy dosing and lowering the risk of adverse drug events.

Therapeutic drug monitoring (TDM) is a process used to optimize drug dosing in individual patients. It is predominantly utilized for drugs with a narrow therapeutic index to avoid both underdosing insufficiently medicating as well as toxic levels. TDM aims to ensure that patients receive the right drug, at the right dose, at the right time, to achieve the desired therapeutic outcome while minimizing adverse effects . The use of AI in TDM has the potential to revolutionize how drugs are monitored and prescribed. AI algorithms can be trained to predict an individual's response to a given drug based on their genetic makeup, medical history, and other factors. This personalized approach to drug therapy can lead to more effective treatments and better patient outcomes .

One example of AI in TDM is using ML algorithms to predict drug-drug interactions. By analyzing large datasets of patient data, these algorithms can identify potential drug interactions. This can help to reduce the risk of adverse drug reactions, and cost and improve patient outcomes . Another application of AI in TDM using predictive analytics to identify patients at high risk of developing adverse drug reactions. By analyzing patient data and identifying potential risk factors, healthcare providers can take proactive steps to prevent adverse events before they occur . Overall, the use of AI in TDM has the potential to improve patient outcomes, reduce healthcare costs, and enhance the accuracy and efficiency of drug dosing. As this technology continues to evolve, AI will likely play an increasingly important role in the field of TDM.

AI Assistance In Population Health Management

Predictive analytics and risk assessment

Population health management increasingly uses predictive analytics to identify and guide health initiatives. In data analytics, predictive analytics is a discipline that significantly utilizes modeling, data mining, AI, and ML. In order to anticipate the future, it analyzes historical and current data , ML algorithms and other technologies are used to analyze data and develop predictive models to improve patient outcomes and reduce costs

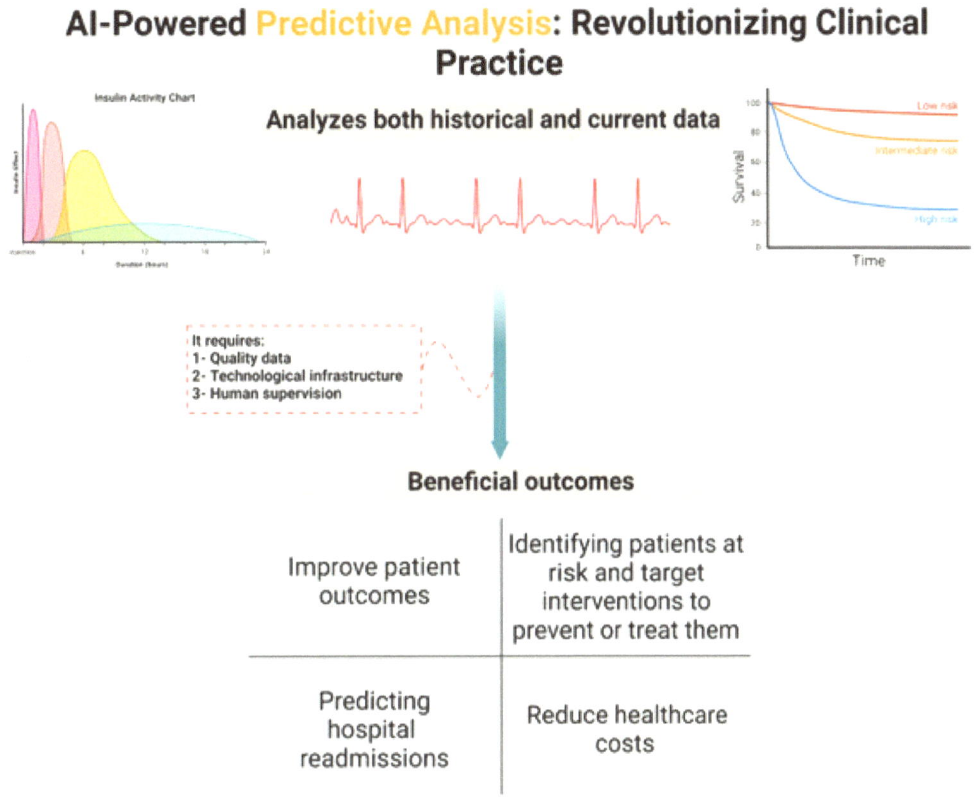

Fig.28.3 Unlocking the Power of Patient Data with AI-Driven Predictive Analytics

One area where predictive analytics can be instrumental is in identifying patients at risk of developing chronic diseases such as endocrine or cardiac diseases. By analyzing data such as medical history, demographics, and lifestyle factors, predictive models can identify patients at higher risk of developing these conditions and target interventions to prevent or treat them . Predicting hospital readmissions is another area where predictive analytics can be applied. By analyzing patient demographics, medical history, and social health factors, predictive models can identify patients at higher risk of hospital readmissions and target interventions to prevent readmissions , this can help reduce healthcare costs and improve patient outcomes which is the reason behind launching new companies such as "Reveal ®"

AI can be used to optimize healthcare by improving the accuracy and efficiency of predictive models. AI algorithms can analyze large amounts of data and identify patterns and relationships that may not be obvious to human analysts; this can help improve the accuracy of predictive models and ensure that patients receive the most appropriate interventions. AI can also automate specific public health management tasks, such as patient outreach and care coordination. Which can help reduce healthcare costs and improve patient outcomes by ensuring patients receive timely and appropriate care. However, it is pivotal to note that the success of predictive analytics in public health management depends on the quality of data and the technological infrastructure used to develop and implement predictive models. In addition, human supervision is vital to ensure the appropriateness and effectiveness of interventions for at-risk patients.

In summary, predictive analytics plays an increasingly important role in population health. Using ML algorithms and other technologies, healthcare organizations can develop predictive models that identify patients at risk for chronic disease or readmission to the hospital . Furthermore, AI is needed to address these challenges regarding vaccine production and supply chain bottlenecks. Testing algorithms on real-time vaccine supply chains can be challenging. To overcome this, investing in research and development is essential to create robust algorithms that can accurately predict and optimize vaccine supply chains. Edge analytics can also detect anomalies and predict Disease X events and associated risks to the healthcare system .

From a Saudi perspective, Sehaa, a big data analytics tool in Saudi Arabia, uses Twitter data to detect diseases, and it found that dermal diseases, heart diseases, hypertension, cancer, and diabetes are the top five diseases in the country .Riyadh has the highest awareness-to-afflicted ratio for six of the fourteen diseases detected, while Taif is the healthiest city with the lowest number of disease cases and a high number of activities. These findings highlight the potential of predictive analytics in population health management and the need for targeted interventions to prevent and treat chronic diseases in Saudi Arabia .AI can optimize health care by improving the accuracy and efficiency of predictive models and automating certain tasks in population health management. However, successfully implementing predictive analytics requires high-quality data, advanced technology, and human oversight to ensure appropriate and effective interventions for patients.

Establishment of working groups, guidelines, and frameworks

AI is transforming how guidelines are established in various fields. In healthcare, guidelines usually take much time, from establishing the knowledge gap that needs to be fulfilled to publishing and disseminating these guidelines. AI can help identify newly published data based on data from clinical trials and real-world patient outcomes within the same area of interest which can then facilitate the first stage of mining information. Then, under the supervision of scientists and experts in the field, AI algorithms can analyze vast amounts of data to identify patterns and trends that can inform the development of evidence-based guidelines in real-time, which allows for a fast exchange of information with essential supervision clinicians for its clinical and ethical implications.

Several professional organizations have developed frameworks for addressing concerns unique to developing, reporting, and validating AI in medicine . Instead of focusing on the clinical application of AI, these frameworks are more concerned with educating the technological creators of AI by providing instructions on encouraging transparency in the design and reporting of AI algorithms . Additionally, regulatory regulation of AI is still in its infancy. The US Food and Drug Administration (FDA) is now developing guidelines on critically assessing real-world applications of AI in medicine while publishing a framework to guide the role of AI and ML in software as medical devices. The European Commission has spearheaded a multidisciplinary effort to improve the credibility of AI , and the European Medicines Agency (EMA) has deemed the regulation of AI a strategic priority . These legislative efforts are meant to shape the healthcare future to be better equipped to be a technology-driven sector. Overall, the role of AI in establishing guidelines is to provide data-driven insights and recommendations based on vast amounts of information, which can lead to more efficient and effective decision-making, better outcomes, and reduced costs. However, it is crucial to ensure that AI-based guidelines are transparent, fair, unbiased, and informed by human expertise and ethical considerations.

AI in drug information and consultation

AI would propose a new support system to assist practical decision-making tools for healthcare providers. in recent years, healthcare institutions have provided a greater leveraging capacity of utilizing automation-enabled technologies to boost workflow effectiveness and reduce costs while promoting patient safety, accuracy, and efficiency . By introducing advanced technologies like NLP, ML, and data analytics, AI can significantly provide real-time, accurate, and up-to-date information for practitioners at the hospital. According to the McKinsey Global Institute, ML and AI in the pharmaceutical sector have the potential to contribute approximately $100 billion annually to the US healthcare system . Researchers claim that these technologies enhance decision-making, maximize creativity, increase the effectiveness of research and clinical trials, and produce new tools that benefit healthcare providers, patients, insurers, and regulators . AI enables quick and comprehensive retrieval of drug-related information from different resources through its ability to analyze the current medical literature, drug databases, and clinical guidelines to provide accurate and evidence-based decisions for healthcare providers. Using automated response systems, AI-powered virtual assistants can handle common questions and provide detailed medical information to healthcare providers . AI-powered chatbots help reduce the workload on healthcare providers, allowing them to focus on more complicated cases that require their expertise. Also, AI algorithms can generate specific recommendations for individual patients, considering factors like health conditions, past medical and medication history, and social/lifestyle preferences, allowing healthcare professionals to optimize medication choices and dosages.

AI-Powered Patient Care

AI virtual healthcare assistance

With continuously increasing demands of health care services and limited resources worldwide, finding solutions to overcome these challenges is essential Virtual health assistants are a new and innovative technology transforming the healthcare industry to support healthcare professionals. It is designed to simulate human conversation to offer personalized patient care based on input from the patient . These digital assistants use AI-powered applications, chatbots, sounds, and interfaces. Virtual assistants can help patients with tasks such as identifying the underlying problem based on the patient's symptoms, providing medical advice, reminding patients to take their medications, scheduling doctor appointments, and monitoring vital signs. In addition, digital assistants can collect information daily regarding patients' health and forward the reports to the assigned physician. By taking off some of these responsibilities from human healthcare providers, virtual assistants can help to reduce their workload and improve patient outcomes.

Furthermore, these tools can always be available, making it easier for patients to access healthcare when needed . Another medical service that an AI-driven phone application can provide is triaging patients and finding out how urgent their problem is, based on the entered symptoms into the app. The National Health Service (NHS) has tested this app in north London, and now about 1.2 million people are using this AI chatbot to answer their questions instead of calling the NHS non-emergency number . In addition, introducing intelligent speakers into the market has a significant benefit in the lives of elderly and chronically ill patients who are unable to use smartphone apps efficiently . Overall, virtual health assistants have the potential to significantly improve the quality, efficiency, and cost of healthcare delivery while also increasing patient engagement and providing a better experience for them.

AI mental health support

AI has the potential to revolutionize mental health support by providing personalized and accessible care to individuals .Several studies showed the effectiveness and accessibility of using Web-based or Internet-based cognitive-behavioral therapy (CBT) as a psychotherapeutic intervention . Even though psychiatric practitioners rely on direct interaction and behavioral observation of the patient in clinical practice compared to other practitioners, AI-powered tools can supplement their work in several ways. AI-powered mental health applications can assist in the early detection and diagnosis of mental health conditions, as well as provide tailored treatment and support . These applications can also offer round-the-clock support, reducing the need for in-person appointments and wait times. Furthermore, these digital tools can be used to monitor patient progress and medication adherence, providing valuable insights into treatments' effectiveness

The current published studies addressing the applicability of AI in mental health concluded that depression is the most commonly investigated mental disorder . Moreover, AI-powered apps prove their benefits in patients with substance use disorder. A recent study evaluated the utility of a mental health digital app called Woebot in patients with substance use disorders. This study found that using Woebot was significantly associated with improved substance use, cravings, depression, and anxiety . While AI-powered mental health diagnosis holds promise, some significant limitations must be addressed. One of the main limitations is the risk of bias in the data and algorithms used in AI-powered diagnosis. If the data used to train AI algorithms does not represent diverse populations, it can lead to biased and inaccurate results. Additionally, AI-powered diagnosis may not take into account the complexity of mental health conditions, which can present differently in different people. Finally, there is a risk that AI-powered diagnosis may lead to a lack of personalization and empathy in mental health care, which is an important aspect of successful treatment .Therefore, while AI-powered diagnosis can be a valuable tool in mental health care, it should be used as a supplement to, rather than a replacement for, professional diagnosis and treatment.

AI in enhancing patient education and mitigating healthcare provider burnout

One of the emerging applications of AI is patient education .AI-powered chatbots are being implemented in various healthcare contexts, such as diet recommendations , smoking cessation, and cognitive-behavioral therapy. Patient education is integral to healthcare, as it enables individuals to understand their medical diagnosis, treatment options, and preventative measures . Informed patients are more likely to adhere to their treatment regimens and achieve better health outcomes . AI has the potential to play a significant role in patient education by providing personalized and interactive information and guidance to patients and their caregivers . For example, in patients with prostate cancer, introducing a prostate cancer communication assistant (PROSCA) chatbot offered a clear to moderate increase in participants' knowledge about prostate cancer .Researchers found that ChatGPT, an AI Chatbot founded by OpenAI, can help patients with diabetes understand their diagnosis and treatment options, monitor their symptoms and adherence, provide feedback and encouragement, and answer their questions . AI technology can also be applied to rewrite patient education materials into different reading levels. This suggests that AI can empower patients to take greater control of their health by ensuring that patients can understand their diagnosis, treatment options, and self-care instructions .However, there are also some challenges and limitations that need to be addressed, such as ensuring the accuracy, reliability, and transparency of the information provided by AI, respecting the privacy and confidentiality of the patients' data, and maintaining a human touch and empathy in the communication . The use of AI in patient education is still in its early stages, but it has the potential to revolutionize the way that patients learn about their health. As AI technology continues to develop, we can expect to see even more innovative and effective ways to use AI to educate patients.

Are individuals more inclined towards AI than human healthcare providers

Public perception of the benefits and risks of AI in healthcare systems is a crucial factor in determining its adoption and integration. People's feelings about AI replacing or augmenting human healthcare practitioners, its role in educating and empowering patients, and its impact on the quality and efficiency of care, as well as on the well-being of healthcare workers, are all important considerations. . In medicine, patients often trust medical staff unconditionally and believe that their illness will be cured due to a medical phenomenon known as the placebo effect. In other words, patient-physician trust is vital in improving patient care and the effectiveness of their treatment . For the relationship between patients and an AI-based healthcare delivery system to succeed, building a relationship based on trust is imperative .

Research on whether people prefer AI over healthcare practitioners has shown mixed results depending on the context, type of AI system, and participants' characteristics .Some surveys have indicated that people are generally willing to use or interact with AI for health-related purposes such as diagnosis, treatment, monitoring, or decision support . However, other studies have suggested that people still prefer human healthcare practitioners over AI, especially for complex or sensitive issues such as mental health, chronic diseases, or end-of-life care . In a US-based study, 60% of participants expressed discomfort with providers relying on AI for their medical care. However, the same study found that 80% of Americans would be willing to use AI-powered tools to help manage their health . In another survey, responders' comfort with AI varied based on clinical application, and most patients felt that AI would improve their healthcare, which suggests that people are generally willing to use AI for healthcare-related purposes and that patient education, concerns, and comfort levels should be accounted for when planning for integration of AI .Moreover, people's trust and acceptance of AI may vary depending on their age, gender, education level, cultural background, and previous experience with technology .

Future Directions And Considerations For Clinical Implementation

Obstacles and solutions

AI has the potential to revolutionize clinical practice, but several challenges must be addressed to realize its full potential. Among these challenges is the lack of quality medical data, which can lead to inaccurate outcomes. Data privacy, availability, and security are also potential limitations to applying AI in clinical practice. Additionally, determining relevant clinical metrics and selecting an appropriate methodology is crucial to achieving the desired outcomes. Human contribution to the design and application of AI tools is subject to bias and could be amplified by AI if not closely monitored . The AI-generated data and/or analysis could be realistic and convincing; however, hallucination could also be a major issue which is the tendency to fabricate and create false information that cannot be supported by existing evidence .This can be particularly problematic regarding sensitive areas such as patient care. Thus, the development of AI tools has implications for current health professions education, highlighting the necessity of recognizing human fallibility in areas including clinical reasoning and evidence-based medicine . Finally, human expertise and involvement are essential to ensure the appropriate and practical application of AI to meet clinical needs and the lack of this expertise could be a drawback for the practical application of AI.Addressing these challenges and providing constructive solutions will require a multidisciplinary approach, innovative data annotation methods, and the development of more rigorous AI techniques and models. Creating practical, usable, and successfully implemented technology would be possible by ensuring appropriate cooperation between computer scientists and healthcare providers. By merging current best practices for ethical inclusivity, software development, implementation science, and human-computer interaction, the AI community will have the opportunity to create an integrated best practice framework for implementation and maintenance . Additionally, a collaboration between multiple health care settings is required to share data and ensure its quality, as well as verify analyzed outcomes which will be critical to the success of AI in clinical practice. Another suggestion is to provide appropriate training and education that starts from the undergraduate level of all the health care practitioners and proceeds to the continuous development and improvement for the practitioners working in the current practice to ensure the proper adaptation which provides the best patient care and avoid any legal or ethical issues or misinterpretation of the outcomes without verifying the results . Medical schools are encouraged to incorporate AI-related topics into their medical curricula. A study conducted among radiology residents showed that 86% of students agreed that AI would change and improve their practice, and up to 71% felt that AI should be taught at medical schools for better understanding and application . This integration ensures that future healthcare professionals receive foundational knowledge about AI and its applications from the early stages of their education.

Legal, ethical, and risk associated with AI in healthcare system

Converting AI and big data into secure and efficient practical applications, services, and procedures in healthcare involves significant costs and risks. Consequently, safeguarding the commercial interests of AI and data-driven healthcare technologies has emerged as an increasingly crucial subject .In the past, only medical professionals could measure vital signs such as blood pressure, glucose levels, and heart rate . However, contemporary mobile applications now enable the continuous collection of such information. Nevertheless, addressing the ethical risks associated with AI implementation is imperative, particularly concerning data privacy and confidentiality violations, informed consent, and patient autonomy . Given the prominence of big data and AI in healthcare and precision medicine, robust data protection legislation becomes paramount to safeguarding individual privacy. Countries around the world have introduced laws to protect the privacy of their citizens, such as the Health Insurance Portability and Accountability Act (HIPAA) in the United States and the General Data Protection Regulation (GDPR) in Europe.While HIPAA protects only relevant health information produced by covered entities, the GDPR has implemented extensive data protection law within the EU, creating a significant global shift in data protection .

One of the major causes that can compromise patient data, disrupt critical healthcare operations, and jeopardize patient safety with the use of AI in the healthcare system is increased cyberattacks.Predictive algorithms can be employed to detect and prevent these cyber threats. To safeguard data privacy and maintain system integrity, it's essential to deeply investigate cybersecurity and the cyber risk landscape of healthcare systems. By implementing a variety of robust AI algorithms, the risk associated with relying on a singular solution can be mitigated While data privacy and security breaches are challenges associated with AI in healthcare . it offers significant advantages such as task streamlining, enhanced efficiency, time and resource savings, research support, and reduced physician stress . In the context of ethical considerations, an epistemological framework for ethical assessment has been proposed to prioritize ethical awareness, transparency, and accountability when evaluating digital technology's impact on healthcare supply chain participants .

Research ,Significance ,Results and Conclusion

The integration of AI in healthcare has immense potential to revolutionize patient care and outcomes. AI-driven predictive analytics can enhance the accuracy, efficiency, and cost-effectiveness of disease diagnosis and clinical laboratory testing. Additionally, AI can aid in population health management and guideline establishment, providing real-time, accurate information and optimizing medication choices. Integrating AI in virtual health and mental health support has shown promise in improving patient care. However, it is important to address limitations such as bias and lack of personalization to ensure equitable and effective use of AI.

Several measures must be taken to ensure responsible and effective implementation of AI in healthcare.

Firstly, comprehensive cybersecurity strategies and robust security measures should be developed and implemented to protect patient data and critical healthcare operations.

Collaboration between healthcare organizations, AI researchers, and regulatory bodies is crucial to establishing guidelines and standards for AI algorithms and their use in clinical decision-making. Investment in research and development is also necessary to advance AI technologies tailored to address healthcare challenges.AI algorithms can continuously examine factors such as population demographics, disease prevalence, and geographical distribution. This can identify patients at a higher risk of certain conditions, aiding in prevention or treatment. Edge analytics can also detect irregularities and predict potential healthcare events, ensuring that resources like vaccines are available where most needed.Public perception of AI in healthcare varies, with individuals expressing willingness to use AI for health purposes while still preferring human practitioners in complex issues. Trust-building and patient education are crucial for the successful integration of AI in healthcare practice. Overcoming challenges like data quality, privacy, bias, and the need for human expertise is essential for responsible and effective AI integration.

Collaboration among stakeholders is vital for robust AI systems, ethical guidelines, and patient and provider trust. Continued research, innovation, and interdisciplinary collaboration are important to unlock the full potential of AI in healthcare. With successful integration, AI is anticipated to revolutionize healthcare, leading to improved patient outcomes, enhanced efficiency, and better access to personalized treatment and quality care.

Healthcare systems are complex and challenging for all stakeholders, but artificial intelligence (AI) has transformed various fields, including healthcare, with the potential to improve patient care and quality of life. Rapid AI advancements can revolutionize healthcare by integrating it into clinical practice. Reporting AI's role in clinical practice is crucial for successful implementation by equipping healthcare providers with essential knowledge and tools.

This review chapter provides a comprehensive and up-to-date overview of the current state of AI in clinical practice, including its potential applications in disease diagnosis, treatment recommendations, and patient engagement. It also discusses the associated challenges, covering ethical and legal considerations and the need for human expertise. By doing so, it enhances understanding of AI's significance in healthcare and supports healthcare organizations in effectively adopting AI technologies

Integrating AI into healthcare holds excellent potential for improving disease diagnosis, treatment selection, and clinical laboratory testing. AI tools can leverage large datasets and identify patterns to surpass human performance in several healthcare aspects. AI offers increased accuracy, reduced costs, and time savings while minimizing human errors. It can revolutionize personalized medicine, optimize medication dosages, enhance population health management, establish guidelines, provide virtual health assistants, support mental health care, improve patient education, and influence patient-physician trust

Bibliography and Acknoledgement

- Abdel-Hameed Al-Mistarehi M, Mijwil M. ; Youssef Filali; Mariem Bounabi; Guma Ali; Mostafa Abotaleb. Artificial Intelligence Solutions for Health 4.0: Overcoming Challenges and Surveying Applications. MJAIH 2023, 2023, 15–20.
- Abubaker Bagabir S, Ibrahim NK, Abubaker Bagabir H, Hashem Ateeq R. Covid-19 and Artificial Intelligence: genome sequencing, drug development and vaccine discovery. J Infect Public Health. 2022;15(2):289–96. https://doi.org/10.1016/j.jiph.2022.01.011.
- Aggarwal A, Tam CC, Wu D, Li X, Qiao S. Artificial Intelligence-Based chatbots for promoting health behavioral changes: systematic review. J Med Internet Res. 2023;25:e40789. https://doi.org/10.2196/40789.
- Amarasingham R, Patzer RE, Huesch M, Nguyen NQ, Xie B. Implementing electronic health care predictive analytics: considerations and challenges. Health Aff (Millwood). 2014;33(7):1148–54. https://doi.org/10.1377/hlthaff.2014.0352.
- Artificial Intelligence and Machine Learning in Software as a Medical Device. US Food and Drug Administration. Released 2021. FDA website: https://www.fda.gov/medical-devices/software-medical-device-samd/artificial-intelligence-and-machine-learning-software-medical-device. Accessed 6.20.2023.
- Artificial Intelligence in Healthcare. 39 Examples Improving the Future of Medicine. Emerj. https://emerj.com/ai-sector-overviews/artificial-intelligence-in-healthcare-39-examples-improving-the-future-of-medicine/. Published September 21, 2021. Accessed June 19, 2023.
- Beam YuK, Kohane AL. Artificial intelligence in healthcare. Nat Biomed Eng. 2018;2(10):719–31. https://doi.org/10.1038/s41551-018-0305-z.
- Becker J, Decker JA, Römmele C, Kahn M, Messmann H, Wehler M, et al. Artificial intelligence-based detection of pneumonia in chest radiographs. Diagnostics. 2022;12(6):1465. https://doi.org/10.3390/diagnostics12061465.
- Berlyand Y, Raja AS, Dorner SC, Prabhakar AM, Sonis JD, Gottumukkala RV, et al. How artificial intelligence could transform emergency department operations. Am J Emerg Med. 2018;36(8):1515–7. https://doi.org/10.1016/j.ajem.2018.01.017.
- Buch VH, Ahmed I, Maruthappu M. Artificial intelligence in medicine: current trends and future possibilities. Br J Gen Pract. 2018;68(668):143–4. https://doi.org/10.3399/bjgp18X695213.
- Burgess M. The NHS is trialling an AI chatbot to answer your medical questions. Wired. 2017. Jan 5, http://www.wired.co.uk/article/babylon-nhs-chatbot-app. Accessed 20 June 2023.
- Chatbots. Medicine Delivery.; Available from: https://hellotars.com/chatbot-templates/healthcare/Hk8N4h/medicine-ordering-chatbot. Accessed 6.20.2023.
- Chew HSJ. The Use of Artificial Intelligence-Based conversational agents (Chatbots) for weight loss: scoping review and practical recommendations. JMIR Med Inform. 2022;10(4):e32578. https://doi.org/10.2196/32578.
- Collins GS, Dhiman P, Andaur Navarro CL, Ma J, Hooft L, Reitsma JB, et al. Protocol for development of a reporting guideline (TRIPOD-AI) and risk of bias tool (PROBAST-AI) for diagnostic and prognostic prediction model studies based on artificial intelligence. BMJ Open. 2021;11(7):e048008. https://doi.org/10.1136/bmjopen-2020-048008.
- Crossnohere NL, Elsaid M, Paskett J, Bose-Brill S, Bridges JFP. Guidelines for Artificial Intelligence in Medicine: Literature Review and Content Analysis of Frameworks. J Med Internet Res. 2022;24(8):e36823. https://doi.org/10.2196/36823.
- Dasta J. Application of artificial intelligence to pharmacy and medicine. Hosp Pharm. 1992;27(4):312–5.
- Davenport T, Kalakota R. The potential for artificial intelligence in Healthcare. Future Healthc J. 2019;6(2):94–8. https://doi.org/10.7861/futurehosp.6-2-94.
- Davoudi A, Malhotra KR, Shickel B, Siegel S, Williams S, Ruppert M et al. The intelligent ICU pilot study: using artificial intelligence technology for autonomous patient monitoring. https://doi.org/10.48550/arXiv.1804.10201.
- deBurca S. The learning health care organization. Int J Qual Health Care. 2000;12(6):457–8. https://doi.org/10.1093/intqhc/12.6.457.
- Donzé J, Aujesky D, Williams D, Schnipper JL. Potentially avoidable 30-day hospital readmissions in medical patients: derivation and validation of a prediction model. JAMA Intern Med. 2013;173:632–8.
- Esmaeilzadeh P. Use of AI-based tools for healthcare purposes: a survey study from consumers' perspectives. BMC Med Inform Decis Mak. 2020;20(1):170. Published 2020 Jul 22. https://doi.org/10.1186/s12911-020-01191-1.
- Esteva A, Kuprel B, Novoa RA, Ko J, Swetter SM, Blau HM, et al. Dermatologist-level classification of skin cancer with deep neural networks. Nature. 2017;542(7639):115–8. https://doi.org/10.1038/nature21056.
- Fitzpatrick KK, Darcy A, Vierhile M. Delivering cognitive behavior therapy to young adults with symptoms of depression and anxiety using a fully automated conversational agent (woebot): a randomized controlled trial. JMIR Mental Health. 2017;4(2):e19.
- Gandhi SO, Sabik L. Emergency department visit classification using the NYU algorithm. Am J Manag Care. 2014;20(4):315–20.
Gerke S, Minssen T, Cohen G. Ethical and legal challenges of artificial intelligence-driven healthcare. Artif Intell Healthc. 2020;295–336. https://doi.org/10.1016/b978-0-12-818438-7.00012-5.
- Ghosh PK, Jain P, Wankhede S, Preethi M, Kannan MK. Virtual nursing Assistant. J Geog Sci. 2021;8:279–85. 20.18001.GSJ.2021.V8I3.21.36690.
- Görtz M, Baumgärtner K, Schmid T, Muschko M, Woessner P, Gerlach A, et al. An artificial intelligence-based chatbot for prostate cancer education: designandpatientevaluationstudy.DigitHealth. 2023;9:20552076231173304. https://doi.org/10.1177/20552076231173304.
- Graham S, Depp C, Lee EE, Nebeker C, Tu X, Kim HC, et al. Artificial Intelligence for Mental Health and Mental Illnesses: an overview. Curr PsychiatryRep.2019;21(11):116.https://doi.org/10.1007/s11920-019-1094-0.
- Han SS, Park I, Eun Chang S, Lim W, Kim MS, Park GH, et al. Augmented Intelligence Dermatology: deep neural networks Empower Medical Professionals in diagnosing skin Cancer and Predicting Treatment Options for 134 skin Disorders. J Invest Dermatol. 2020;140(9):1753–61. https://doi.org/10.1016/j.jid.2020.01.019.
- Haug CJ, Drazen JM. Artificial Intelligence and Machine Learning in Clinical Medicine, 2023. N Engl J Med. 2023;388(13):1201–8.
Hautz WE, Kämmer JE, Hautz SC, Sauter TC, Zwaan L, Exadaktylos AK, et al. Diagnostic error increases mortality and length of hospital stay in patients presenting through the emergency room. Scand J Trauma Resusc Emerg Med. 2019;27(1):54. https://doi.org/10.1186/s13049-019-0629-z.
- IOM (Institute of Medicine). Measuring the impact of Interprofessional Education on collaborative practice and patient outcomes. Washington, DC: The National Academies Press; 2015. p. 182.
- irchner GJ, Kim RY, Weddle JB, Bible JE. Can Artificial Intelligence improve the readability of Patient Education Materials? Clin Orthop Relat Res 2023 Apr 28. https://doi.org/10.1097/CORR.0000000000002668. Jiang F, Jiang Y, Zhi H, Dong Y, Li H, Ma S, et al. Artificial intelligence in healthcare: past, present and future. Stroke Vasc Neurol. 2017;2(4):230–43.

- Johnson KB, Wei WQ, Weeraratne D, Frisse ME, Misulis K, Rhee K, et al. Precision Medicine, AI, and the future of Personalized Health Care. Clin Transl Sci. 2021;14(1):86–93. https://doi.org/10.1111/cts.12884.
- Jordan MI, Mitchell TM. Machine learning: Trends, perspectives, and prospects.Science.2015;349(6245):255–60.https://doi.org/10.1126/science.aaa8415.
- Khullar D, Casalino LP, Qian Y, Lu Y, Krumholz HM, Aneja S. Perspectives of patients about Artificial Intelligence in Health Care. JAMANetwOpen.2022;5(5):e2210309.https://doi.org/10.1001/jamanetworkopen.2022.10309. Published 2022 May 2.
- Lee EE, Torous J, De Choudhury M, Depp CA, Graham SA, Kim HC, et al. Artificial Intelligence for Mental Health Care: clinical applications, barriers, facilitators, and Artificial Wisdom. Biol Psychiatry Cogn Neurosci Neuroimaging. 2021;6(9):856–64. https://doi.org/10.1016/j.bpsc.2021.02.001.
- Lee H, Kim HJ, Chang HW, Kim DJ, Mo J, Kim JE. Development of a system to support warfarin dose decisions using deep neural networks. Sci Rep. 2021;11(1):14745. Published 2021 Jul 20. https://doi.org/10.1038/s41598-021-94305-2.
- Liu Y, Chen PC, Krause J, Peng L. How to read articles that use machine learning: users' guides to the medical literature. JAMA. 2019;322(18):1806–16.https://doi.org/10.1001/jama.2019.16489.2754798.
- Martin GL, Jouganous J, Savidan R, Bellec A, Goehrs C, Benkebil M, et al. Validation of Artificial Intelligence to support the automatic coding of patient adverse drug reaction reports, using Nationwide Pharmacovigilance Data. Drug Saf. 2022;45(5):535–48.
- Nakhleh A, Spitzer S, Shehadeh N. ChatGPT's response to the diabetes knowledge questionnaire: implications for Diabetes Education. Diabetes Technol Ther. 2023 Apr;16. https://doi.org/10.1089/dia.2023.0134.
- Nelson KM, Chang ET, Zulman DM, Rubenstein LV, Kirkland FD, Fihn SD. Using Predictive Analytics to Guide Patient Care and Research in a National Health System. J Gen Intern Med. 2019;34(8):1379–80. https://doi.org/10.1007/s11606-019-04961-4.
- Panch T, Szolovits P, Atun R. Artificial Intelligence, Machine Learning and Health Systems. J Global Health. 2018;8(2). https://doi.org/10.7189/jogh.08.020303.
- Pinto dos Santos D, Giese D, Brodehl S, Chon SH, Staab W, Kleinert R, et al. Medical students' attitude towards Artificial Intelligence: a multicentre survey. Eur Radiol. 2018;29(4):1640–6.
- Pulley JM, Denny JC, Peterson JF, Bernard GR, Vnencak-Jones CL, Ramirez AH, et al. Operational implementation of prospective genotyping for personalized medicine: the design of the Vanderbilt PREDICT project. Clin Pharmacol Ther. 2012;92(1):87–95. https://doi.org/10.1038/clpt.2011.371.
- Quazi S. Artificial intelligence and machine learning in precision and genomic medicine. Med Oncol. 2022;39(2):120. https://doi.org/10.1007/ Radanliev P, De Roure D, Ani U, Carvalho G. The ethics of shared Covid-19 risks: an epistemological framework for ethical health technology assessment of risk in vaccine supply chain infrastructures. Health Technol (Berl).2021;11(5):1083–91.
- Rivera SC, Liu X, Chan A, Denniston AK, Calvert MJ, SPIRIT-AICONSORT-AI. Working Group Guidelines for clinical trial protocols for interventions involving artificial intelligence: the SPIRIT-AI extension. BMJ.2020;370:m3210.https://doi.org/10.1136/bmj.m3210.
- Sheu YH, Magdamo C, Miller M, Das S, Blacker D, Smoller JW. AI-assisted prediction of differential response to antidepressant classes using electronic health records. npj Digit Med. 2023;6:73. https://doi.org/10.1038/s41746-023-00817-8.
- Singh DP, Kaushik B. A systematic literature review for the prediction of anticancer drug response using various machine-learning and deep-learning techniques. Chem Biol Drug Des. 2023;101(1):175–94. https://doi.org/10.1111/cbdd.14164.
- Topol EJ. High-performance medicine: the convergence of human and Artificial Intelligence. Nat Med. 2019;25(1):44–56. https://doi.org/10.1038/s41591-018-0300-7.
- Tran TTV, Surya Wibowo A, Tayara H, Chong KT. Artificial Intelligence in Drug Toxicity Prediction: recent advances, Challenges, and future perspectives. J Chem Inf Model. 2023;63(9):2628–43. https://doi.org/10.1021/acs.jcim.3c00200.
- Undru TR, Uday U, Lakshmi JT, et al. Integrating Artificial Intelligence for ClinicalandLaboratorydiagnosis- a review. Maedica (Bucur).2022;17(2):420–6.https://doi.org/10.26574/maedica.2022.17.2.420.
- Vandenberg O, Durand G, Hallin M, Diefenbach A, Gant V, Murray P, et al. Consolidation of clinical Microbiology Laboratories and introduction of Transformative Technologies. Clin Microbiol Rev. 2020;33(2). https://doi.org/10.1128/cmr.00057-19.
- VanLEHN K. The relative effectiveness of human tutoring, intelligent tutoring systems, and other tutoring systems. Educational Psychol. 2011;46(4):197–221.https://doi.org/10.1080/00461520.2011.611369.
- Vollmer S, Mateen BA, Bohner G, Király FJ, Ghani R, Jonsson P, et al. Machine learning and artificial intelligence research for patient benefit: 20 critical questions on transparency, replicability, ethics, and effectiveness. BMJ.2020;368:l6927.https://doi.org/10.1136/bmj.l6927.
- Wang H, Avillach P. Diagnostic classification and prognostic prediction using common genetic variants in autism spectrum disorder: genotype-based Deep Learning. JMIR Med Inf. 2021;9(4). https://doi.org/10.2196/24754.
- Wang H, Zhang Z, Ip M, Lau J. T.F. Social media–based conversational agents for health management and interventions. J Med Internet Res. 2018;20(8):e261.https://doi.org/10.2196/jmir.9275.
- Weis CV, Jutzeler CR, Borgwardt K. Machine learning for microbial identification and antimicrobial susceptibility testing on MALDI-TOF mass spectra: a systematic review. Clin Microbiol Infect. 2020;26(10):1310–7. https://doi.org/10.1016/j.cmi.2020.03.014.
- West SM, Whittaker M, Crawford K. Discriminating Systems: gender, race andpowerinAI.AINowInstitute;2019.
- White Paper on Artificial Intelligence, European Commission. A European approach to excellence and trust. 2020. Feb 19, https://ec.europa.eu/info/publications/white-paper-artificial-intelligence-european-approach-excellence-and-trust_en.Accessed6.20.2023.
- Widen E, Raben TG, Lello L, Hsu SDH. Machine learning prediction of biomarkers from SNPs and of Disease risk from biomarkers in the UK Biobank. Genes (Basel). 2021;12(7):991. https://doi.org/10.3390/genes12070991.Published2021Jun29.
- Williams AD, Andrews G. The effectiveness of internet cognitive behavioural therapy (iCBT) for depression in primary care: a quality assurance study. PLoSONE.2013;8(2):e57447.
- Wong CK, Yeung DY, Ho HC, Tse KP, Lam CY. Chinese older adults' internet use for health information. J Appl Gerontol. 2014;33(3):316–35. https://doi.org/10.1177/0733464812463430.
- Young AT, Amara D, Bhattacharya A, Wei ML. Patient and general public attitudes towards clinical artificial intelligence: a mixed methods systematic review. Lancet Digit Health. 2021;3(9):e599–e611.
- Yuan B, Li J. The policy effect of the General Data Protection Regulation (GDPR) on the digital public health sector in the European Union: an empirical investigation. Int J Environ Res Public Health. 2019;16(6):1070.https://doi.org/10.3390/ijerph16061070.
- Zhang J, Oh YJ, Lange P, Yu Z, Fukuoka Y. Artificial Intelligence Chatbot Behavior Change Model for Designing Artificial Intelligence Chatbots to promote physical activity and a healthy Diet: viewpoint. J Med Internet Res. 2020;22(9):e22845. https://doi.org/10.2196/22845.

CHAPTER

29

Artificial Intelligence in the Differential Diagnosis of Cardiomyopathy Phenotypes

Cardiomyopathy is defined as abnormal myocardial structure and function in the absence of coronary artery disease, hypertension, valvular disease, or congenital heart diseases . According to the recent European Society of Cardiology (ESC) guidelines, cardiomyopathies are now divided into five major subtypes, namely: hypertrophic cardiomyopathy (HCM), dilated cardiomyopathy (DCM), arrhythmogenic right ventricular cardiomyopathy (ARVC), non-dilated left ventricular cardiomyopathy (NDLVC), and restrictive cardiomyopathy (RCM)

Early detection, diagnosis, and treatment are significant in slowing the progression of cardiomyopathy to advanced diseases and improving overall outcomes, not only for the individual patient, but also for the family as a whole . Patients with cardiomyopathy may access health services through a heterogeneous clinical presentation or incidental findings, such as electrocardiogram abnormalities during routine sports visits or family screening . A multidisciplinary approach is required in order to evaluate this complex cardiac condition, aiming to establish and characterize the cardiomyopathy phenotypes and the underlying etiological diagnosis [3]. This phenotype-based etiological diagnosis necessitates the integration of various data, including personal and family history, clinical examination, electrocardiography, and laboratory investigations, as well as multimodality imaging .

Novel approaches based on artificial intelligence (AI), and on the subsets of machine learning (ML) and deep learning (DL).could provide more accurate stratification and typing for patients with cardiomyopathy, presenting a potential solution to overcome the limitations associated with traditional approaches and optimize personalized medicine..Indeed, one of the many applications of AI and its subsets is to create models that consider a large amount of data, including laboratory information and clinical, molecular, and imaging data, for the superior diagnostic and prognostic stratification of patients. Developing effective knowledge systems that integrate different layers of data is critical to maximizing the impact on translational research and personalized medicine. Currently, there is limited research that directly investigates the integration of these algorithms into clinical practice and verifies their positive impact on clinical outcomes. Additionally, few reviews have analyzed the impact of AI in the classification of cardiomyopathies, and, to the best of our knowledge, none have focused on the impact of AI models in the differential diagnosis of cardiomyopathy phenotypes.The purpose of this review is to provide an overview of AI models developed to discriminate between cardiomyopathy phenotypes, following the recent ESC guidelines for the management of cardiomyopathies, and to highlight the benefits of their application in clinical practice. Finally, we discuss the current limitations of these AI models and their potential future development.

Notion of AI

From the invention of the term "artificial intelligence" in 1956 by John McCarthy, the research and development of AI have not stopped. AI is a broad term encompassing a variety of methods that enable machines to gain knowledge through experience and replicate human cognitive functions .Several subfields of AI exist, namely, machine learning (ML) and deep learning (DL

Machine Learning

ML refers to the ability of AI systems to extract patterns in raw data without being explicitly programmed to do so. It involves training a model through the utilization of data with known ground-truths to subsequently generate predictions for new, unseen inputs . ML models can be broadly classified into different classes according to the type of experience which they are authorized to undergo throughout their training processes, including supervised, unsupervised, and hybrid paradigms such as semi-supervised learning, weakly supervised learning, and self-supervised learning .Supervised learning requires annotated data, also known as "labels". These labeled data are usually evaluated by an expert physician and represent the ground truth data used in the training process. The algorithm involves iteratively adjusting to minimize the disparity between predicted outputs and actual labels, with the aim of understanding the relationship between input data and output labels. The inclusion of expert evaluation and annotation makes these models more time-consuming and resource-intensive compared to

Identifying HCGs to ML based diagnosis of cardiomyopathies.

The next step of this study was to further select HCGs, as potential candidate biomarkers, from the top 1,000 high-variance gene features. This step was considered to be the second step of feature selection to further decrease the dimensionality of the feature space. To perform this task, we calculated variable importance scores of the genes, and the top 50 genes with the highest scores were selected for each model present the top genes and their scores for each model and experiment

Given that the importance scores (ranging from 0 to 100) are relative and specific to each model, only a few genes were scored more than 0 in the DT model, which is why we have a limited number of genes . A, F, K. HCGs were selected if they were shared among at least two models .Since the final number of selected HCGs depended on the shared HCGs among different ML models, the number of HCGs selected for each classification experiment is different . Selected HCGs, including 50 genes for DCM-NF, 68 genes for ICM-NF, and 59 genes for DCM-ICM, are presented

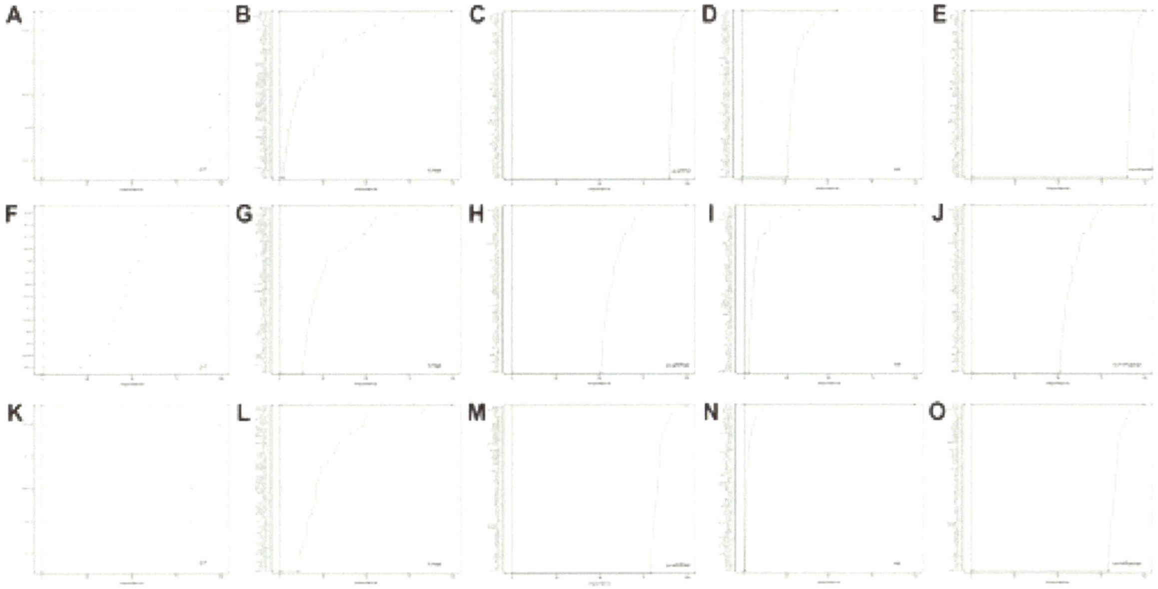

Fig. 29.1 Variable importance scores of top gene features highly contributing to classifications of dilated cardiomyopathy (DCM), ischemic cardiomyopathy (ICM), and nonfailure control (NF) in each ML algorithm. A–E: NF vs. DCM, F–J: NF vs. ICM, K–O: DCM vs. ICM. DT, decision tree; ENet, elastic net; pcaNNet, neural networks with principal component analysis; RF, random forest; svmRadial, support vector machine with radial kernel

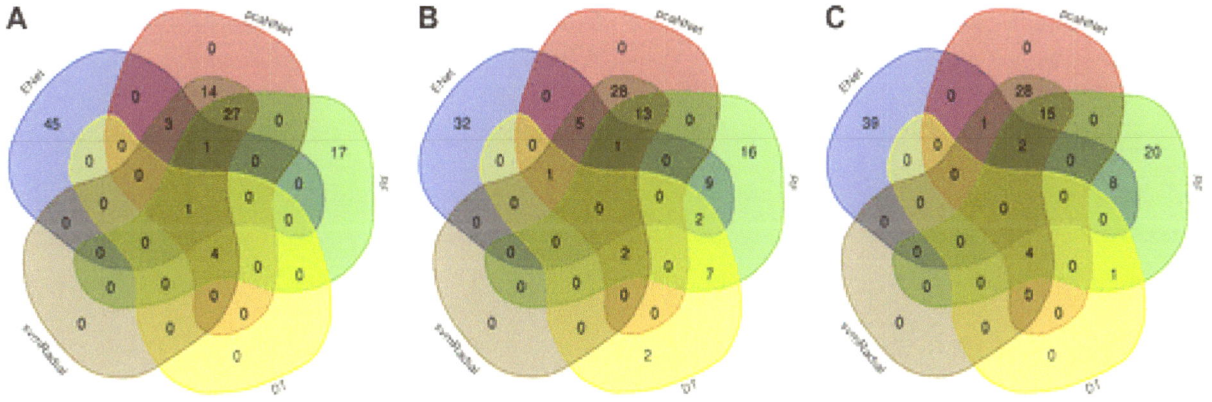

Fig.29.2 Venn diagrams of shared highly contributing genes among different machine learning models in each classification. A: nonfailure controls (NF) vs. dilated cardiomyopathy (DCM), B: NF vs. ischemic cardiomyopathy (ICM), C: DCM vs. ICM. DT, decision tree; ENet, elastic net; pcaNNet, neural networks with principal component analysis; RF, random forest; svmRadial, support vector machine with radial kernel.

Retraining ML models using HCGs.

After selecting the HCGs for each classification experiment, we reimplemented five ML algorithms for training and testing using the only selected HCGs present performance measures of different ML models evaluated on the testing data sets for classifications of different types of cardiomyopathies by using HCGs. In the case of classifying DCM and NF, ~90% accuracy was achieved by using RF, and >85% accuracy was achieved .

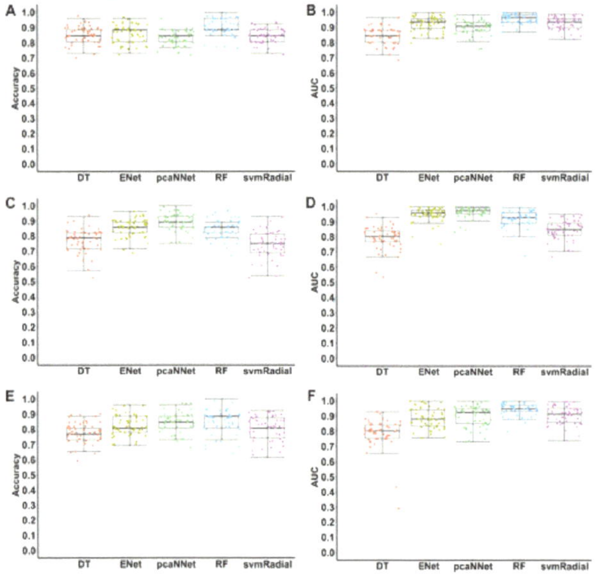

Fig.29.3 .Accuracies and areas under the receiver operating characteristic curve (AUCs) of different machine learning algorithms in classifications of dilated cardiomyopathy (DCM), ischemic cardiomyopathy (ICM), and nonfailure control (NF) samples using only selected highly contributing genes. Each point represents one iteration (total 50 iterations) using each algorithm in each classification. A, B: NF vs. DCM; C, D: NF vs. ICM; E, F: DCM vs. ICM. DT, decision tree; ENet, elastic net; pcaNNet, neural networks with principal component analysis; RF, random forest; svmRadial, support vector machine with radial kernel.

with other models In terms of AUC, four algorithms (ENet, pcaNNet, RF, and svmRadial) achieved ≥0.90 AUC in classifying DCM and NF . RF outperformed other ML models regarding all the performance measures Compared with initial classification using the top 1,000 high-variance genes, an increased prediction accuracy was observed in the RF and DT models using the only selected HCGs.However, all the measurements in ENet, pcaNNet, and svmRadial decreased with only using the selected HCGs .

Pathophysiological pathway analysis.

Furthermore, IPA pathway analyses were performed to examine if any selected HCGs, as the potential biomarkers, were enriched in pathophysiological pathways related to HF. Integrated networks of top five diseases and their corresponding genes in each classification experiment are presented in Fig. 5. The selected HCGs from the DCM-NF classification were clearly involved in cardiac dysfunctions, such as DCM, familial DCM, left ventricular dysfunction, primary DCM, and enlargement of heart, and thegenes DES, DSP, MYH6, MYL3, PKP2, RYR2, TPM1, and TTN were shared among these top five cardiac dysfunctions .Similarly, using the selected HCGs for classifying ICM and NF, fibrosis of heart, hypertrophy of heart, enlargement of heart, primary DCM, and DCM were identified as the top five cardiac dysfunctions, and the genes TNNT2, MYH6, and DES were shared among all these top five cardiac dysfunctions . Finally, in the case of subtype differentiation (DCM vs. ICM), the goal was to identify the distinct dysfunctions between the two cardiomyopathies. Interestingly, none of the pathways related to the heart were detected, and the top five dysfunctional indexes were cell death of kidney cells, cell death of kidney cell lines, disorder of coronary artery, liver tumor, and liver cancer .

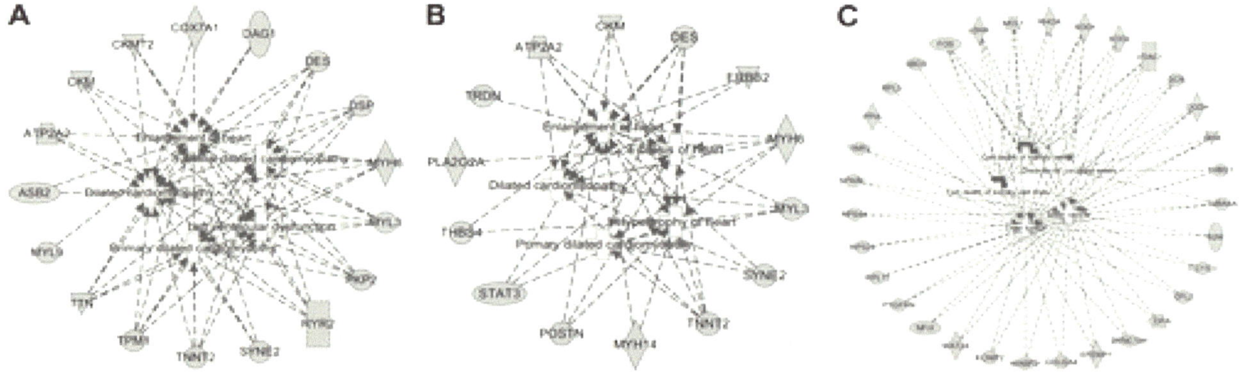

Fig.29.4 Integrated networks of the top 5 pathophysiological dysfunctions and their associated genes. A: NF vs. DCM, B: NF vs. ICM, C: DCM vs. ICM. DCM, dilated cardiomyopathy; ICM, ischemic cardiomyopathy; NF, nonfailure controls

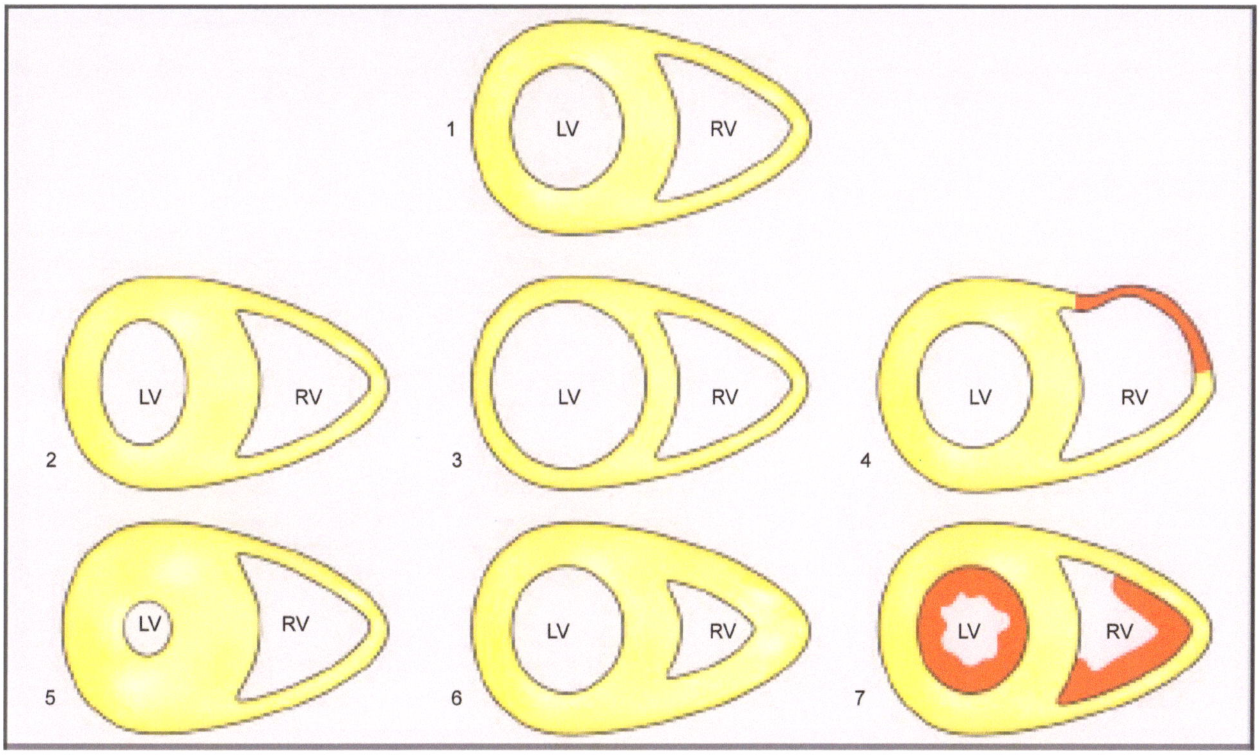

Fig. 29.5 Diagrammatic representation of different types of cardiomyopathies at short axis views and right and left ventricles at mid septal levels. (1), Normal. (2), HCM, nonobstructive hypertrophic cardiomyopathy. (3), DCM,dilated cardiomyopathy. (4), ARVD, arrhythmogenic right ventricular dysplasia. (5), HOCM, hypertrophic obstructive cardiomyopathy. (6), RCM. restrictive cardiomyopathy (7), EMF, endomyocardial fibrosis or obliterative cardiomyopathy.

unsupervised and hybrid paradigms in machine learning. Examples of supervised learning algorithms include logistic regression (LR), support vector machine (SVM), random forest (RF), and nearest-neighbor algorithms .

Conversely, unsupervised learning does not require annotated data for training. Instead, these models utilize unlabeled data to uncover patterns that facilitate the identification of clustering or associations. Some examples of unsupervised learning include k-means, hierarchical clustering, and generative adversarial networks .

Finally, hybrid paradigms are represented by semi-supervised, weakly-supervised, and self-supervised learning approaches as a bridge between supervised and unsupervised learning. For instance, when labeled data are scarce, semi-supervised learning can integrate both labeled and unlabeled data during the training process, utilizing annotated data to guide the learning process and unlabeled data to capture additional information, thus promoting more effective generalization .Weakly supervised learning models are designed to learn from partially or noisily annotated data, rather than complete and accurate labels, and make predictions or classifications based on this information . Instead, in self-supervised learning, only unlabeled data are available, and the algorithm formulates its own learning tasks by creating surrogate tasks from the input data, such as deriving pseudolabels from the intrinsic attributes of the data

Deep Learning

Traditional ML algorithms require hand-crafted features for the learning process, which is often a complex, time-consuming process. DL, a subset of ML, addresses this challenge by allowing algorithms to autonomously learn and extract pertinent features. The architecture of DL systems comprises input, hidden, and output neurons organized into multiple layers, enabling the automatic extraction of features without the need for human intervention or explicit guidance. Most DL models employed in the field of medical imaging, as discussed in this review, rely on convolutional neural networks (CNN). CNNs are specialized DL models tailored to process visual data, such as images and videos. They excel by exploiting the spatial relationships between adjacent pixels to effectively and quantitatively interpret and analyze the content. These networks comprise multiple layers of interconnected artificial neurons, referred to as convolutional layers. These layers are designed to learn filters (or kernels), which process input data and facilitate the extraction of a hierarchy of features, ranging from basic to increasingly abstract and high-level. This hierarchical feature extraction enables the network to discern not only low-level features, like edges and textures, but also high-

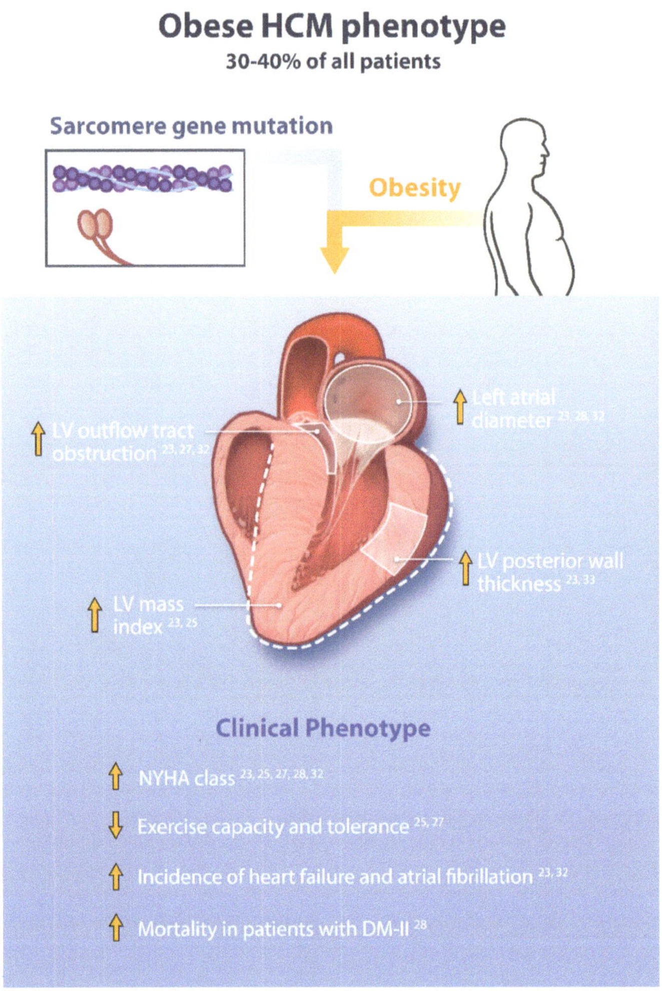

Fig.29.6 Summary of structural and clinical features of the obese hypertrophic cardiomyopathy (HCM) phenotype.

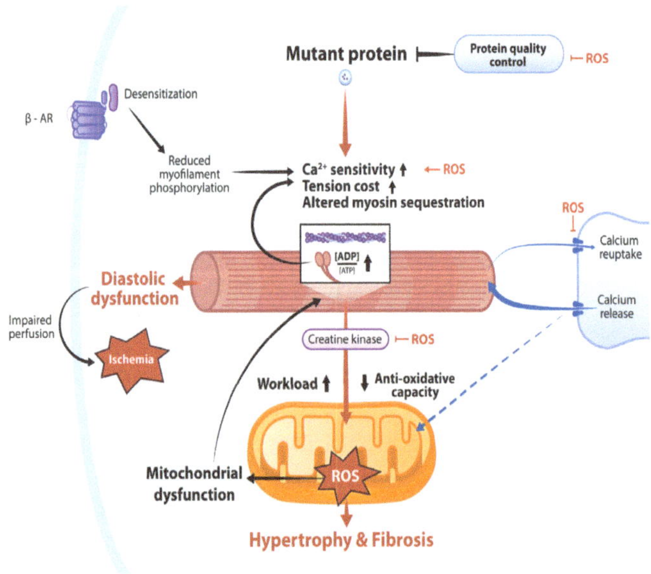

Fig.29.7 Proposed pathophysiology of hypertrophic cardiomyopathy.

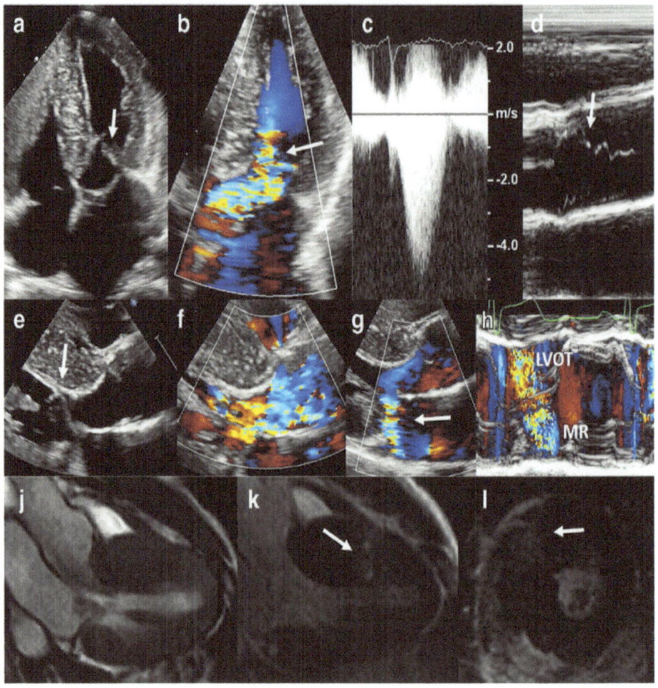

Fig 29.8 Hypertrophic obstructive cardiomyopathy. Asymmetric hypertrophy causing dynamic obstruction of the LV outflow tract by a combination of septal thickening and anterior movement of the anterior mitral valve leaflet (arrow, a = apical 4-chamber view, e = parasternal long axis) during systole. LVOT obstruction causes turbulence (arrow, b), flow acceleration up to nearly 5 m/s (c), as well as fluttering of the aortic valve leaflets on M-mode echocardiography(d). In addition to LV outflow obstruction (e), systolic displacement of the anterior mitral leaflet also causes eccentric, often mid-late systolic, mitral regurgitation as visualized on color-flow 2D (arrow, g) and color-flow M-mode echocardiography (h). CMR confirms hypertrophy of the LV septum (J), but also demonstrates a discrete region of late-enhancement (arrow) where the RV free connects to the left ventricle (K, L)

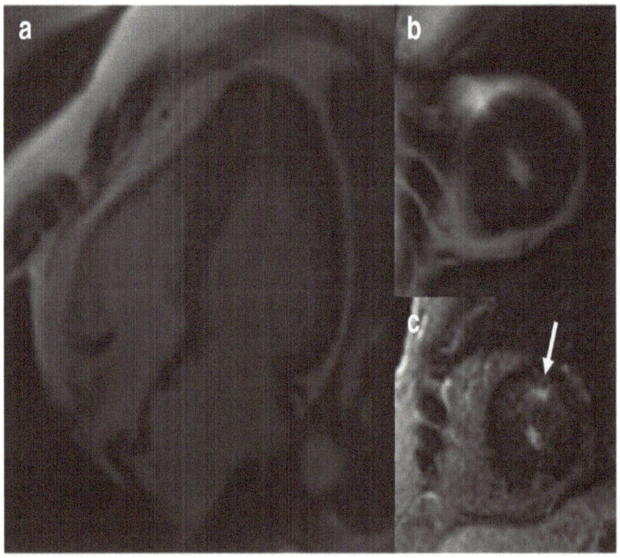

Fig.29.9 Apical hypertrophy. LV hypertrophy grossly limited to the apical segments (a, b) with a discrete region of late enhancement (arrow) on CMR

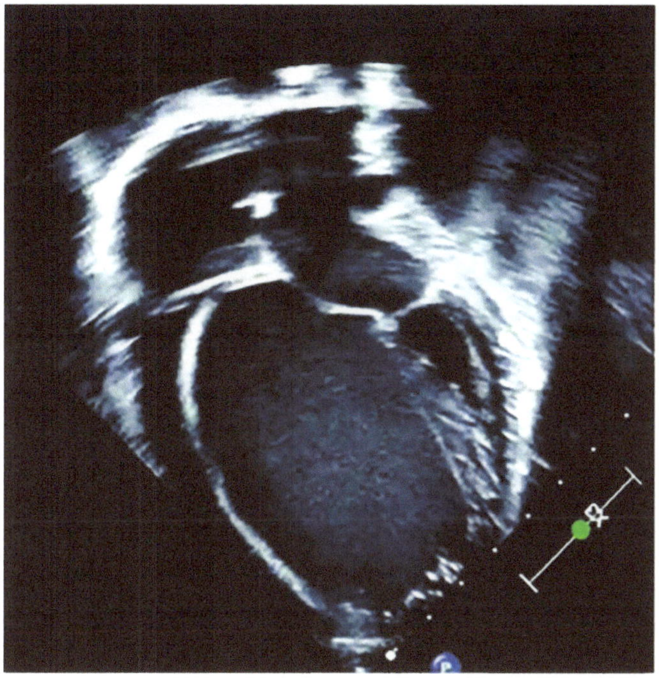

Fig.29.10 Two-dimensional, apical 4-chamber echocardiographic image depicting an enlarged ventricle with spherical geometry and bilateral atrial enlargement in a patient harboring dilated cardiomyopathy secondary to a pathogenic gene variant in the TTN gene

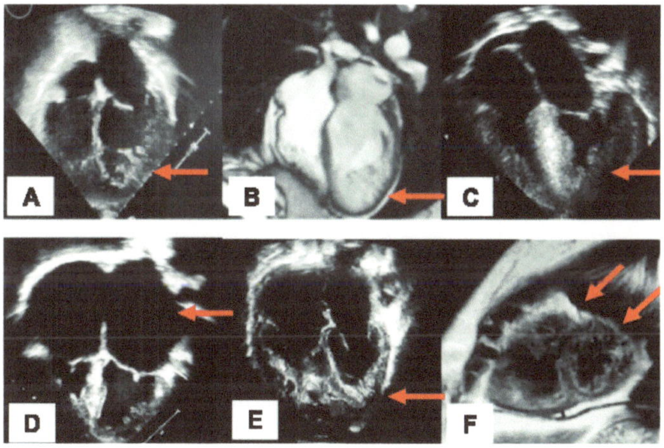

Fig.29.11 Distinct phenotypes of non-compaction cardiomyopathy. (A) Echocardiographic 4-chamber view displays the isolated type of LVNC illustrated by the cardinal feature of left ventricular trabeculations (arrow) with normal anatomy and function; (B) from a cardiac magnetic resonance imaging (CMRi), a 4-chamber view displays the dilated sun-type of LVNC, denoting the enlargement of the LV and the presence of inferolateral trabeculations (arrow); (C) echocardiographic 4-chamber view shows the hypertrophic type of LVNC represented by asymmetric hypertrophy of the interventricular septum and the presence of lateral LV trabeculations (arrow); (D) display of the restrictive type of LVNC, significant bilateral atrial enlargement (arrows) and the presence of left ventricular trabeculations; (E) biventricular hypertrabeculations (arrows); (F) cMRI in a short axis view displays a mixed LVNC phenotype represented by dilated and dysfunctional ventricles in a patient with ventricular arrhythmias and biventricular trabeculations secondary to a pathogenic variant in the PRDM16 gene (arrows).

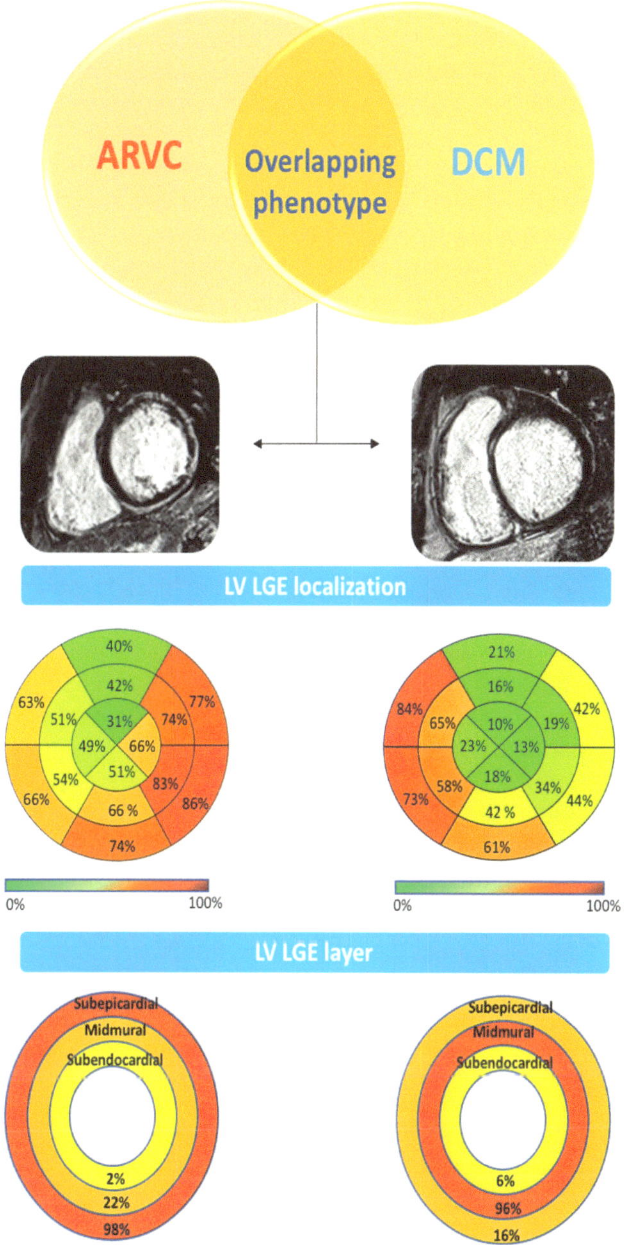

Fig.29.12 Left ventricular regional and wall layer distribution of LGE in ARVC- and DCM-LV phenotype. Comparison between CMR findings in the subgroup of ARVC (left) and DCM (right) patients with overlapping LV phenotypes (ie, combination of LV systolic dysfunction and LV LGE). Patients with ARVC-LV phenotype had lower LV volume and mass, less depressed LVEF (not shown) and greater amount of LV LGE (ie, "hypokinetic, non-dilated and fibrotic left ventricle") compared with DCM patients. LV LGE predominately affected the infero-lateral segments in ARVC-LV phenotype and septal segments in DCM. Compared with DCM, in ARVC the LV LGE significantly more often appeared as a stria pattern than a spot/patchy pattern and more frequently affected the subepicardial layers. ARVC indicates arrhythmogenic right ventricular cardiomyopathy; CMR, cardiac magnetic resonance; DCM, dilated cardiomyopathy; LGE, late gadolinium enhancement; LV, left ventricular; LVEF, left ventricular ejection fraction.

level semantic features, such as complex structures and shapes .Additionally, the architecture of the final layers of CNNs varies based on the specific tasks performed. For example, in a classification task, which could be applied in the differential diagnosis of cardiomyopathy phenotypes, the final layer comprises one or more fully connected layers followed by a softmax activation function. This configuration enables the network to generate probabilistic outputs for each class in this case, each class represents a different pathology involved in the differential diagnosis. Furthermore, multimodal neural networks can be devised to integrate visual data from various imaging modalities with other types of information, such as demographics, family history, clinical examination findings, laboratory results, and electronic health records . In these networks, each data modality is processed through independent branches, each yielding a partial result. These partial results are then merged and fed into the final layers of the network to produce a comprehensive outcome. Consequently, these networks can conduct a more holistic evaluation of a patient, learning to effectively assign probabilities to different pathologies. This may lead to enhanced accuracy in medical diagnoses, as the networks consider a wide array of patient-specific data. Recently, a distinct type of neural architecture known as transformers has emerged as a popular approach, enabling the incorporation of surrounding context in the interpretation of specific portions of images or data

Application of AI in Cardiomyopathies

Technical advancement in the use of AI within the cardiac imaging field has opened up the potential to use extensive datasets to develop models that can automatically interpret data . These algorithms can support the diagnosis and treatment of patients with cardiomyopathies, allowing for early detection, outcome prediction, and prognosis evaluation . AI-based algorithms have proven useful in different cardiac imaging areas, including automated image acquisition, reconstruction, and analysis . In addition, AI approaches can contribute to a more efficient and standardized interpretation of coronary plaque burden, ruling out ischemic etiologies..

With regards to CMR, non-contrast CMR examinations combined with AI have shown promising results, enabling faster, more accessible, and cost-effective CMR images that unquestionably offer advantages in the clinical assessment of cardiomyopathy . This becomes particularly relevant in light of the anticipated exponential rise in CMR examinations in accordance with the recent ESC guidelinesAI models can merge different data, including demographic, clinical, genetic, ECG, echocardiography, CMR, and nuclear imaging parameters, allowing for a more comprehensive assessment of cardiomyopathy phenotypes . In recent years, radiomics features have been suggested as an additional tool to characterize features of cardiomyopathies, extracting voxel-based information from images and capturing the inherent complexity and heterogeneity of pixels in relation to their spatial “neighbors” . Radiomics analysis generates a high number of features from each medical image, and can be coupled with AI thanks to its ability to handle a massive amount of data compared to traditional statistical analysis. AI is rising as a leading component in cardiovascular medicine, and some studies have attempted to generate AI models for the differential diagnosis of cardiomyopathy phenotypes .

Hypertrophic Cardiomyopathy

HCM is defined by the presence of elevated LV wall thickness or mass, with potential concomitant involvement of the right ventricle. Myocardial hypertrophy cannot be exclusively attributed to abnormal loading conditions (e.g., hypertension and valve disease).

LV hypertrophy can arise from numerous etiologies, and the differential diagnosis of “unexplained” hypertrophy is crucial for patient management and outcomes. Indeed, some LV hypertrophy etiologies may require family screening and the implantation of a cardioverter–defibrillator. AI models have demonstrated potential in classifying the underlying causes of ventricular hypertrophy, facilitating efficient diagnosis and prognosis, and preventing morbidity .

Haimovich et al. trained a CNN model using both 12-lead and single-lead electrocardiogram waveform data to differentiate between cardiac diseases associated with LV hypertrophy. The authors retrospectively analyzed 50,709 patients from the Enterprise Warehouse of Cardiology dataset, which were divided into groups characterized by cardiac amyloidosis (n = 304), HCM (n = 1056), hypertension (n = 20,802), aortic stenosis (n = 446), and other causes (n = 4766) . The DL model based on 12-lead electrocardiograms, trained with a derivation cohort of 34,258 individuals and validated with a cohort of 16,451 individuals, achieved an AUROC of 0.95 [95% CI, 0.93–0.97] for cardiac amyloidosis, 0.92 [95% CI, 0.90–0.94] for HCM, 0.90 [95% CI, 0.88–0.92] for aortic stenosis, 0.76 [95% CI, 0.76–0.77] for hypertensive LV hypertrophy, and 0.69 [95% CI 0.68–0.71] for other LV hypertrophy etiologies. In addition, the CNN model trained on single-lead waveforms could also accurately discriminate between LV hypertrophy, with an AUROC of 0.90 [95% CI, 0.88–0.92] for cardiac amyloidosis and 0.90 [95% CI, 0.88–0.92] for HCM. Similarly, an AI model based on electrocardiograms was proposed to identify pediatric patients with HCM. The CNN model was tested in 300 pediatric patients with both echocardiographic and clinical diagnoses of HCM and 18,439 healthy controls, achieving competitive diagnostic performance with an AUC of 0.98 (95% CI 0.98–0.99), sensitivity of 92%, specificity of 95%, positive predictive value of 22%, and negative predictive value of 99%. In a subgroup analysis, the DL models demonstrated a robust diagnostic performance in both sexes, as well as in genotype-positive and genotype-negative HCM patients .

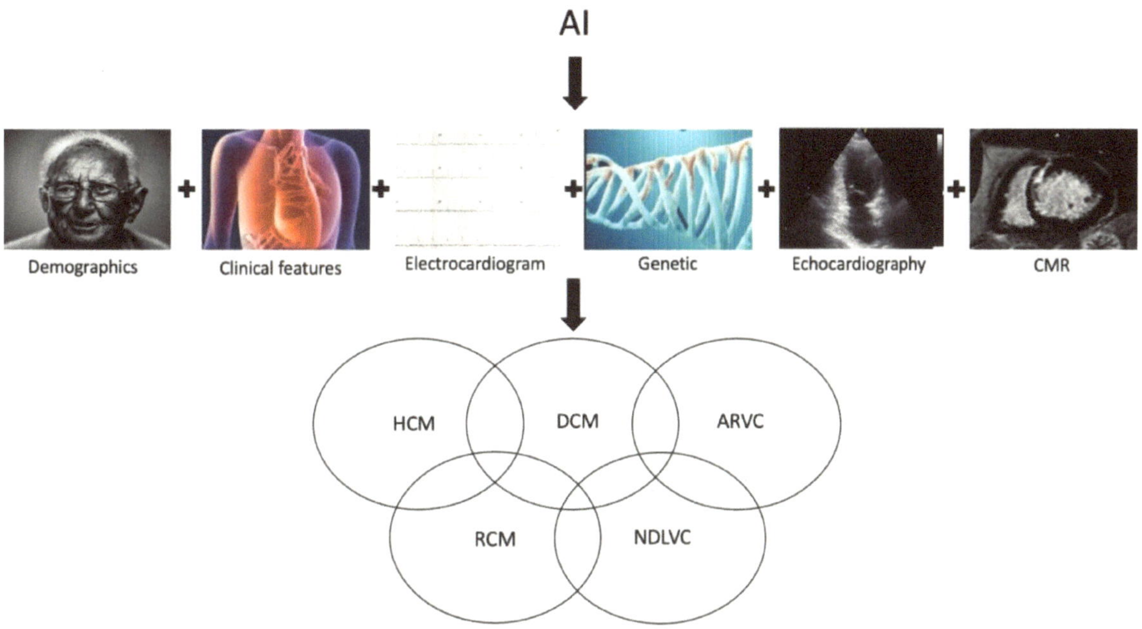

Fig. 29.13 Graphical overview of an AI-based model that integrates various data, including demographic, clinical, genetic, ECG, and cardiac imaging features, to enhance the identification of a phenotype-based etiological diagnosis. AI: artificial intelligence; ARVC: arrhythmogenic right ventricular cardiomyopathy; DCM: dilated cardiomyopathy; HCM: hypertrophic cardiomyopathy; NDLVC: non-dilated left ventricular cardiomyopathy; RCM: restrictive cardiomyopathy.

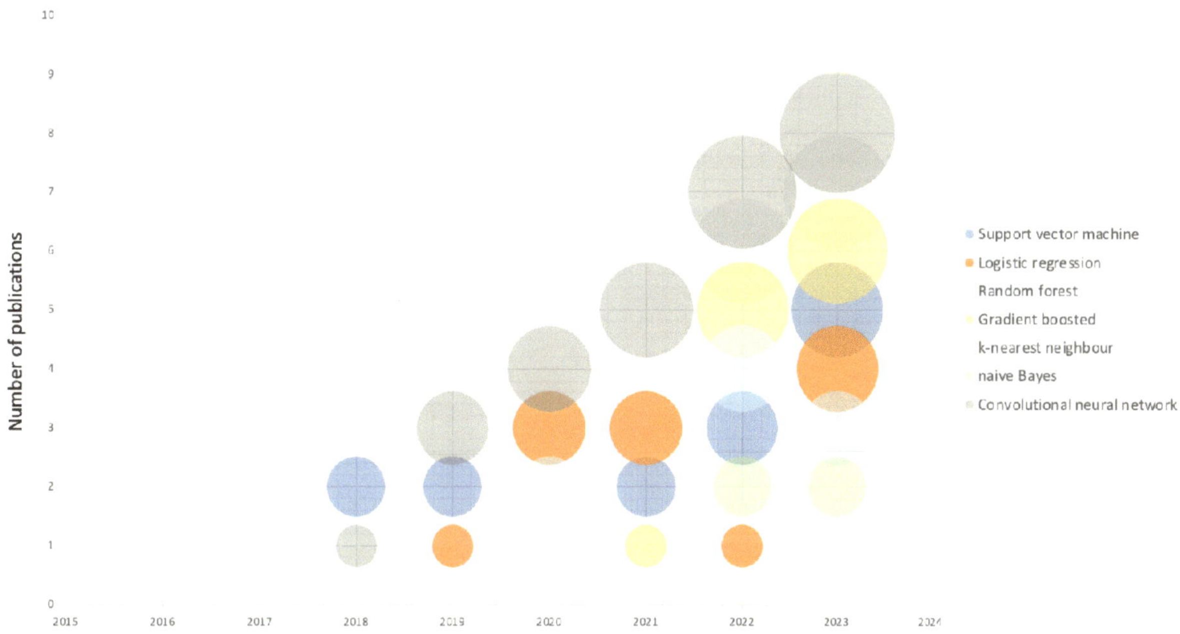

Fig. 29.14 Bubble chart illustrating publications on AI-based models for the differential diagnosis of cardiomyopathy, categorized by the types of machine learning models used. Data were collected from PubMed spanning from 2016 to 2023, as of 31 December 2023. Keywords used were "cardiomyopathy", "artificial intelligence", "machine learning", and "deep learning".

Table29.1 An overview of AI models with brief descriptions.

Algorithm	Overview	Advantages	Disavantages
Support vector machine	A supervised ML model used for both classification and regression. It works by finding an hyperplane that maximally separates data points of different classes in a high-dimensional space, aiming to maximize the margin between the classes.	• Effectively handles unstructured and semi-structured data • Low generalization error	• Requires long training time for large datasets • Results may be difficult to interpret
Logistic regression	A supervised ML algorithm used for binary classification. It models the probability of an instance belonging to a particular class using the logistic function, and the decision boundary is a linear combination of input features.	• Provides insight into feature relevance • Efficient for small datasets • Rapid training	• Assumption of linearity • Sensitivity to outliers
Random forest	A supervised ML algorithm used for classification and regression tasks. It builds multiple decision trees during training and merges their predictions to improve accuracy and robustness. Each tree is trained on a random subset of the data, and the final prediction is determined by a majority vote (for classification) or an average (for regression).	• High accuracy in capturing complex relationships in data • Efficient on large datasets • Provides insight about feature relevance	• Sensitive to small changes in data • Bias towards dominant classes
Gradient-boosted decision tree	An ensemble learning technique used for both classification and regression. It builds a series of decision trees sequentially, with each tree correcting the errors of the previous ones. It combines the predictions of individual trees to create a strong predictive model.	• High accuracy in capturing complex relationships in data • Provides insight into feature relevance • Effective on structured and unstructured data	• Requires long training time for large datasets • Complex interpretability
k-nearest neighbour	A supervised ML algorithm for classification and regression that predicts a data point's label or value based on the majority of its nearby neighbors in the dataset. The "k" represents the number of neighbors considered for the prediction.	• No training period • Supports dynamic data addition • Efficient for small datasets	• Poor performance with large datasets • Impact of irrelevant features • Sensitivity to outliers and missing data
Naive Bayes	A supervised ML algorithm for classification. It is based on Bayes' theorem and assumes independence between features. The algorithm calculates the probability of a data point belonging to a particular class by considering the probabilities of its individual features.	• Simple and fast • Requires small amount of training data • Less sensitive to irrelevant features	• Assumption of feature independence • "Zero Probability" issue • Sensitivity to outliers and missing data
Convolutional neural network	A DL algorithm designed for image and video recognition. It uses convolutional layers to automatically and adaptively learn spatial hierarchies of features from input data.	• Learns hierarchical features from spatial data • Allows parameter sharing, reducing overfitting • Automated feature learning	• Large datasets needed • Requires long training time • Complex interpretability

The prediction of LV hypertrophy was also explored by an ML model that combined clinical, laboratory, and echocardiographic data. In their retrospective monocentric study, the authors evaluated 591 LV hypertrophy patients, and after splitting them into training and testing sets (75%:25%), developed three different ML models, namely, decision tree, RF, and SVM. The SVM model displayed the better diagnostic performance, with an AUROC of 0.90 (0.85–0.94), sensitivity of 0.31 (0.17–0.44), specificity of 0.96 (0.91–0.99), and accuracy of 0.80 (0.75–0.85) in the testing set.

Hwang et al. also developed a CNN long short-term memory DL algorithm to aid in the differentiation of common etiologies of LV hypertrophy (i.e., hypertensive heart disease, HCM, and cardiac amyloidosis) .They achieved average AUC values of 0.962, 0.982, and 0.996 in the test set for hypertensive heart disease, HCM, and cardiac amyloidosis, respectively, and the diagnostic accuracy for the DL algorithm was significantly higher (92.3%) than for echocardiography specialists (80.0% and 80.6%) .

Conversely, Baeßler et al. developed a ML model using radiomics data from CMR images to detect myocardial tissue alterations in HCM. The authors retrospectively evaluated radiomics features from T1 mapping images in 32 patients with known HCM, comparing them to 30 healthy individuals. The proposed ML-based model achieved an AUC of 0.95, with a diagnostic sensitivity of 91% and a specificity of 93% .

Finally, Soto et al. developed a multimodal fusion network by integrating both electrocardiogram and echocardiogram data for the determination of the etiology of LV hypertrophy. The model was trained on more than 18,000 combined instances of examinations from 2728 patients. The proposed fusion model achieved an AUC of 0.92 (95% CI [0.862–0.965]), an F1-score of 0.73 (95% CI [0.585–0.842]), a sensitivity of 0.73 (95% CI [0.562–0.882]), and a specificity of 0.96 (95% CI [0.929–0.985])

Dilated Cardiomyopathy

DCM is defined as the presence of LV dilatation and systolic dysfunction that cannot solely be explained by coronary artery disease or altered loading conditions (e.g., hypertension, congenital heart disease, and valve disease) .DCM is a heterogenous myocardial disease with a variable natural history and patient outcomes. The application of AI has shown the ability to define the underlying cause of LV dilatation and stratify patients according to distinct pathophysiological mechanisms .

The performance of an AI-based model using electrocardiogram data as a screening tool was tested by Shrivastava et al. .The authors evaluated 16,471 individuals, who were divided into DCM patients (n = 421) and control subjects (n = 16,025), using a CNN model trained with 12-lead electrocardiograms. The diagnostic performance of the proposed DL models yielded an excellent diagnostic performance, with an AUC of 0.955, a sensitivity of 98.8%, a specificity of 44.8%, a negative predictive value of 100%, and a positive predictive value of 1.8% for the detection of ejection fractions ≤45% .A radiomics-based ML approach to discriminate between DCM, HCM, and healthy patients was recently explored. Among the various ML models tested, RF minimum redundancy maximum relevance achieved the best performance, with an accuracy of 91.2% and average AUC values of 0.962, 0.982, and 0.996 in the test set for HCM, DCM, and healthy controls, respectively.

Tayal et al. proposed a ML-based approach with profile regression mixture modeling to classify patients with DCM into different sub-phenotypes. They used multiparametric data that included demographic, clinical, genetic, CMR, and proteomics parameters . The proposed ML model was tested in a derivation cohort comprising 426 patients who had been prospectively enrolled in the National Institute for Health Research Royal Brompton Hospital Cardiovascular Biobank project, identifying three novel subtypes: profibrotic metabolic, mild nonfibrotic, and biventricular impairment. The DCM clusters were validated with a cohort of 239 DCM patients prospectively enrolled in the Maastricht Cardiomyopathy Registry.The profibrotic metabolic cluster demonstrated the presence of mid-wall LGE in all cases (100%); 20% had diabetes, and their NYHA functional classification was predominantly class II. Conversely, among the 249 patients in the mild nonfibrotic group, none displayed myocardial fibrosis according to LGE. These patients had milder illnesses, with a significant number falling into NYHA functional class I. A separate group, consisting of 27 patients, was identified as the biventricular impairment group. These patients were notably sicker, with half of them experiencing NYHA functional class III or IV symptoms .

In addition, discrimination between ischemic and non-ischemic etiologies is crucial in patient management. Zhou et al. developed an ML model based on clinical and echocardiography data to discriminate between ischemic and non-ischemic LV dilatation .The authors evaluated 299 patients with dilated LV, and, after splitting them into training and testing sets, developed four different ML models, namely, RF, LR, neural network, and XGBoost. The XGBoost model demonstrated the best accuracy, with a sensitivity of 72%, specificity of 78%, accuracy of 75%, F-score of 0.73, and AUC of 0.934. In addition, the ML model demonstrated good accuracy in terms of discriminating between different etiologies in an external validation cohort, with a sensitivity of 64%, a specificity of 93%, and an AUC of 0.804 .

Non-Dilated Left Ventricular Cardiomyopathy and Arrhythmogenic Right Ventricular Cardiomyopathy

ARVC is characterized by the presence of right ventricle dilatation and/or dysfunction, along with histological involvement and/or electrocardiographic abnormalities, according to the Task Force criteria .Conversely, NDLVC is a newly proposed category of cardiomyopathy

It is defined by the presence or absence of left ventricular systolic impairment, either regionally or globally, along with non-ischemic myocardial scarring or the presence of fatty replacement. This includes a heterogenous group of patients previous described as having dilated cardiomyopathy without dilated LV, arrhythmogenic left ventricular cardiomyopathy, left-dominan tarrhythmogenic cardiomyopathy,orarrhythmogenic dilated cardiomyopathy. These patients do not fulfill the Task Force criteria . AI-based models promise to facilitate the diagnosis of these cardiomyopathy subtypes .

Zhang et al. developed an algorithm for distinguishing between arrhythmogenic cardiomyopathy and dilated cardiomyopathy based on ML algorithms from two public datasets containing myocardial samples. Several ML models were tested, including SVM, naive Bayes, decision tree, K147 nearest neighbor, gradient boosting machine, extreme gradient boosting, and RF, to identify key candidate genes with which to construct a predictive model for favoring separation between arrhythmogenic cardiomyopathy and dilated cardiomyopathy. The RF model achieved the best performance, with an AUC of 0.86 . Similarly, Bleijendaal et al. developed ML and DL models based on typical electrocardiographic features to diagnose Phospholamban p.Arg14del cardiomyopathy, a well-known mutation associated with the development of dilated and/ or arrhythmogenic cardiomyopathy .The authors compared the proposed AI models with an expert cardiologist, demonstrating that the AI models outperformed the expert cardiologist in term of accuracy and sensitivity in both the training and testing datasets. In addition, T-wave morphology was identified as the most important electrocardiographic feature used to classify PLN p.Arg14del carriers .

Another ML model based on electrocardiograms was recently developed by Papageorgiou et al. to discriminate patients with ARVC. The authors proposed the utilization of a CNN for the detection of arrhythmogenic heart disease, achieving 99.98% accuracy, 99.96% specificity, and 99.98% sensitivity during the training phase and 98.6% accuracy, 98.25% specificity, and 98.9% sensitivity when tested .

Restrictive Cardiomyopathy

RCM is defined by the presence of non-dilated left or right restrictive pathophysiology, with normal ventricular wall thickness and normal or reduced diastolic and/or systolic volume in one or both ventricles .The distinction between RCM and constrictive pericarditis could be challenging because of the overlap in clinical presentation and restrictive flow patterns with diastolic dysfunction .Chao et al., by using an apical four-chamber view from transthoracic echocardiography studies, trained a ResNet50 deep learning model, achieving a performance with an area under the curve of 0.97, to differentiate constrictive pericarditis from cardiac amyloidosis .Sengupta et al. designed a ML approach that combines clinical parameters, conventional echocardiographic, and speckle tracking echocardiography data to discriminate between RCM and constrictive pericarditis.. The associative memory classifier demonstrated the best diagnostic performance, with an accuracy of 93.7% and an AUC of 96.2% .

Another cardiac condition that can result in a restrictive pattern is thalassemia. AI-based models have been proposed to identify and measure iron deposits in the heart, enabling early recognition of myocardial dysfunction and subsequent prompt treatment. Taleie et al. proposed a ML model to discriminate between beta-thalassemia major patients with myocardial iron overload from those without myocardial iron overload based on radiomic features extracted from echocardiography images. Among the various ML models tested, maximum relevance–minimum redundancy–extreme gradient boosting achieved the best performance, with an AUC of 0.73, accuracy of 0.73, specificity of 0.73, and sensibility of 0.73 .. Similarly, a ML model to evaluate heart iron overload was proposed by Asmarian et al. achieving an AUC of 0.68 (95% CI 0.60, 0.75) .

Among RCM, Fabry diseases should be taken into account. Due to the heterogenous and multisystemic clinical presentation, this diagnosis could be challenging. An AI-based approach was recently proposed to identify patients affected by Fabry diseases using health record data from 4978 patients with Fabry diseases and 1,000,000 healthy controls. The AI model was trained using a training cohort comprising 75% of all patients, who were selected at random to construct a statistical "phenotypic biomarker" for Fabry disease. Then, the authors predicted the likelihood of having Fabry disease for each patient in the testing cohort, which included 25% of all patients. This method achieved a strong analytic performance, with an AUC of 0.82 .

Eckstein et al. developed a supervised ML model that integrates various strain parameters from the right atrium, left atrium, and right ventricle, as well as cardiac function metrics, to identify cardiac amyloidosis using multiple machine learning classifier algorithms, including k-nearest neighbor, linear and non-linear SVM, and decision trees. The non-linear SVM exhibited the best performance, achieving an accuracy rate of 90.9% and an AUC of 0.996, outperforming other machine learning algorithms in their study .

Other Cardiac Syndromes Associated with Cardiomyopathy Phenotypes

In accordance with the recent ESC guidelines, this category encompasses LV hypertrabeculation and Takotsubo syndrome.Theterm "LV hypertrabeculation" is recommended over LV non-compaction, especially if this phenomena is transient or if it clearly occurs during adulthood .. Takotsubo syndrome is defined as a peculiar pattern of LV dysfunction that presents, in its most typical variant, as apical ballooning and hyperkinesis of LV basal segments in the absence of obstructive coronary disease . AI models have been applied to identify these cardiac syndromes associated with cardiomyopathy phenotypes .

Cau et al. designed an ML model that combines CMR parameters and demographics factors to identify patients with Takotsubo syndrome among individuals with acute chest pain. The authors retrospectively enrolled three groups of patients: those with Takotsubo cardiomyopathy, patients with acute myocarditis, and healthy individuals. To assess the model's performance, they employed five different tree-based ensemble learning algorithms, specifically RF, extremely randomized Trees, bagging of trees, adaptive boosting, and extreme gradient boosting. The extremely randomized trees ML algorithm showcased a sensitivity of 92% (with a 95% confidence interval of 78–100), a specificity of 86% (95% CI: 80–92), and an AUC of 0.94 (95% CI: 0.90–0.99) in the diagnosis of Takotsubo syndrome. Furthermore, the proposed model outperformed clinical reader diagnoses, exhibiting an average increase in AUC of 0.42 (representing an 80% improvement), an increase in sensitivity of 0.08 (equivalent to a 10% boost), and an increase in specificity of 0.618 (indicating a 257% enhancement). Importantly, this improved diagnostic performance was achieved with a significantly shorter duration of analysis, taking only 0.26 s compared to 560 s for the clinical reader.

An ML approach based on radiomics data was developed to automatically differentiating LV non-compaction from other cardiomyopathy phenotypes, including HCM and DCM . The authors extracted a set of 420 radiomics features from 118 patients (including 37 DCM, 25 HCM, and 35 left ventricle non-compaction patients, as well as 21 healthy control individuals).The radiomics model to discriminate cardiomyopathy phenotypes was built with different consecutive steps, namely,

(1) removing radiomics features that were highly correlated;

(2) normalization to introduce the features into ML models;

(3) feature selection, selecting the best features based on univariate statistical tests; and

(4) training and testing different ML models, such as SVM, multi-class RF, and multi-class LR, for classification. The radiomics models for the automated diagnosis of left ventricle non-compaction achieved excellent diagnostic performance, with AUC values of 0.95

Limitations and Future Directions

AI has the potential to reduce costs and save physicians' time by analyzing complex data and enabling phenotype-based etiological diagnosis, but several challenges must be addressed for its effective implementation in real-world clinical practices. These challenges include the heterogeneity of collected data, issues related to reproducibility, the necessity of internal and external validation, interpretability concerns, and ethical and legal considerations.

Data Heterogeneity and Reproducibility

First, building robust AI algorithms demands a significant amount of data, along with complex software and infrastructure. To ensure the reliability and generability of AI models, an ample supply of annotated data from different centers is essential. It is also crucial to homogenize data in terms of their formats, definitions, and quality control protocols, as well as standardize data acquisition across different imaging modalities. Indeed, insufficient data can lead to overfitting or underfitting, resulting in inaccurate predictions. As the array of AI algorithms continues to expand, there is a pressing need for research standardization to ensure the reproducibility of the proposed models. Reproducibility, in this context, refers to the ability to duplicate prior results using the same methods employed in the original work. Achieving technical reproducibility in AI studies is contingent on the release of both the code and dataset by the study group . For this reason, open-access datasets and algorithm codes are foundational to advancing the field of AI in healthcare by providing the necessary resources for training, external validation, and reproducibility, as well as mirroring real-world data.

Ethical and Legal Issues

Second, ethical and legal concerns regarding the implementation of AI in healthcare encompass the use of patient data for the development of AI-based models. The generation of large and homogeneous datasets gives rise to significant issues, particularly in the domains of data privacy and security. A notable area of apprehension pertains to informed consent, surveillance, and the violation of individuals' data protection rights. This concern extends to the possibility of undisclosed uses of the data by entities distinct from the individual from whom the data were obtained Moreover, the vulnerability of information collected for and by AI systems to hacking attempts introduces an additional layer of worry. Instances of unauthorized access and data breaches pose threats to the integrity and confidentiality of sensitive medical information Privacy and data protection laws have taken proactive steps to address these concerns. These efforts aim to establish frameworks ensuring transparency, safety, and ethical standards in the handling, processing, and sharing of data related to healthcare . Ensuring the fairness of AI models is a critical concern, particularly due to the potential for biases to be embedded in these models, especially when training data exhibit imbalances. This imbalance can lead to significant variations in the performance of AI models across demographic groups, such as sex and race, potentially worsening existing healthcare disparities. A comprehensive examination of fairness and equity in the development and deployment of AI in healthcare is essential. Addressing these challenges is vital for unlocking the full potential of AI while safeguarding privacy, promoting transparency, and ensuring equitable healthcare outcomes for all

Model Transparency, Explainability, and Validation

Third, some AI-generated models, especially those based on DL, are considered "black box" systems that do not offer any insight or explanations about how the output is obtained, limiting clinical applicability due to their lack of transparency and interpretability. To overcome the significant challenges presented by "black box" models, recent studies have focused on developing AI models that are both explainable and interpretable . Specifically, interpretability refers to the human ability to understand cause and effect within an AI model. Conversely, explainability refers to the capability to elucidate an AI-generated decision-making process using language that is intelligible to humans, enabling an understanding of why a model produces a specific outcome . Many ML models are designed to be intrinsically interpretable (e.g., LR, linear regression, decision trees, K-nearest neighbors) due to their simple structure and inherent logical relationships to their components .In models of greater complexity, the direct interpretation process becomes intricate and rapidly extends beyond quick logical comprehension, requiring post-modeling explainability . Additionally, an interpretable model should undergo clinical validation through an evaluation of whether the interpretations provided by the model are as effective enough to support healthcare decision making as expert advice.

Moreover, when a dataset is available, internal .and external validation of the model, as well as studies conducted in real-world settings, are also crucial to assessing the practical utility of deployed models . Indeed, a significant barrier to the widespread adoption of AI algorithms is the lack of an evaluation of their clinical impacts through prospective studies, leaving the benefits of AI approaches largely theoretical. Similarly, there are no studies assessing the economic or health system advantages associated with population-level approaches to cardiomyopathy using AI algorithms.

Future Directions

Randomized trials are crucial for assessing the application of AI models to the differential diagnosis of cardiomyopathy phenotypes across different centers, minimizing bias through sex and minority representation. To enhance the applicability of these models, it is mandatory not only to collect extensive, homogenous datasets with external validation, quality controls, and explainable and interpretable approaches, but also to inform physicians about the usefulness of these models. Additionally, developing a privacy protection algorithm with encryption and AI techniques is necessary for secure and

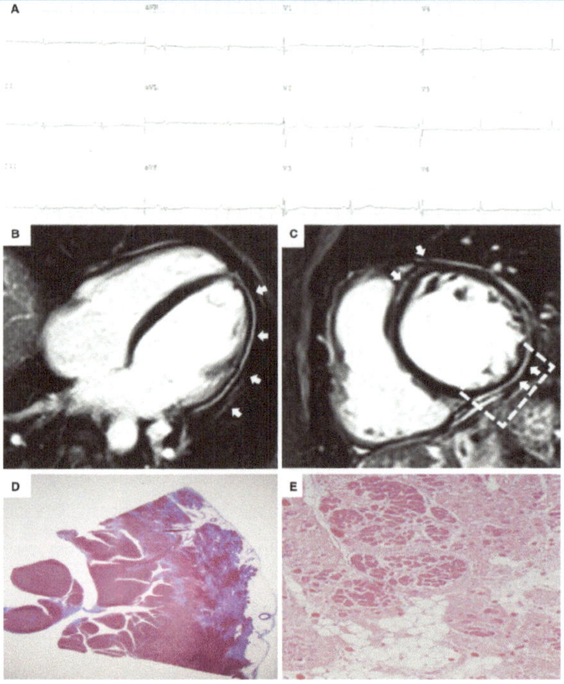

Fig.29.15 Electrocardiographic, CMR imaging, and histological features of a representative patient with ARVC undergoing cardiac transplantation. Basal ECG showing low voltages in limb leads and flattened T-waves in the inferolateral leads (A). Post-contrast CMR images in long-axis (B) and short-axis (C) views showing normal LV cavity size and subepicardial LGE (white arrows) involving the LV free wall (boxed area) and septum, from basal to apical regions (white arrows). Histologic examination of the boxed area showing fibro-fatty myocardial replacement affecting the subepicardial LV layer (Heidenhain trichrome stain) (D); close up detailing residual myocytes embedded within fibrous and fatty tissue (E.E stain) (E). ARVC indicates arrhythmogenic right ventricular cardiomyopathy; CMR, cardiac magnetic resonance; LGE, late gadolinium enhancement; LV, left ventricular.

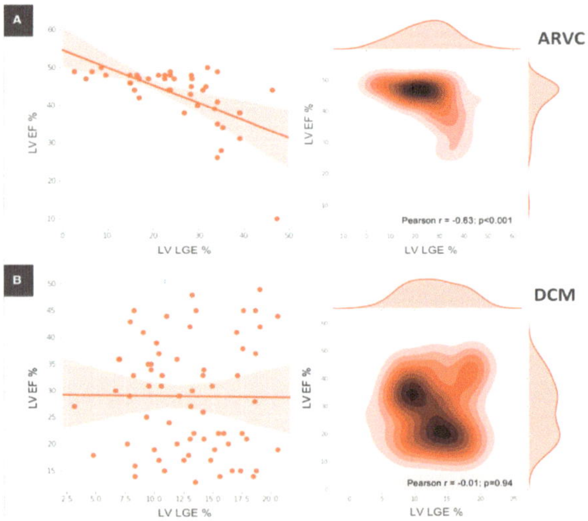

Fig. 29.16 Relationship between the amount of LV LGE and LVEF. Graphs (regression plot—left, joint plot—right) showing the relationship between the amount of LV LGE and LVEF in ARVC- (A) and DCM-LV phenotype (B). LGE indicates late gadolinium enhancement; LV, left ventricular; LVEF, left ventricular ejection fraction.

generalizable models.AI models used in cardiomyopathy-oriented approaches with multiparametric data may represent a potential advancement in cardiomyopathy management. This includes disease classification, early diagnosis, risk stratification, and early detection of complications, as well as prognosis and tailored treatment. Additionally, AI imaging pre-processing and post-processing approaches are undoubtedly useful in clinical practice to optimize clinical workflows and reduce the cost of cardiovascular healthcare, providing a solution to the exponential increase in cardiovascular examinations .

AI algorithms exhibit the capacity to manage larger and more intricate datasets in comparison with traditional medical models, and do not require the pre-specification of predictors or interactions, thereby facilitating the identification of novel relationships . These AI-based models allow us to bridge the gap between the pathogenesis of diseases, genotypes, and phenotypes of cardiomyopathies, enabling personalized medicine not only for the individual, but for the entire family.

Conclusions

The implementation of AI-based models for the differential diagnosis of cardiomyopathy phenotypes holds promise in terms of significantly enhancing daily clinical practice in cardiovascular healthcare. The multiparametric approach to evaluating and discriminating patients with suspected cardiomyopathy has been demonstrated to be crucial in identifying the cardiomyopathy phenotypes and the underlying etiological diagnoses. AI models have the potential to create composite algorithms that include demographics and laboratory data, clinical parameters, molecular, and cardiac imaging features to automate the detection and diagnosis of cardiomyopathies. Despite the potential advantages of these AI algorithms in cardiovascular healthcare, their applicability is currently limited due to several challenges. These concerns include the lack of homogenous datasets with external validation and real-world evaluations, the limited interpretability and robustness of the models, and lingering issues regarding trust in AI-generated approaches. To expedite the clinical implementation of these models as valuable tools in cardiomyopathy diagnosis, it is crucial to design future multicenter trials with homogenous and open-access datasets to achieve universal applicability of these AI models.

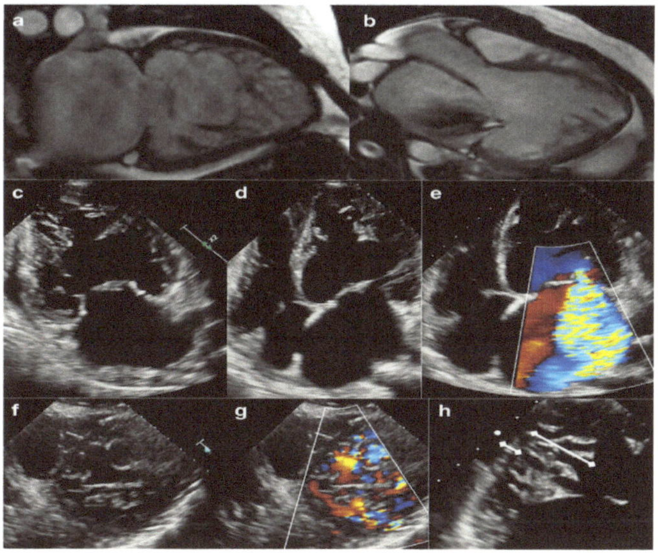

Fig.29.17 Non-compaction cardiomyopathy. Dilated LV with prominent trabeculation (a) and functional mitral regurgitation (b) visualized by CMR, as well as echocardiography (c, d, e). Using color-flow Doppler blood flow can be demonstrated between the extensive trabeculae on short-axis LV cross-sections (f, g). Thickness of the non-compacted layer largely exceeds that of the compacted myocardial layer (h).

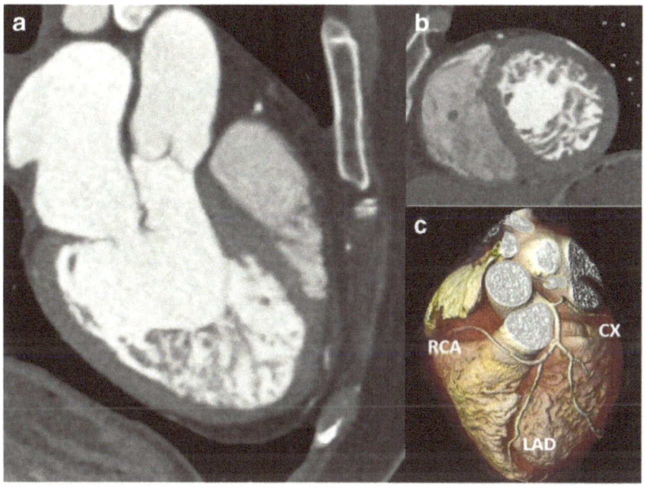

Fig.29.18 Non-compaction cardiomyopathy. Extensive trabeculation as observed by contrastenhanced ECG-synchronized CT (a, b). There is a single coronary artery originating from the left coronary sinus supplying the left anterior descending (LAD) and left circumflex coronary artery (CX) as well as the right coronary artery (RCA) (in c)

SUMMARY

Artificial intelligence (AI) is rapidly being applied to the medical field, especially in the cardiovascular domain. AI approaches have demonstrated their applicability in the detection, diagnosis, and management of several cardiovascular diseases, enhancing disease stratification and typing. Cardiomyopathies are a leading cause of heart failure and life-threatening ventricular arrhythmias. Identifying the etiologies is fundamental for the management and diagnosticpathway of these heart muscle diseases, requiring the integration of various data, including personal and family history, clinical examination, electrocardiography, and laboratory investigations, as well as multimodality imaging, making the clinical diagnosis challenging. In this scenario, AI has demonstrated its capability to capture subtle connections from a multitude of multiparametric datasets, enabling the discovery of hidden relationships in data and handling more complex tasks than traditional methods. This review aims to present a comprehensive overview of the main concepts related to AI and its subset. Additionally, we review the existing literature on AI-based models in the differential diagnosis of cardiomyopathy phenotypes, and we finally examine the advantages and limitations of these AI approaches.

Biliography and Acknowledgement

- Acosta, J.N.; Falcone, G.J.; Rajpurkar, P.; Topol, E.J. Multimodal biomedical AI. Nat. Med. 2022, 28, 1773–1784. [Google Scholar] [CrossRef]
- Adadi, A.; Berrada, M. Peeking Inside the Black-Box: A Survey on Explainable Artificial Intelligence (XAI). IEEE Access 2018, 6, 52138–52160. [Google Scholar] [CrossRef]
- Allen, B. The Role of the FDA in Ensuring the Safety and Efficacy of Artificial Intelligence Software and Devices. J. Am. Coll. Radiol. 2019, 16, 208–210. [Google Scholar] [CrossRef]
- Alloghani, M.; Al-Jumeily, D.; Mustafina, J.; Hussain, A.; Aljaaf, A.J. A systematic review on supervised and unsupervised machine learning algorithms for data science. Supervised unsupervised Learn data science. Supervised Unsupervised Learn. Data Sci. 2020, 3–21. [Google Scholar]
- Antoniades, C.; Oikonomou, E.K. Artificial intelligence in cardiovascular imaging—Principles, expectations, and limitations. Eur. Heart J. 2021, ehab678. [Google Scholar] [CrossRef]
- Arbelo, E.; Protonotarios, A.; Gimeno, J.R.; Arbustini, E.; Barriales-Villa, R.; Basso, C.; Bezzina, C.R.; Biagini, E.; Blom, N.A.; de Boer, R.A.; et al. 2023 ESC Guidelines for the management of cardiomyopathies: Developed by the task force on the management of cardiomyopathies of the European Society of Cardiology (ESC). Eur. Heart J. 2023, 44, 3503–3626. [Google Scholar] [CrossRef]
- Asmarian, N.; Kamalipour, A.; Hosseini-Bensenjan, M.; Karimi, M.; Haghpanah, S. Prediction of Heart and Liver Iron Overload in β-Thalassemia Major Patients Using Machine Learning Methods. Hemoglobin 2022, 46, 303–307. [Google Scholar] [CrossRef]
- Baeßler, B.; Mannil, M.; Maintz, D.; Alkadhi, H.; Manka, R. Texture analysis and machine learning of non-contrast T1-weighted MR images in patients with hypertrophic cardiomyopathy—Preliminary results. Eur. J. Radiol. 2018, 102, 61–67. [Google Scholar] [CrossRef]
- Barragán-Montero, A.; Javaid, U.; Valdés, G.; Nguyen, D.; Desbordes, P.; Macq, B.; Willems, S.; Vandewinckele, L.; Holmström, M.; Löfman, F.; et al. Artificial intelligence and machine learning for medical imaging: A technology review. Phys. Med. 2021, 83, 242–256. [Google Scholar] [CrossRef]
- Bellamy, R.K.E.; Dey, K.; Hind, M.; Hoffman, S.C.; Houde, S.; Kannan, K.; Lohia, P.; Martino, J.; Mehta, S.; Mojsilovic, A.; et al. AI Fairness 360: An extensible toolkit for detecting and mitigating algorithmic bias. IBM J. Res. Dev. 2019, 63, 4:1–4:15. [Google Scholar] [CrossRef]
- Beneyto, M.; Ghyaza, G.; Cariou, E.; Amar, J.; Lairez, O. Development and validation of machine learning algorithms to predict posthypertensive origin in left ventricular hypertrophy. Arch. Cardiovasc. Dis. 2023, 116, 397–402. [Google Scholar] [CrossRef]
- Benjamens, S.; Dhunnoo, P.; Meskó, B. The state of artificial intelligence-based FDA-approved medical devices and algorithms: An online database. npj Digit. Med. 2020, 3, 118. [Google Scholar] [CrossRef] [PubMed]
- Bleijendaal, H.; Ramos, L.A.; Lopes, R.R.; Verstraelen, T.E.; Baalman, S.W.; Pool, M.D.O.; Tjong, F.V.; Melgarejo-Meseguer, F.M.; Gimeno-Blanes, F.J.; Gimeno-Blanes, J.R.; et al. Computer versus cardiologist: Is a machine learning algorithm able to outperform an expert in diagnosing a phospholamban p.Arg14del mutation on the electrocardiogram? Heart Rhythm. 2021, 18, 79–87. [Google Scholar] [CrossRef]
- Cademartiri, F.; Balestrieri, A.; Cau, R.; Punzo, B.; Cavaliere, C.; Maffei, E.; Saba, L. Insight from imaging on plaque vulnerability: Similarities and differences between coronary and carotid arteries—Implications for systemic therapies. Cardiovasc. Diagn. Ther. 2020, 10, 1150–1162. [Google Scholar] [CrossRef]
- Cau, R.; Bassareo, P.; Cademartiri, F.; Cadeddu, C.; Balestrieri, A.; Mannelli, L.; Suri, J.S.; Saba, L. Epicardial fat volume assessed with cardiac magnetic resonance imaging in patients with Takotsubo cardiomyopathy. Eur. J. Radiol. 2023, 160, 110706. [Google Scholar] [CrossRef]
- Cau, R.; Bassareo, P.; Caredda, G.; Suri, J.S.; Esposito, A.; Saba, L. Atrial Strain by Feature-Tracking Cardiac Magnetic Resonance Imaging in Takotsubo Cardiomyopathy. Features, Feasibility, and Reproducibility. Can. Assoc. Radiol. J. 2021, 73, 573–580. [Google Scholar] [CrossRef] [PubMed]
- Cau, R.; Bassareo, P.; Deidda, M.; Caredda, G.; Suri, J.S.; Pontone, G.; Saba, L. Could CMR Tissue-Tracking and Parametric Mapping Distinguish Between Takotsubo Syndrome and Acute Myocarditis? A Pilot Study. Acad. Radiol. 2021, 29, S33–S39. [Google Scholar] [CrossRef] [PubMed]
- Cau, R.; Cherchi, V.; Micheletti, G.; Porcu, M.; Mannelli, L.; Bassareo, P.; Suri, J.S.P.; Saba, L. Potential Role of Artificial Intelligence in Cardiac Magnetic Resonance Imaging. J. Thorac. Imaging 2021, 36, 142–148. [Google Scholar] [CrossRef]
- Cau, R.; Faa, G.; Nardi, V.; Balestrieri, A.; Puig, J.; Suri, J.S.; SanFilippo, R.; Saba, L. Long-COVID diagnosis: From diagnostic to advanced AI-driven models. Eur. J. Radiol. 2022, 148, 110164. [Google Scholar] [CrossRef]
- Cau, R.; Flanders, A.; Mannelli, L.; Politi, C.; Faa, G.; Suri, J.S.; Saba, L. Artificial intelligence in computed tomography plaque characterization: A review. Eur. J. Radiol. 2021, 140, 109767. [Google Scholar] [CrossRef]
- Cau, R.; Pisu, F.; Muscogiuri, G.; Mannelli, L.; Suri, J.S.; Saba, L. Applications of artificial intelligence-based models in vulnerable carotid plaque. Vessel. Plus 2023, 7, 20. [Google Scholar] [CrossRef]
- Cau, R.; Pisu, F.; Porcu, M.; Cademartiri, F.; Montisci, R.; Bassareo, P.; Muscogiuri, G.; Amadu, A.; Sironi, S.; Esposito, A.; et al. Machine learning approach in diagnosing Takotsubo cardiomyopathy: The role of the combined evaluation of atrial and ventricular strain, and parametric mapping. Int. J. Cardiol. 2022, 373, 124–133. [Google Scholar] [CrossRef] [PubMed]
- Cau, R.; Pisu, F.; Suri, J.S.; Mannelli, L.; Scaglione, M.; Masala, S.; Saba, L. Artificial Intelligence Applications in Cardiovascular Magnetic Resonance Imaging: Are We on the Path to Avoiding the Administration of Contrast Media? Diagnostics 2023, 13, 2061. [Google Scholar] [CrossRef]
- Chao, C.-J.; Jeong, J.; Arsanjani, R.; Kim, K.; Tsai, Y.-L.; Yu, W.-C.; Farina, J.M.; Mahmoud, A.K.; Ayoub, C.; Grogan, M.; et al. Echocardiography-Based Deep Learning Model to Differentiate Constrictive Pericarditis and Restrictive Cardiomyopathy. JACC Cardiovasc. Imaging 2023, in press. [Google Scholar] [CrossRef] [PubMed]
- Davis, A.; Billick, K.; Horton, K.; Jankowski, M.; Knoll, P.; Marshall, J.E.; Paloma, A.; Palma, R.; Adams, D.B. Artificial Intelligence and Echocardiography: A Primer for Cardiac Sonographers. J. Am. Soc. Echocardiogr. 2020, 33, 1061–1066. [Google Scholar] [CrossRef]
- Dey, D.; Slomka, P.J.; Leeson, P.; Comaniciu, D.; Shrestha, S.; Sengupta, P.P.; Marwick, T.H. Artificial Intelligence in Cardiovascular Imaging: JACC State-of-the-Art Review. J. Am. Coll. Cardiol. 2019, 73, 1317–1335. [Google Scholar] [CrossRef]
- Doshi-Velez, F.; Kim, B. Towards A Rigorous Science of Interpretable Machine Learning. arXiv 2017, arXiv:1702.08608. [Google Scholar]
- Eckstein, J.; Moghadasi, N.; Körperich, H.; Valdés, E.W.; Sciacca, V.; Paluszkiewicz, L.; Burchert, W.; Piran, M. A Machine Learning Challenge: Detection of Cardiac Amyloidosis Based on Bi-Atrial and Right Ventricular Strain and Cardiac Function. Diagnostics 2022, 12, 2693. [Google Scholar] [CrossRef] [PubMed]
- Faes, L.; Sim, D.A.; van Smeden, M.; Held, U.; Bossuyt, P.M.; Bachmann, L.M. Artificial Intelligence and Statistics: Just the Old Wine in New Wineskins? Front. Digit. Health 2022, 4, 833912. [Google Scholar]

- Gunzer, F.; Jantscher, M.; Hassler, E.M.; Kau, T.; Reishofer, G. Reproducibility of artificial intelligence models in computed tomography of the head: A quantitative analysis. Insights Into Imaging 2022, 13, 173. [Google Scholar] [CrossRef] [PubMed]
- Haibe-Kains, B.; Adam, G.A.; Hosny, A.; Khodakarami, F.; Shraddha, T.; Kusko, R.; Sansone, S.-A.; Tong, W.; Wolfinger, R.D.; Mason, C.E.; et al. Transparency and reproducibility in artificial intelligence. Nature 2020, 586, E14–E16. [Google Scholar] [CrossRef]
- Haimovich, J.S.; Diamant, N.; Khurshid, S.; Di Achille, P.; Reeder, C.; Friedman, S.; Singh, P.; Spurlock, W.; Ellinor, P.T.; Philippakis, A.; et al. Artificial intelligence–enabled classification of hypertrophic heart diseases using electrocardiograms. Cardiovasc. Digit. Health J. 2023, 4, 48–59. [Google Scholar] [CrossRef]
- He, K.; Gan, C.; Li, Z.; Rekik, I.; Yin, Z.; Ji, W.; Gao, Y.; Wang, Q.; Zhang, J.; Shen, D. Transformers in medical image analysis. Intell. Med. 2023, 3, 59–78. [Google Scholar] [CrossRef]
- Hwang, I.-C.; Choi, D.; Choi, Y.-J.; Ju, L.; Kim, M.; Hong, J.-E.; Lee, H.-J.; Yoon, Y.E.; Park, J.-B.; Lee, S.-P.; et al. Differential diagnosis of common etiologies of left ventricular hypertrophy using a hybrid CNN-LSTM model. Sci. Rep. 2022, 12, 20998. [Google Scholar] [CrossRef]
- Izquierdo, C.; Casas, G.; Martin-Isla, C.; Campello, V.M.; Guala, A.; Gkontra, P.; Rodríguez-Palomares, J.F.; Lekadir, K. Radiomics-Based Classification of Left Ventricular Non-compaction, Hypertrophic Cardiomyopathy, and Dilated Cardiomyopathy in Cardiovascular Magnetic Resonance. Front. Cardiovasc. Med. 2021, 8, 764312. [Google Scholar] [CrossRef] [PubMed]
- Jaiswal, A.; Babu, A.R.; Zadeh, M.Z.; Banerjee, D.; Makedon, F. A Survey on Contrastive Self-Supervised Learning. Technologies 2020, 9, 2. [Google Scholar] [CrossRef]
- Jefferies, J.L.; Spencer, A.K.; Lau, H.A.; Nelson, M.W.; Giuliano, J.D.; Zabinski, J.W.; Boussios, C.; Curhan, G.; Gliklich, R.E.; Warnock, D.G. A new approach to identifying patients with elevated risk for Fabry disease using a machine learning algorithm. Orphanet J. Rare Dis. 2021, 16, 518. [Google Scholar] [CrossRef] [PubMed]
- Jiang, T.; Gradus, J.L.; Rosellini, A.J. Supervised Machine Learning: A Brief Primer. Behav. Ther. 2020, 51, 675–687. [Google Scholar] [CrossRef]
- John-Mathews, J.-M.; Cardon, D.; Balagué, C. From Reality to World. A Critical Perspective on AI Fairness. J. Bus. Ethics 2022, 178, 945–959. [Google Scholar] [CrossRef]
- Kim, K.-H.; Kwon, J.-M.; Pereira, T.; Attia, Z.I.; Pereira, N.L. Artificial Intelligence Applied to Cardiomyopathies: Is It Time for Clinical Application? Curr. Cardiol. Rep. 2022, 24, 1547–1555. [Google Scholar] [CrossRef]
- Krishnan, R.; Rajpurkar, P.; Topol, E.J. Self-supervised learning in medicine and healthcare. Nat. Biomed. Eng. 2022, 6, 1346–1352. [Google Scholar] [CrossRef] [PubMed]
- LeCun, Y.; Bengio, Y.; Hinton, G. Deep learning. Nature 2015, 521, 436–444. [Google Scholar] [CrossRef]
- Leighton, S.P.; Upthegrove, R.; Krishnadas, R.; Benros, M.E.; Broome, M.R.; Gkoutos, G.V.; Liddle, P.F.; Singh, S.P.; Everard, L.; Jones, P.B.; et al. Development and validation of multivariable prediction models of remission, recovery, and quality of life outcomes in people with first episode psychosis: A machine learning approach. Lancet Digit. Health 2019, 1, e261–e270. [Google Scholar] [CrossRef]
- Leiner, T.; Rueckert, D.; Suinesiaputra, A.; Baeßler, B.; Nezafat, R.; Išgum, I.; Young, A.A. Machine learning in cardiovascular magnetic resonance: Basic concepts and applications. J. Cardiovasc. Magn. Reson. 2019, 21, 61. [Google Scholar] [CrossRef
- Li, Y.-F.; Guo, L.-Z.; Zhou, Z.-H. Towards Safe Weakly Supervised Learning. IEEE Trans. Pattern Anal. Mach. Intell. 2019, 43, 334–346. Linardatos, P.; Papastefanopoulos, V.; Kotsiantis, S. Explainable AI: A Review of Machine Learning Interpretability Methods. Entropy 2021, 23, 18. [Google Scholar] [CrossRef]
- Marcus, F.I.; McKenna, W.J.; Sherrill, D.; Basso, C.; Bauce, B.; Bluemke, D.A.; Calkins, H.; Corrado, D.; Cox, M.G.; Daubert, J.P.; et al. Diagnosis of arrhythmogenic right ventricular cardiomyopathy/dysplasia: Proposed Modification of the Task Force Criteria. Eur. Heart J. 2010, 31, 806–814. [Google Scholar] [CrossRef]
- Maron, B.J.; Towbin, J.A.; Thiene, G.; Antzelevitch, C.; Corrado, D.; Arnett, D.; Moss, A.J.; Seidman, C.E.; Young, J.B. Contemporary definitions and classification of the cardiomyopathies: An American Heart Association scientific statement from the council on clinical cardiology, heart failure and transplantation committee; quality of care and outcomes research and functio. Circulation 2006, 113, 1807–1816.
- Minh, D.; Wang, H.X.; Li, Y.F.; Nguyen, T.N. Explainable artificial intelligence: A comprehensive review. Artif. Intell. Rev. 2022, 55, 3503–3568. [Google Scholar] [CrossRef]
- Moassefi, M.; Rouzrokh, P.; Conte, G.M.; Vahdati, S.; Fu, T.; Tahmasebi, A.; Younis, M.; Farahani, K.; Gentili, A.; Kline, T.; et al. Reproducibility of Deep Learning Algorithms Developed for Medical Imaging Analysis: A Systematic Review. J. Digit. Imaging 2023, 36, 2306–2312. [Google Scholar] [CrossRef]
- Molinaro, A.M.; Simon, R.; Pfeiffer, R.M. Prediction error estimation: A comparison of resampling methods. Bioinformatics 2005, 21, 3301–3307. [Google Scholar] [CrossRef]
- Molnar, C. Interpretable Machine Learning. 2020. Available online: lulu.com (accessed on 30 December 2023).
- Murphy, K.; Di Ruggiero, E.; Upshur, R.; Willison, D.J.; Malhotra, N.; Cai, J.C.; Malhotra, N.; Lui, V.; Gibson, J. Artificial intelligence for good health: A scoping review of the ethics literature. BMC Med. Ethics 2021, 22, 14. [Google Scholar] [CrossRef] [PubMed]
- Muscogiuri, G.; Volpato, V.; Cau, R.; Chiesa, M.; Saba, L.; Guglielmo, M.; Senatieri, A.; Chierchia, G.; Pontone, G.; Dell'aversana, S.; et al. Application of AI in cardiovascular multimodality imaging. Heliyon 2022, 8, e10872. [Google Scholar] [CrossRef]
- Onnis, C.; Muscogiuri, G.; Bassareo, P.P.; Cau, R.; Mannelli, L.; Cadeddu, C.; Suri, J.S.; Cerrone, G.; Gerosa, C.; Sironi, S.; et al. Non-invasive coronary imaging in patients with COVID-19: A narrative review. Eur. J. Radiol. 2022, 149, 110188. [Google Scholar] [CrossRef] [PubMed]
- Papageorgiou, V.E.; Zegkos, T.; Efthimiadis, G.; Tsaklidis, G. Analysis of digitalized ECG signals based on artificial intelligence and spectral analysis methods specialized in ARVC. Int. J. Numer. Methods Biomed. Eng. 2022, 38, e3644. [Google Scholar] [CrossRef] [PubMed]
- Petch, J.; Di, S.; Nelson, W. Opening the Black Box: The Promise and Limitations of Explainable Machine Learning in Cardiology. Can. J. Cardiol. 2022, 38, 204–213. [Google Scholar] [CrossRef]
- Petersen, S.E.; Abdulkareem, M.; Leiner, T. Artificial Intelligence Will Transform Cardiac Imaging—Opportunities and Challenges. Front. Cardiovasc. Med. 2019, 6, 133. [Google Scholar] [CrossRef]
- Puyol Anton, E.; Ruijsink, B.; Piechnik, S.K.; Neubauer, S.; Petersen, S.E.; Razavi, R.; King, A.P. Fairness in AI: Are deep learning-based CMR segmentation algorithms biased? Eur. Heart J. 2021, 42 (Suppl. 1), ehab724-3055. [Google Scholar] [CrossRef]
- Quinn, T.P.; Jacobs, S.; Senadeera, M.; Le, V.; Coghlan, S. The three ghosts of medical AI: Can the black-box present deliver? Artif. Intell. Med. 2022, 124, 102158. [Google Scholar] [CrossRef] [PubMed]
- Radanliev, P.; De Roure, D. Epistemological and Bibliometric Analysis of Ethics and Shared Responsibility—Health Policy and IoT Systems. Sustainability 2021, 13, 8355. [Google Scholar] [CrossRef]

- Rajula, H.S.R.; Verlato, G.; Manchia, M.; Antonucci, N.; Fanos, V. Comparison of Conventional Statistical Methods with Machine Learning in Medicine: Diagnosis, Drug Development, and Treatment. Medicina 2020, 56, 455. [Google Scholar] [CrossRef]
- Rapezzi, C.; Aimo, A.; Barison, A.; Emdin, M.; Porcari, A.; Linhart, A.; Keren, A.; Merlo, M.; Sinagra, G. Restrictive cardiomyopathy: Definition and diagnosis. Eur. Heart J. 2022, 43, 4679–4693. [Google
- Rapezzi, C.; Arbustini, E.; Caforio, A.L.; Charron, P.; Gimeno-Blanes, J.; Heliö, T.; Linhart, A.; Mogensen, J.; Pinto, Y.; Ristic, A.; et al. Diagnostic work-up in cardiomyopathies: Bridging the gap between clinical phenotypes and final diagnosis. A position statement from the ESC Working Group on Myocardial and Pericardial Diseases. Eur. Heart J. 2013, 34, 1448–1458. [Google Scholar] [CrossRef]
- Richardson, M.L.; Garwood, E.R.; Lee, Y.; Li, M.D.; Lo, H.S.; Nagaraju, A.; Nguyen, X.V.; Probyn, L.; Rajiah, P.; Sin, J.; et al. Noninterpretive Uses of Artificial Intelligence in Radiology. Acad. Radiol. 2020, 28, 1225–1235. [Google Scholar] [CrossRef]
- Rodrigues, R. Legal and human rights issues of AI: Gaps, challenges and vulnerabilities. J. Responsible Technol. 2020, 4, 100005. [Google Scholar] [CrossRef]
- Saba, L.; Cau, R.; Murgia, A.; Nicolaides, A.N.; Wintermark, M.; Castillo, M.; Staub, D.; Kakkos, S.K.; Yang, Q.; Paraskevas, K.I.; et al. Carotid Plaque-RADS, a novel stroke risk classification system. JACC Cardiovasc. Imaging 2023, 17, 62–75. [Google Scholar] [CrossRef]
- Sengupta, P.P.; Huang, Y.M.; Bansal, M.; Ashrafi, A.; Fisher, M.; Shameer, K.; Gall, W.; Dudley, J.T. Cognitive Machine-Learning Algorithm for Cardiac Imaging: A Pilot Study for Differentiating Constrictive Pericarditis from Restrictive Cardiomyopathy. Circ. Cardiovasc. Imaging 2016, 9, e004330. [Google Scholar] [CrossRef]
- Shrivastava, S.; Cohen-Shelly, M.; Attia, Z.I.; Rosenbaum, A.N.; Wang, L.; Giudicessi, J.R.; Redfield, M.; Bailey, K.; Lopez-Jimenez, F.; Lin, G.; et al. Artificial Intelligence-Enabled Electrocardiography to Screen Patients with Dilated Cardiomyopathy. Am. J. Cardiol. 2021, 155, 121–127. [Google Scholar] [CrossRef]
- Siegersma, K.R.; Leiner, T.; Chew, D.P.; Appelman, Y.; Hofstra, L.; Verjans, J.W. Artificial intelligence in cardiovascular imaging: State of the art and implications for the imaging cardiologist. Neth. Heart J. 2019, 27, 403–413. [Google Scholar] [CrossRef] [PubMed]
- Singh, A.; Thakur, N.; Sharma, A. A review of supervised machine learning algorithms. In Proceedings of the 2016 3rd International Conference on Computing for Sustainable Global Development (INDIACom), New Delhi, India, 16–18 March 2016; pp. 1310–1315.
- Siontis, K.C.; Liu, K.; Bos, J.M.; Attia, Z.I.; Cohen-Shelly, M.; Arruda-Olson, A.M.; Farahani, N.Z.; Friedman, P.A.; Noseworthy, P.A.; Ackerman, M.J. Detection of hypertrophic cardiomyopathy by an artificial intelligence electrocardiogram in children and adolescents. Int. J. Cardiol. 2021, 340, 42–47. [Google Scholar] [CrossRef]
- Soffer, S.; Ben-Cohen, A.; Shimon, O.; Amitai, M.M.; Greenspan, H.; Klang, E. Convolutional Neural Networks for Radiologic Images: A Radiologist's Guide. Radiology 2019, 290, 590–606. [Google Scholar]
- Soto, J.T.; Hughes, J.W.; Sanchez, P.A.; Perez, M.; Ouyang, D.; Ashley, E.A. Multimodal deep learning enhances diagnostic precision in left ventricular hypertrophy. Eur. Heart J. Digit. Health 2022, 3, 380–389. [Google Scholar] [CrossRef] [PubMed
- Taleie, H.; Hajianfar, G.; Sabouri, M.; Parsaee, M.; Houshmand, G.; Bitarafan-Rajabi, A.; Zaidi, H.; Shiri, I. Left Ventricular Myocardial Dysfunction Evaluation in Thalassemia Patients Using Echocardiographic Radiomic Features and Machine Learning Algorithms. J. Digit. Imaging 2023, 36, 2494–2506. [Google Scholar] [CrossRef]
- Tang, A.; Tam, R.; Cadrin-Chênevert, A.; Guest, W.; Chong, J.; Barfett, J.; Chepelev, L.; Cairns, R.; Mitchell, J.R.; Cicero, M.D.; et al. Canadian Association of Radiologists White Paper on Artificial Intelligence in Radiology. Can. Assoc. Radiol. J. 2018, 69, 120–135. [Google Scholar] [CrossRef]
- Tayal, U.; Verdonschot, J.A.; Hazebroek, M.R.; Howard, J.; Gregson, J.; Newsome, S.; Gulati, A.; Pua, C.J.; Halliday, B.P.; Lota, A.S.; et al. Precision Phenotyping of Dilated Cardiomyopathy Using Multidimensional Data. J. Am. Coll. Cardiol. 2022, 79, 2219–2232. [Google Scholar] [CrossRef] [PubMed]
- Usama, M.; Qadir, J.; Raza, A.; Arif, H.; Yau, K.-L.A.; Elkhatib, Y.; Hussain, A.; Al-Fuqaha, A. Unsupervised Machine Learning for Networking: Techniques, Applications and Research Challenges. IEEE Access 2019, 7, 65579–65615. [Google Scholar] [CrossRef]
- Van Assen, M.; Muscogiuri, G.; Caruso, D.; Lee, S.J.; Laghi, A.; De Cecco, C.N. Artificial intelligence in cardiac radiology. Radiol. Medica 2020, 125, 1186–1199. [Google Scholar] [CrossRef]
- Van Kolfschooten, H. EU regulation of artificial intelligence: Challenges for patients' rights. Common Mark. Law Rev. 2022, 59, 81–112. [Google Scholar] [CrossRef]
- Van Timmeren, J.E.; Cester, D.; Tanadini-Lang, S.; Alkadhi, H.; Baessler, B. Radiomics in medical imaging-"how-to" guide and critical reflection. Insights Imaging 2020, 11, 91. [Google Scholar] [CrossRef]
- Wachter, S.; Mittelstadt, B. A right to reasonable inferences: Re-thinking data protection law in the age of big data and AI. Columbia Bus. Law Rev. 2019, 2, 494–620. [Google Scholar]
- Xu, B.; Kocyigit, D.; Grimm, R.; Griffin, B.P.; Cheng, F. Applications of artificial intelligence in multimodality cardiovascular imaging: A state-of-the-art review. Prog. Cardiovasc. Dis. 2020, 63, 367–376. [Google Scholar] [CrossRef]
- Youssef, A.; Pencina, M.; Thakur, A.; Zhu, T.; Clifton, D.; Shah, N.H. External validation of AI models in health should be replaced with recurring local validation. Nat. Med. 2023, 29, 2686–2687. [Google Scholar] [CrossRef] [PubMed]
- Zhang, X.; Cui, C.; Zhao, S.; Xie, L.; Tian, Y. Cardiac magnetic resonance radiomics for disease classification. Eur. Radiol. 2023, 33, 2312–2323. [Google Scholar] [CrossRef]
- Zhang, Y.; Xie, J.; Wu, Y.; Zhang, B.; Zhou, C.; Gao, X.; Xie, X.; Li, X.; Yu, J.; Wang, X.; et al. Novel algorithm for diagnosis of Arrhythmogenic cardiomyopathy and dilated cardiomyopathy: Key gene expression profiling using machine learning. J. Gene Med. 2023, 25, e3468. [Google Scholar] [CrossRef]
- Zhou, J.; Chen, F.; Holzinger, A. Towards explainability for AI fairness. In International Workshop on Extending Explainable AI Beyond Deep Models and Classifiers; Springer: Berlin/Heidelberg, Germany, 2020; pp. 375–386. [Google Scholar]
- Zhou, M.; Deng, Y.; Liu, Y.; Su, X.; Zeng, X. Echocardiography-based machine learning algorithm for distinguishing ischemic cardiomyopathy from dilated cardiomyopathy. BMC Cardiovasc. Disord. 2023, 23, 476. [Google Scholar] [CrossRef] [PubMed]
- Zhou, Z.-H. A brief introduction to weakly supervised learning. Natl. Sci. Rev. 2018, 5, 44–53. [Google Scholar] [CrossRef]
- Zhu, X.J. Semi-Supervised Learning Literature Survey; University of Wisconsin: Madison, WI, USA, 2005. [Google Scholar]

Artificial Intelligence in Cardiovascular Medicine: Current Insights and Future Prospects. Review

CHAPTER

30

Cardiovascular disease (CVD) is the leading cause of death in the world and poses an ever-growing challenge.Citation1 The global prevalence of CVD is rapidly rising, increasing from 271 million in 1990 to 523 million in 2019, accompanied by rising mortality, from 12.1 million to 18.6 million during the same period.Citation1 Moreover, the cost of treating CVD is projected to increase from 863 billion United States Dollars (USD) in 2010 to more than 1.044 trillion USD by 2030.Citation2 Cost-effective and scalable solutions are needed to help mitigate CVD burden, and artificial intelligence (AI) can play a critical role.

AI is a rapidly evolving transdisciplinary field which integrates computer science, statistics, psychology, neuroscience, material science, mechanical engineering and computer hardware design to develop algorithms that aim to simulate human intuition, decision-making and object recognition.Citation3 The overarching aims of AI in cardiovascular medicine are threefold: to optimize patient care, improve efficiency and improve clinical outcomes.Citation3 In cardiology, there has been a growth in the potential sources of new patient data, as well as advances in investigations and therapies, which position the field well to uniquely benefit from AI.Citation4

In this review, we introduce the core AI techniques, their historical development and contemporary applications in cardiology. The future prospects and challenges of AI are also discussed.

AI Techniques

Machine learning (ML) refers to a set of techniques which enable AI, and these techniques vary in their objectives, applications and architectures . ML is an iterative process which involves approximating complex mathematical relationships between inputs and outputs by learning from a large data set to predict values from new, unseen data. Supervised, unsupervised, semi-supervised and deep learning are terms describing the ways in which ML algorithms learn from data .Supervised learning refers to algorithms learning rules between a set of inputs and outputs using a labelled training data set (referred to as mapping) in order to predict outcomes for new inputs. The labelled training data set typically consists of predictor variables, features and labeled outcomes.. Features refer to pieces of information that make up data and the quality, accuracy and richness of features determines the overall effectiveness of supervised ML algorithms..Supervised ML algorithms are especially useful when the research question involves classification or regression-based analysis. A well-labelled training data set can be reused if the pre-specified features do not need to be changed. However, the drawbacks of supervised learning include the often timely and costly process of accurately labelling a large data set. Deep learning is another subfield of ML and refers to algorithms which are modelled on the neural structures of the brain, consisting of inter-connected perceptrons . Compared to traditional ML algorithms, deep learning requires minimal data arbitration or feature engineering .An example of supervised learning is a study which used 91,232 single-lead ECGs from 55,549 patients to train an ML algorithm to classify the ECGs into 12 distinct rhythm classes. The ECGs contained features suggestive of different arrhythmias and were manually labelled by a consensus committee of board-certified cardiologists before the supervised ML algorithm was trained..When compared with the consensus committee of cardiologists, the algorithm had an AUC of 0.97.

Unsupervised learning is a different form of learning which uses unlabeled data to discover underlying relationships and is often referred to as knowledge discovery. Examples of unsupervised learning include principal component analysis, cluster analysis and deep learning..In principal component analysis, large, multidimensional datasets are broken into simpler data sets with a smaller number of dimensions through the identification of correlated variables. Cluster analysis involves dividing objects into groups that share similar characteristics with the aim of finding subgroups within a larger data set. Unsupervised learning is extremely useful in clinical practice where manually labelling large datasets is unfeasible.Moreover, unsupervised learning has reduced scope for incorporating human error. An example is an ML algorithm using principal component and cluster analysis to successfully differentiate heart failure with preserved ejection fraction (HFpEF) from healthy subjects by analyzing LV long axis myocardial velocity patterns on stress echocardiography.The study trained an unsupervised ML algorithm from 156 patients using 22 descriptors with 300 features collected from tissue Doppler-derived longitudinal myocardial velocity traces at rest and during exercise.

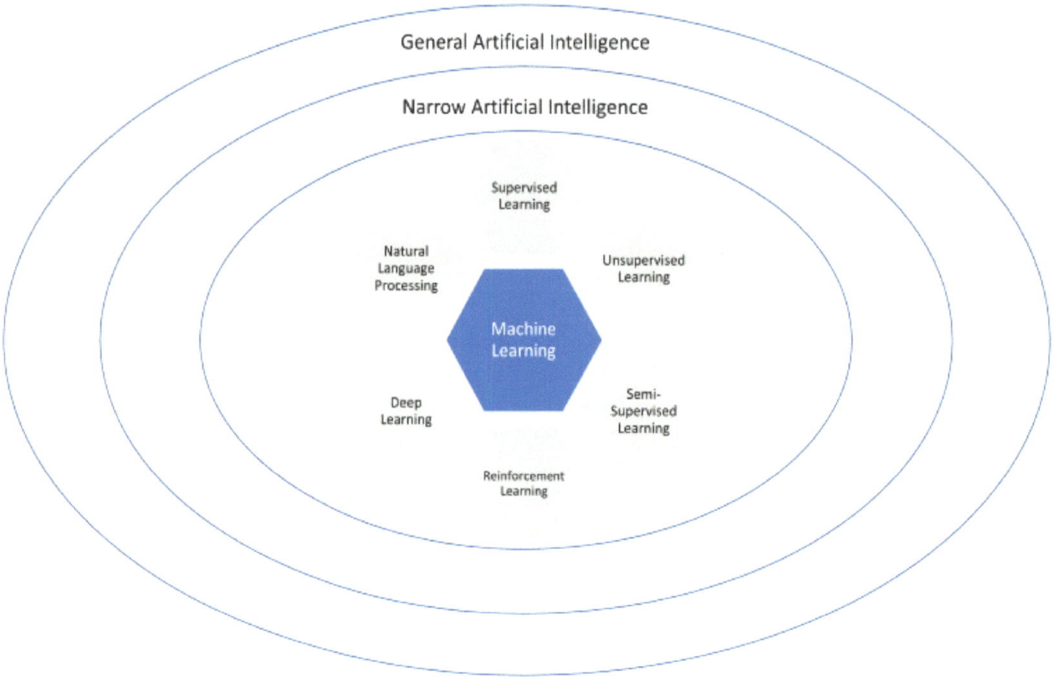

Fig.30.1 Relationships between artificial intelligence (AI) and machine learning (ML) techniques.

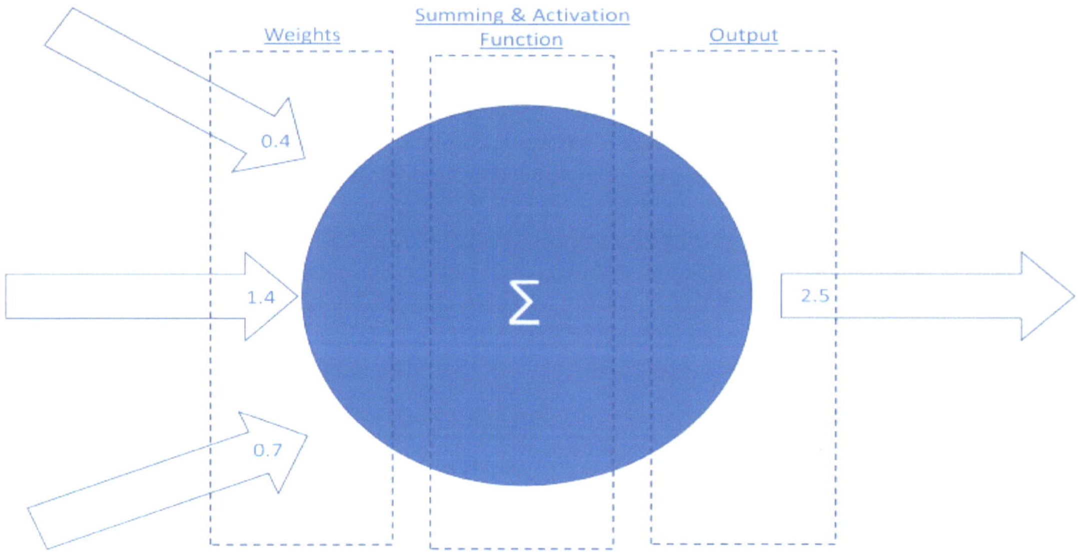

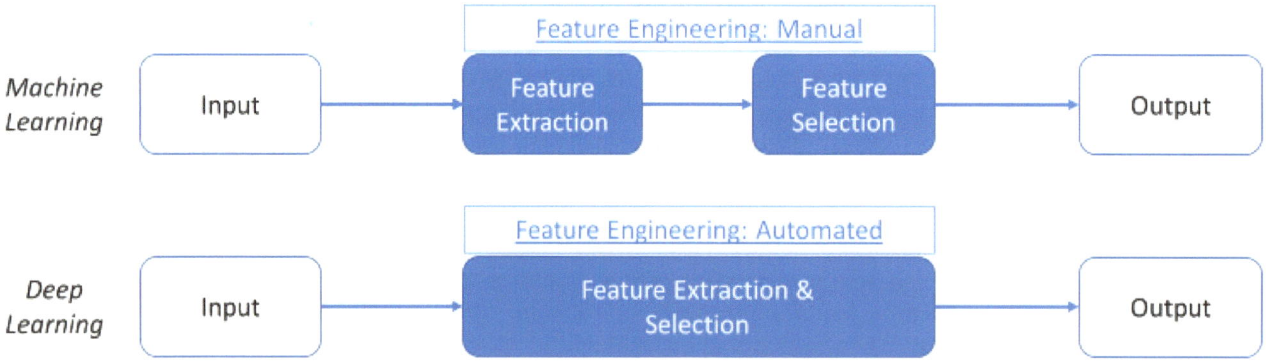

Fig.30.3 Comparing the stepwise approach of machine learning (ML) and deep learning (DL) approaches with respect to feature extraction and selection.

The algorithm found naturally occurring patterns and relationships within the details to identify a continuum of disease from normal cardiac function to patients with HFpEF. The spectrum varied in their age, body mass index, left ventricular mass index and left ventricular filling pressure and symptom burden as measured by the 6-minute walk test. Semi-supervised learning combines supervised and unsupervised learning techniques. It provides the ability to extrapolate and label a large data set from a smaller, manually labelled data set. This is performed by manually labelling a small portion of data and then employing unsupervised learning algorithms to extrapolate from this data.

Historical Perspectives of AI in Cardiology

The origins of AI can be traced to Alan Turing who explored the mathematical possibility of AI and described how to build and test intelligent machines in the early 1950s. However, computers lacked the functional capabilities to implement this theoretical knowledge at the time. As computing power improved and information could be stored, processed and extracted, ML algorithm development flourished in the 1970s and 1980s Early work focused on AI applications in computer gaming, but its role in clinical decision-making only began taking shape in the 1990s.

In cardiology, the first applications of AI were the development of self-learning neural networks applied to electrocardiography (ECG). One of the earliest works in 1990 trained a self-learning neural network using 60 ECGs to localize the atrioventricular accessory pathway in patients with Wolff-Parkinson-White Syndrome by using the polarity of the delta waves as an input. In a testing cohort of 25 ECGs, the algorithm correctly localized the atrioventricular pathway in 23 patients As AI techniques developed and computing power continued to improve, applications of AI in cardiology expanded to other fields, including cardiac imaging, electrophysiology, heart failure and interventional procedures. In 1999, a study applied artificial neural networks to echocardiography to segment images into either blood or tissue regions..The study trained the ML algorithm using 279 images and compared the algorithm to manual segmentation by two independent investigators and found good agreement (R = 0.93). More recently, the development of big-data analytical techniques has further opened the field of cardiology. Big-data analytical techniques have focused on integrating and synthesizing various multimodality imaging data points, including various omics data, imaging, ECG and unstructured free text

Over the intervening years, AI advancements in cardiology have led to wide-ranging applications, which encompass precise disease stratification, integration of multi-modality imaging, continuous remote monitoring and diagnostics, therapy selection and AI-aided diagnosis .In this review, we distill the broad applications of AI in cardiology into four clinical areas relevant for the practicing cardiologist: heart failure, electrophysiology, valvular heart disease and coronary artery disease .

Contemporary Applications of AI in Cardiology

Heart Failure

Heart failure (HF) is a complex and progressive clinical syndrome characterized by the heart's inability to pump sufficient blood to meet the body's demand. Heart failure can be categorized into three subgroups based on left ventricular ejection fraction (LVEF): HF with reduced EF (HFrEF; EF < 40%), HF with mid-range EF (HFmrEF; EF 40–49%), and preserved EF (EF ≥ 50%) The etiologies are often multifactorial but lead to a combination of elevated intracardiac pressure and impaired cardiac output. There is a growing appreciation for the role of AI in helping guide clinicians manage patients with HF. A broad range of AI applications revolve around augmenting diagnostic capabilities and clinical decision-making through automated cardiac function measurements and AI-based predictive modeling.

Heart failure is a clinical diagnosis, but echocardiography plays a pivotal role in evaluating underlying cardiac structure and function However, echocardiography is highly dependent on the experience of the sonographer for image acquisition, and precise interpretation by an expert reader. As a result, ML-based platforms are being developed, tested and validated, aiming to augment echocardiography. One recent example is the "HeartModel A.I." which uses AI segmentation algorithms and 3D echocardiography to automatically measure cardiac volumes and function. Medvedofsky et al performed a multicenter study validating this technology and including 180 patients from six different sites The algorithm correlated strongly with manual tracings with R-values of 0.97 when measuring left ventricular (LV) end-diastolic volume, 0.97 when measuring LV end-systolic volume, 0.88 when measuring LV ejection fraction (EF) and 0.96 when measuring left atrial volume. Another similar example is a CNN-based algorithmic tool developed by Ouyang et al using 10,030 echocardiograms from a single center. The testing cohort included 2895 echocardiograms and the study found the algorithm accurately segmented the LV with a Dice similarity coefficient of 0.92, predicted LV ejection fraction (EF) with a mean absolute error of 4.1%, and was able to classify patients with HF with reduced EF with an area under the curve (AUC) of 0.97. Identifying LV dysfunction using echocardiography has also been augmented by incorporating 12-lead electrocardiograms (ECGs). Sun et al developed a CNN to identify LV dysfunction and used 12,732 ECG-TTE pairs for training, 2530 pairs for validation and 2530 pairs for testing. The authors found the CNN-based model detected LV dysfunction with an accuracy of 73.9%, sensitivity of 69.2%, specificity of 70.5% and AUC of 0.713. The positive and negative predictive values of the model were 70.1% and 69.9%, respectively. AI algorithms have also been developed and validated for risk stratification and predicting mortality, medication adherence and recurrent hospitalizations in patients with HF. An ANN studied by Ortiz et al in 95 patients found the AI tool was able to predict 1-year all-cause mortality in patients with HFrEF with an accuracy of 90%, specificity of 93% and a sensitivity of 71.4%. Son et al used an SVM-based model to predict medication adherence. Electronic health record data was collected from 76 patients with HFrEF, and an SVM model was developed to identify variables which best predicted medication adherence. The variables included in the model were gender, daily frequency of medications, New York Heart Association (NYHA) class, medication knowledge, and presence of a spouse; the highest detection accuracy for the model was 77.6%. Another example is Kang et al who used a combination of decision trees and metaheuristic approaches from 552 patients to predict HF hospital admission., 382 patients were included in the training dataset and 184 patients in the validation dataset. The study found that the algorithm was able to predict HF admission with a C-statistic of 0.59, a true-positive rate of 0.65 and a false-positive rate of 0.49 with a final accuracy of 77%. Further studies have also applied ML algorithms to telemetry data from non-invasive wearable technology to predict HF re-hospitalization. The LINK-HF study used a disposable multisensor patch placed on the chest of 100 study subjects over 3 months. The study found that multivariate physiological data points could accurately predict HF hospitalizations with a sensitivity of 76% to 88% and a specificity of 85%. AI-based algorithms have also been used to predict the future development of HF. Akbilgic et al developed a CNN-based ECG-AI model using 14,618 patients from a nationwide perspective study to predict the likelihood of HF development within 10 years using standard 12-lead ECG. With an AUC of 0.818, the model output, when combined with clinical variables including age, gender, race, BMI, smoking status, coronary heart disease, diabetes mellitus, systolic blood pressure, and heart rate, outperformed traditional HF risk calculators such as ARIC with an AUC of 0.802 and the Framingham Heart Study with an AUC of 0.780. Another example is Choi et al who developed a recurrent neural network using 3884 patients with HF and 18,903 patients without HFrEF to predict a future diagnosis of HFrEF using traditional electronic health record system data points. The study used a 12-month observation window and found that the algorithm had an AUC of 0.747 for predicting HFrEF.

Cardiomyopathy

Hypertrophic cardiomyopathy (HCM) is a genetic disorder that occurs when the walls of the heart muscle thicken, resulting in the heart's reduced ability to pump out and take in blood. Though the condition is rare, affecting around 1 in 200 to 500 people, it is a leading cause of death among younger individuals and is associated with serious morbidity in all age groups. Given that more than 90% of patients with HCM have ECG abnormalities, ECGs can provide excellent screening for this condition, and AI can be used to detect HCM in imaging.

Recent studies have shown the efficacy of AI in detecting HCM in both adults and children. Ko et al trained a CNN model on ECGs from 46,901 adult patients, including a majority of controls and a minority of confirmed HCM cases. When tested on 12-lead ECGs from 13,400 patients, again with a majority of controls, the model was able to discriminate HCM cases from non-HCM control cases with an AUC of 0.96. Siontis et al also used a CNN trained on ECGs from 300 pediatric patients with HCM and 18,439 non-HCM pediatric controls. The model detected HCM from 12-lead ECGs with an AUC of 0.98 and a corresponding sensitivity and specificity of 92% and 95%, respectively.

Electrophysiology

Cardiac arrhythmias refer to abnormal atrial or ventricular rhythms and are estimated to affect 1.5–5% of the general population, with atrial fibrillation (AF) being the most prevalent arrhythmia in an ageing population. ECGs remain a key diagnostic tool for the timely diagnosis and management of arrhythmias. AI is increasingly being applied to the ECGs to garner new insights with respect to diagnosis, risk stratification and prediction.

Several recent studies have trained neural networks on single, 3 and 12-lead ECGs to accurately differentiate and diagnose arrhythmias. Hannun et al used 92,000 single-lead ECG tracings from 53,877 patients wearing adhesive patches to train a deep neural network (DNN) to classify an ECG into 12 rhythm classes. The algorithm was validated against a group of board-certified cardiologists and found to have an AUC of 0.837. Similarly, Raghunath et al trained a DNN to predict 1-year all-cause mortality from an ECG. The study trained the algorithm using 1,169,662 resting ECGs from 253,397 patients and tested the model on a sample of 168,914 patients. The algorithm was found to have an AUC of 0.88 when predicting all-cause mortality at 1-year from a single ECG

Electrolyte derangements can alter cardiac membranes and lead to arrhythmias. These derangements are often manifested with subtle ECG changes. Recent studies have developed and validated algorithms to help diagnose electrolyte derangements from the ECG. A recent study trained a DNN using 1,576,581 ECGs from 449, 380 patients to detect serum potassium levels of 5.5 mEq/l or less. The algorithm was validated using 61,965 patents with stage 3 or greater chronic kidney disease (CKD) and was found to have an AUC of 0.853 to 0.883. Another study trained a separate algorithm using 83,449 ECGs from 48,356 patients to diagnose various electrolyte derangements. The study was comprised of internal and external validation groups with the AUCs for predicting hyperkalemia, hypokalemia, hypernatremia, hyponatremia, hypercalcemia, and hypocalcemia being 0.873, 0.857, 0.839, 0.856, 0.831, and 0.813, respectively.

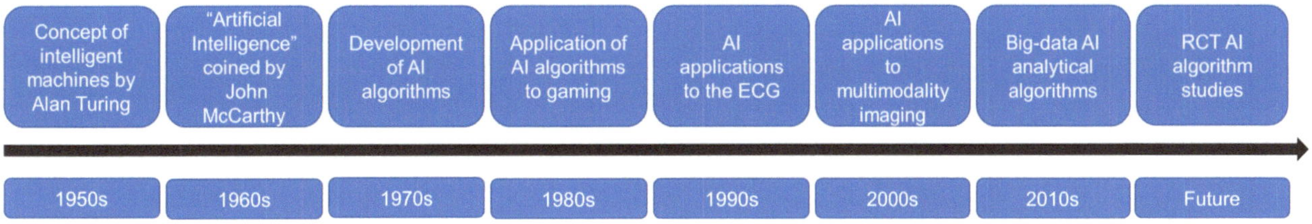

Fig.30.4 .The historical development of artificial intelligence (AI) in cardiology.Abbreviations: ECG, electrocardiogram; RCT, randomized controlled trial.

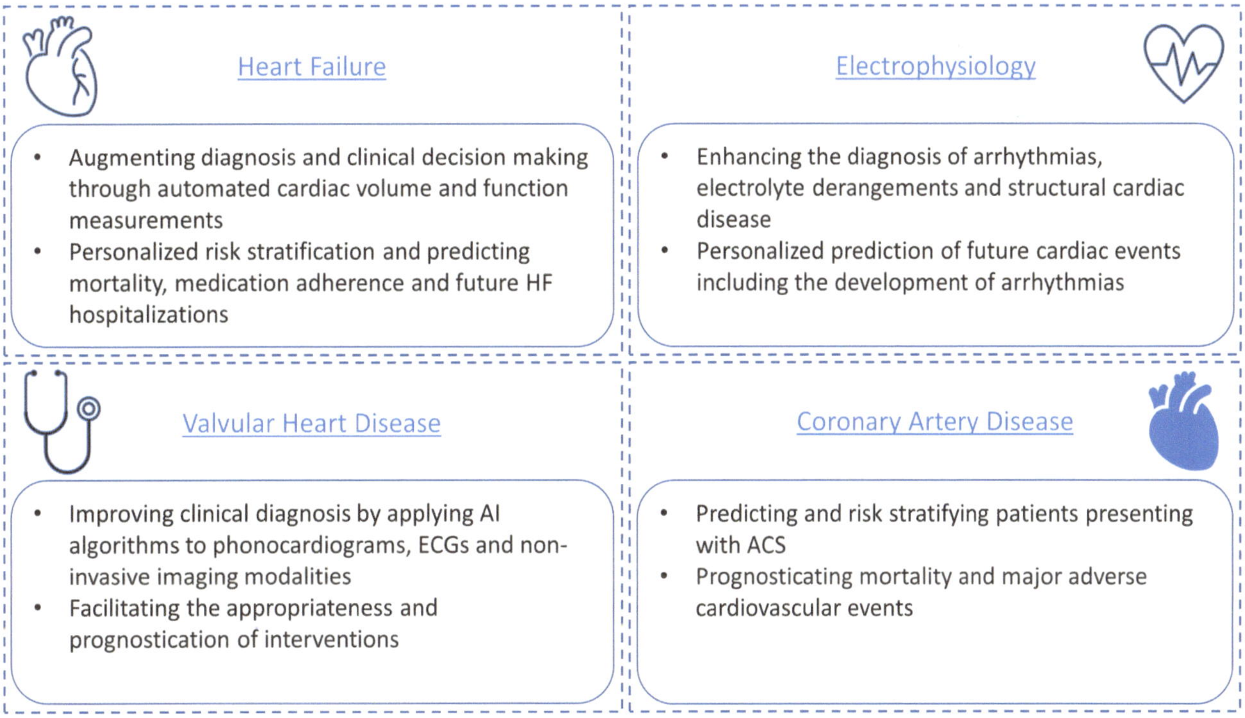

Fig.30.5 *Selected applications of artificial intelligence (AI) in cardiovascular medicine.Abbreviation: ACS, acute coronary syndrome.*

ML algorithms have also been applied to the ECG to predict the future onset of arrhythmias. Attia et al developed a CNN-based algorithm using 649,931 ECG traces from 180,922 patients to predict the future development of AF. The study found a single AI-enabled ECG was able to identify AF with an AUC of 0.87, sensitivity of 79.0%, specificity of 79.5%, and an overall accuracy of 79.4%. The hypothesis proposed for this AI-powered insight is that cardiac substrate modulations such as atrial dilation often precede the onset of AF. Hence, these substrate changes result in subtle ECG changes, which can be detected by the DL algorithms to predict the future onset of AF. The notion of AI-ECG being able to detect occult and manifest structural changes has been studied in patients with LV dysfunction, hypertrophy, amyloid heart disease and peripartum cardiomyopathy. For example, Grogan et al trained a neural network using 12-lead ECG data from 2541 patients to predict the presence of cardiac amyloidosis, and found the CNN had an AUC of 0.91 (CI, 0.90 to 0.93), with a positive predictive value of 0.86.

Valvular Heart Disease

Valvular heart disease (VHD) encompasses many important cardiovascular conditions related to the heart's valvular apparatus, and accounts for 10–20% of all cardiac procedures in the US. AI supported algorithms have been developed and validated to enhance the diagnosis, prognostication and treatment of patients with valvular heart disease.

VHD gives rise to characteristic murmurs, and recent studies have applied AI algorithms to phonocardiograms obtained from digital stethoscopes to augment clinical decision-making. A recent study developed an SVM classifier using 49 patients with VHD, and 325 healthy controls to help classify abnormal heart sounds The algorithm was proven to successfully classify aortic regurgitation, mitral regurgitation and pulmonary stenosis with an accuracy of 98.8%, 98.4% and 98.7%, respectively. Another example is a study which used an automated batch processing protocol to classify heart sounds. The authors trained the algorithm using 3180 heart sounds from 603 outpatient visits, and found the algorithm had a sensitivity, specificity and accuracy of 93% (95% confidence intervals (CI): 90–95%), 81% (CI: 75–85%) and 88% (CI: 85–91%), respectively.

AI algorithms are capable of identifying subtle changes and patterns in pixel density and have increasingly been applied to echocardiography. A recent study developed and tested an ML algorithm in 52 patients with aortic stenosis (AS) undergoing transcatheter aortic valve replacement (TAVR), which aimed to measure the aortic annulus dimensions. When compared with measurements obtained from cardiac computed tomography (CT), the study found that there was less than 10% variability in the ML derived measurements. Another study compared an ML-based algorithm with manual tracings for measuring the mitral annulus area. The study found that the ML algorithm had a good correlation with manual measurements, but the time for analysis was significantly shorter (260 ± 65 vs 381 ± 68 seconds, $P < 0.001$). Measuring valvular dimensions has extended beyond echocardiography, and recent studies have shown its applicability to cardiac CT. A recent study compared a semi-automated ML algorithm with manual measurements for measuring the aortic annulus in 74 patients. The study found that the ML algorithm was highly correlated with manual annulus measurements in both systole ($r = 0.94$) and diastole ($r = 0.93$).

AI-based algorithms have also been developed to help guide clinicians on the prognosis of patients with VHD who undergo intervention. A recent study used a combination of artificial neural network, logistic regression, and random forest machine learning algorithms to predict in-hospital mortality after TAVR using patient data from 10,883 patients from 2012 to 2015. All models showed a good AUC for predicting in-hospital mortality (AUC = 0.92 (95% CI: 0.89–0.95); 0.85 (95% CI: 0.82–0.88); 0.90 (95% CI: 0.88–0.92) and 0.90 (95% CI: 0.87–0.93)), respectively.

Coronary Artery Disease

Coronary artery disease (CAD) is the most common type of heart disease and was the cause of death in 360,900 people in 2019. ML algorithms play a far-reaching role in the risk stratification, diagnosis, prognostication and management of patients with CAD.

Recent research has focused on applying AI algorithms to patients in the emergency department (ED) presenting with acute coronary syndrome (ACS). A recent study developed and validated a CNN algorithm to predict which patients presenting to the ED with ACS would require invasive angiography. The study retrospectively evaluated 2204 patients and developed a CNN using 40 variables including the patient's ECG, cardiac biomarkers and clinical history. The ML network was found to have a sensitivity of 88.1% (95% CI: 84.8% to 91.4%) and a specificity of 86.2% (95% CI: 84.6% to 87.7%) in predicting which patients presenting to the ED with chest pain had cardiac ischemia. Another study included 269 patients presenting with chest pain to predict which patients were likely to have a non-ST elevation myocardial infarct (NSTEMI) using a CNN derived from 42 demographic and clinical features The sensitivity, specificity, positive predictive value and negative predictive value of the CNN model to predict which patients had a NSTEMI were 90.91%, 93.33%, 76.92%, and 97.67%, respectively.

AI algorithms have also been studied to predict short- and long-term mortality in patients with ACS. A recent study developed an SVM to predict in-hospital mortality in patients admitted with ACS. A total of 4871 patients were included in the analysis and 668 in-hospital deaths occurred; the receiver operating characteristic (ROC) scores for discrimination of the SVM ranged from 0.71 to 0.99. In a larger, registry-based, study of 9066 consecutive ACS patients, models were developed to predict 6-month mortality using two ML methods: logistic regression and extreme gradient boosting. The XBboost and logistic regression had better performance compared to the GRACE score: AUCs of 0.890 (95% CI: 0.864–0.916) and 0.867 (95% CI: 0.837–0.897), respectively, versus 0.822 (95% CI: 0.785–0.859).

AI-based algorithms are also being applied to noninvasive cardiac imaging to help risk stratify patients. A recent study developed a random forest ML model to automatically quantify coronary artery calcification (CAC) from non-contrast cardiac CT scans and tested the algorithm on 530 images. Compared to manual measurements, the ML algorithm demonstrated a high level of correlation with a correlation coefficient of 0.95. When stratified by coronary anatomy, the correlation coefficients were 0.98, 0.69 and 0.95, for the left anterior descending artery (LAD), left circumflex artery (LCx) and right coronary artery (RCA), respectively. Importantly, the algorithm also shortened processing times when compared with manual interpretation (45 vs 128 seconds). Another example is a similar study by Van Velzen et al which employed two consecutive CNNs to quantify CAC from 7240 CT scans with the algorithm having a correlation coefficient of 0.9 when compared to manual scoring. Studies have also applied similar ML-based algorithms to quantify epicardial adipose tissue. A recent multicenter study trained a CNN-based ML algorithm on 850 CT scans to quantify epicardial adipose tissue, and tested the algorithm on 141 CT scans. Compared to three expert radiologists, the ML algorithm was found to be quicker (1.57 seconds ± 0.49 seconds vs 15 mins for manual expert review) and showed a strong correlation with expert opinion ($r = 0.974$; $P < 0.001$). AI algorithms have also been developed to assess plaque morphology to identify high-risk features. In a recent study, a CNN was compared with an expert reader in detecting luminal area, stenosis and contrast density in 716 diseased coronary segments in 156 patients. The study found an excellent correlation for all values (R = 0.98, 0.96, 0.97, respectively).

Recent advances in AI have also enabled algorithms to be developed to predict obstructive CAD. In a recent study, a boosted ensemble ML algorithm (LogitBoost) was used to analyze myocardial perfusion single-photon emission CT (SPECT) images of 713 consecutive cases with suspected CAD and 468 with low likelihood of CAD (<5%)The diagnostic accuracy of the model for prediction of obstructive CAD ≥70% was compared to standard prone/supine quantification and to visual analysis by two experienced readers utilizing all imaging, quantitative, and clinical data. The diagnostic accuracy of ML (87.3% ± 2.1%) was similar to Expert 1 (86.0% ± 2.1%), but superior to combined supine/prone total perfusion defect (82.8% ± 2.2%) and Expert 2 (82.1% ± 2.2%) (P < 0.01).

There is a growing appreciation of AI algorithms for prognosticating outcomes for patients with ACS. In a study of 2619 patients who underwent exercise or a pharmacological stress test with SPECT myocardial perfusion imaging, 239 patients developed major adverse cardiovascular events (MACE) during a mean follow-up of 3.2 years The study found that the ML-based algorithm had a higher predictive accuracy compared to conventional physician-diagnosis (AUC 0.81 vs 0.62, P < 0.01). Another study trained an ML algorithm using 25 clinical variables and 44 cardiac CT angiography parameters on 10,030 patients to predict 5-year all-cause mortality. The study found that the ML score (AUC: 0.79) outperformed the Framingham risk score (AUC: 0.61; P < 0.001).

Future Prospects

Cardiac disease remains an important cause of global morbidity and mortality. Timely and effective diagnosis, management, and follow-up are essential in improving patient outcomes and ensuring effective use of health resources. Fortunately, the data-driven nature of managing many complex cardiac diseases, and the abundant use of cardiac imaging techniques including ECG, echocardiography, CT and nuclear imaging make cardiovascular medicine a prime field for AI. As with all interventions, clinical trials are the cornerstones for demonstrating clinical utility. As such, the bulk of studies thus far have been developed in silico, using single-center homogenous study groups. There will invariably be a shift from initial validation studies to external validation using multicenter clinical trials. The first AI-ECG prospective clinical trial was recently published to study the real-world application of AI-ECG algorithms. The study randomized 120 primary care teams to a control arm, which utilized an AI ECG algorithm to predict LV dysfunction in a control arm without access to the AI algorithm, and found that the study arm had increased diagnostic accuracy.. Apart from AI applications in ECG, published literature in the cardiology is largely restricted to current research context, rather than routine clinical use. Increased funding for AI research studies coinciding with a rapid growth in clinical databases, medical smartphone applications and wearable devices provides a perfect environment for widening the study of AI platforms in cardiology.

Challenges

Despite the promise of AI in cardiology, there are a number of inherent challenges to this technology which need to be addressed before AI models become integrated into clinical care pathways.

AI algorithms require large volumes of accurately labelled training data sets to extract the most value and overcome the variety, complexity and potential noise involved in applying algorithms to external patient cohorts.Such datasets arehard to curate and data-sharing agreements often restrict multicenter collaborations. Additionally, storing and sharing sensitive datasets needed for multi-center trials is challenging with data privacy, compliance and potential data breaches representing real risks Naturally, current frameworks and guidelines are limited due to the novelty of this technology, and updated guidelines are needed to enable larger multicenter studies and collaborations. The lack of standardization and heterogeneity of AI techniques employed in studies raises the additional challenge of systematically comparing and critiquing AI research studies.

The aim of ML algorithms is to optimize their generalizability such that the model defines the underlying relationship but not to the extent of introducing inadvertent bias from poorly curated data sets. Hence, a variance-bias trade-off exists where variance refers to how well the model performs with new, subtly different data, and bias refers to how well the model fits to the training data. Overfitting refers to a model that has a high bias and a low variance. In other words, a model is overfitted when it struggles to adapt to new, subtly different data. This represents a significant challenge for AI research in cardiology, as the majority of existing studies have only been trained and tested in research settings. The introduction of biases in curating data sets for AI is another challenge. Specifically, DNNs are vulnerable to adversarial attacks, in which algorithms are presented with inputs that looks "normal" to humans but cause misclassification by models due to minute differences both during and after training. Fortunately, researchers have developed a regularization method that reduces the impact of adversarial noise upon the output of a DNN model. Beyond such solutions, regular feedback from clinicians and potential operators is essential in the development of a balanced and robust model, which is not just applicable to a selected subgroup of potential patients. However, machine learning algorithms are designed and modified by human experts whose proficiency may significantly differ among centers, affecting the robustness of the model. At some level, all AI algorithmic applications in cardiology are susceptible to the "black-box" phenomenon. This refers to the notion that despite the input and output variables being known, knowledge about how the AI/ML algorithm works is often obscure to the clinician While a model may be very accurate, its operations may be difficult to interpret by a clinician On the other hand, a model that has easily interpretable features within its algorithm may be less accurate, fostering a debate about AI/ML algorithm adoption in clinical practice. Finally, current DNNs are not robust to out-of-distribution inputs, which are samples that are not similar to those in the training set. Since AI models are limited in what they can evaluate, they may not replace human experts in the near future

This review highlights the key advances in AI algorithms within cardiovascular medicine with respect to heart failure, electrophysiology, valvular heart disease and coronary artery disease. The use of multicenter, heterogeneous patient populations, the wider adoption of AI technology in cardiovascular medicine seems eventually inevitable in the digital world of 21st century healthcare.

Bibliography and Acknowledgement

- Adedinsewo D, Carter RE, Attia Z, et al. Artificial intelligence-enabled ECG algorithm to identify patients with left ventricular systolic dysfunction presenting to the emergency department with dyspnea. Circ Arrhythm Electrophysiol. 2020;13:e008437. doi:10.1161/CIRCEP.120.008437
- Adedinsewo DA, Johnson PW, Douglass EJ, et al. Detecting cardiomyopathies in pregnancy and the postpartum period with an electrocardiogram-based deep learning model. European Heart Journal - Digital Health. 2021;2(4):586–596. doi:10.1093/ehjdh/ztab078
  Akbilgic O, Butler L, Karabayir I, et al. ECG-AI: electrocardiographic artificial intelligence model for prediction of heart failure. Eur Heart J Digit Health. 2021;2:626–634. doi:10.1093/ehjdh/ztab080
- Arsanjani R, Dey D, Khachatryan T, et al. Prediction of revascularization after myocardial perfusion SPECT by machine learning in a large population. J Nucl Cardiol. 2015;22:877–884. doi:10.1007/s12350-014-0027-x
- Attia ZI, Noseworthy PA, Lopez-Jimenez F, et al. An artificial intelligence-enabled ECG algorithm for the identification of patients with atrial fibrillation during sinus rhythm: a retrospective analysis of outcome prediction. Lancet. 2019;394:861–867. doi:10.1016/S0140-6736(19)31721-0
- Baxt WG, Shofer FS, Sites FD, Hollander JE. A neural network aid for the early diagnosis of cardiac ischemia in patients presenting to the emergency department with chest pain. Ann Emerg Med. 2002;40:575–583. doi:10.1067/mem.2002.129171
- Betancur J, Otaki Y, Motwani M, et al. Prognostic value of combined clinical and myocardial perfusion imaging data using machine learning. JACC Cardiovasc Imaging. 2018;11:1000–1009. doi:10.1016/j.jcmg.2017.07.024
- Binder T, Sussner M, Moertl D, et al. Artificial neural networks and spatial temporal contour linking for automated endocardial contour detection on echocardiograms: a novel approach to determine left ventricular contractile function. Ultrasound Med Biol. 1999;25:1069–1076. doi:10.1016/S0301-5629(99)00059-9
- Choi E, Schuetz A, Stewart WF, Sun J. Using recurrent neural network models for early detection of heart failure onset. J Am Med Inform Assoc. 2017;24:361–370. doi:10.1093/jamia/ocw112
- Commandeur F, Goeller M, Razipour A, et al. Fully Automated CT quantification of epicardial adipose tissue by deep learning: a multicenter study. Radiol Artif Intell. 2019;1:e190045. doi:10.1148/ryai.2019190045
- Dassen WR, Mulleneers R, Smeets J, et al. Self-learning neural networks in electrocardiography. J Electrocardiol. 1990;23:200–202. doi:10.1016/0022-0736(90)90102-8
- Dassen WR, Mulleneers RG, Den Dulk K, et al. An artificial neural network to localize atrioventricular accessory pathways in patients suffering from the Wolff-Parkinson-White syndrome. Pacing Clin Electrophysiol.1990;13:1792–1796.doi:10.1111/j.1540-8159.1990.tb06892.x
- Galloway CD, Valys AV, Shreibati JB, et al. Development and validation of a deep-learning model to screen for hyperkalemia from the electrocardiogram. JAMA Cardiol. 2019;4:428–436. doi:10.1001/jamacardio.2019.0640
  Google Scholar
- Grogan M, Lopez-Jimenez F, Cohen-Shelly M, et al. Artificial intelligence-enhanced electrocardiogram for the early detection of cardiac amyloidosis. Mayo Clin Proc. 2021;96:2768–2778. doi:10.1016/j.mayocp.2021.04.023
- Guez D, Boroumand G, Ruggiero NJ, Mehrotra P, Halpern EJ. Automated and manual measurements of the aortic annulus with ECG-gated cardiac CT angiography prior to transcatheter aortic valve replacement: comparison with 3D-transesophageal echocardiography. Acad Radiol. 2017;24:587–593. doi:10.1016/j.acra.2016.12.008
- Hannun AY, Rajpurkar P, Haghpanahi M, et al. Cardiologist-level arrhythmia detection and classification in ambulatory electrocardiograms using a deep neural network. Nat Med. 2019;25:65–69. doi:10.1038/s41591-018-0268-3
- Haq IU, Haq I, Xu B. Artificial intelligence in personalized cardiovascular medicine and cardiovascular imaging. Cardiovasc Diagn Ther. 2021;11:911–923. doi:10.21037/cdt.2020.03.09
- Hernandez-Suarez DF, Kim Y, Villablanca P, et al. Machine learning prediction models for in-hospital mortality after transcatheter aortic valve replacement. JACC Cardiovasc Interv. 2019;12:1328–1338. doi:10.1016/j.jcin.2019.06.013
- Hernesniemi JA, Mahdiani S, Tynkkynen JA, et al. Extensive phenotype data and machine learning in prediction of mortality in acute coronary syndrome - the MADDEC study. Ann Med. 2019;51:156–163. doi:10.1080/07853890.2019.1596302
- Hong Y, Commandeur F, Cadet S, et al. Deep learning-based stenosis quantification from coronary CT Angiography. Proc SPIE Int Soc Opt Eng. 2019;10949:643–651.
- Hopkins CB, Suleman J, Cook C. An artificial neural network for the electrocardiographic diagnosis of left ventricular hypertrophy. Crit Rev BiomedEng.2000;28:435–438.doi:10.1615/CritRevBiomedEng.v28.i34.140
- January CT, Wann LS, Calkins H, et al. 2019 AHA/ACC/HRS focused update of the 2014 AHA/ACC/HRS guideline for the management of patients with atrial fibrillation: a report of the American College of Cardiology/American Heart Association task force on clinical practice guidelines and the heart rhythm society in collaboration with the society of thoracic surgeons. Circulation. 2019;140:e125–e151. doi:10.1161/CIR.0000000000000665
- Johnson KW, Torres Soto J, Glicksberg BS, et al. Artificial intelligence in cardiology. J Am Coll Cardiol. 2018;71:2668–2679. doi:10.1016/j.jacc.2018.03.521
- Kagiyama N, Toki M, Hara M, et al. Efficacy and accuracy of novel automated mitral valve quantification: three-dimensional transesophageal echocardiographic study. Echocardiography. 2016;33:756–763. doi:10.1111/echo.13135
- Kang Y, McHugh MD, Chittams J, Bowles KH. Utilizing home healthcare electronic health records for telehomecare patients with heart failure: a decision tree approach to detect associations with Rehospitalizations. Comput Inform Nurs. 2016;34:175–182. doi:10.1097/CIN.0000000000000223
- Kaul V, Enslin S, Gross SA. History of artificial intelligence in medicine. Gastrointest Endosc. 2020;92:807–812. doi:10.1016/j.gie.2020.06.040
  Ko WY, Siontis KC, Attia ZI, et al. Detection of hypertrophic cardiomyopathy using a convolutional neural network-enabled electrocardiogram. J Am Coll Cardiol. 2020;75:722–733. doi:10.1016/j.jacc.2019.12.030
- Kwon JM, Jung MS, Kim KH, et al. Artificial intelligence for detecting electrolyte imbalance using electrocardiography. Ann Noninvasive Electrocardiol. 2021;26:e12839. doi:10.1111/anec.12839
- Ma L, Liang L. A regularization method to improve adversarial robustness of neural networks for ECG signal classification. Comput Biol Med. 2022;144:105345. doi:10.1016/j.compbiomed.2022.105345
- Marian AJ, Braunwald E. Hypertrophic cardiomyopathy: genetics, pathogenesis, clinical manifestations, diagnosis, and therapy. Circ Res. 2017;121:749–770. doi:10.1161/CIRCRESAHA.117.311059
- McDonagh TA, Metra M, Adamo M, et al. 2021 ESC Guidelines for the diagnosis and treatment of acute and chronic heart failure. Eur Heart J. 2021;42:3599–3726. doi:10.1093/eurheartj/ehab368
- Mediratta A, Addetia K, Medvedofsky D, et al. 3D echocardiographic analysis of aortic annulus for transcatheter aortic valve replacement using novel aortic valve quantification software: comparison with computed tomography. Echocardiography. 2017;34:690–699. doi:10.1111/echo.13483

- Medvedofsky D, Mor-Avi V, Amzulescu M, et al. Three-dimensional echocardiographic quantification of the left-heart chambers using an automated adaptive analytics algorithm: multicentre validation study. Eur Heart J Cardiovasc Imaging. 2018;19:47–58. doi:10.1093/ehjci/jew328
- Mela A, Rdzanek E, Poniatowski LA, et al. Economic costs of cardiovascular diseases in Poland Estimates for 2015–2017 Years. Front Pharmacol. 2020;11:1231. doi:10.3389/fphar.2020.01231
- Motwani M, Dey D, Berman DS, et al. Machine learning for prediction of all-cause mortality in patients with suspected coronary artery disease: a 5-year multicentre prospective registry analysis. Eur HeartJ.2017;38:500–507.doi:10.1093/eurheartj/ehw188
- Nabi W, Bansal A, Xu B. Applications of artificial intelligence and machine learning approaches in echocardiography. Echocardiography. 2021;38:982–992. doi:10.1111/echo.15048
- Nichols JA, Herbert Chan HW, Baker MAB. Machine learning: applications of artificial intelligence to imaging and diagnosis. Biophys Rev. 2019;11:111–118. doi:10.1007/s12551-018-0449-9
- Ortiz J, Ghefter CG, Silva CE, Sabbatini RM. One-year mortality prognosis in heart failure: a neural network approach based on echocardiographic data. J Am Coll Cardiol. 1995;26:1586–1593.doi:10.1016/0735-1097(95)00385-1
- Otto CM, Nishimura RA, Bonow RO, et al. 2020 ACC/AHA guideline for the management of patients with valvular heart disease: a report of the American College of Cardiology/American Heart Association joint committee on clinical practice guidelines. Circulation.2021;143:e72–e227.doi:10.1161/CIR.0000000000000923
- Ouyang D, He B, Ghorbani A, et al. Video-based AI for beat-to-beat assessment of cardiac function. Nature. 2020;580:252–256. doi:10.1038/s41586-020-2145-8
- Pinaire J, Chabert E, Aze J, Bringay S, Landais P. Sequential pattern mining to predict medical in-hospital mortality from administrative data: application to acute coronary syndrome. J Healthc Eng. 2021;2021:5531807.
- Quer G, Arnaout R, Henne M, Arnaout R. Machine learning and the future of cardiovascular care: JACC State-of-the-art review. J Am Coll Cardiol. 2021;77:300–313. doi:10.1016/j.jacc.2020.11.030
- Raghunath S, Ulloa Cerna AE, Jing L, et al. Prediction of mortality from 12-lead electrocardiogram voltage data using a deep neural network. Nat Med. 2020;26:886–891.doi:10.1038/s41591-020-0870-z
- Romiti S, Vinciguerra M, Saade W, Anso Cortajarena I, Greco E. Artificial Intelligence (AI) and cardiovascular diseases: an unexpected alliance. Cardiol Res Pract. 2020;2020:4972346.
- Roth GA, Mensah GA, Johnson CO, et al. Global burden of cardiovascular diseases and risk factors, 1990–2019: update from the GBD 2019 study. J Am Coll Cardiol. 2020;76:2982–3021.Sanchez-
- Martinez S, Duchateau N, Erdei T, et al. Machine learninganalysis of left ventricular function to characterize heart failure with preserved ejection fraction. Circ Cardiovasc Imaging. 2018;11:e007138. doi:10.1161/CIRCIMAGING.117.007138
- Siontis KC, Liu K, Bos JM, et al. Detection of hypertrophic cardiomyopathy by an artificial intelligence electrocardiogram in children and adolescents. Int J Cardiol. 2021;340:42–47.doi:10.1016/j.ijcard.2021.08.026
- Son YJ, Kim HG, Kim EH, Choi S, Lee SK. Application of support vector machine for prediction of medication adherence in heart failure patients. Healthc Inform Res. 2010;16:253–259. doi:10.4258/hir.2010.16.4.253
- Stehlik J, Schmalfuss C, Bozkurt B, et al. Continuous wearable monitoring analytics predict heart failure hospitalization: the LINK-HF multicenter study. Circ Heart Fail. 2020;13:e006513. doi:10.1161/CIRCHEARTFAILURE.119.006513
- Sun JY, Qiu Y, Guo HC, et al. A method to screen left ventricular dysfunction through ECG based on convolutional neural network. J Cardiovasc Electrophysiol. 2021;32:1095–1102. doi:10.1111/jce.14936
- Sun S, Huang T, Zhang B, et al. A novel intelligent system based on adjustable classifier models for diagnosing heart sounds. Sci Rep. 2022;12:1283.doi:10.1038/s41598-021-04136-4
- Thompson WR, Reinisch AJ, Unterberger MJ, Schriefl AJ. Artificial intelligence-assisted auscultation of heart murmurs: validation by virtual clinical trial. Pediatr Cardiol. 2019;40:623–629. doi:10.1007/s00246-018-2036-z
- van Velzen SGM, Lessmann N, Velthuis BK, et al. Deep learning for automatic calcium scoring in CT: validation using multiple cardiac CT and Chest CT Protocols. Radiology. 2020;295:66–79. doi:10.1148/radiol.2020191621
- Virani SS, Alonso A, Aparicio HJ, et al. Heart disease and stroke statistics-2021 update: a report from the American Heart Association. Circulation. 2021;143:e254–e743. doi:10.1161/CIR.0000000000000950
- Wolterink JM, Leiner T, Takx RA, Viergever MA, Isgum I. Automatic coronary calcium scoring in non-contrast-enhanced ECG-Triggered Cardiac CT with ambiguity detection. IEEE Trans Med Imaging. 2015;34:1867–1878. doi:10.1109/TMI.2015.2412651
- Wu CC, Hsu WD, Islam MM, et al. An artificial intelligence approach to early predict non-ST-elevation myocardial infarction patients with chest pain. Comput MethodsProgramsBiomed.2019;173:109–117
- Xu B, Kocyigit D, Grimm R, Griffin BP, Cheng F. Applications of artificial intelligence in multimodality cardiovascular imaging: a state-of-the-art review. Prog Cardiovasc Dis. 2020;63:367–376. doi:10.1016/j.pcad.2020.03.003
- Yao X, Rushlow DR, Inselman JW, et al. Artificial intelligence-enabled electrocardiograms for identification of patients with low ejection fraction: a pragmatic, randomized clinical trial. Nat Med. 2021;27:815–819. doi:10.1038/s41591-021-01335-4

CHAPTER

31

AI Embeded Advances In Cardiovascular Medicine-Brief Notes.

10 Latest Innovations in Artificial Intelligence (AI)

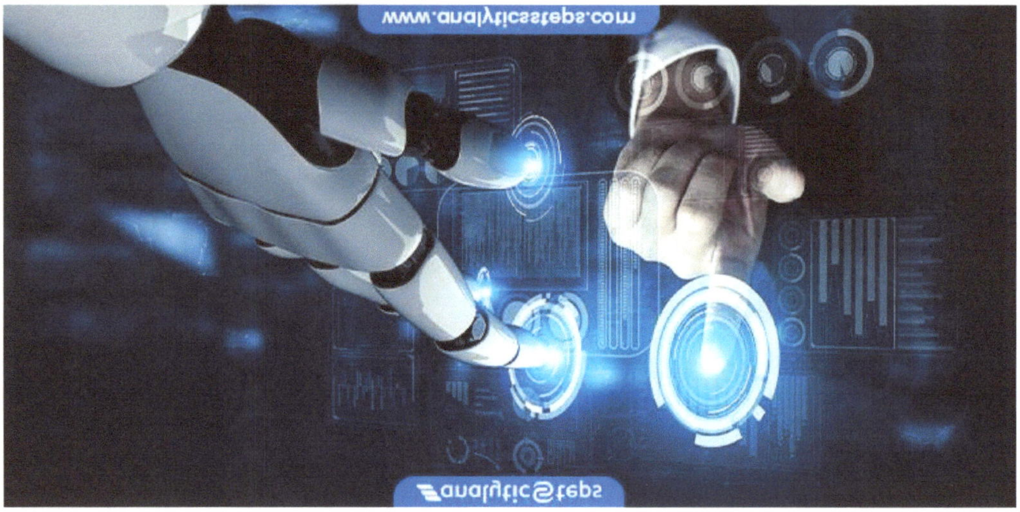

Fig. 31.1 Latest Innovations in Artificial Intelligence (AI)

The replication of human intellectual processes by machines, particularly computer systems, is known as Artificial Intelligence, and it is one of the modern world's fastest developing technologies. Also, discover emerging technologies. The various creative Artificial Intelligence initiatives in various sectors such as Finance, Healthcare, Business, Marketing, Security, Automation, and so on are creating promising trends in the market. These developments are reshaping the world, altering people's perceptions about technology.

Let us look at the Top 10 latest innovations in the field of Artificial Intelligence that are currently trending in 2021.

1.Intelligent Process Automation (IPA)

Companies may automate the processing of unstructured data using a feature called Intelligent Process Automation in Artificial Intelligence. Unstructured data is more difficult for machines to understand than structured data, yet unstructured data makes up the majority of data received from the actual world.

In the banking and financial industries, IPA is utilized with other technologies such as Machine Learning, Cognitive Automation, and Robotic Process Automation.IPA is used by investment bankers to spot discrepancies in data collection that are practically impossible to spot with human eyes.

2.AI in the Healthcare industry

The Healthcare industry is one of the most important working industries in the world. With the passing days, technology is having a huge impact in the healthcare field and AI is currently supporting the healthcare business in a meaningful and precise way.

Some of the latest innovations of AI, according to health it analytics are:

- AI has helped in narrowing the gaps in mental healthcare. There are many smart-phone based AI applications that recognize different problems one might be facing with their mental health and offer cognitive behavioral therapy for them.
- By identifying damage patterns and studying the types of fractures depicted on x-rays, AI is utilized to detect any symptoms of domestic abuse that may be experienced by

individuals. This will allow medical personnel to approach the patient without fear of offending the patient's partner/ spouse.

- AI can recognize the sort of stroke a patient is having and determine where the clotting or bleeding is occurring. This aids detection since every second matters when someone is having a stroke.
- AI has also made it possible to monitor brain health in real-time. The brain is one of the most complex organs of the human body and it produces a lot of complex data and is harder to treat. But, with the help of AI, many things like predicting seizures, identifying early stages of dementia, reading EEG, etc, are possible now.

3.AI with the Internet of Things (IoT)

The Internet of Things (IoT) is a method of connecting a large number of physical objects over the Internet in order to gather and share data. IoT has done miracles in the world of technology, alongside AI.

Many products, such as smart locks, smart plugs, Google Nest, and others, have taken automation to the next level. It is a business solution and a powerful technology in the sphere of business. It is assumed that it comprehends and meets the basic needs of humans.

IoT devices function with instructions, but when combined with AI, they can foresee the requirements of the user and start equipment without the need for human interaction.

4.AI in Smart Money

Artificial Intelligence is proving itself to be revolutionary in the field of finance. According to appen, the fast advancing applications of AI are as follows:

- 60% of the companies are now using Natural Language Processing (NLP), which is a subfield of machine learning that helps computers understand and manipulate the natural language spoken by humans.
- 70% of the firms are now actively using machine learning for business solutions.
- Leading financial services businesses are seeing a 19% increase in overall income as a result of their AI projects.
- 49% of frontrunners have a full AI adoption plan in place, with departments expected to follow, providing them an instant size and speed advantage over competitors.
- Today, 45 % of AI frontrunner companies are investing more than $5 million in AI projects, which is three times the amount of early or late adopters

5.AI in Automobiles

Artificial Intelligence has made vehicles Autonomous now. Cars are now able to operate themselves without the need for any driver's intervention. There are six levels of automation that can be installed within the vehicle.

- At level 0, the car requires human control.
- At level 1, the advanced driver assistance system (ADAS) in the car may aid the driver with navigation, acceleration, and brakes.
- In some circumstances, the ADAS can handle steering, acceleration, and braking at level 2, but the human driver must maintain total attention to the driving environment during the travel while also completing the other responsibilities.
- In some circumstances, the ADS (advanced driving system) can execute all aspects of the driving duty at level 3, but the human driver must be able to restore control when the ADS requests it.
- In the remaining cases, the human driver performs the required tasks. In some circumstances where human attention is not required, the vehicle's ADS can execute all driving duties autonomously at level 4.
- Finally, level 5 entails complete automation, in which the vehicle's ADS is capable of performing all duties in all situations and no human driver assistance is necessary.

The use of 5G technology will enable full automation by allowing cars to communicate not just with one another, but also with traffic signals, signage, and even the roadways themselves.

6.AI for Virtual Assistants and Chatbots

We've all heard of voice assistants like Alexa, Siri, and Google Assistant, as well as chatbots that are embedded into many websites to aid and advise new users. A voice assistant is a piece of software that employs NLP, Artificial Intelligence, and speech recognition to interpret and respond to a user's spoken instructions.

Chatbots, on the other hand, are programs that are meant to help a user 24 hours a day, seven days a week, and to reply correctly and answer any questions that the user may have. Most Chatbots and Virtual Assistants have pre-programmed response systems that respond in accordance with particular rules and patterns.

Some voice assistants can now communicate with the user and reply properly thanks to powerful AI. They even improve as they are used more. Siri and Alexa, for example, may converse with the user just like a normal human being!

7.AI in Processors

Because of the abundance of low-cost processors on the market, it is relatively simple to incorporate Artificial Intelligence and related technologies into projects and tasks.

AI-enabled processors or chips are offered from a variety of firms, including NVIDIA, AMD, and Qualcomm, and aid in the improvement of all business operations.

These chips are utilized in facial recognition and object detecting features. Biometrics are widely used in many devices since they improve security and restrict access to any system to only registered users.

8.Quantum AI

Artificial Intelligence has been playing a very important role in the progress of quantum computing. With classical computers, artificial intelligence creates usable applications; nevertheless, it is restricted by the computing capabilities of classical computers.

Quantum computing can provide artificial intelligence a computational boost, allowing it to solve more difficult tasks. The use of quantum computing for the calculation of machine learning algorithms is known as quantum AI. Because of the processing benefits of quantum computing, quantum AI can assist in achieving outcomes that are not achievable with traditional computers.

It is slowly but steadily expanding as firms embrace technology that allows them to solve problems more quickly. This can aid in the analysis and processing of large amounts of data, allowing the pattern to be quickly retrieved. Quantum AI is improving the sectors of banking and healthcare

9. AI for Cybersecurity

Cybersecurity is very essential nowadays as most of the important data is stored on the internet by companies and businesses. Even as an individual one might have many personal data stored on the internet like passwords, photos, documents, etc. It is convenient and easier to find but with it comes the risk of data breach and leaking.

Every business requires internet security since all of their company's key databases, including financial data, plans, and private information, are housed online. Cybersecurity is a must-have for all businesses, making it one of the most essential uses of AI.

Cyber professionals can use Artificial Intelligence to identify and eliminate undesirable noise or data that they may notice. It enables them to be aware of any unusual activity or viruses and to be ready for any assault. In order to decrease cyber risks, it also analyses large volumes of data and improves the system accordingly.

10. Robotic Process Automation (RPA)

Robotic process automation (RPA) is a technology that allows the creation, installation, and management of software robots that mimic human movements while dealing with digital systems and software. Many businesses are turning to RPA to improve their operations.

RPA is capable of handling and automating repetitive activities. It can help in the repetition of any task multiple times each day, freeing up human time for other useful pursuits.

RPA is widely utilized in the insurance business, but by incorporating AI into typical insurance RPA procedures, automation can employ image recognition to access and process claims with minimum human intervention

Conclusion

With the passing days, Artificial Intelligence is advancing more and more in its domain and setting new trends every day. In this article, we have discussed some of the latest innovations that have been possible with the help of AI. AI has now taken over many fields and has become a very essential part of businesses, healthcare, and other industries.

Expert panel recommends coronary CTA as first choice when evaluating for stable CAD

Coronary computed tomography angiography (CTA) should be the first test clinicians use to evaluate stable coronary artery disease (CAD), according to a group of specialists assembled by the American College of Cardiology (ACC). The ACC Summit on Technology Advances in Coronary Computed Tomography Angiography held a roundtable event in September 2019 to discuss this topic. The group's report has been published in full in the Journal of the American College of Cardiology. The report's authors noted that recent evidence—including studies in both the United States and the United Kingdom—suggests a coronary CTA-first strategy can improve outcomes and "does not result in more cardiac catheterizations andrevascularization."

Getting more specialists to commit to a coronary CTA-first strategy may prove difficult at first, the authors explained, because SPECT myocardial perfusing imaging is currently much much more common. "Transition to 'coronary CTA first' requires revising training programs in coronary CTA and advanced technologies to cover both coronary artery stenosis and atherosclerotic plaque, strong leadership from industry experts, and expanded certification of imaging skills to ensure consistent performance, the group wrote. "Capital investment will be critical. A national registry to monitor scan quality and medical and financial outcomes is advised." The ACC Summit Team also shared nine specific recommendations related to coronary CTA:

1. Begin with coronary CTA when evaluating patients with stable chest pain and "low-to-intermediate pre-test probability of obstructive CAD." When patients have a high pre-test probability, staring with coronary CTA can also help rule out the presence of left main CAD, "particularly when a conservative treatment strategy is selected."
2. Move cardiac CT services to the Ambulatory Payment Classification group and increase the overall payment for coronary CTA exams.
3. Consider bundled payment options for cardiac testing.
4. Investigate ways to increase the number of coronary CTA providers available to the public.
5. Update training guidelines for cardiovascular fellows, technologists and other staff members to improve overall provider competency when it comes to coronary CTA exams.
6. Begin work on a coronary CTA registry for the evaluation of chest pain.
7. Work with CMS, Congress and other applicable bodies to improve coronary CTA advocacy.
8. Engage and educate commercial providers about the importance of these exams, potentially convincing them to end required pre-approvals for coronary CTA exams.
9. Educate cardiologists and primary care physicians so that hey gain a better understanding of when—and when not—to consider coronary CTA.

Breaking Studies On Pulsed-field Ablation technology

The new cardiac electrophysiology technology of pulsed field ablation may be a safer option that the current standard of care using cryoablation and radiofrequency ablation techniques, according to the late-breaking PULSED-AF trial presented at ACC.23. The technology is widely expected to replace current technologies ablation technologies in the treatment at atrial fibrillation (AFib).

The PULSED-AF trial looking at the Medtronic pulsed field ablation system was the first big pivotal trial to report results. Biosense Webster announced in early March the first cases with its investigational Dual Energy Catheter for cardiac ablation, which uses both pulsed field ablation (PFA) and radiofrequency (RF) ablation. Boston Scientific is also conducting the ADVENT trial for its Farapulse pulsed ablation technology.

Atul Verma, MD, director of cardiology with the McGill University Health Centre in Montreal, presented the late-breaking trial data on Medtronic's pulsed-field ablation technology in patients with paroxysmal or persistent AFib. He spoke with Cardiovascular Business at ACC about the PULSED-AF trial results and what it takes to use this new technology.

The new technology delivers short-duration electrical pulses to the cardiac tissue that causes pores, or holes, to form in the cellular walls of the myocytes. This irreversible electroporation process kills the cells without excess heat or cold, which can adversely effect healthy underlying tissues. This has a lot of appeal for electrophysiologists, because existing technologies can damage the esophagus, phrenic nerve, or cause pulmonary vein stenosis. Verma said anatomical structures around the right atrium are much more resistant to damage from electroporation. This fact alone makes it very appealing to electrophysiology to help avoid these major adverse events.

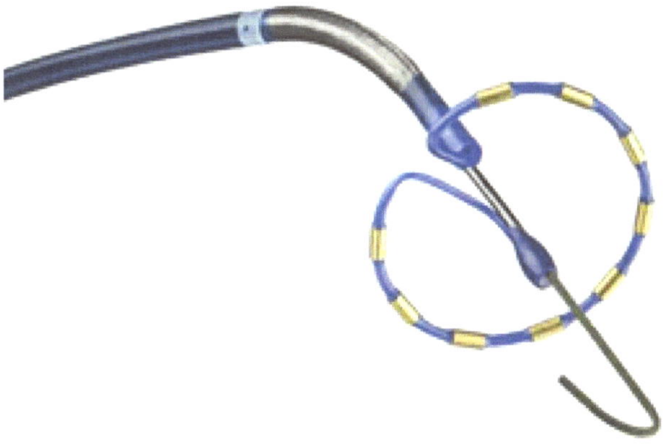

Fig.31.2 Medtronic's PulseSelect Pulsed Field Ablation System. Image courtesy of Medtronic.

PULSED-AF clinical trial outcomes

The PULSED-AF trial treated both paroxysmal AFib and persistent AFib patients, and all of the patients were resistant to anti-arrhythmic drugs. The success rates were 66% among paroxysmal patients and about 55% in the persistent AFib cohort. Verma noted that this was using a very rigid definition of treatment endpoints. This included very rigorous monitoring and a definition of freedom or 30 seconds or more of atrial arrhythmia, no further ablation and no adjustment in anti-arrhythmic drugs.

"If we look at more traditional endpoints, which is freedom from any atrial arrhythmia of more than 30 seconds, the success was about 70% paroxysmal group and 62% in the persistent group," Verma said.

It was the efficiency and the safety of the technology that really had the most impact.

"What was really impressive was efficiency and the safety," Verma explained. "The overall safety event rate was less than 1%. It was just 0.7%, which is one of the lowest complication rates of any AFib ablation trial."

In terms of efficiency, he said the dwell time in the right atrium was about 60 minutes. This is a far cry from the usually dwell time of a couple hours in traditional AFib ablation procedures.

"If you take out the mandatory 20-minute waiting period, these procedures were being done within about 40 minutes or so," Verma said. "And most of these operators had only used the catheter once before they started enrolling in the trial, so it is pretty impressive."

Comparison of success of pulsed field vs. cryo and RF ablation

Overall, Verma said the success rate of pulsed field ablation was about the same at traditional thermal ablation. So about a third of patients did not have their AFib resolved by the therapy during the first attempt procedure. But, he said the number of repeats procedures were very low.

"The biggest advance here is a the speed and safety," Verma stressed. "Over time, I think we are going to see even better outcomes in terms of efficacy."

How does pulsed-field ablation work?

The investigational Medtronic PulseSelect pulsed field ablation system is a round catheter with nine electrodes that create pulsed fields. It was designed to be placed around the ostium of the pulmonary veins. An operator can rotate the catheter two or three times to apply energy to create a a pulmonary vein isolation.

"That was part of the instructions for use we gave to operators to overlap the leasing. We told operators to not worry too much about over applying the energy because it is a very safe energy source, so we actually encouraged the use of repetitive applications to make sure we got lesions as deep as possible," Verma explained.

Each treatment takes a fraction of a second. Unlike tradition catheter ablation, which requires a certain amount of pressure or force to be applied to ensure a good scar in the tissue, Verma said you just need to have contact with the tissue and contact force is not a factor. Then the operator rotates the catheter and repeats the therapy to create a lesion that isolates any electrical activity from the pulmonary vein to the rest of the heart. The total application of energy for a full treatment in these patients was less than 30 seconds, Verma said.

"As long as you can visualize that contact with the catheter and the tissue on X-ray or intra-cardiac ultrasound, that is good enough," Verma explained.

What is the future of pulsed-field ablation?

Based on the results on the PULSED-AF trial, Verma said he believes there will be a rapid adoption rate of the technology once it gains U.S. FDA clearance.

"I think over the next five years, we are really going to see pulsed field take up a lot of there thermal ablation space, especially for AFib," he explained. "And I think this being one of the first global, pivotal trial results, it certainly is baring out in that direction."

He expects to see pulsed field on a variety of platforms in the near future, including different types of catheter

Cardiac CT Soft Plaque Assessment May Offer Paradigm Shift For Coronary Disease Screening

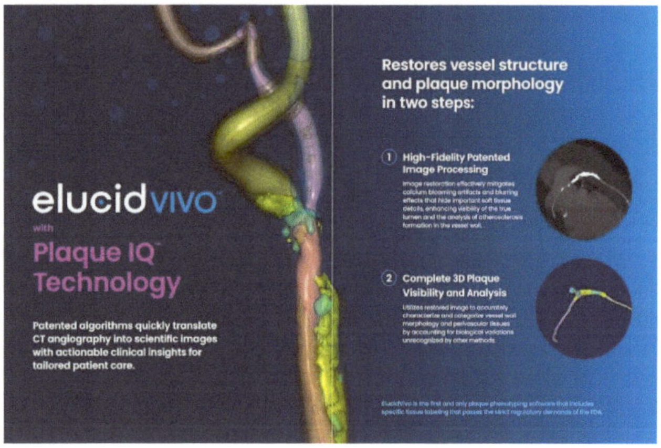

Fig.31.3 Elucid's AI analysis software in action. The left image shows coronary CT angiography of a vessel showing plaque heavy calcium burden. The right image, processed by Elucid's software, highlights the various types of plaque morphology of these lesions.

The ability to use artificial intelligence (AI) to automatically assess soft coronary plaques in the coronary arteries was by far the biggest technology advance in cardiovascular computed tomography (CT) presented at the Society of Cardiovascular Computed Tomography (SCCT) 2022 meeting. Several top cardiac CT experts said this has the potential to change the practice of cardiology by enabling a sort of "mammogram for the heart" type serial screening in the years to come.

Numerous session speakers detailed how soft plaque characterization and accurate quantification could be used as a baseline, followed by future serial, noninvasive CT angiograms (CTA). Similar to mammography, new exams could be compared to priors to assess progression of disease and the need for more aggressive drug therapy or lifestyle changes. This data could potentially be used as a justification for high-cost drugs to lower cholesterol in select patients. Serial CT scans showing detailed plaque information can also show regression of plaques due to effective medical therapy and lifestyle changes.

"Soft plaque evaluation is something we have been talking about for nearly two decades, but the limitations always have been how to overcome the large amount of post-processing times," explained SCCT President Eric Williamson, MD, MSCCT, associate chair for radiology informatics at Mayo Clinic Rochester, supervisor of the radiology artificial intelligence program and professor of radiology at Mayo Clinic. "Previously, it was very time and labor intensive. But, with the advent of AI and machine learning, this process can be automated."

For more than a decade, CT system and advanced visualization software vendors have offered tools to assess soft plaque, but it only showed plaque listed by various Hounsfield units (HU) densities and did not offer a definitive description of what this meant. To quantify the plaque, radiologists or cardiologists had to decide what these units meant and and then contour each part of the plaques in the vessel segments by manually drawing lines around these areas, calculating the area they occupied and then adding all these numbers up. Williamson said it was not feasible for physicians to spend time doing that, so imagers generally just offer a broad overview language to eyeball an assessment of the plaques. Williamson said the AI removed the large amount time and variability between image readers, and allows for reproducible analysis.He said at least four vendors showed new plaque assessment technologies at SCCT this year, and two of them now have U.S. Food and Drug Administration (FDA) clearance. These advances led to several sessions at this year's meeting on the importance and evaluation of soft plaque. Several speakers said this technology will likely be the way of the future and move cardiology toward the long-sought goal of preventive care, rather than reactionary care to advanced disease and acute coronary events."We have developed a lot of new technologies that are driving down CT radiation dose levels, and we are getting to the point where we could certainly do a coronary CT angiography — maybe not quite at mammogram doses — but close," Williamson said. "When you think about the success of our cancer screening programs, as we start to think about our risk and benefits, coronary atherosclerosis kills a lot more people than these other diseases."

Creating a cardiac screening program similar to several cancer screening programs now in use could enable much earlier preventive care, long before it develops into symptomatic disease. While cancer is the focus of current imaging screening programs for breast cancer, lung cancer and colon cancer, cardiovascular disease is actually the largest cause of death in world. Cardiovascular disease kills close to 700,000 Americans per year, while cancer deaths are just over 600,000, according to Centers for Disease Control and Prevention (CDC) statistics.

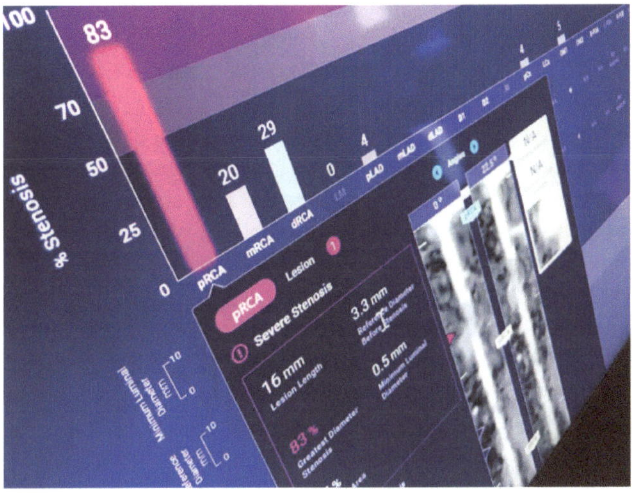

Fig. 31.4 One of several pages of an artificial intelligence report on the coronary plaque from a patient's CTA scan. The FDA-cleared software developed Cleerly enables rapid soft plaque AI assessment, overcoming the previously tedious and time consuming manual task of making these calculations. These types of reports may enable a new level of preventive care in cardiology, treating patients long before they have symptomatic disease.

AI can overcome complexity and time involved in evaluating coronary artery plaques

Several coronary CT angiography (CCTA) experts echoed the need for AI to perform the complex and time-consuming task of soft plaque assessment.

"Soft plaque composition is quite complex and the whole process of evaluating these plaques is becoming complex for imagers as well, and that is where the AI comes in," explained former European Society of Cardiology (ESC) President Prof. Jeroen Bax, director of noninvasive imaging and director of the echo laboratory, Department of Cardiology at the Leiden University Medical Center in The Netherlands. "Looking at the products from these vendors, it becomes clear that visual analysis on the plaques is not enough. We need need to have a better understanding of the composition on the plaques and the only way to do that is through quantification. It will become important that we can assess the extent of the non-calcified lesion."Automated plaque analysis can quantify the amount of plaque and the specific kids of soft plaque much faster and more accurately than a human. This may enable better patient care and earlier interventions.

"This is a really excited area right now, where we can use AI to process the CT images and pull in a new wealth in data," said Ron Blankstein, MD, SCCT, associate director, cardiovascular ima-nag program, director of cardiac CT, and professor of medicine, Harvard Medical School, Brigham and Woman's Hospital. "This is something that today takes a long time to do manually, which is why nobody really uses this in clinical care. But this is going to be the future, where with every coronary CTA, we will be able to provide a very detailed report about how much plaque someone has. Ultimately, this will tell us the amount of risk a patient has and the amount of benefit a patient might get from preventive therapies."

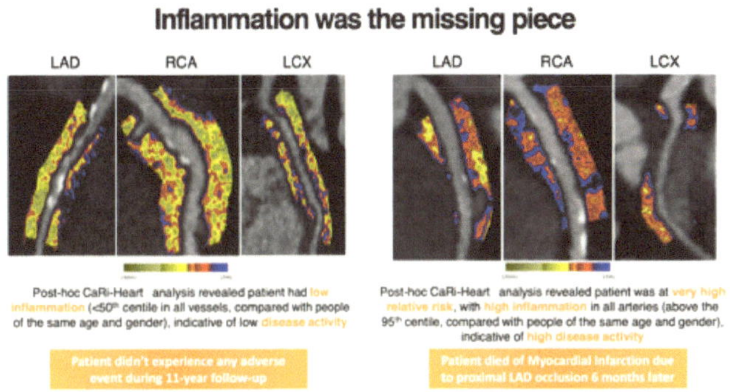

Fig. 31.5 Examples of Caristo's fat attenuation index (FAI) CT imaging of coronary vessel fat to show inflammation.

Analyzing coronary inflammation using CT fat attenuation index (FAI) imaging

Beyond soft plaques, Blankstein was also excited about a new AI technology from Caristo at SCCT, which uses an algorithm to analyze CTA scans for the tiny layers of fat surrounding coronary arteries. Using a scale of fat attenuation index (FAI) on the CT scan, the technology visualizes inflammation of the vessel wall. This can confirm if a soft plaque is inflammed, which can accelerate plaque progression and rupture. This technology was cited as one of the most exciting new advances discussed at both the 2020 and 2021 virtual SCCT meetings.

"We can see inflammation in the vessel wall, so this may allow us to look at risk assessments even before a patient develops plaque," Blankstein said. "Or, this can be used to tell us if a patient does have plaque, if it is stable or do they have a significant amount of ongoing inflammation, where we expect a faster plaque progression."

FDA-cleared AI technology to assess soft coronary plaques

Two companies currently have FDA for AI coronary soft plaque assessments — Cleerly and Elucid. Cleerly maintains its plaque assessment goes beyond traditional measures of heart disease, with a comprehensive assessment of each coronary artery and branch.

The AI identifies, characterizes and quantifies plaque buildup in each vessel to generate a comprehensive report. The company says this data can help determine a patient's risk of a heart attack and developing a treatment plan. Speakers on this technology at SCCT said it could be leveraged for personalized medicine rather than the usual one-size fits all approach in cardiovascular disease prevention.

Cleerly includes an automated coronary tree model made from the scan that color codes area of different types of plaques and flags areas of interest for the radiologist or cardiologist. It also auto segments and reformats the coronary vessels to show the plaque on the CT MIP images. A detailed report offers a list of automated quantifications.

Elucid's technology analyzes CT angiography using AI computer algorithms that were developed using expert histologic examination of thousands of tissue samples. It can objectively quantify the extent and stability of arterial plaque to develop a tailored patient care plan. The system color codes the various types of plaque inside a vessel for easier interpretation of the image and to pinpoint high risk lesions.

The company said the new 2021 Chest Pain Evaluation Guidelines[2] will increase the number of cardiac CT exams where this technology will be able to offer additional information of the patient's disease and risk factors for future events.

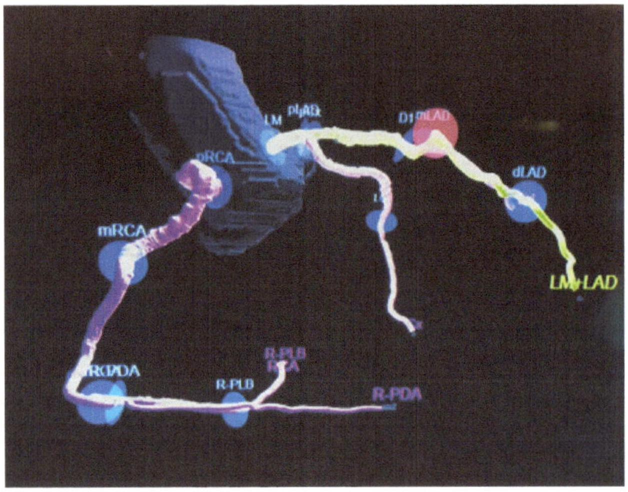

Fig.31.6 AI-generated coronary tree from a patient's CT scan showing a color code of areas of interest for plaque burden from the Cleerly software shown at SCCT 2022.

Two key CTA thought leaders left clinical practice to help new plaque AI startups

The two vendors that recently gained FDA clearance for their AI plaque assessment software have been taken more seriously, because two key cardiac CTA experts, both former presidents of the SCCT, left or will soon be leaving their academic and clinical posts to work for these companies full time.

CTA pioneer James Min, MD, said he saw the large opportunity in the technology to advance cardiology. He felt strongly enough to leave his job last year as professor of radiology and medicine at Weill Cornell Medical College and the director of the Dalio Institute of Cardiovascular Imaging at NewYork-Presbyterian. He is now the founder and CEO of Cleerly.

Min said the development, validation and dissemination of Cleerly's technology offers him an opportunity to translate the large-scale clinical trial research he has worked on over the last 17 years into daily clinical practice. He said this type of innovative solution for coronary heart disease has not existed in the marketplace to date.

Fellow past SCCT President Todd Villines, MD, also announced in a session at SCCT 2022 that he is soon leaving his post as an endowed professor and clinical researcher at the University of Virgina to take over as chief medical officer of Elucid.

"Our current paradigm relies too much on atherosclerotic symptoms and ischemia," explained Villines. He said cardiology largely bases patient care on these factors rather than looking at the root cause of the disease with the soft plaques. Villines said "our future paradigm" will be AI-based plaque assessments to enable much earlier detection of disease.

He noted in his SCCT presentation the Elucid AI algorithm has been validated against real-life histology. Villines also presented the results of a recent study using Elucid's technology, which showed regression of plaques from optimized medical therapy.

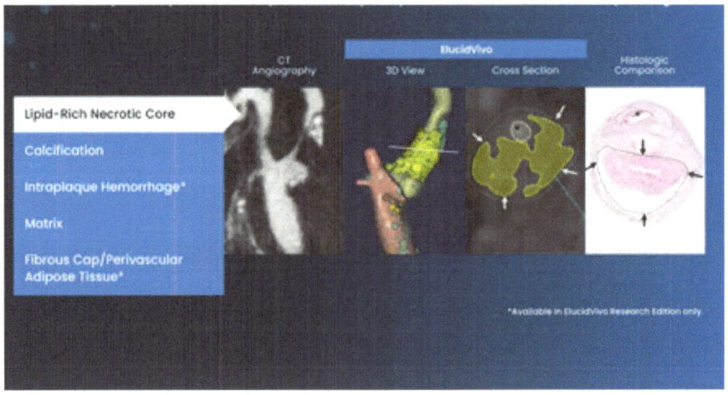

Fig.31.7 Example of the CT image, AI plaque assessment, cross section of a coronary plaque AI assessment and the matching histology for comparison from the same vessel segment from testing of the Elucid AI soft plaque analysis software.

Taking coronary risk assessments beyond calcium scoring to wider cardiovascular disease prevention

CT calcium scoring (CAC) is a common imaging exam that assesses a patient's risk of further coronary events by looking at the amount of calcium in the coronary vessels.Today, calcium scoring is largely automated by AI and it is considered a primary cardiac risk assessment and is recommended in the 2018 Guideline on the Management of Blood Cholesterol

However, Bax said calcium is formed when a plaque ruptures and the vessel repairs itself, so it shows past history. Soft plaque analysis can show the future, and help track regression of plaque due to drug therapy, he explained.

"Through retrospective analysis where we did a CT and later the patient got an event, we linked back that event to soft plaque on the CT. We noticed that in most patients who had a coronary event, most of the culprit plaques were not calcified lesions. That is what put us on the direction that noncalcified lesions are the ones that are dangerous," Bax explained. "These are the ones that develop into vulnerable plaques that rupture and cause myocardial infarction. That was a breakthrough when we realized that."

However, the plaque makeup can be very complex with different components and not all soft plaques are dangerous or will rupture, Bax added. He said more data was needed to understand the variations in plaque makeup to figure out which patients were high risk or not. Today, much more is known about the progression of plaque and the role of inflammation. With the new AI assessments, he said cardiology may be able to go in a new direction. He said this also comes at a time when cardiac CT has drastically reduced radiation dose for the exams over the past decade through new techniques and better detector technology and image reconstruction software. "The dose of cardiac CT has gone down so significantly, it has become possible for us to treat patients with medications, perform a CT scan and do the AI quantifications with serial exams over time to see what the influence of our treatment is."Bax believes the potential for CTA screening and followup serial exams with AI assessment offers a tool to help cardiology finally reach a long sought goal of completely preventing coronary disease in patients, and possibly even eventual eradication of the disease over time

Colchicine Treatment Reduces Coronary Plaque Following ACS

Low-dose colchicine therapy can favorably remodel coronary plaque following acute coronary syndrome (ACS), reducing one of the major predictors of future cardiovascular events, according to a new study in JACC: Cardiovascular Imaging.

Kaivan Vaidya, MBBS, with the department of cardiology at Royal Prince Alfred Hospital in Sydney, and colleagues studied 80 nonrandomized patients who had presented with ACS within the previous month. Half of the patients received optimal medical therapy (OMT) plus 0.5 milligrams per day of colchicine, while the other half received OMT alone.All of the patients—who were 77.5 percent men and 57 years old on average—were assessed via coronary CT angiography at baseline and one year later .The group on colchicine therapy showed a 40.9 percent reduction in low attenuation plaque volume (LAPV) and a 37.3 percent reduction in high-sensitivity C-reactive protein (hsCRP). The control group experienced reductions of 17.0 percent and 14.6 percent, respectively, for LAPV and hsCRP. Reductions in total atheroma volume and low-density lipoprotein levels were comparable in both groups.

"Our findings suggest, for the first time, that low-dose colchicine therapy favorably modifies coronary plaque, independent of high-dose statin intensification therapy and substantial low-density lipoprotein reduction," Vaidya and colleagues wrote. "The improvements in plaque morphology are likely driven by the anti-inflammatory properties of colchicine, as demonstrated by reductions in hsCRP, rather than changes in lipoproteins. Colchicine may be beneficial as an additional secondary prevention agent in patients post-ACS if validated in future studies."

Colchicine, an anti-inflammatory medication most often used to treat or prevent gout, has been hypothesized to reduce adverse cardiovascular events following ACS. But this is the first study to associate the drug with reductions in LAPV, the authors note.

"Additional large, randomized clinical trials are required to evaluate whether low-dose colchicine therapy results in lower rates of future adverse cardiovascular events," Vaidya et al. wrote.

The future of cardiology: 5 potentially game-changing AI studies from AHA 2023

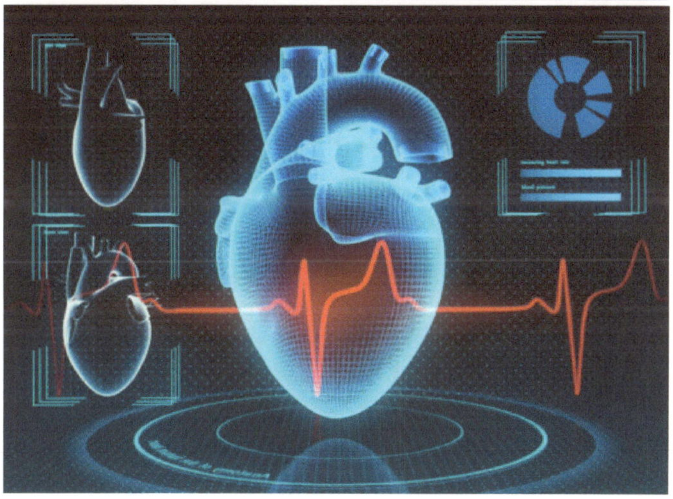

Fig.31.8. potentially game-changing AI studies from AHA 2023

The use of artificial intelligence (AI) to evaluate and treat heart disease has been one of the biggest stories at the American Heart Association's Scientific Sessions 2023 conference in Philadelphia.

After years of hype about AI, and some significant breakthroughs along the way, is it finally time for more and more cardiologists to start using these advanced algorithms on a daily basis?

"Computational methods to develop novel predictors of health and disease—'artificial intelligence'—are becoming increasingly sophisticated," Dan Roden, MD, a professor with Vanderbilt University Medical Center and chair of the AHA's Council on Genomic and Precision Medicine, said ahead of the three-day event. These are just some of the big AI studies presented during the first few days of AHA 2023:

1. AI shows potential to accelerate heart attack diagnosis, treatment

According to new data out of Taiwan, advanced AI can help shave nearly 10 minutes off of the total time needed to diagnose and treat a ST-elevation myocardial infarction (STEMI). The ARISE trial focused on more than 43,000 patients. AI-powered electrocardiogram (ECG) evaluations were used to evaluate approximately one-half of the study's patients, and the others were treated without any AI assistance. The full abstract was presented during AHA 2023.

The AI-ECG algorithm used in the analysis achieved a positive predictive value of 88%, a negative predictive value of 99.9% and helped reduce the median time from ECG to cath lab from 52.3 minutes to 43.3 minutes."Hospitals can use AI tools more to help front-line doctors, especially those with less experience," lead author Chin-Sheng Lin, MD, PhD, vice dean at the School of Medicine at the National Defense Medical Center in Taiwan, said in a statement. "This could lead to faster treatment and less mistakes when it comes to treating patients who are experiencing heart attacks." Lin also emphasized that the algorithm was proven to be especially helpful when treating hospitalized patients, calling its impact "astonishing.""This tells us that there's a lot we can do to improve how we diagnose STEMI in hospitalized patients," he said.

2. Smartphone-based AI monitors voices of heart failure patients for signs of trouble

Another abstract presented at AHA 2023 explored AI's ability to detect key differences in a heart failure patient's voice that could suggest they face an increased risk of hospitalization. The study focused on Cordio Medical's smartphone-based speech analysis software, the HearO system. HearO was designed to evaluates the pitch, volume, dynamics and other characteristics of a patient's speech pattern, alerting specialists when it believes worse heart failure symptoms could be on the horizon. The algorithm built into HearO was trained using data from 263 patients and then validated with data from another 153 patients.

Overall, the application was able to predict worsening heart failure symptoms in 76% of patients nearly a month before hospitalization. The AI offering did generate an average of three unnecessary alerts per year for each patient, and the study included a relatively low number of patients, but researchers were encouraged by these findings."Speech analysis is novel technology that may be a useful tool in remote monitoring of heart failure patients, providing early warning of worsening heart failure that frequently results in hospitalization," lead author William T. Abraham, MD, a professor with The Ohio State University Wexner Medical Center, said in a statement. "This technology has the potential to improve patient outcomes, keeping patients well and out of the hospital, through the implementation of proactive, outpatient care in response to voice changes."

3. AI can reduce number of false alerts from insertable cardiac monitors

Advanced AI models can make a significant impact on the number of false alerts associated with insertable cardiac monitors (ICMs), according to one abstract presented at AHA 2023. The research focused on Medtronic's LINQ II ICM, an implantable device approved by the U.S. Food and Drug Administration for multiple indications. Medtronic wanted the study to measure the impact of using its AccuRhythm AI algorithm enhancements to improve the performance of the LINQ II ICM.

Overall, researchers determined that the AccuRhythm algorithms helped reduce false atrial fibrillation alerts associated with the LINQ II by more than 91%. According to Medtronic, this could save physicians more than 400 hours of time over the course of a single year.

"What this validation dataset suggests is that AI algorithms can help device clinics better manage their ICM patients, saving time and minimizing data review burden," lead author Jagmeet Singh, MD, a professor of medicine at Harvard Medical School and Resynchronization and Advanced Cardiac Therapeutics Program at the Massachusetts General Hospital Heart Center, said in a statement from Medtronic. "When we apply AI, we observed that on average, a LINQ II ICM patient will now have about one false, or non-clinically relevant alert per year related to AF or pause, which is a manageable number for most clinics."The combination of Eko Health's AI-powered SENSORA platform and its digital stethoscope technology achieved a sensitivity of 94.1% and specificity of 84.5% when it came to identifying valvular heart disease

4. AI-supported digital stethoscope detects valvular heart disease

Yet another key abstract presented during AHA 2023 focused on the combination of Eko Health's AI-powered SENSORA platform and its digital stethoscope technology. According to the analysis, which included 369 patients with no prior diagnosis of valvular heart disease (VHD), the SENSORA platform achieved a sensitivity of 94.1% and specificity of 84.5% when it came to identifying VHD.

"The implications of undiagnosed or late diagnosis of valvular heart disease are dire, as well as costly to our health system," lead author Moshe Rancier, MD, senior medical director of Mass General Brigham Community Physicians in Lawrence, Massachusetts, said in a statement from Eko Health. "This study demonstrates that patients can be more effectively

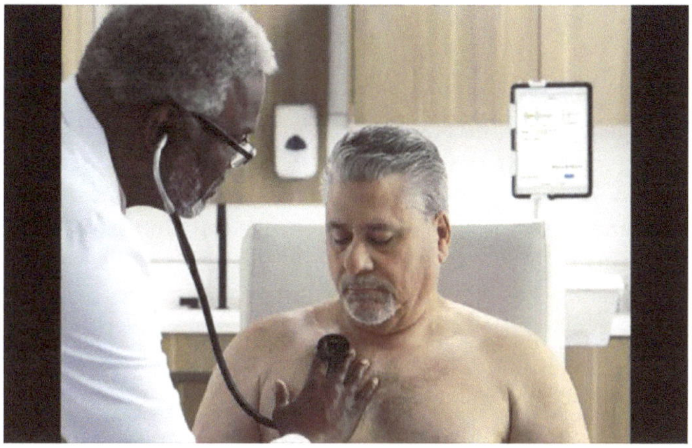

Fig.31.9 The combination of Eko Health's AI-powered SENSORA platform and its digital stethoscope technology achieved a sensitivity of 94.1% and specificity of 84.5% when it came to identifying valvular heart disease.

evaluated for VHD in primary care by augmenting the standard cardiac exam with AI-enabled technology."

5. AI boosts cardiomyopathy detection during, and after, pregnancy

A second study presented during the conference examined how AI algorithms can potentially work together with Eko Health's digital stethoscopes. SPEC-AI Nigeria included nearly 1,200 pregnant or recently pregnant women in Nigeria. The area is known for an especially high number of peripartum cardiomyopathy cases. Patients were randomly selected to either receive an ECG using an AI-powered digital stethoscope or receive an ECG using traditional methods.

Overall, pregnancy-related cardiomyopathy was detected in 4% of patients treated with AI and 1.8% of patients treated with usual care.

"While we expected AI-guided screening to improve the diagnosis of cardiomyopathy, we did not anticipate the frequency of cardiomyopathy diagnosis would be doubled," lead author Demilade A. Adedinsewo, MD, a professor at Mayo Clinic in Jacksonville, Florida, said in a statement. "Additional large trials enrolling a diverse group of women in other geographic locations are needed to evaluate the impact of AI-guided screening on cardiomyopathy diagnosis as well as its impact on adverse maternal outcomes."

AI model for predicting sudden cardiac death more accurate than expected

Artificial intelligence (AI) models can be trained to identify warning signs of sudden cardiac death (SCD) in electronic health records (EHRs), according to new research to be presented at Resuscitation Science Symposium 2023, a two-day international meeting presented by the American Heart Association (AHA).

The advanced AI algorithm was designed to detail a patient's risk of SCD based on a long list of factors, providing a snapshot of their overall heart health.

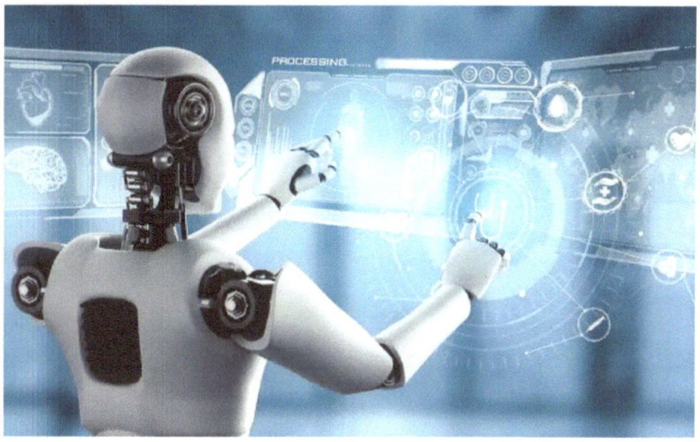

Fig.31.10 Artificial intelligence (AI) models can be trained to identify warning signs of sudden cardiac death (SCD) in electronic health records (EHRs)

If the patient's EHR said they had been diagnosed with hypertension, for instance, the AI model would highlight this detail and explain just how much this increased their risk of SCD within a specific timeframe. The AI model was built using data from more than 12,000 SCD cases and a matched control group of patients who did not experience SCD. The model was then validated with data from more than 11,000 additional SCD cases. Overall, the model was able to build personalized SCD prediction models that achieved an area under the curve (AUC) of 0.80, a positive predictive value of 77% and a sensitivity of 68%. "We have been working for almost 30 years in the field of SCD prediction, however, we did not expect to reach such a high level of accuracy," lead author Xavier Jouven, MD, PhD, a professor of cardiology and epidemiology at the Paris Cardiovascular Research Center, said in a statement. "We also discovered that the personalized risk factors are very different between the participants and are often issued from different medical fields (a mix of neurological, psychiatric, metabolic and cardiovascular data) – a picture difficult to catch for the medical eyes and brain of a specialist in one given field. While doctors have efficient treatments such as correction of risk factors, specific medications and implantable defibrillators, the use of AI is necessary to detect in a given subject a succession of medical information registered over the years that will form a trajectory associated with an increased risk of sudden cardiac death."

For AI-powered risk assessments to work, the researchers noted, consistency would be required from one EHR to the next; an algorithm trained to extract data from one resource may not be reliable if using input from a completely difference resource.

ChatGPT tackles hypertension: Popular AI model a helpful resource for patients with high blood pressure

"Previous research has highlighted that ChatGPT provided largely appropriate responses to queries related to the prevention of cardiovascular diseases,"

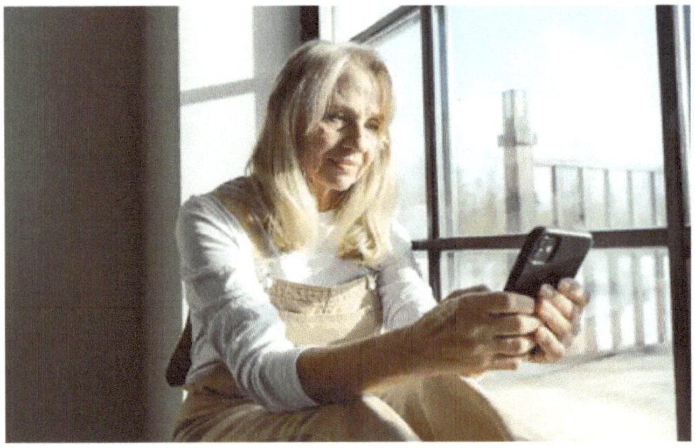

Fig.31.11 ChatGPT-4, the latest version of Open AI's massively popular dialogue-based artificial intelligence (AI) model,

wrote first author Yuichiro Yano, MD, PhD, a researcher with the department of family medicine and community health at Duke University and the department of advanced epidemiology at Shiga University of Medical Science in Japan, and colleagues. "However, these questions were formulated by experts in preventive cardiology and grounded in established guidelines. The evaluators assessing GPT's responses were cognizant of the fact that they originated from ChatGPT, introducing a possible bias."Yano et al. took a different approach with this analysis, instructing ChatGPT to come up with the questions it would be answering—"Please provide a list of frequently asked questions from patients with hypertension"—and then asking it to provide its information in both English and Japanese.

After interacting with ChatGPT several times in both English and Japanese, the researchers agreed on 20 final questions to include in their analysis. Three hypertension or nephrology specialists were then brought in to grade the AI model's answers as either appropriate or inappropriate. The reviewers were also asked to decide if the English or Japanese answer was "superior in terms of accuracy, comprehensiveness, professionalism and level of detail." Overall, the three reviewers determined that ChatGPT-4's answers were appropriate for 17 of the 20 questions. Also, they all agreed that the English answers were superior to the Japanese answers to 11 of the 20 questions.

"Notably, ChatGPT-4 demonstrated superior performance in English compared with Japanese, which is likely because OpenAI's models, including GPT-4, predominantly train on English data sets, thereby resulting in more precise and nuanced English responses," the authors wrote. "Furthermore, the intricacies and nuances of Japanese grammar are distinctively complex. Capturing these subtleties may pose challenges for natural language processing models."

The study did have certain limitations. Twenty questions may not be enough to truly evaluate ChatGPT's abilities, for instance, and the three reviewers did not have an established criteria for what makes an answer appropriate or inappropriate. The group also emphasized that ChatGPT was not specifically designed to be a healthcare resource and "should not supplant professional medical consultation, diagnosis or therapy." With all of those things in mind, however, ChatGPT's performance was still impressive."The present study indicates that a prominent online dialogue-based AI model, when evaluated by certified hypertension and nephrology specialists, offers largely suitable answers to hypertension-related inquiries," the authors concluded.

FDA Grants Breakthrough Device Designation to AI-powered, Retinal imaging-based CVD Assessment.

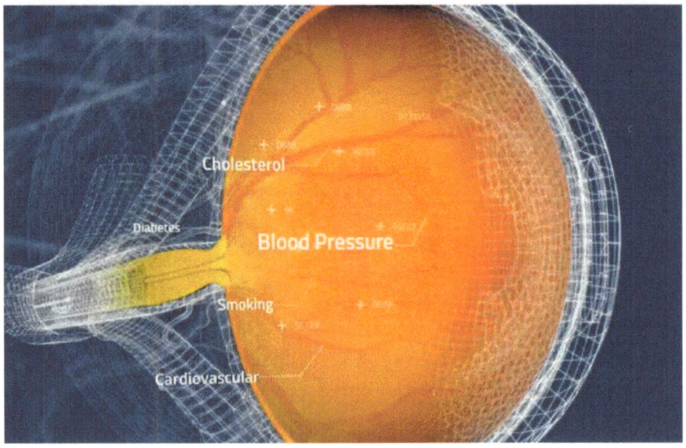

Fig.31.12 Toku, a New Zealand-based medical device company focused on retinal imaging technology, has received a breakthrough device designation from the U.S. Food and Drug Administration (FDA) for its CLAiR platform.

CLAiR offers physicians a new away to evaluate a patient's cardiovascular health using non-invasive retinal images captured during routine eye exams. Because the retina represents the only transparent part of the human vascular system, Toku began focusing on ways to photograph it quickly and easily.

CLAiR uses advanced artificial intelligence (AI) algorithms to provide real-time cardiovascular disease assessments, examining retinal images for signs of high cholesterol, hypertension or other risk factors. The technology was designed to be integrated with the retinal imaging cameras eye doctors already have equipped in their offices.

"Toku's mission is to make identifying disease accessible for everyone, everywhere, all the time," Ehsan Vaghefi, CEO and co-founder of Toku, said in a statement. "The breakthrough device designation that the FDA has granted to our CLAiR technology platform is a validation of the tremendous potential our CLAiR AI technology can provide to the tens of millions of patients who may unknowingly be at risk of a devastating cardiovascular condition. This designation greatly de-risks our clinical development and regulatory pathway for the technology, as the FDA's breakthrough devices program offers medical device companies accelerated review processes, enhanced guidance, and prioritized evaluation, facilitating quicker market access for innovative technologies and encouraging the development of devices that significantly improve patient care."

"Predictive analytics technology, provided it has been proven to be accurate and applicable to the population using it, has tremendous potential to benefit patients by identifying those at highest risk so treatments and preventive measures can be initiated quickly," added April Maa, MD, a professor of ophthalmology with Emory University School of Medicine. "The medical literature has published many examples using different types of eye imaging to predict risk of other systemic conditions beyond cardiovascular disease, such as neurologic or kidney disease. Therefore, further developing this type of technology is very exciting as cardiovascular disease remains a significant cause of morbidity and mortality in the whole country,"

Siemens Healthineers unveils 'truly revolutionary' AI-enabled echo system

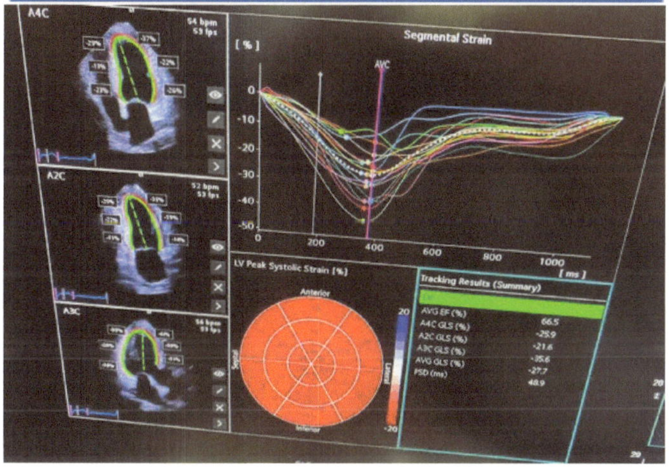

Fig.31.13 Example of the Siemens Origin AI-automated cardiac ultrasound system performing auto contours and measurements after the AI sees what is being imaged and the operator hits the AI button on the console. The system is designed to be an assistant to the operator and knows the next steps in the exams.

Siemens Healthineers has unveiled Acuson Origin, a new cardiovascular ultrasound system with robust artificial intelligence (AI) capabilities that allow it to identify the anatomy being imaged and anticipate the next steps needed to advance patient care. The new system includes AI algorithms to automate approximately 500 different measurements.

The system was unveiled Friday, Aug. 25, at ESC Congress 2023, the annual meeting of the European Society of Cardiology (ESC)."This is truly revolutionary. Most of the time with a technology advancement, you can't say that because it is just a new feature on an old system, but this is a completely new creature. For the first time, the machine knows what it is looking at, so it knows what the next three steps are to help you do them," explained Robert Burke, MD, director of noninvasive cardiovascular diagnostic imaging for HonorHealth in Phoenix.

Burke has tested the Origin system to evaluate and follow up with patients undergoing heart valve and left atrial appendage occlusion (LAAO) procedures. He also tested the system using transesophageal echo (TEE) during transcatheter aortic valve replacement (TAVR) procedures.

According to Burke, the system's AI detects and understands the anatomy in real time. He said this prevents the need for a sonographer or echocardiographer to search for the AI measurement tools in submenus, which can waste valuable time. Burke said a single AI button on the system can perform hundreds of measurements with the AI just looking at the current image on screen.

The vendor said this is the replacement for the SC2000, its long-time premium echocardiography system. While the company has offered various AI algorithms on the SC2000 over the past decade, these required humans to tell the machine what algorithms to use on each image to automate quantification. The company said the Acuson Origin has AI that detects all the cardiac anatomy immediately after the transducer is placed on the patient, and it knows what the next steps in exams are based on what it is looking at when the AI button on the console is pressed.Siemens Healthineers said the Acuson Origin will addresses the entire continuum of cardiovascular patient care, including diagnostic, structural heart, electrophysiological, and pediatric procedures.

The number and complexity of cardiovascular disease patients is growing rapidly worldwide. At the same time, patient volumes are increasing while there is a growing shortage of cardiologists and sonographers. The demand for structural heart cases is also expected to increase rapidly with new transcatheter tricuspid and mitral valve devices being introduced. To address the rising demands, Siemens Healthineers said the AI-enabled Acuson Origin can help greatly speed workflows, while at the same time greatly improving accuracy and eliminating variability and issues with reproducibility in measurements between operators.

Siemens said the Origin is designed to minimize the cognitive and ergonomic workload of cardiac exams and procedures, potentially allowing for greater consistency and efficiency for the user.

"Siemens Healthineers is committed to shaping the future of ultrasound imaging by empowering healthcare professionals with the latest cutting-edge tools," Ajay Gannerkote, president of ultrasound for Siemens Healthineers said in a statement. "The Acuson Origin is the latest example of that steadfast commitment, with its vast array of new AI features and its potential to enhance diagnostic accuracy, elevate patient care and revolutionize the way we approach cardiovascular imaging."The Acuson Origin's AI features have been trained on what Siemens says is the the world's largest cardiac image database of more than 80 million cardiac ultrasound exams.

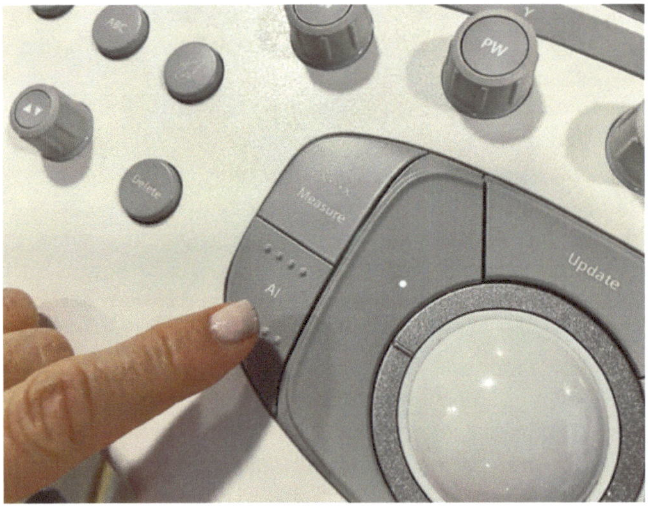

Fig.31.14.The Siemens Acuson Origin features an AI button on the console. When pressed, the artificial intelligence looks at the image on screen and knows the anatomy and the view, as well as the next steps to process the image and will automatically perform contouring and measurements for the user to assess.

The system delivers automated contouring and quantification of all four cardiac chambers without the need for an ECG via the 2D and 4D HeartAI features. The 2D HeartAI opens up auto tracking on contrast images, distinguishing the Acuson Origin as the only commercially available system with this capability. 4D HeartAI is a dual modality advancement for 4D auto contouring of all four chambers in 4D transthoracic echo (TTE) and both ventricles in 4D TEE, averaging up to 5 beats with or without ECG.

Additionally, Siemens said the system is the first in the industry to provide real-time cardiac view recognition. AI Assist, a new AI-driven feature specific to TEEs, recognizes cardiac structures the moment the transducer makes contact with the chest wall.

The system was also designed to be lightweight and easy to maneuver, with an ergonomic that requires less repetitive motion than other ultrasound systems. In addition, the most frequently used controls are positioned closest to the user's hands. "Some of the exciting things the system can do are strain in the 3D volume and with contrast, which historically we have not been able to do," Burke explained. "The AI Doppler is also incredibly fast and accurate."

He said the Acuson Origin has helped him with TEE during structural heart procedures. The AI automatically defaults to a multiplaner reconstruction view and Burke said it easily tracks the catheters without the need to look at different screens.

The Acuson Origin is pending both European CE mark and U.S. FDA clearance.

AI could be a game-changer for TAVR, but cardiologists remain 'irreplaceable'

The continued rise of transcatheter aortic valve replacement (TAVR) as a go-to treatment option for aortic stenosis (AS) has been one cardiology's biggest trends for several years now. Long-term patient outcomes continue to impress, and other transcatheter therapies are even starting to gain significant momentum.

Can artificial intelligence (AI) help TAVR outcomes get even better? A new analysis written by two cardiologists, and published in full in Diagnostics, explored that very question.

"Within the realm of cardiology, AI plays a significant role by assisting in the interpretation of medical imaging, such as echocardiograms and cardiac MRIs," wrote first author Mina M. Benjamin, MD, a cardiologist with Saint Louis University Hospital, and co-author Mark G. Rabbat, MD, a cardiologist with Loyola Medicine. "Additionally, AI-powered wearable devices and remote monitoring systems can continuously track cardiac parameters, providing real-time insights and facilitating remote patient management for better overall cardiovascular health. Moreover, AI-driven predictive models can analyze patient data and identify individuals at higher risk of cardiac events, enabling early intervention and better preventive care strategies. The application of AI in TAVR procedures is being explored in order to improve patient selection and procedural planning and optimize patient outcomes and post-implantation valve monitoring."

4 key ways AI can improve TAVR outcomes

1. Improve the diagnosis of severe aortic stenosis

Diagnosing AS can present certain challenges, the authors wrote, particularly because it may be asymptomatic at first and its symptoms are often linked to other conditions. AI has already shown potential to help clinicians evaluate patients for AS with a number of imaging modalities, including electrocardiography, cardiac CT and echocardiography. AI's potential to help clinicians during echo exams is especially strong; researchers have found that it can reduce the issues often caused by interobserver variability and overworked echo labs.

"By assisting with echocardiography interpretation, AI can also play a vital role in situations or locations where qualified individuals may not be readily accessible," the authors wrote. "Deep learning models have demonstrated efficacy in identifying left ventricular hypertrophy, which is associated with AS, and also in accurately measuring left ventricular volumes and dysfunction."

2. Improve the patient selection process for TAVR procedures

Should a patient with severe AS undergo TAVR? Would surgical aortic valve replacement (SAVR) be a better choice? These are just some of the decisions care teams face on a regular basis, and AI has already shown potential to make those choices more straightforward than ever before.

The authors pointed to one AI technique, for instance, that used variables such as a patient's heart failure data and the presence of peripheral vascular disease to anticipate who should be chosen for TAVR and who may be a better fit for SAVR.

3. Assist with pre-TAVR planning

Benjamin and Rabbat highlighted AI's ability to help cardiologists with pre-TAVR FFRCT evaluations, noting that advanced algorithms can measure the patient's aortic valve annular plane, determine the ideal access route and even assist with device sizing.

AI could even help care teams "virtually implant" different device types from different depths, simulating how blood might flow and how the patient's anatomy may respond in these different scenarios. Many of these algorithms are "not currently ready for prime-time application," the authors wrote, but they highlight yet another way advanced AI can ensure patients are receiving the best care possible.

4. Predicting a TAVR patient's mortality risk

"Predicting mortality before TAVR is of paramount importance as it allows clinicians to assess the potential risks and benefits of the procedure for individual patients, aiding in informed decision-making," the authors wrote. "Accurate mortality prediction helps optimize patient selection, enhance procedural planning, and improve patient outcomes by tailoring treatment strategies based on individual risk profiles."

Typical cardiovascular risk scores are not necessary as helpful when focusing on TAVR, the authors noted, and AI has helped several research teams develop their own risk scores for this specific purpose. One machine learning-based risk score tracked data from more than 10,000 patients, for instance, and had an area under the ROC curve of 0.92 when it came to predicting in-hospital mortality after TAVR. In addition, AI models can be developed to anticipate the risk of other specific patient outcomes, including bleeding events or heart failure hospitalizations. Research teams have been working on these algorithms for many years now, helping ensure the care teams of the future will be able to click a single button and suddenly gain access to a wide variety of predictions they can confidently use to make treatment decisions.

A word of caution about AI vs. trained specialists

"While AI holds immense potential for advancing TAVR procedures, challenges must be addressed to ensure its safe and responsible integration," the authors wrote. Some of the current challenges clinicians still face when trying to use AI include data privacy, publication bias, selection bias, the use of outdated data and the "unintentional continuance of historical biases/stereotypes in the data that can lead to inaccurate conclusions Benjamin and Rabbat also noted that the innerworkings of many of these AI algorithms are still "only partially understood."

While these algorithms may go on to be game-changers for the diagnosis and treatment of severe AS, it is still relatively early. They said there is still much more TAVR research that needs to be done before cardiologists and other cardiology professionals can truly know how this technology will impact patient care.

"The advanced artificial intelligence algorithms described in this paper are promising tools that have, and will, further enhance the planning, execution and postoperative follow up of TAVR procedures," Benjamin and Rabbat concluded. "However, the authors also believe that nuanced clinical judgment by skilled physician teams will remain irreplaceable."

FDA clears advanced AI model for detecting, quantifying bleeding strokes

Viz.ai, the San Francisco-based healthcare company focused on artificial intelligence (AI) technologies, has gained U.S. Food and Drug Administration (FDA) approval for an advanced AI model designed to guide the treatment of intracranial hemorrhage (ICH) patients. ICHs, commonly referred to as "bleeding strokes," can be life-threatening if not treated in a timely manner.

The newly approved algorithm, Viz ICH Plus, is capable of identifying, labeling and quantifying brain bleeds in noncontrast CT images. It can evaluate intracranial hyperdensities, lateral ventricles and midline shift, delivering users with immediate volume measurements. This helps monitor the brain bleed for any changes and guide the care team's plan moving forward. "The ability and mobility to obtain accurate and quantifiable measurements of intracerebral hemorrhages through Viz ICH Plus significantly enhances our decision-making process," Peter Kan, MD, professor and chair of the department of neurosurgery at the University of Texas Medical Branch, said in a statement. "This technology, which marries precision with AI, is poised to transform how we approach intracerebral hemorrhage cases."

"Viz ICH Plus exemplifies our dedication to enhancing patient care by leveraging technology," added Jayme Strauss, chief clinical officer at Viz.ai. "We are excited to introduce a product that bridges the gap between AI capabilities and improved patient outcomes." Viz.ai, which started as a neurosurgeon-founded startup in 2016, has been a leading player in the AI space for years now. The company's algorithm for identifying hypertrophic cardiomyopathy (HCM) received a de novo approval from the FDA in August 2023, and the all-in-one Viz.ai Platform now includes more than a dozen different FDA-approved AI models.

According to Viz.ai, more than 1,500 U.S. hospitals are actively using at least one of the AI models available through Viz.ai Platform. The platform runs on its own, assessing medical images as they are captured and alerting physicians immediately when sings of a significant problem are detected.

Regulatory Roundup: FDA clears AI model for RV/ LV ratios, approves calcium-blocking TAVR valve and much more

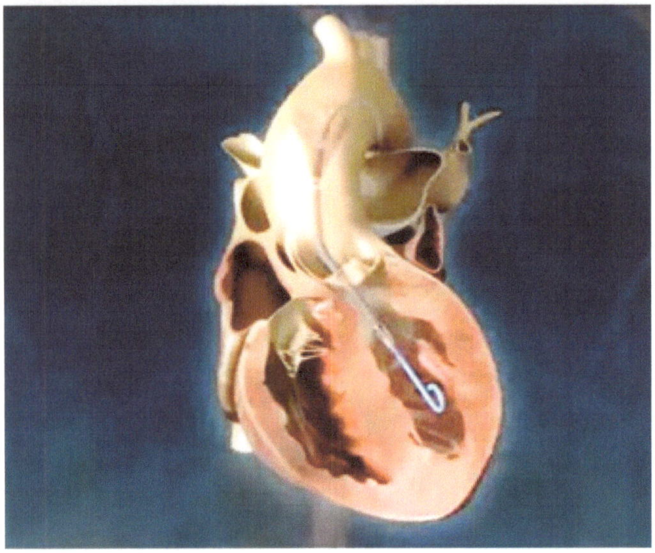

Fig.31.15 Impella Heart Pump image courtesy of Abiomed.

The U.S. Food and Drug Administration (FDA) has stayed busy these past few weeks, clearing multiple structural heart devices, overseeing a significant recall and approving a new contrast agent for MRI exams. FDA Commissioner Robert Califf, MD, even made headlines, delivering a passionate speech about innovation and misinformation at TCT 2022 in Boston. That's just the tip of the iceberg, however. Here is a review of some of the biggest FDA-related stories to hit the cardiology since the last Regulatory Roundup was published August 24:

1. FDA clears new AI algorithm for RV/LV ratio from Viz.ai

Viz.ai announced that its new advanced artificial intelligence (AI) algorithm for measuring RV/LV ratios has gained FDA clearance. The algorithm measures the diameters of a patient's right ventricle and left ventricle, alerting users when it identifies a potential case of right ventricle dilation.

The newly-cleared algorithm is now part of the company's Viz PE solution, which uses AI-based alerts to help clinicians identify early signs of pulmonary embolism.

"With AI-powered enhanced image interpretation that dramatically improves the quality and speed of mobile image viewing—and caregiver communication—Viz PE already helps identify suspected pulmonary embolisms in under two minutes," Jayme Strauss, Viz.ai chief clinical officer, said in a statement. "The addition of the RV/LV algorithm is expected to further aid care teams to quickly make the right clinical decision for their patients, improving outcomes and saving lives."

2. FDA approves a new calcium-blocking TAVR valve from Edwards Lifesciences

Edwards Lifesciences announced that its new Sapien 3 Ultra Resilia transcatheter aortic valve replacement (TAVR) valve, which combines the company's Resilia tissue technology with its Sapien 3 Ultra TAVR device, was approved by the FDA. This updated tissue, expected to be a key building block of the next generation of Edwards valves, was designed to reduce the risk of reintervention among TAVR patients.

"The Resilia tissue's anti-calcification technology addresses one of the primary causes of reintervention following heart valve replacement," Larry Wood, Edwards' corporate vice president of TAVR, said in a statement. "The Sapien 3 Ultra Resilia valve is a prime example of Edwards' continued focus on innovating to meet the current and future needs of patients to help them live longer, healthier and more productive lives."

Edwards also announced it is officially launching the new-look TAVR valve. It is expected to be available in the United States in a limited capacity soon.

3. FDA approves new RCT focused on Abiomed's Impella heart pump

Abiomed announced the FDA has approved a new randomized controlled trial (RCT) focused on the use of its Impella heart pumps among acute myocardial infarction (AMI) cardiogenic shock patients. The RECOVER IV RCT will randomize patients to either undergo percutaneous coronary intervention (PCI) with Impella support prior to the procedure or without Impella support. The primary endpoint will be all-cause mortality after 30 days, and secondary endpoints will include major adverse cardiovascular events after 30 days, LV function recovery and more.

"This landmark trial will be the culmination of over 20 years of research in the interventional therapy of AMI and will apply all the clinical advancements we have made to improve survival and heart recovery for AMI patients with cardiogenic shock as demonstrated in multiple prospective studies," William O'Neil, MD, RECOVER IV national co-principal investigator and medical director of the center for structural heart disease at Henry Ford Health, said in a statement.

4. FDA approves a new indication for Medtronic's Onyx Frontier drug-eluting stent

Medtronic announced that the treatment of non-left main bifurcation lesions using the Onyx Frontier drug-eluting stent (DES) has been approved by the FDA. According to Medtronic, this newest approval will help the company develop new training resources for interventional cardiologist who perform PCI in patients with bifurcation lesions"As the first and only medical device company to offer this indication to U.S. interventional cardiologists, Medtronic remains committed to investing in DES

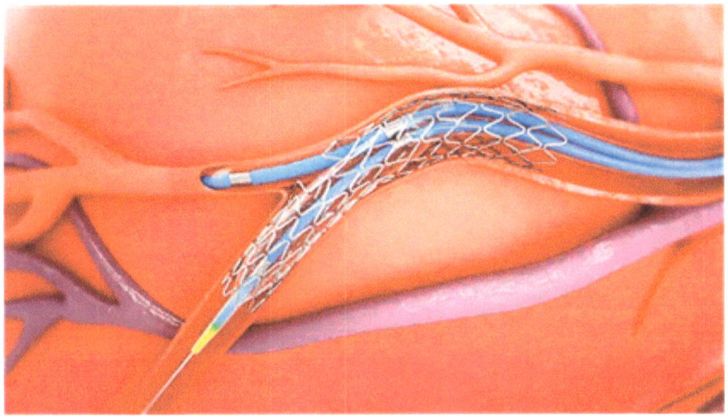

Fig.31.16 Bifurcation using the Onyx Frontier DES. Image courtesy of Medtronic.

technology, clinical evidence and physician education," Jason Weidman, senior vice president and president of Medtronic's coronary and renal denervation business, said in a statement. "We are looking forward to helping even more physicians access the tools they need to give their patients best-in-class care."

Key trends in transcatheter tricuspid and mitral valve technologies

After the stunning success of transcatheter aortic valve replacement (TAVR), many healthcare professionals hoped transcatheter interventions for the mitral valve would follow a similar path to approval. That never happened. In fact, it now seems clear that transcatheter tricuspid valve interventions are more likely to be cleared by the FDA in the next year or so. Kendra Grubb, MD, surgical director of the Emory Structural Heart and Valve Center and associate professor of surgery with the Emory University School of Medicine, spoke with Cardiovascular Business at TCT 2023 about this and other ongoing trends in mitral valve and tricuspid valve care.

Mitral valve innovations

The mitral valve has long been a challenging target for transcatheter interventions due to its complex anatomy and diverse failure modes. Despite the success of the MitraClip in addressing mitral regurgitation over the past nine years since FDA clearance, the field has been slow to commercialize additional solutions. Grubb emphasizes that a one-size-fits-all approach is unlikely to work.

"The first MitraClip procedure was in 2002, the same year as the first TAVR. We haven't made as much progress. This is because of the diversity of ways a mitral valve fails," Grubb said. She believes a variety of tools are needed in the toolbox to be able to treat the atrial valve with minimally invasive approaches. One promising development in the mitral valve space is the emergence of newer replacement technologies. These innovations build upon lessons learned from previous failures the past several years, with a focus on creating better-designed valves that can adapt to the dynamic nature of the mitral annulus. While progress is being made, it is acknowledged that it will be a long road before these technologies reach the market."I'm actually really excited about some of the newer mitral replacement technologies as we've learned from the failures as well. I'm really encouraged that with some of the newer designs and the thinking around it. Fortunately, what we learn from a lot of those mitral devices is that with just a small bit of engineering, they actually work in the tricuspid space," Grubb explained.

Tricuspid valve advancements

In contrast to the mitral valve, the tricuspid valve has seen remarkable progress in transcatheter interventions. It is sometimes referred to as the "forgotten valve" because often it is not treated for stenosis or regurgitation due to historically poor surgical outcomes and a lack of options. But that is now all about to change as cardiology is clearly gearing up with conferences on new approaches to treat the tricuspid valve. Early trial results have shown very good improvements in quality of life in these patients, who often present with right side heart failure.

"The tricuspid valve has presented a lower surgical bar, making it more accessible for innovation. Patients suffering from tricuspid regurgitation have limited treatment options, and even modest improvements in their quality of life can be considered a significant success," Grubb explained.

The TRILUMINATE trial, for instance, has demonstrated that tricuspid leaflet clips can lead to substantial reductions in regurgitation and a notable improvement in patients' overall well-being, despite not showing a difference in death rates or rehospitalization. Unlike the aortic and mitral valves, the goal of treatment is not to eliminate the valve regurgitation, but to improve the patient's quality of life.

This is a big shift in terms of perspective, and the focus is actually enhancing patients' daily lives.

"The patients feel better. For me, that was the win. So that's oftentimes what we look for in heart failure trials, so maybe instead of thinking about just the tricuspid valve, we have to think about treating heart failure with these devices," Grubb said.

Timing interventions and surgery have been the handicap in tricuspid valve care

The main issue for poor outcomes in tricuspid interventions may be the timing of treatment. Patients often receive interventions too late, when they have already developed severe right-sided heart failure. Grubb said this likely led to poor outcomes in trials for surgery in the past and if surgery was performed when the patient was healthier, the results might have been much different. Grubb said this mirrors the historical experience with aortic valve interventions, where earlier treatment has shown better outcomes. Addressing tricuspid valve disease at an earlier stage could dramatically improve results and transform the field.

"I think in the past there was never a huge commitment to the treatment of tricuspid regurgitation or tricuspid valve disease other than in patients with endocarditis. Oftentimes, we were getting the patients so late. And so if somebody has hepatic congestion from their tricuspid valve, we have waited too long. And I think that's going to possibly be the Achilles heel to a lot of the tricuspid trials is that we're not intervening early enough," Grubb stressed.

A similar issue with timing of procedures was realized with the aortic valve, which has led to the TAVR trials focused on low-risk and asymptomatic patients with moderate to severe aortic stenosis that are happening now.

"If we intervene earlier, do the patients do even better? I think that it's going to be a good lesson, because I am suspicious that in the surgical literature, the reason that our tricuspid patients did so poorly was because we were really dealing with in-stage, tricuspid valve disease and end-stage right-sided heart failure. We just needed to get to them earlier and our results would've been dramatically different, in my opinion," Grubb said.

Two late-breaking trials for mitral and tricuspid valves at TCT

The late-breaking data from the Tendyne SUMMIT pivotal trial included results from the study roll-in and mitral annular calcification (MAC) arm for the Tendyne transcatheter mitral valve replacement (TMVR) system. The data for the first 100 patients showed 100% procedural survival, few procedural complications, and mitral regurgitation elimination sustained through one year. The data also show improved heart failure symptoms and quality of life at one year.

Early outcomes of 103 subjects using a transapical TMVR system for severe MAC and MR/mitral stenosis showed procedural success was high with a 30-day mortality rate of 6.8%. MR elimination (100% mild or less) was associated with meaningful changes in cardiac output and forward stroke volume, with reduced heart failure symptoms.

The second study was the TRILUMINATE pivotal trial for the Abbott TriClip, a modified version of the MitraClip, to treat tricuspid regurgitation (TR). The primary cohort analysis results were first presented at the ACC.23. At TCT, the outcomes of all randomized and the single-arm patients with tricuspid TEER were reported. Despite the complex anatomies present in the single-arm cohort, outcomes between single-arm and randomized cohorts were comparable, including 30-day safety, sustained TR reduction, and 12-month improvements in KCCQ-OS scores.

TRILUMINATE trial may pave the way for FDA clearance for tricuspid valve clip device

Edwards shares new one-year data on transcatheter tricuspid valve replacement

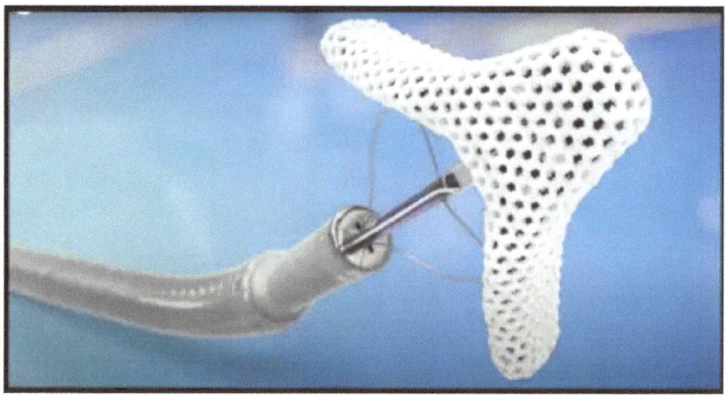

Fig.31.17 FDA advisory panel votes in favor of Abbott's TriClip device for tricuspid regurgitation

Paul Sorajja, MD, director, Center for Valve and Structural Heart Disease, Minneapolis Heart Institute, Abbott Northwestern Hospital, was the principal investigator for the late-breaking TRILUMINATE pivotal trial at the American College of Cardiology (ACC) 2023 meeting and explains details of this landmark trial.

TRILUMINATE was a randomized study of transcatheter tricuspid valve edge-to-edge (TEER) repair for tricuspid regurgitation (TR). Surgical outcomes in these patients are not the best and only about 500 tricuspid surgical replacements are performed each year in the United States, Sorajja explained. This has left most patients to be treated medically, and interventions for this valve have largely been absent.

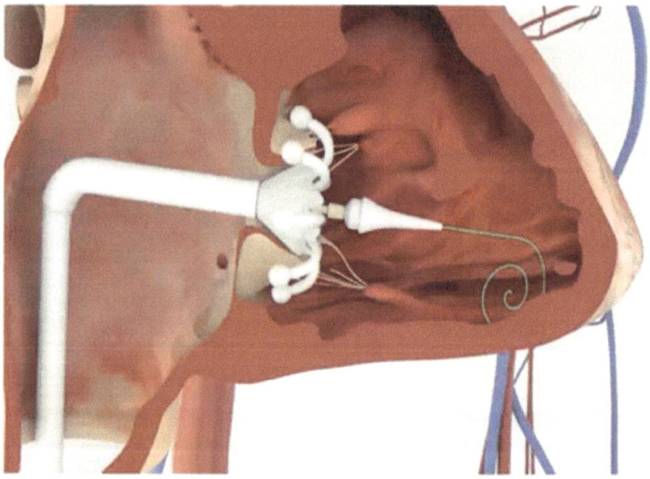

Fig.31.18 Image courtesy of Edwards Lifesciences Corporation study of transcatheter tricuspid valve edge-to-edge (TEER) repair for tricuspid regurgitation (TR).

Paul Sorajja, MD, director, Center for Valve and Structural Heart Disease, Minneapolis Heart Institute, Abbott Northwestern Hospital, was the principal investigator for the late-breaking TRILUMINATE pivotal trial at the American College of Cardiology (ACC) 2023 meeting and explains details of this landmark trial.

TRILUMINATE was a randomized study of transcatheter tricuspid valve edge-to-edge (TEER) repair for tricuspid regurgitation (TR). Surgical outcomes in these patients are not the best and only about 500 tricuspid surgical replacements are performed each year in the United States, Sorajja explained. This has left most patients to be treated medically, and interventions for this valve have largely been absent. With the success of the MitraClip device over the past decade for mitral regurgitation, a similar device, the TriClip, was developed for the tricuspid position. The positive data from this trial will be used for U.S. Food and Drug Administration (FDA) device review.

"It's an exciting therapy, to be honest, because when you look at these patients with TR, they have had very few options for so many years," Sorajja explained. "For the first time we now have a solution that works. It is highly effective, it is safe and leads to a lot of improvement in quality of life." The data show TR was reduced using TriClip from the categories of severe, massive and torrential, down to moderate or below in 87% of patients. The reduction in the control group who were treated with medical therapy alone was only 4.8%.

The safety in the procedure was also a big improvement over surgical risks in these patients. The overall major adverse cardiovascular event (MACE) rate was 1.7%, with a death rate of 0.6% and a pacemaker rate of 0.6%.

"This is an incredibly safe procedure, and that is really important because the alternative of surgery in these patients really carry significant risk," Sorajja explained.

Tricuspid regurgitation is not the same as MR or AR

The surgical risk is much higher in these patients, unlike the much better surgical valve replacement outcomes seen in mitral and aortic valve replacements. Many times physicians make comparisons with the mitral regurgitation (MR) and aortic regurgitation (AR) to the tricuspid, but it has much different functionality and its own specific traits on the right side of the heart.

For example, Sorajja said unlike residual MR or AR, tricuspid patients can endure residual TR levels much better. For thls reason, any improvement in TR, even with residual regurgitant jets, make the patient feel much better.

"Residential TR is actually something that patients tolerate in a much different way, and we need to get away from trying to extrapolate that what we see on the left side of the heart is what we should see on the right side, because it is not. There are a lot of patients that live with moderate or severe TR for many years, and our data actually sheds light on the fact that when they are well managed medically, they can also go a long time as well.," Sorajja said.

With the higher risks associated with tricuspid valve replacement, repair now looks like the best option in TR patients. "It is always better to have what nature gave you and try to work with that rather than replace everything," he explained.

Use of 4D ICE to navigate tricuspid procedures

Five to seven years ago most interventional operators and echiocardiographers did not have any idea of how to get the best transesophageal echo (TEE) views of the tricuspid valve, and a lot has been learned in the just the past few years. Since the valve is on the side of the heart closest to the chest wall, TEE has to image through a lot of tissue and blood to view the valve and its surrounding anatomy, which is not ideal. Transgastric TEE views have also been developed to help image the valve.

Another advancement helping transcatheter tricuspid valve procedures is intra-cardiac echo (ICE). With the introduction of 3D/4D ICE imaging catheters over the past few years, this technology has been very helpful to guide TriClip procedures.

"I think this is one of the most amazing things that we teach the field of medicine is how to image the tricuspid valve in ways that we haven't been able to before," Sorajja said. "ICE is a really interesting way to look at the valve. When coming up from the IVC, the ICE catheter is right on top of the tricuspid valve."

He said right now he does not believe 4D ICE can replace TEE completely, but said it is an "amazing" complement to TEE.

"We have had a lot of experience with ICE, and it has saved us in a number of cases where the TEE could not see what we needed to see," Sorajja said.

What TriClip means to the future of tricuspid regurgitation patients

He said quality of life appears to be much more of a factor for patients with right side valve disease that in left side valve diseases. From that standpoint, he does see TEER as a major step forward to help these patients. "It would be one thing if the safety and effectiveness in the trial were just marginal. But the effectiveness and safety were out of this world, and the improvements for the quality of life were highly meaningful. So while we did not see differences in survival or hard endpoints, to me it fits with what these patients want," Sorajja explained. "The average age of these patients is 79. They do not come in asking to live longer, they ask about feeling better tomorrow." The complexity of the anatomy and treating the tricuspid valve is also much easier that that of the mitral valve. After the success of transcatheter aortic valve replacement (TAVR), there was wide expectation that the mitral valve was going to be the next great frontier. While that is how things started out several years ago, tricuspid valve device therapies and trials have been able to speed past mitral devices in development.

The TriClip and a couple other tricuspid valve now appear to be of the verge of regulatory clearance in the next couple years. The fact that they are few treatment options for tricuspid patients and surgical outcomes are poor also has raised interest in finding new tricuspid solutions.

"Tricuspid valve therapies will likely pass mitral in that way, because there is no good alternatives. In mitral, we have great alternatives. Recent surgical data for mitral shows it has a mortality risk of just 0.6%, I mean, who can argue with that safety margin," he said.

Sorajja said transcatheter mitral valve repair and replacement still has a ways to go to catch up with surgical outcomes, but the story is very different in the tricuspid valve.

"The surgical risks in tricuspid are so much higher, but transcatheter tricuspid is so much different and the alternatives with medical therapy are just not there," Sorajja concluded.

Paul Sorajja, MD, director, Center for Valve and Structural Heart Disease, Minneapolis Heart Institute, Abbott Northwestern Hospital, was the principal investigator for the late-breaking TRILUMINATE pivotal trial at the American College of Cardiology (ACC) 2023 meeting and explains details of this landmark trial.

TRILUMINATE was a randomized study of transcatheter tricuspid valve edge-to-edge (TEER) repair for tricuspid regurgitation (TR). Surgical outcomes in these patients are not the best and only about 500 tricuspid surgical replacements are performed each year in the United States, Sorajja explained. This has left most patients to be treated medically, and interventions for this valve have largely been absent.

Paul Sorajja, MD, director, Center for Valve and Structural Heart Disease, Minneapolis Heart Institute, Abbott Northwestern Hospital, was the principal investigator for the late-breaking TRILUMINATE pivotal trial at the American College of Cardiology (ACC) 2023 meeting and explains details of this landmark trial.

TRILUMINATE was a randomized study of transcatheter tricuspid valve edge-to-edge (TEER) repair for tricuspid regurgitation (TR). Surgical outcomes in these patients are not the best and only about 500 tricuspid surgical replacements are performed each year in the United States, Sorajja explained. This has left most patients to be treated medically, and interventions for this valve have largely been absent.

With the success of the MitraClip device over the past decade for mitral regurgitation, a similar device, the TriClip, was developed for the tricuspid position. The positive data from this trial will be used for U.S. Food and Drug Administration (FDA) device review.

"It's an exciting therapy, to be honest, because when you look at these patients with TR, they have had very few options for so many years," Sorajja explained. "For the first time we now have a solution that works. It is highly effective, it is safe and leads to a lot of improvement in quality of life."

The data show TR was reduced using TriClip from the categories of severe, massive and torrential, down to moderate or below in 87% of patients. The reduction in the control group who were treated with medical therapy alone was only 4.8%. The safety in the procedure was also a big improvement over surgical risks in these patients. The overall major adverse cardiovascular event (MACE) rate was 1.7%, with a death rate of 0.6% and a pacemaker rate of 0.6%.

"This is an incredibly safe procedure, and that is really important because the alternative of surgery in these patients really carry significant risk," Sorajja explained.

The Key Technology Advances In Echocardiography

Ultrasound is the most widely used cardiac imaging modality and it has witnessed several advances in recent years that are making echocardiography more accessible, accurate and efficient. Advances in computer processing have also made a quantum jump in the past decade, allowing much more of the data collected by ultrasound to be processed and presented in a usable format to bolster patient care.

Cardiovascular Business discussed these recent trends with William A. Zoghbi, MD, MACC, FAHA, FASE, chair of the Department of Cardiology at Houston Methodist DeBakey Heart and Vascular Center, and past president of both the American College of Cardiology (ACC) and the American Society of Echocardiography (ASE). He also was the course director for the ASE State-of-the-Art Echocardiography 2022 course that took place in late February, which

Zoghbi said the top 5 cardiac ultrasound trends include:

- Artificial Intelligence (AI)
- Strain imaging
- 3D echo systems
- Point of care ultrasound systems (POCUS)
- Structural heart interventions, and
- The impact of COVID-19 on ultrasound

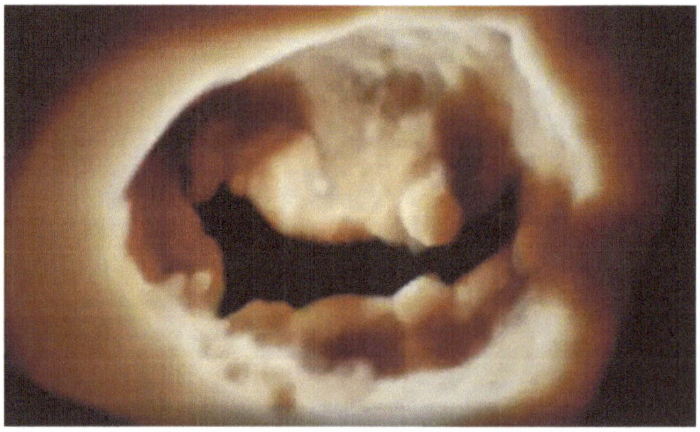

Fig.31.19 The mitral valve seen on 3D cardiac ultrasound offers a noninvasive surgeon's view of the valve for better diagnostics and pre-planning of structural heart procedures.

William Zoghbi: Well, actually the field of echo has never been stagnant. And I think this year has not been any different, with some very exciting, newer aspects of ultrasound. The basics of ultrasound have not changed, but what has changed is how do you process this, and what kind of information do you get. You hear about the use of strain for the left ventricle and global longitudinal strain, but also there is use of strain for the assessment of the right ventricle and left atrial function. This improves our diastolic function assessment in patients such as those with heart failure and patients with shortness of breath. The right ventricle has always been more problematic for echocardiography, so having this technology to assess the right ventricle function, is really a significant advancement.

Have you seen a wider adoption of myocardial strain in recent years? This was a pretty hot topic at the 2019 ASE meeting.

William Zoghbi: I think there is much more adoption now. People are much more comfortable with it. The technology is better now, more robust. There is still a little bit of variability among vendors, but overall, adoption is much better than before. People are using it to compliment their overall interpretation of the echocardiograms.

I think it also can help use with the ventricle to look for certain patterns that alert us to infiltrative diseases like amyloidosis. Nowadays, amyloidosis has a treatment as opposed to the past. So I think having this in our armamentarium will certainly help us navigate and help patients in much better ways.

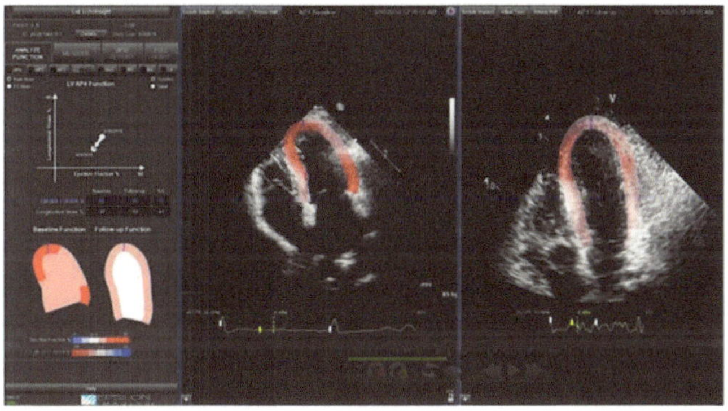

Fig.31.20 An example of myocardial strain strain imaging, which is becoming more widely used to complement overall interpretation of echo exams and to help identify infiltrative heart diseases.

AI for cardiac ultrasound has now been commercialized. How is this helping cardiology?

William Zoghbi: I think the big excitement right now is the applications of AI and machine learning. For example, AI can enhance the accuracy of acquiring images. In echocardiography, as opposed to other technologies, it is the individual who is acquiring the images with the transducer in their hand that can influence the adequacy of the images, and therefore the interpretation. So nowadays, with AI, it can give you a signal while you're acquiring these images as to whether they're appropriate and in the best format for different views of the parasternal long axis or the apical views of the heart.And the amazing thing is that these are available now in portable ultrasound, and even the handheld devices that can really help you at the bedside wherever you are. And they've been tested in individuals who have not had significant training before. I think that is very helpful.On the display and interpretation side, meanwhile, I think the echocardiography field is gradually moving toward enhancing the display of various images since they can be obtained in multiple fashions, to put them together in a way to enhance the interpreter. For example, if you want to look at the left ventricle, the machine would recognize all the acquired images would know these are to emphasize the left ventricle. So you have all the views that relate to the left ventricle. If you want to assess the right ventricle, if you assess aortic valve or the mitral valve, I think this is where the field is going to give you as much information as an interpreting physician to collate all these, and come up with a better, and hopefully more accurate diagnosis.The third trend I'm seeing in AI is automation. The automation of measurements, of ventricular volumes, of ejection fraction, of 3D volumes, you will see quite a bit of that. The field needed something like this to enhance the process and basically put all these various parameters that may be quite complex at the fingertips of the interpreting physician. So I think that this is a significant advance for echocardiography. One of our international attendees in the ASE program last week said they can't wait for AI to be implemented in our world because it brings all the technology and knowledge to our fingertips.

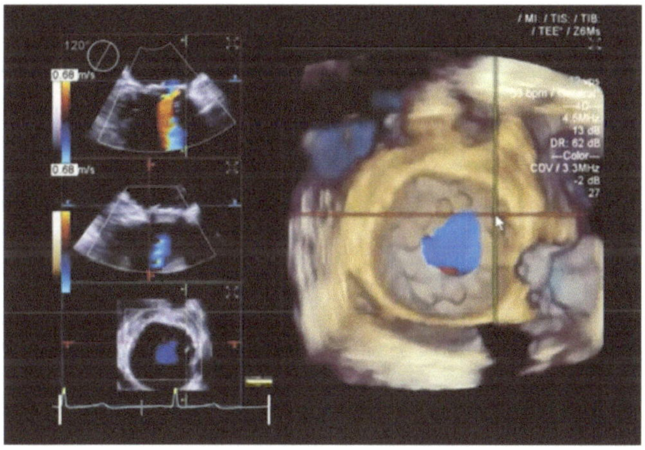

Fig.31.21 An example of 3D echocardiography showing the addition of advanced visualization aids overlaying the aortic valve for a structural heart evaluation of the mitral valve. The 3D/4D imaging also shows a mitral regurgitation jet.

There appears to be a much wider adoption of 3D echo acquisition systems over the past few years. Is this a trend that you've been seeing?

William Zoghbi: I think you will see the majority of systems nowadays already have 3D incorporated in them. What we need there is more educational formats. But I think 3D is going to be very important in certain situations. One situation where it really matters is if you have somebody with a lot of regional abnormalities of the heart, previous infractions, etc., this is where the estimation of an ejection fraction or volumes may be difficult. The impact of 3D echo could be felt the most in these situations where accuracy becomes more difficult. It will be very helpful for us.

In valvular heart disease, obviously 3D with transesophageal echo has been crucial for mitral valve disease, particularly in visualizing in real time the various scallops of the mitral valve and where the abnormalities are.

Structural heart has become a big focus of echo. What are some advances in echo that are helping improve workflow?

William Zoghbi: When we talk about structural heart, we emphasize mostly valvular heart disease, but there are also the occluder devices that interventional cardiologists use, be it inter-atrial septum or left atrial appendage. But for valvular heart disease, a really big focus nowadays is really much more on the mitral valve, and particularly the tricuspid valve. These have been areas where people have not focused as much in the past, because obviously it's a little more challenging. But nowadays, I think we have the technology to be able to help in pre-procedural evaluation when it comes guiding the interventional cardiologist for the assessment of regurgitation and severity of stenosis. I think the role of an interventional imager nowadays is particularly on the mitral and tricuspid disease.

In the aortic realm, I think most institutions nowadays are using a quick transthoracic examination during the procedure. So we feel less of an urgent need to do a transesophageal, unless you have an unusual situation or maybe complications. But I think it is crucial for the use of echo to guide the procedure. You need an interventional imager who is very adapt in acquiring the images and interacting with the interventional cardiologists to see the deployment of either a repair clip or a total valve deployment. And I think you're going to see this grow tremendously in the near future.

What are the impacts of these technologies in terms of helping patients or aiding workflow?

William Zoghbi: We have more and more information that is coming from the usual echocardiographic examination. I think if you compare what we were doing 20 years ago, 15 years ago, to what we're doing now, the information that you're getting from the same examination is so much more. To serve patients well, you have to look at structure, function, diastolic assessment, and everything else, and all that takes time. So most often, patients are scheduled for almost an hour examination or so. Yes, you can cut it down a bit, but you don't want to short change getting as much the information that is needed. The beauty of ultrasound is it is very versatile and can be taken to the bedside, and this is where it's implications are.

Everybody is cognizant of the value of their time. But if it helps you make a quick diagnosis at the bedside to initiate therapy.

What has the impact of COVID-19 been on echocardiography?

William Zoghbi: During the early phases of the pandemic, echo was impacted in two ways. One, there was lesser utilization early on where we had to be cognizant of what to do and how to do it. But at the same time, there was much more stress on the echocardiography field because it is a technology that is available at the bedside. So therefore the sonographers were on the front line. Really my hat is off to our sonographers throughout the nation and the world. Early on during the pandemic, we were not doing stress testing. We took patients to the catheterization laboratory only if they were unstable or were unusual, but all the diagnostics on heart failure, and the shortness of breath, and understanding the heart function, and the right ventricular function that was affected so much because of the COVID pulmonary disease, that actually increased utilization of echocardiography. We are still doing that because we've had four or five phases of this pandemic come through.

But currently I think we're close to back to where we were prior to COVID when it comes to utilization. Or maybe utilization is up a bit. Patients are much more comfortable with the precautions that we use and everything else.

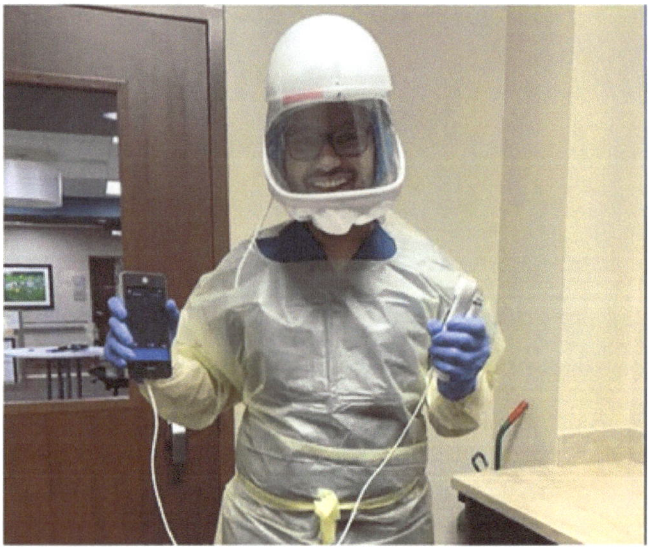

Fig.31.22 An example of the GE point-of-care ultrasound (POCUS) vScan system being used to scan severely ill COVID patients in the ICU. The small device makes it easier to sterilize

Point-of-care ultrasound (POCUS) appears to have exploded over the last two years due to COVID. Are you still seeing this?

William Zoghbi: The portability is one of the advantages of echocardiography, and there are even handheld devices that you could now use. But there are some other things to remember as well. One is that, in difficult patients who are attached to a lot of instrumentation, very short of breath or really critically ill, you have to be cognizant of the limitations of such miniaturized devices. They may still give you the information you need, but you don't want to shortchange the patient. If you are really unsure about what you see, you really want a full examination with a more powerful instrument. There's no question about it. Two, I think we have to be cognizant of difficult patients. With these people who are more difficult to interpret, you may need the full power of a larger ultrasound system. And what I mean by that is good Doppler, spectral, CW, color, good penetration.

I'm not downgrading the importance of smaller, portable systems; I think they are going to be very important in our bedside management of critically ill patients. But my message is, if you're not satisfied with what you get, and if you're not satisfied with interpretation and overall diagnosis of such a patient, I would not hesitate to bring in a more powerful machine.

Can intracardiac echo replace TEE during structural heart procedures?

With the introduction of 3D/4D intracardiac echo (ICE) catheters in recent years, there has been growing use of this imaging modality for structural heart periprocedural imaging to simplify procedures and potentially lower costs. Some interventional operators see 3D ICE imaging as good enough to guide transcatheter edge-to-edge repair (TEER) of valves and left atrial appendage occlusions without the need for transesophageal echo (TEE).

TEE has been used to guide most transcatheter structural heart cases over the past decade, but 3D ICE is changing how some centers image these cases. The biggest advantage of ICE is that it can eliminate the need for an anesthesiologist to fully sedate patients so the TEE probe can be inserted down the esophagus. Anesthesiologists add cost to the procedure and an extra body in the procedure room. Using conscious sedation also helps facilitate faster patient recovery. ICE also offers views inside the heart that can sometimes be difficult to image with TEE. There is the possibility of eliminating the need for an echocardiographer in the procedure, since the interventionist is the person controlling the ICE catheter. However, some centers still believe an interventional echocardiographer is needed because they are an internal part of the heart team and can manipulate the image view on screen and help interpret the image.

At recent cardiology conferences, the role of 3D ICE has been highlighted in atrial appendage occlusion (LAAO) and transcatheter tricuspid valve repairs.There is growing interest in using 3D ICE for mitral and tricuspid TEER valve procedures, mainly as an adjunct to TEE, Rebecca Hahn, MD, professor of Medicine at Columbia University Irving Medical Center, chief scientific officer of the echo core lab at the Cardiovascular Research Foundation (CRF) and director of interventional echocardiography at the Columbia Structural Heart and Valve Center, told Cardiovascular Business. 3D ICE offers an additional tool to image transcatheter procedures and overcome issues with suboptimal TEE imaging. TEE has a wider field of view, deeper tissue imaging capability and can obtain views that ICE cannot. For these reasons, 3D ICE is often used in conjunction with TEE in complex procedures. However, some speakers at the Transcatheter Valve Therapies (TVT) structural heart summit said they have moved mainly to ICE only for certain procedures. "With ICE you don't need the anesthesiologist, you could do an awake case," Hahn said. "At Columbia, depending on the procedure, we are using ICE in conjunction with TEE. In addition, TEE can give you different types of images that ICE has difficulty getting," Hahn explained. "But there are procedures where you might not need TEE."

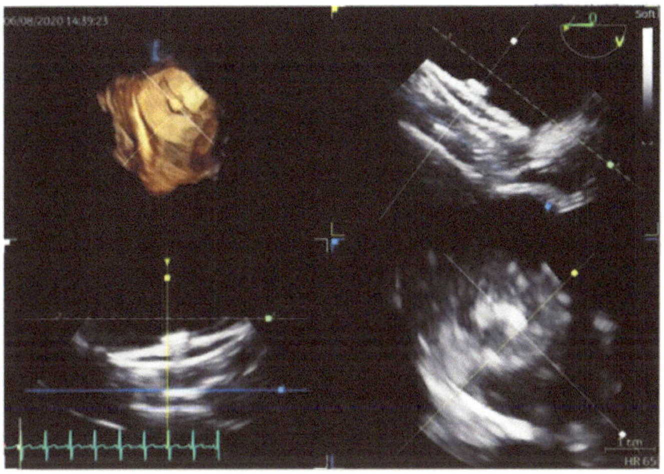

Fig.31.23 An Amulet LAA closure device visualized using 3D intracardiac echo (ICE) imaging using the Biosense Webster NuVision Ultrasound Catheter.

Using 3D ICE to guide LAA occlusion

Devi Nair, MD, FACC, FHRS, director of cardiac electrophysiology at St. Bernard's Healthcare in Jonesboro, Arkansas, said there is a movement toward using 3D ICE for LAAO in conjunction with or as an alternative to TEE. "Years ago when we did 2D TEE, we never thought we would get to 3D TEE, and now we are so dependent on 3D TEE. There is something to be said about seeing things in three dimensions. The left atrial appendage is a three-dimensional structure. We are moving away from TEE-guided procedures to ICE-guided procedures, and I think it is important for us to step to the next technology," Nair explained. However, Nair did said a key barrier to wider ICE adoption is the higher cost of the ICE catheters, in the range of $3,400 per catheter. This is something centers need to consider, as it is possible costs might be offset if ICE can eliminate extra staff or equipment needed during the procedures. "3D ICE is definitely one step forward, but there are nuances to cost, nuances to acquiring the technology and the need to fine tune the technology, but the future is bright I would say," Nair said.

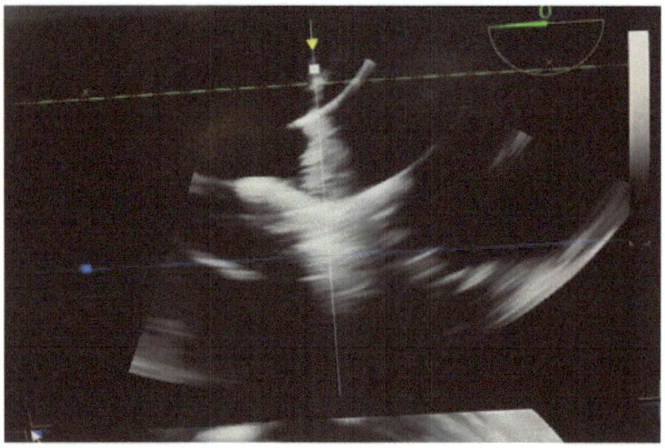

Fig.31.24 A MitraClip transcatheter mitral valve repair device visualized by a NuVision 4D intra-cardiac echo (ICE) catheter. The Biosense Webster catheter was co-developed with GE. It also can be used in place of TEE in procedures to eliminate the need for an interventional echocardiography.

She also explained how she uses ICE during LAA procedures and the ease of use of the newer systems. "There are now three 3D/4D ICE catheters that allow us to image the appendage without doing much manipulation. You cannot image the left atrium from the right atrium, so you do need to go into the left atrium with the catheter. But once you are in the left atrium, you don't really have to manipulate the ICE catheter so much," Nair explained.

3D ICE allows Nair to get multiplanar renderings (MPR) and do a full volumetric analysis of the appendage and measure the ostium."I would not dare to measure the ostium using 2D ICE and size off of that, but 3D is a different story," Nair said.

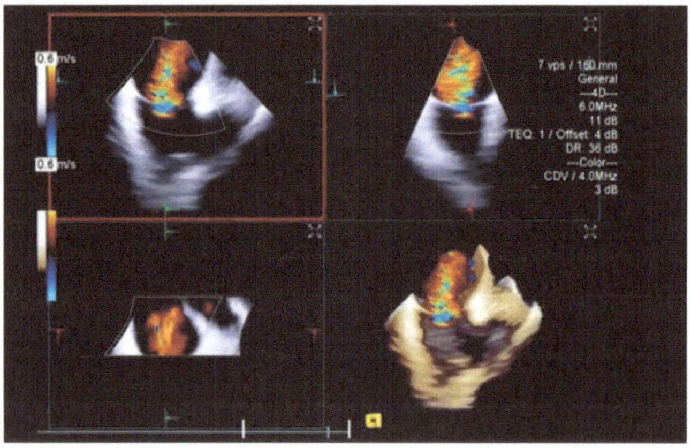

Fig.31.25 Color flow Doppler 3D ICE showing mitral regurgitation during a MitraClip procedure using Siemens ICE system.

New generation 3D ICE probes can overcome suboptimal TEE

In recent years, the U.S. Food and Drug Administration (FDA) has cleared three next-generation matrix array intra-cardiacecho probes that enable 3D and 4D imaging. Hahn and Nair said these new technologies have increased interest in 3D ICE in recent years because it better shows the anatomical structures and the relation of devices in live procedural imaging over 2D imaging. These newer ICE probes do offer 2D views and multiplayer reconstruction imaging as well

The image quality of these probes is absolutely fantastic," Hahn explained. "It really has changed how we deal with difficult imaging by TEE."

The need for ICE arises for a variety of reasons, according to Hahn. For example, during one MitraClip case, the patient had a very large hiatal hernia which prevented clinicians from getting good TEE images. They used an ICE probe concomitantly with the TEE to navigate the procedure. Imaging the tricuspid valve can be challenging in some patients with TEE because of the need to image through the right side of the heart, and ICE can offer another approach to seeing the anatomy.

The ICE system Columbia is using has the same functionality as their TEE probes, so it is easier for interventional imagers to switch between the two modalities.

New LAA occluder technology and the debate on echo vs. CT image guidance

There are now two transcatheter left atrial appendage (LAA) occlusion devices cleared by the U.S. Food and Drug Administration (FDA) and a couple more are expected to soon enter FDA investigational device exemption (IDE) trials. Experts presenting in LAA occlusion (LAAO) sessions at the 2022 Transcatheter Valve Therapeutics (TVT) Structural Heart in June said this offers patients more options to treat a large variety of anatomies.

LAA sessions at TVT include discussions on new devices in development, issues frequently encountered and how to over come them, and what type of imaging is best for pre-planning and procedural guidance.

In atrial fibrillation (AFib) patients, the LAA, a pocket the extends off the left atrium, has been implicated as the main source of clots that form embolisms and cause strokes. While anticoagulation therapy is the standard-of-care in AFib, there are many patients who are at a higher risk of bleeding. LAAO uses a transcatheter device implant to close the LAA in select AFib patients so they can reduce or eliminate anticoagulation drugs or other blood thinners.

The two FDA-clear LAA occluder devices in the U.S.

There are now two next generation FDA-cleared LAA occlusion (LAAO) devices – the Boston Scientific Watchman FLX and the Abbott Amulet. Both use small barbs to offer better device anchoring than the first generation LAA occluder on the market. "These devices set a new bar," explained Devi Nair, MD, FACC, FHRS, director of cardiac electrophysiology at St. Bernard's Healthcare, Jonesboro, Arkansas. "The safety of this therapy is extremely good, and the efficacy rates are extremely good, and stroke rates are extremely low in patients who cannot tolerate anticoagulation therapy."

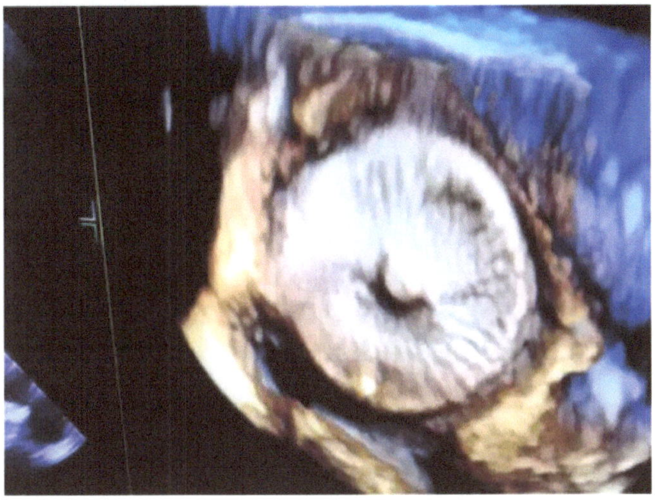

Fig.31.26 View of an Amulet left atrial appendage (LAA) occluder on 4D intra-cardiac echo (ICE). Since ICE is operated by the interventionalist, it can be used to reduce the number of people needed to perform an LAA occlusion procedure and help eliminate the need for anesthesia.

The first generation Watchman was cleared by the FDA in March 2015. This device has the largest amount of clinical data gathered to date. Based on operator feedback, the device was redesigned and replaced in 2020 by the new Watchman FLX. The redesign includes a better seal and anchoring for the device.

The Amulet gained FDA in August 2021. It was designed with two sealing components to better close off the LAA, rather than the single seal competent used on the Watchman. The Watchman requires the patient to continue taking anticoagulation drugs, while the Watchman's screen is endothelialized to ensure a complete closure of the LAA.

Abbott says the double sealing components of the Amulet are designed to enable patient discharge after the procedure without the need for anticoagulation. The device fits in a broad range of anatomies and has the widest range of occluder sizes on the market. It also is recapturable and repositionable to ensure optimal placement.

Remaining issues with LAA occlusion devices

Despite the good performance of the latest generation LAAO devices, some problems remain. These include peri-device leaks and device related thrombus formation. These have led to new designs for occluders working their way through pre-clinical and clinical trials. There are also issues involving imaging to properly size the devices needed for the procedure. Sometimes devices end up being undersized, which can embolism, or the device will form a poor seal.

Why pre-procedural imaging is important for LAA occluder device implants

One of the debates in sessions at TVT was whether computed tomography (CT) imaging is needed for preplanning these procedures, when transesophegeal echo (TEE) can be used for sizing and live procedural guidance. A few experts said the CT measurements are more accurate, so the cost and extra time involved for the CT is worth while.

Nair said between the two FDA-cleared devices, one might fit a patient's anatomy better than the other to achieve an optimal seal, so it is good to be able to understand the anatomy better before going into a procedure. "Some of the software allows you to perform a virtual implant with the devices to see which one fits better and how the device sits within the appendage," she said. These include the TruePlan and FEOPS software.

If a patient can get a CT scan, there are many computational algorithms that help make these procedures so simple, Nair said. "It almost takes the surprises away, so you walk into the case knowing what anatomy you are going for, you know the dimensions, you know if the patient has a thrombus, and you know what the ideal landing zone is needed for transeptal punctures, and you know which device is a better option." If a procedure can be pre-planned prior to getting into the cath or EP lab, she said it can cut procedure time and help eliminate the need for general anesthesia.

Having CT images of the anatomy also makes it easier to use catheter-based 3D intracardiac echo (ICE) rather than needing TEE.

She said 3D/4D ICE is more expensive, but the higher image quality is needed to perform transcatheter procedures in 3D anatomy. There are three of these devices now on the market being used to guide structural heart and EP procedures, including MitraClip and LAAO procedures. Nair said you need to access the left atrium to image the LAA, but once there, she said there is not much manipulation of the catheter needed. She said 3D ICE also allows for sizing of the device, which Nair said she would never try to do using 2D ICE.

However, cost is the main issue. At $3,400 for each imaging catheter, it is just not cost effective, said Rahul Sharma, MBBS, director of structural interventions at Stanford Healthcare. He said they size off of TEE.

Brijeshwar Maini, MD, regional medical director of structural heart, Tenet Florida Health, presented a case of a patient where the echo clearly was showing the wrong sizing for the occluder. In the case, they tried three different sizes until they found the actual size that proper fit. He advocated for pre-procedural CT scans.

However, if an operator is very experience and does a lot of LAA cases each year, they are probably comfortable enough and look at TEE or ICE and properly size the appendage. However, for operators that only do a small number, like five a year, they would be better off with the CT imaging.

CT has the added advantage of showing if a patient has a thrombus in the LAA prior to the procedure. This raises concerns that the clot can embolism during the procedure once catheters are inserted into the appendage. This is why CT is a standard-of-care for Jacqueline Saw, MD, interventional cardiologist at Vancouver General Hospital and St Paul's Hospital, and clinical assistant professor at

Coastal Health Research Institute. She said it offers additional information on the patient and she also conducts all of her sizing depth measurements from the CT.

Next generation LAA occlusion devices in trials

There are several new LAAO devices in development that will try to overcome some of the issues with the current technology. A few of these are already in trials. These include the CLAAS Conformal, Laminar, LAmbre and devices that may combine ablation with LAAO. Some devices being developed are for specific LAA anatomies, she said.

Nair was involved in the early feasibility study of the Conformal device, implanting 10 of them. The device is expected to enter an FDA pivotal trial soon. "The beauty of the device is that it comes in just two sizes, regular and large, so the sizing is very easy," Nair explained. She added the device is also more fluoro dependent, so there is less reliance on TEE. She said the LAmbre device is also expected to begin its FDA pivotal trial soon. "Having one device that fits all appendages would be great, but I think it will be challenging with the different variations of anatomies, with different take offs and different orientations within the left atrium," Nair explained. "But, if we can get a device that offers complete closure without having to go into the more distal parts of the appendage and is more conformable, we would be in a good place."

TAVR valve deterioration lower that surgical valves

A long standing question has been the durability of transcatheter aortic valve replacement (TAVR) systems compared to traditional surgical aortic valve replacement (SAVR) devices. It has always been assumed SAVR would out-perform TAVR, but new data from a late-breaking review of the CoreValve U.S. pivotal and SURTAVI trials showed this was not the case, making it one of the key take-away trials presented at ACC this year.

Patients who received a transcatheter supra-annular, self-expanding, CoreValve had significantly less structural valve deterioration (SVD) after five years compared with similar patients who had the biologic SAVR valve. TAVR is now approved by the U.S. Food and Drug Administration (FDA) for use in patients of all ages and risk levels who need a replacement heart valve. But, heart teams often refer younger patients for surgery because of increased durability. "For moderate and greater regurgitation patients, TAVR did better than surgery," said Michael J. Reardon, MD, professor of cardiothoracic surgery and Allison Family Distinguished chair of cardiovascular research at Houston Methodist DeBakey Heart and Vascular Center and the study's senior author. "We know these TAVR valves have superior hemodynamics compared to surgical valves in every randomized trial and timepoint we tested. And this might be why surgery is behind the 8-ball when it begins, and why TAVR has a head start."

SVD is only an issue with bioprosthetic valves and is the most frequent cause of valve failure. SVD includes problems such as scarring, thickening/calcification of the leaflets hardening, and fracturing of the valve frame. Reardon said 10-year data on the intermediate and low risk trials is being collected to determine the valve deterioration level in these patients using TAVR and SAVR. "We will get 10 year data in a lower risk, younger group of patients that are going to live longer and we are going to find out which valves last longer," he said.

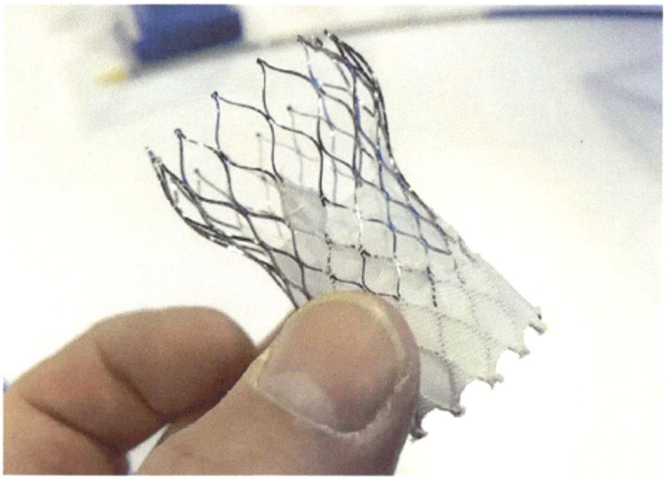

Fig 31.27 showing the Medtronic Evolut TAVR valve on display .

There is still a lot of apprehension on heart teams about sending younger patients, since they will likely live much longer than elderly patients who are more of the typical candidates for TAVR. The metal support frame used in TAVR valves gets embedded in the wall of the heart and can complicate later open heart surgical valve replacement procedures. However, if TAVR valves show they can last longer than surgical valves in most patients, there will likely be a shift toward a younger TAVR population.

"Heart surgeons tend to worry that in younger, lower-risk patients, replacement valves inserted using TAVR may fail more quickly than surgically inserted valves," Reardon said. "The results of this study suggest exactly the opposite — that at five years, the TAVR-inserted valve has less structural deterioration than the surgically inserted one."

NCDR LAAO Registry: Clinical impact of residual leaks following LAA occlusion

This analysis of the National Cardiovascular Data Registry (NCDR) Left Atrial Appendage Occlusion (LAAO) Registry was the first study to show that peri-device leak is associated with increased stroke risk. The ACC late-breaking data showed peri-device leak is associated with increased stroke risk, so LAAO operators should assess devices carefully for leak and strive to leave no leak, explained Andrew M. Goldsweig, MD, MSc, RPVI, FSCAI, associate cath lab director for structural heart disease, University of Nebraska Medical Center and associate editor for the Journal of the Society of Cardiovascular Angiography and Interventions (SCAI). The study examined rates of a primary endpoint composite of stroke, transient ischemic attack, and systemic embolism among LAAO patients stratified by no leak, small leak (less than 5 mm), and large leak (more than 5 mm). Among 51,333 patients undergoing LAAO with the Watchman 2.5 device (Boston Scientific, Marlborough, MA) from 2016 through 2019, 37,696 (73.4%) had no leak, 13,258 (25.8%) had small leaks (<5 mm), and 379 (0.7%) had large leaks (>5 mm). The presence of a small leak was associated with a slightly higher rate of the primary endpoint (adjusted HR 1.152, 95% confidence interval [CI] 1.025-1.294), major bleeding (HR 1.11, 95% CI 1.029-1.120), and any major adverse events (HR 1.102, 95% CI 1.048-1.160).

Large leaks were not statistically associated with adverse events, although more patients with large leaks continued anticoagulation.

The NCDR LAAO Registry is the largest LAAO dataset in the world, including every commercial LAAO procedure performed in the U.S. However, Goldsweig said the study was subject to the usual cadre of biases inherent when performing a retrospective analysis of a large data registry, particularly information bias.

Tricuspid valve repair with the Edwards Pascal transcatheter clip at 1 year — CLASP TR

Severe symptomatic tricuspid regurgitation (TR) is prevalent and causes significant morbidity. This prospective, single-arm multicenter early feasibility study was designed to evaluate the safety and performance of the Pascal transcatheter valve repair clip system in symptomatic severe TR. The device is similar to the functionality of the MitraClip, in that its arms clasp the leaflets to the valve to perform a transcatheter edge-to-edge repair (TEER).

Surgical intervention is not commonly utilized in TR, compared to left sided valve disease and there are questions regarding outcomes with surgical intervention in advanced stages, explained Kalkidan Bishu, MD, MS, FSCAI, an interventional cardiologist at Essential Health St. Mary's-Heart and Vascular Center, and an SCAI Council member. He said there is a need for, and a lot of interest in, a percutaneous intervention for native valve TR. The study included 65 patients (mean age 77; 55% women) with severe symptomatic TR despite medical therapy underwent treatment using Ewards Pascal Transcatheter Repair System. Primary endpoint was the composite of major adverse events at 30 days with follow up at six months and then annually. One-year follow up results were reported for 46 out of 65 patients in whom follow-up data was available (loss of follow up attributed to COVID-19 pandemic). Mortality was 10.8%. About 18 % were hospitalized for heart failure and 16.9% experienced a major adverse event, the most common adverse event was bleeding at 9.2%. The majority of patients improved. Heart failure severity, six-minute walk test and quality of life were improved.

"Tricuspid valve regurgitation is a big and growing problem for us, and there is about a 30% mortality rate," said Adam Greenbaum, MD, co-director, Structural Heart and Valve Center, Emory University, who presented the study at ACC. "We don't have good therapies to offer these patients other than diuretics, and surgery is associated with high rates of morbidity and mortality because the patients are so sick, frail and elderly.

However, he said this opens the door for minimally invasive procedures such as the Pascal and MitraClip in these patients. "We were able to achieve a reduction of 86% in TR, reducing it to moderate for less, and most patients had a two grade reduction," Greenbaum said.

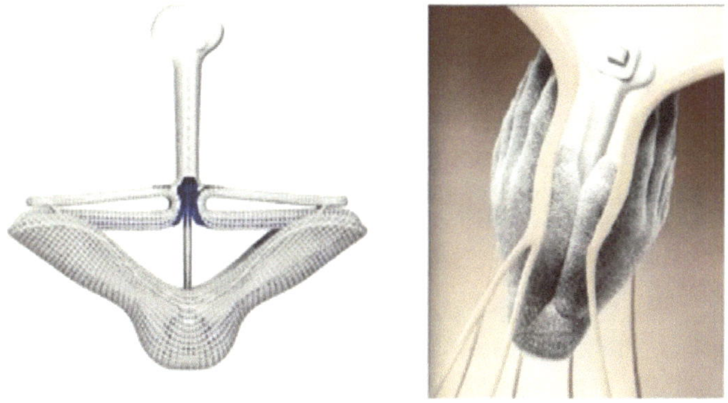

Fig.31.28 The Edwards Lifesciences Pascal edge-to-edge repair (TEER) device showed safety and efficacy in a trial looking at its use in elderly, severe tricuspid regurgitation patients at ACC22.

Trends and final results of the North American COVID-19 Myocardial Infarction (NACMI) Registry

NACMI was established in 2020 to characterize the presentation profiles, treatment and outcomes for patients who were hospitalized with ST-elevated myocardial infarction (STEMI) in the context of confirmed COVID-19 infection. A significant drop in in-hospital mortality was observed in the 2021 cohort as compared with the 2020 cohort. The investigators also found a significant drop in the secondary composite endpoint of death, stroke, or a repeat myocardial infarction from 35% in 2020 to 25% in 2021. Reductions were largely associated COVID vaccinations.

In 2020, it quickly became apparent that COVID-19 infection also encompasses a variety of cardiac and vascular manifestations, including hypercoagulability with extensive formation of venous and arterial thrombus, acute coronary syndromes (ACS), elevated risk for STEMI and sudden cardiac death. The risk for STEMI is now known to persist for several weeks after the onset of clinical COVID-19 infection, explained Sandeep Nathan, MD, MSc, FSCAI, co-director, cardiac cath lab, University of Chicago. He NACMI was created as a collaboration between the SCAI, the ACC Interventional Council, and the Canadian Association of Interventional Cardiology (CAIC).The NACMI Investigators analyzed data from 586 patients: n=227 in the 2020 cohort and n=359 in the 2021 cohort.

In April 2021, Garcia et al. reported that the primary endpoint of in-hospital mortality for COVID-19 infection complicated by STEMI was 33% (75/227) in 2020, a figure which dropped to 23% (83/359) in 2021.

The notable reduction in COVID-19 STEMI mortality was likely related to the lower incidence of cardiogenic shock and concomitant pulmonary manifestations in 2021, both of which significantly increased mortality when present.

Vaccination data was available for 54% (193/359) of the 2021 cohort and found that 0% of vaccinated patients suffered in-hospital mortality while 22% of unvaccinated patients died in 2021, a value which is significantly higher than historical (pre-COVID-19) estimates of in-hospital STEMI mortality. There was a significant drop in in-hospital mortality (the primary endpoint) observed in the 2021 cohort as compared with the 2020 cohort. The investigators also found a significant drop in the secondary composite endpoint of death, stroke, or a repeat myocardial infarction from 35% in 2020 to 25% in 2021.

FAME 3 Quality of life after FFR-guided stunting vs. coronary bypass

This study compared multi-vessel coronary artery disease treated with coronary artery bypass graft (CABG) to fractional flow reserve (FFR)-guided percutaneous coronary intervention (PCI). The data show these have similar quality of life, angina relief and return to work outcomes. But, FFR-guided PCI resulted in a faster improvement in quality of life than CABG during the first year after revascularization, and improved working status in patients younger than 65 years old, explained Luai Tabaza, MD, an interventional cardiologist at Virtua Health in Philadelphia, which summarizing the study for SCAI members.

This quality-of-life sub study showed that FFR-guided PCI have similar quality of life and angina relief compared to CABG at one year, in the younger than 65 year-old group, CABG was associated with less return to work compared to PCI at 1, 6 and 12 months, Tabaza said.

Management of patients with multi-vessel coronary disease is a clinical challenge we face every day, FAME-3 compares the two main treatment options, FFR-guided PCI and CABG," Tabaza said. The primary end point was major adverse cardiac and cerebral events (MACCE) and repeat revascularization, PCI did not meet non-inferiority at one year as presented at TCT in November 2021. Both study arms had low event rates, and the differences between PCI and CABG narrowed compared to previous studies, which prompted the quality-of-life sub-study to further aid in clinical decision making.

Comparison of FFR-guided and IVUS-guided PCI in intermediate coronary artery stenosis — FLAVOUR randomized trial

FFR guided vs. intravascular ultrasound (IVUS)-guided PCI for intermediate coronary lesions.

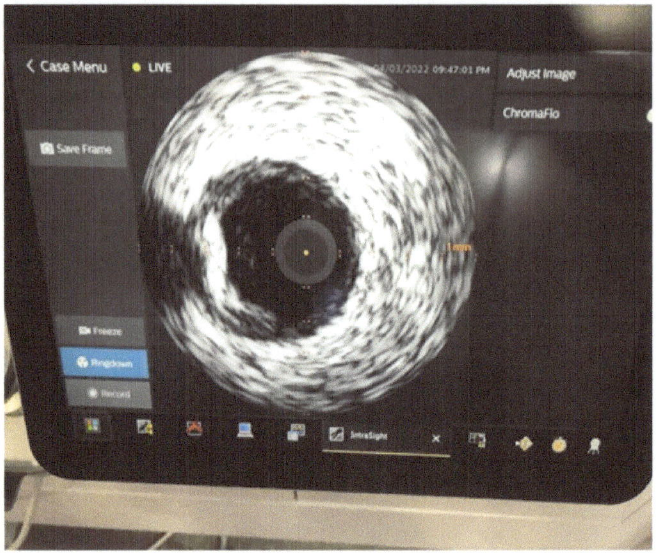

Fig.31.29 FFR and IVUS were compared for the first time in a trial at ACC22, which found both are good at determining if a stent was needed in the cath lab in intermediate risk patients.

The study showed both are an appropriate initial strategy for intermediate lesions and results in reduced resource utilization for coronary stenting.

FFR is an appropriate initial strategy to evaluate intermediate stenosis , which makes up between 40-70% lesions. When FFR was compared to IVUS, there were fewer stents placed (44.5 vs. 65.3%), summarized Tanveer Rab, MD, FSCAI, a professor and an interventional cardiologist at Emory University, and an SCAI committee member. He said there were no statistically significant differences in the rates of death, myocardial infarction or repeat revascularization in either the FFR or IVUS group (8.1 vs. 8.5% (p< 0.001 for non-inferiority).

Cardiac CT now in the spotlight thanks to chest pain guidelines

Advocates for cardiac computed tomography (CT) have been saying for the past decade that CT offers many advantages for the evaluation of chest pain. This was officially recognized last October with the release of the American College of Cardiology (ACC) and American Heart Association (AHA) 2021 Chest Pain Evaluation Guidelines. In the guidelines, cardiac CT was elevated to a top 1A, front-line test indication.

While some hospitals were already using CT in emergency departments (ED) for triage, a large number of new centers are now looking to begin more comprehensive cardiac CT angiography (CTA) programs. The guidelines focused on hospitals on the fence about creating CTA programs, and it is very clear interest is rising rapidly. Vendors with CTA technologies at the 2022 ACC meeting in April said they were swamped with serious conversations with physicians and cardiology department administrators.

The Society of Cardiovascular Computed Tomography (SCCT) broke all previous attendance records at its 2022 meeting in July,

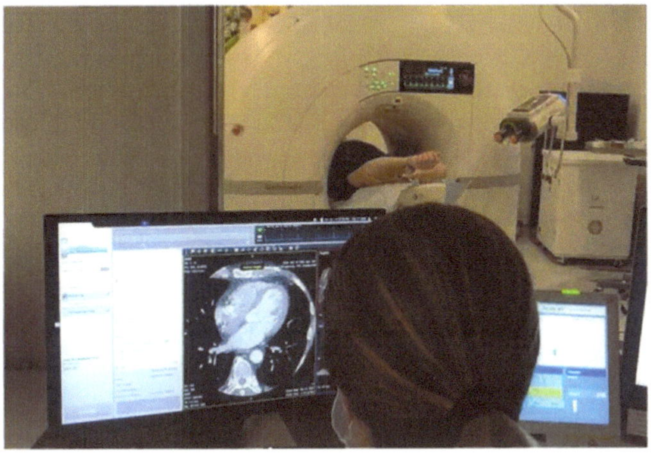

Fig. 31.30 A cardiac CT scan being performed at Duly Healthcare in suburban Chicago in the spring of 2022. This is one of the first outpatient cardiology clinics in the U.S. to implement a CCTA program for screening non-acute chest pain patients and for structural heart evaluations.

despite attendance being lower at most in-person medical conferences as COVID-19 restrictions continue to wane. Vendors exhibiting at the SCCT meeting also said they had much higher engagement with attendees compared to previous years. A CTA accreditation company exhibiting at SCCT also said they have seen a massive increase in cardiologists and radiologists looking to get certified in CTA since the guidelines were released.

Eric Williamson, MD, MSCCT, 2021-22 SCCT president and professor of radiology at Mayo Clinic, said there has been a 60% increase in CCTA exams at Mayo over the past year or so. He said this was partly fueled by COVID-19, where a CT scan that is almost contactless was seen as an advantage over other tests with closer or prolonged contact with patients. He said the change in guidelines and a movement toward multi-specialty care teams also helped fuel this rise.

He said there has been close coordination between emergency department (ED) physicians, cardiologists and radiologists at many hospitals in recent years to take a care-team approach to address chest pain presentations in the ED.

"The guidelines give a new 1A indication for cardiac CT for the evaluation of stable and acute chest pain," Williamson said. "We believe in our community this is long overdue. But it is nice to see the broader medical community of medical care acknowledging and understanding the strengths of this technology."

Many key academic cardiology centers have been using CTA for years as a first-line test. Massachusetts General Hospital has been using CT angiography as a primary test to evaluate chest pain since 2014, explained SCCT President Brian Ghoshhajra, MD, MBA, division chief, cardiovascular imaging, at Mass General, and associate professor of radiology, Harvard Medical School.

"It's a disruptive technology," Ghoshhajra said. "It can certainly obliviate the need for invasive tests. What is well codified in the new guidelines is that there are many first-line tests for different types of patients, and sometimes there are choices. We strongly feel CT is often a first-line test, more so than what prior guidelines had reflected. I would say the first-line indication is highly appropriate in a large and ever growing number of patients." Details of the 2021 chest pain guidelines

"There are many tests with a Class 1A recommendation, and cardiac CT is not always going to be the right test for everyone," explained Ron Blankstein, MD, MSCCT, associate director, cardiovascular imaging program, director, cardiac computed tomography, Brigham and Women's Hospital, and professor of medicine, Harvard Medical School. He also was a co-author on the 2021 Chest Pain Guidelines.

"In particular, coronary CTA would be useful in patients who do not have known coronary artery disease (CAD) who have an intermediate to high pre-test probability of having obstructive disease," Blankstein explained

While not always the first test choice, he said these factors favor use of coronary CTA (CCTA):

- Younger patients who are not on preventive therapies.
- Individuals where the objective of testing is to identify non-obstructive or obstructive coronary artery disease.
- This includes scanning patients where there was a previously inconclusive stress test.

The guidelines also put a new emphasis on non-obstructive coronary artery disease.

"This guideline is the first time ever that non-obstructive CAD is now classified as coronary disease, and there is a Class 1 to optimize preventive therapies for those patients," Blankstein said. "Coronary CT gives us an opportunity to identify non-obstructive disease, which we might not identify on other types of stress test imaging."

CTA also can be used as a gatekeeper to decide which patients get sent for diagnostic angiograms in the cath lab.

"In the new guidelines, particularly for patients with stable chest pain, there is no longer a category of patients who should go directly to invasive angiography," he said. "The use of imaging in general, including coronary CTA, should always be done, and this is why those intermediate- and high-risk patients are both grouped as a single group when we are deciding whether to do further testing." The guidelines state CCTA has a 1A recommendation for anatomical imaging for intermediate-risk patients with acute chest pain and no known CAD eligible for diagnostic testing after a negative or inconclusive evaluation for ACS, CCTA is useful for exclusion of atherosclerotic plaque and obstructive CAD. CCTA had a 2A recommendation for intermediate-risk patients with acute chest pain with evidence of previous mildly abnormal stress test results (within one year), CCTA is reasonable for diagnosing obstructive CAD. The guidelines also recommended the use of non-invasive fractional flow reserve-CT (FFR-CT) in select patients. More information on this technology is in the subsections below.

Large amount of clinical evidence led to change in guidelines for CCTA

"In the last iteration of the guidelines, cardiac CT got a 2A or 2B, which is a lower indication, but the 1A in these guidelines is the highest level indication that you can get for any type of testing, and that is a byproduct of the evidence," explained Leslee Shaw, PhD, FACC, MASNC, FAHA, FSCCT, clinical scientist and director of The Blavatnik Family Women's Health Research Institute, Mount Sinai Hospital, New York. She is a former president of both the SCCT and the American Society of Nuclear Cardiology (ASNC), and was a co-author on the 2021 Chest Pain Guidelines.

Many cardiac CT imagers have believed for a decade or more that CCTA should be a first-line imaging modality for chest pain because it offers more information than other modalities, it is noninvasive, and has the potential for faster discharge. But Shaw said CCTA advocates were told they needed to gather large amounts of clinical trial evidence to show the modality has benefits before guidelines committees would recommend it as a front-line imaging modality. So CT investigators, along with support from the SCCT, sponsored a large number of trials since 2000 to gather that evidence. Collecting this data has been one of the main priorities of SCCT over the past decade.

"I think the recent chest pain guidelines are proof positive of what can happen when a field dedicates itself to providing better evidence to guide clinical care," Shaw explained. "I think CT really has a tremendous amount of evidence, and in the guidelines we included 19 randomized trials, which is a lot."

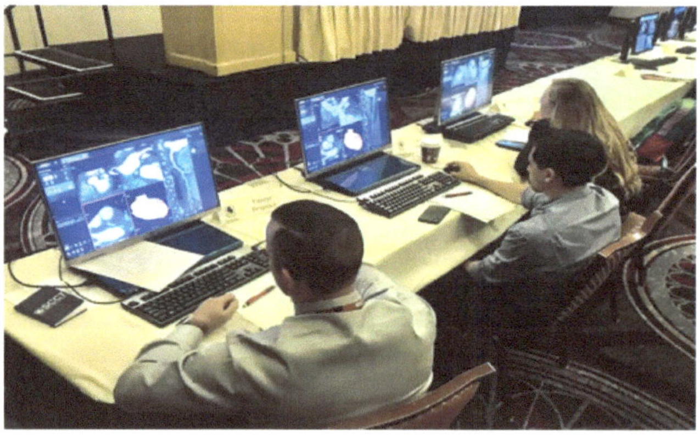

Fig. 31.31 A SCCT 2022 meeting pre-conference, all-day training course for the Coronary CTA Academy: Cases from Basic to Intermediate. CTA experts explained step-by-step how to review cardiac CT scans and how to do basic post-processing of the datasets.

Getting started in cardiac CT

With the elevation of CCTA in the guidelines, Blankstein said there has been a lot more interest since late last fall.

"We are seeing increased interest in coronary CTA, and frankly we say that even before the guidelines, but the guidelines will likely fuel that even more," Blankstein said. "I think there are a lot of hospitals that are looking to invest more in coronary CT, and it does take a lot of investment."

He said hospitals making the investment need to ensure that they have the right equipment, and the right people in terms or radiologists or cardiologists who can read the studies.

In response to the wave of interest, SCCT is building a new website called the SCCT Starter Kit. It will provide materials, resources and advice to centers looking to create or expand their cardiac CT programs.

"If you do have a 64-slice scanner, that is the minimum price of entry into cardiac CT," Ghoshhajra said

He said it's not just the number of slices, but the speed of the scanner, the type of iterative reconstruction the system uses to create images, field of view and the gantry rotation speed. Technologists also need to be proficient in CCTA, able to setting up patients with ECG leads attached to the ECG triggering system on the CT scanner, understand the imaging protocols, and be able to set up and coordinate the contrast injection during the scan.

"Coronary CT angiography is a highly technically demanding sub-speciality exam to both perform and interpret," Ghoshhajra said. "The fact remains that there are not a lot of interpretive skill for this, and the scans don't yet read themselves. It does require expertise to read and acquire these scans."

He said most EDs now have 64-slice and greater CT scanners that are cardiac capable. Creating a cardiac CT program does require expertise, and staff may require additional training. He said there are training resources available through SCCT for technologists, cardiologists and radiologists.

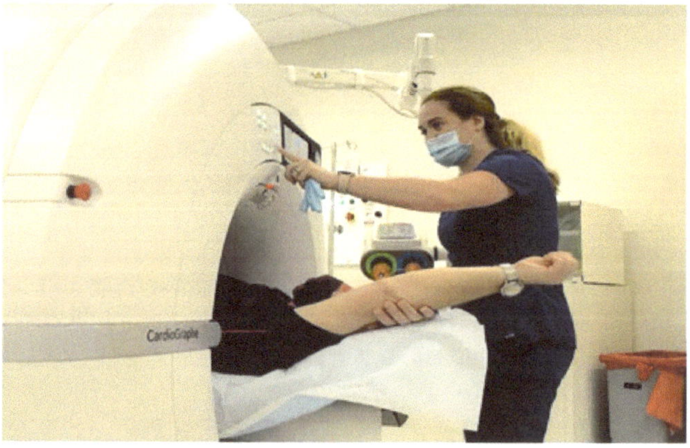

Fig 31.32 photograph showing technician helping patient in getting CT Angiography done

It has been predicted for years by SCCT experts that in the future, cardiac CT could be used in an outpatient setting as a standard-of-care to evaluate non-acute chest pain and offer more detailed coronary risk assessments by looking at soft plaques and calcium scoring. That prediction is now becoming a reality in the wake of the 2021 chest pain guidelines. One of the first outpatient dedicated cardiac CT programs was started in the fall of 2021 by Duly Health and Care, in the Chicago suburb of Lisle. They use the dedicated cardiac CT scanner for stable patient chest pain evaluations and for structural heart evaluations and transcatheter procedural preplanning. "We have been finding that as the technology of CT angiography has improved more and more over the years, we also are finding we are leaning on it more for diagnosis of coronary artery disease and chest pain syndromes in patients. We also found we were sending patients to the hospital environments to obtain that imaging, but we have had such a robust volume of cases for our large practice, we started investigating if it made sense to bring CT imaging in-house," explained Evans Pap¬pas, MD, chair of the Duly Department of cardiology

All patients who are scanned and have at least a 30% blockage in a coronary artery are also evaluated with fractional flow reserve CT (FFR-CT), which also was included in the new chest pain guidelines. This offers physiologic information and serves as a non-invasive version of a diagnostic angiogram and invasive pressure wire FFR used to assess the severity of flow limitation by a blockage. This can also help determine if a patient really needs percutaneous coronary intervention (PCI), or if they can be managed with medication.

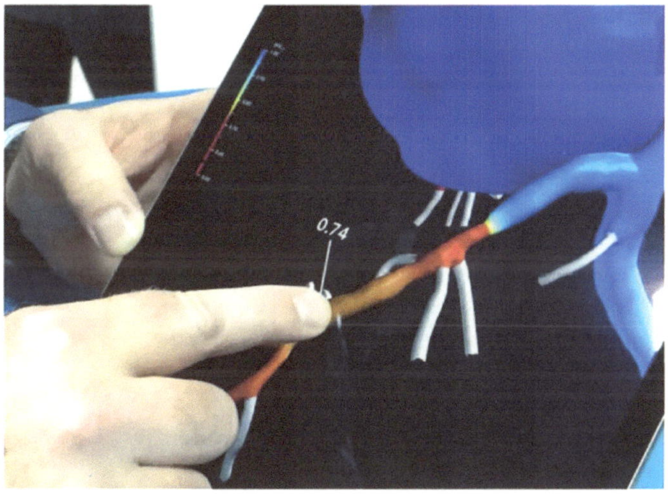

Fig. 31.33 An example of HeartFlow's FFR-CT technology showing the coronary tree of a patient with a color-coded overlay showing critical drops in coronary blood flow. It takes the cardiac CT dataset and uses computational fluid dynamics to create virtual fraction flow reserve values. Photo by Dave Fornell

FFR-CT is included in the 2021 chest pain guidelines

Fractional flow reserve-CT was included in the 2021 chest pain guidelines as a 2A recommendation. It was given a level of clinical evidence of B-NR, which means it has moderate quality evidence from one or more, well-designed and executed nonrandomized studies. The guidelines cite six studies

For intermediate-risk patients with acute chest pain and coronary artery stenosis of 40% to 90% in a proximal or middle segment on CCTA, the guidelines state FFR-CT is reasonable for diagnosis of vessel-specific ischemia and to guide decision-making regarding the use of coronary revascularization. From one large clinical registry, the deferral of coronary revascularization with a normal FFR-CT was safe, with no difference in MACE at 90 days. The guidelines also stated patients with acute chest pain who have coronary artery stenosis from 40% to 90% on CCTA may benefit from measurement of FFR-CT, especially when the stenosis is proximal or mid-coronary artery. Ghoshhajra said FFR-CT is often used when there is an intermediate grade stenosis, and the reader is not sure if it is significant enough for revascularization or not. He said the FFR-CT can show the physiologic consequence of the lesion, which cannot always be determined from anatomical imaging alone.

"And even in the invasive angiography lab, it is not always possible to visually predict the stenosis grading. We have known that for a while through the FAME and the DEFER trials," Ghoshhajra explained. "But what can be done with an invasive flow wire, can be virtually predicted noninvasively with a high level of accuracy using computational fluid dynamics."

Shaw said about half of significant stenosis seen on CT are ischemic and need to be revascularized. The rest may look bad, but are not causing problems for the patient. FFR-CT can help separate out the lesions that are actually an issue and can qualify the amount go severity.

She said there is now a large amount of evidence showing the value and accuracy of FFR-CT, enough that most of the guideline committee members supported its inclusion and elevating its indication. It also offers advantage that a single test can provide both anatomical and physiological assessment.

"With FFR-CT, we have to remember that you don't have to send a patient for another test," Shaw said. "If you are concerned about that stenosis being ischemic, you don't have to stop and re-order another test, send them to stress MRI or stress nuclear, you can send the existing CT for evaluation in one test so we are cognizant of the patient's time. So there are a lot of distinct advantages with FFR-CT. It gives you the physiological significance of that specific stenosis, where as the stress imaging modalities are not that specific."

5 Essential Apps for Doctors and Practice Managers

Technology influences our lives in many different ways, both at home and in the workplace. With the advent of EHRs and a naturally more tech-savvy consumer, there has been a massive push to transform traditional office-based operations into ones that use tech smartly to keep the machine well-oiled.

Today we look at how one piece of technology that almost all of us possess can assist us: the smartphone, and its many applications. Check out these 5 apps / practices that could potentially boost your productivity, and save you both time and money.

Epocrates

This is an all-in-one-type app that does everything from check drug interactions to pill identification to selecting national and regional healthcare insurance formularies for drug coverage information. The app can also perform many calculations such as BMI and GFR, and it provides access to the latest medical news and research. According to their website, 1 out of 2 physicians use Epocrates—a whopping 1 million members of the healthcare community. It is subscription based (with a free trial).

2 Doximity

This is an industry and social platform for communication between doctors and clinicians. According to their description in the Apple app store, "Doximity is the largest medical professional network in the US, with over 60% of clinicians as members. Through both mobile and web platforms, clinicians can use Doximity's free tools for HIPAA-secure communication, electronic faxing, reading custom-curated medical news, and career management...designed exclusively for healthcare professionals."

3 drchrono

This is a subscription-based practice management suite and one of only a few that is simultaneously deployable on tablets, smartphones, desktops, and even the Apple watch. According to their description in the app store, "To date, drchrono's Meaningful Use Stage 1 & 2 compliant platform is used by over 80,000 physicians & 5.5 million patients" and it was "voted the #1 iPad Electronic Health Record three years in a row by 20,000 physicians." This app is ICD-10 ready, has real-time medical speech-to-text, electronic sending of prescriptions and lab requests, and referrals.

4 Electronic Payment Platforms

While this is more on the buyer-side of things, you can ease some of the burden of billing and possibly eliminate waste by making your practice friendly to consumers who wish to pay electronically. Apple Pay, for instance, allows its users to link up their credit cards with their smartphone, so that in many locations they can pay with a swipe of their phone. Millennials in particular are cozy with the idea of paying with their smartphone, as we touched on in a previous blog post, and it could be a great way to tap into this ever-growing market.

5 Quotes

As a physician in a private practice, you are both the brain and the heart of the operation. While Quotes is not specifically tailored to physicians, any leader will find it daily doses of knowledge and wisdom inspiring while having their morning cup of coffee. Take a look at this nice article on Inc.com for a list of 10 apps that may also enhance your leadership skills and help you formulate and realize goals for both your practice and personal life.Give one of our representatives a ring to discuss ideas about how to make technology work for you, or fill out our online, no-hassle free quote. At PracticeProtection, we of course focus on insuring medical professionals, but our philosophy of "by doctors, for doctors" extends to helping our clients navigate the difficult road of practice management so that they can focus on what they do best: helping patients.

AI-powered blood test supports risk stratification of heart disease patients

A blood test powered by artificial intelligence (AI) has shown promise in the assessment of patients with total blockage of a heart artery.

Around 25% of patients with obstructive coronary artery disease on coronary angiography have a fully narrowed coronary artery. The blockage, known medically as chronic total occlusion, is associated with higher rates of major adverse cardiovascular events (MACE). Observational trials suggest that percutaneous coronary intervention improves outcomes, but there is a lack of tools for identifying high-risk patients.

Prevencio, a developer of blood tests for cardiovascular diseases, has developed the HART CVE multibiomarker panel, which uses targeted proteomics and machine learning. The panel incorporates results from N-terminal pro-B type natriuretic peptide and other biomarkers into a weighted algorithm.

To assess the panel, Prevencio worked with Massachusetts General Hospital. In a study of 241 participants, patients with chronic total occlusions for an average of four years were followed for the occurrence of MACE, such as heart attack and stroke. The dataset included 67 MACE and 56 cardiovascular deaths or heart failure hospitalization events.

"The HART CVE panel provided excellent discrimination for predicting such risk throughout the 4-year follow-up period. By 4 years, compared to a referent low-risk population, the high-risk group had a greater than 12-fold higher MACE risk during the 4 years of follow-up and nearly 16-fold higher risk for CV death/HF hospitalization during that same period," the researchers wrote.

Prevencio recently presented the findings at the 2023 Transcatheter Cardiovascular Therapeutics scientific meeting held in San Francisco from October 23-26. The presentation followed the publication of a preprint paper covering the same research.

The panel is currently available as a laboratory-developed test, enabling Prevencio to try to drive sales of the product before it seeks U.S. Food and Drug Administration (FDA) approval. Prevencio is talking to "multiple companies that have large immunoassay platforms placed in hospitals" about developing the panel and other tests on their systems ahead of working through the FDA process, according to 360Dx

Laptop Requirements For AI?

AI (Artificial Intelligence) and machine learning tasks can vary greatly in their system requirements based on the complexity of the project, the size of the dataset, and the specific software and libraries being used. Here are the minimum and maximum system requirements to give you an idea of the range you might need for AI tasks.

Minimum System Requirements for AI:

- Processor (CPU): Intel Core i5 or AMD equivalent, with at least 4 cores.
- Graphics Processing Unit (GPU): Integrated GPU or a basic dedicated GPU, such as NVIDIA GeForce GTX series.
- RAM: 8GB.
- Storage: 256GB Solid State Drive (SSD).
- Operating System: Windows 10, macOS, or Linux (Ubuntu is a popular choice).

Maximum (Recommended) System Requirements for AI:

1. **Processor (CPU): High-end CPU** such as Intel Core i9 or AMD Ryzen 9, with multiple cores and high clock speed.
2. **Graphics Processing Unit (GPU):** High-performance dedicated GPU, ideally with AI-optimized cores. NVIDIA RTX 30 series (or later) or AMD Radeon RX 6000 series (or later) would be excellent choices. For more intensive tasks, consider NVIDIA's GPUs with Tensor cores, designed for AI workloads.
3. **RAM: 32GB or more.**
4. **Storage: 1TB or more Solid State Drive (SSD).** Having additional HDD storage for backup or less frequently accessed data can also be beneficial.
5. **operating System:** Windows 10 Pro, macOS, or Linux (Ubuntu or another AI-friendly distro). Keep in mind that these are general recommendations and the actual requirements can vary based on the specific AI tasks you're planning to carry out. Some tasks can be offloaded to cloud-based servers or AI platforms, which can provide high computational power without the need for high-spec local hardware.

For those planning to run AI workloads primarily on the local machine, investing in the higher end of these requirements can save time and provide a smoother work experience. Always consider the software you plan to use and check its specific system requirements as well.

Moreover, laptops equipped with dedicated graphics cards, such as the NVIDIA GeForce RTX or AMD Radeon RX series, offer accelerated performance for AI-related tasks, including training neural networks and running computationally intensive simulations. The world of artificial intelligence demands laptops that can handle the immense computational requirements of AI workloads.

How To Buy The Top Rated AI Laptops

The right laptop for AI (Artificial Intelligence) needs to have certain specifications that allow it to efficiently handle machine learning, deep learning, and other AI-related tasks. Here are the key requirements:

- Processor (CPU): AI applications are typically CPU-intensive. Therefore, you need a laptop with a strong processor. A high-end Intel Core i7 or i9, or AMD Ryzen 7 or 9, is recommended. Look for models that have multiple cores and high clock speed for the best performance.
- Graphics Processing Unit (GPU): Many AI and machine learning tasks are GPU-accelerated. A dedicated graphics card, such as those from NVIDIA's GeForce RTX series or AMD's Radeon RX series, is highly recommended. For intensive tasks, NVIDIA's GPUs with Tensor cores that are specially designed for AI workloads can provide a significant boost.
- RAM: Machine Learning and AI tasks can be memory intensive, especially when working with large datasets. Aim for at least 16GB of RAM, though 32GB or more would be ideal for more complex tasks.
- Storage: Solid State Drive (SSD) storage is preferable over Hard Disk Drive (HDD) storage because of its speed. SSDs can significantly reduce data read-write times, which is important when dealing with large data sets. A minimum of 512GB SSD is recommended, but 1TB or more would provide more room for data and applications.
- Software Compatibility: Ensure the laptop is compatible with AI software tools and libraries you plan to use such as TensorFlow, PyTorch, Jupyter Notebook, or any other specific IDE or programming language you'll be working with.
- Operating System: Linux is commonly used in AI and machine learning applications because many AI tools are built to be compatible with it. However, Windows and macOS can also be used depending on your comfort level and software requirements.
- Battery Life: If you're planning on using your laptop for AI tasks while on the go, consider the battery life. However, keep in mind that high-performance laptops often have a shorter battery life due to their powerful components.
- Portability: Depending on your needs, you might want a laptop that's easy to carry around. However, high-performance laptops are often heavier and larger due to the hardware they pack.

It's important to note that AI tasks can be extremely resource-intensive, and laptops, while portable and convenient, may not always be the best fit for certain tasks. In such cases, you might want to consider a powerful desktop PC or using cloud-based AI services.

1.Apple MacBook Pro

The Apple MacBook Pro stands out as an exceptional laptop for artificial intelligence. It comes equipped with numerous high-quality features, making it compatible with a variety of AI tasks. The heart of this machine is a formidable 9th Gen 6-core Intel Core i7 processor, which is engineered to handle even the most demanding AI computing tasks.

With a clock speed of 2.6GHz, this laptop delivers lightning-fast performance that ensures smooth multitasking and seamless operations. Whether you're dealing with intricate artificial intelligence tasks or data processing, this powerhouse CPU has got you covered.

One of the unique features of this laptop for artificial intelligence is its immersive 16-inch Retina display. This feature, designed exclusively for the Apple MacBook Pro, provides breathtaking visuals with a resolution of 3070 x 1920 pixels and P3 wide color gamut. With the inclusion of True Tone technology, the display enhances color accuracy and image vibrancy.

Adding to its usability, the MacBook Pro is equipped with a Touch Bar and Touch ID for enhanced navigation and security. The Touch Bar, located at the top of the keyboard, dynamically adapts to the active application, providing context-specific controls. This not only simplifies tasks like volume adjustment and app access but also boosts productivity. The integrated Touch ID sensor in the power button facilitates secure and straightforward login with quick authentication.

When it comes to graphics performance, the MacBook Pro doesn't disappoint. The laptop is armed with AMD Radeon Pro 5300M graphics integrated with GDDR6 memory, delivering excellent graphics performance essential for AI tasks.

In the realm of storage, the MacBook Pro takes it up a notch with ultrafast SSD storage. This high-end innovation surpasses traditional hard drives in data retrieval speed, essential for AI operations.

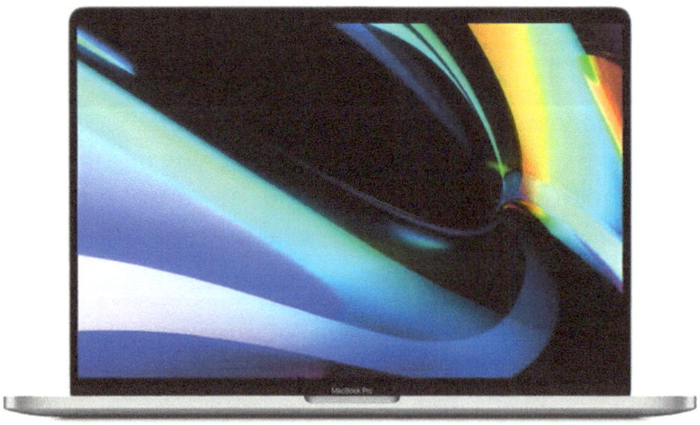

Fig 31..34 Apple MacBook Pro

This laptop for artificial intelligence also boasts versatile connectivity options with 4x Thunderbolt 3 ports. Additionally, the six-speaker system with force-canceling woofers provides crisp and clear sound, enhancing your multimedia experience. In conclusion, the Apple 2019 MacBook Pro sets the bar high as a laptop for artificial intelligence.

Pros:

- Excellent display
- 11 hours battery life
- Powerful Intel core
- AMD Radeon Pro graphics card
- Innovative audio quality

Cons:

- Lack of USB Type-A port

2. MSI P65 Creator-654

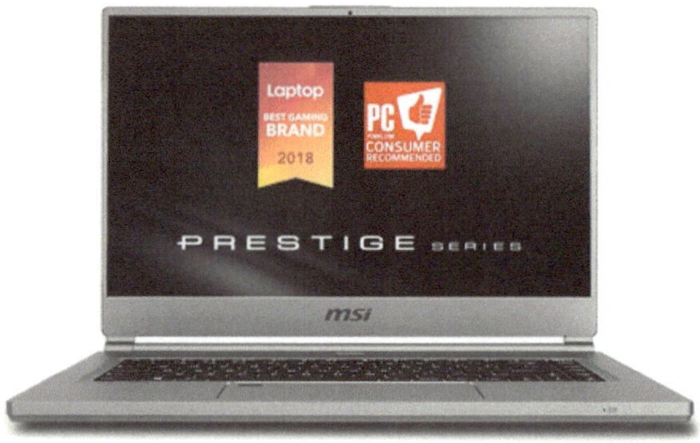

Fig 31..35 Apple MacBook Pro

The MSI P65 Creator-654 is a powerful and versatile laptop that is perfect for AI programming. It features a stunning 15.6-inch UHD display, an NVIDIA GeForce RTX 2070 graphics card, and an Intel Core i9-9800H processor. This combination of hardware makes the MSI P65 Creator-654 ideal for running demanding AI programs and applications. It is also suitable for 3D designers and content creators.

The MSI P65 Creator-654 features a stunning 15.6-inch UHD display that provides breakthrough visuals. With a 3840 x 2160 aspect ratio and anti-glare wide viewing angle, it is incredible.

It is also armed with NVIDIA GeForce RTX 2070 graphics. This card features 8GB GDDR6 memory to handle complex tasks. It delivers smooth gameplay and performs all data-intensive tasks at a fast rate. Allowing you to experience your workload at its best.

Connect the MSI P65 Creator-654 laptop to external peripherals with ease using the HDMI-out port. With support for 4K resolution, you can enjoy crystal-clear visuals. Moreover, increase your productivity and gaming with multi-screen support.

Design-wise, it gives a sleek metallic look with a silver thin bezel. It is styled with a minimal yet aesthetic approach. Likewise, for connectivity, you will find ports like Thunderbolt 3, USB 3.1, and HDMI port on the right side.

Adorned with the solid Intel Core i9-9800H CPU for high-demanding tasks. This core features a boost clock speed of up to 4.8GHz. Moreover, it is also capable of handling multiple tasks with ease.

Another highly notable spec is the wireless connectivity and HD webcam. Stay connected wirelessly with the Intel 9560 Jefferson Peak module. It supports 2×2 802.11ac Wi-Fi connectivity. Thus, you can conveniently connect with other peripherals.

The laptop also comes with pre-installed Microsoft Windows 10 Pro. Thus, you can work in a productive environment with a seamless computing experience. So, no doubt, this laptop is a solid build for every user.

Pros

- Versatile connectivity options
- Intel Core i9-9800H
- Windows 10 Pro
- Stunning screen display
- Solid core performance

Cons

- Not-so-good battery life

3.Lenovo Legion 5 15.6"

The Lenovo Legion 5 stands out as the best laptop for Cricut Explore Air 2, boasting a potent combination of power, versatility, and performance. This gaming laptop is powered by a 6-core Ryzen 5-5600H processor and GeForce RTX 3050 Ti graphics card, allowing for swift handling of demanding tasks beyond gaming, including working with Cricut Explore Air 2.

Its large 32GB RAM and 2TB PCIe SSD offer ample power and storage, accommodating the needs of users dealing with large design files. With a 15.6-inch FHD IPS display featuring a 120Hz refresh rate, this laptop provides a smooth, high-quality visual experience perfect for detailed crafting work.

Featuring a backlit keyboard, it caters to late-night crafting or low-light environments, while Legion Coldfront 3.0 technology ensures it stays cool during intense work sessions. Its comprehensive array of ports allows for easy connectivity to a variety of devices, including your Cricut machine.Beyond crafting, the Lenovo Legion 5 also shines for AI tasks, where its robust gaming features provide powerful performance. It comes with upgraded SSD memory for reliable, fast data retrieval, and a one-year manufacturer warranty for added assurance.

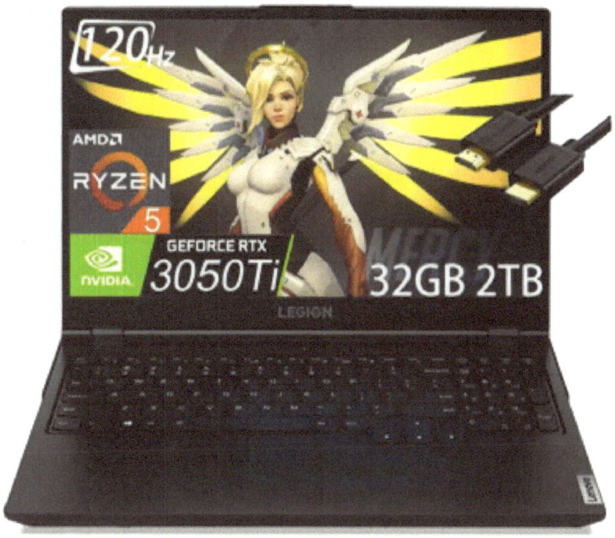

Fig 31..36 Lenovo Legion 5 15.6"

Overall, this laptop is not just ideal for gaming but is also an excellent choice for Cricut Explore Air 2 users and AI professionals.

Pros

- Powerful performance
- Versatile features
- Great price
- Backlit keyboard
- Built-in cooling system
- Multiple ports

Cons

- Not the lightest laptop

4. Acer Predator Helios 300

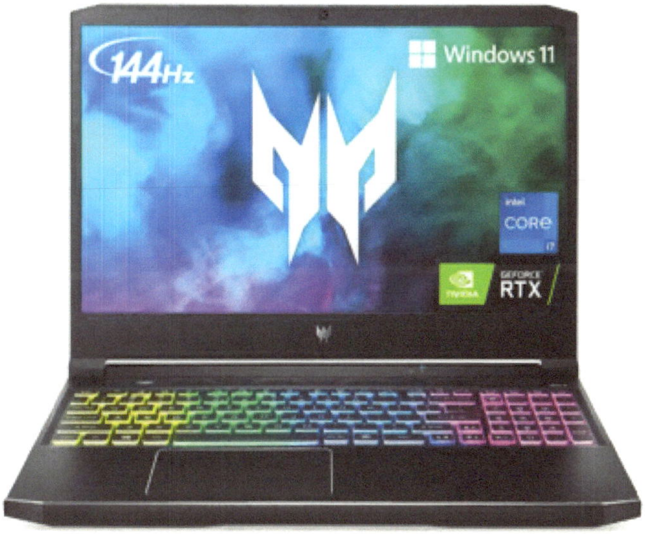

Fig 31..37 Lenovo Legion 5 15.6"

The Acer Predator Helios 300 is an exceptional laptop for AI and machine learning, powered by an 11th Gen Intel Core i7-11800H processor and a cutting-edge NVIDIA GeForce RTX 3060 graphics card. This laptop was crafted not only to dominate gaming but also to handle complex AI and machine learning tasks with ease.

The high-performing Intel Core i7 processor, with its 8 cores and 16 threads, is perfect for multitasking and data-intensive tasks, and its support for DDR4-3200 memory ensures smooth operation. It pairs excellently with the advanced NVIDIA GeForce RTX 3060, which incorporates Ampere architecture for an exceptional visual experience, especially crucial in AI and machine learning applications.

In terms of display, the Acer Predator Helios offers a vibrant 15.6-inch full HD LED backlit screen with a fast 144Hz refresh rate and 3ms response time, reducing blur and providing an immersive viewing experience.

It's armed with 16GB DDR4 memory and supports both Wi-Fi and Ethernet connectivity, ensuring fast data transfers, a crucial factor when handling large datasets typical in AI and machine learning work.

Besides AI and machine learning, the Acer Predator Helios 300 is also ideal for gaming, professional content creation, and other demanding applications, thanks to its robust features and superior performance.

Pros

- 512GB SSD
- Long battery life
- 15.6-inch Full HD display
- 16GB of DDR4 RAM
- RGB backlighting keyboard

Cons . No webcam

5 GIGABYTE G5 GD – 15.6"

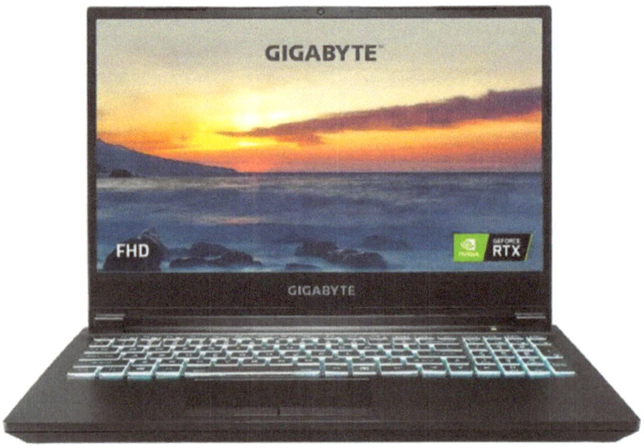

Fig 31..38 GIGABYTE G5 GD – 15.6

The Gigabyte G5 GD is an ideal laptop for AI students, offering robust performance at a budget-friendly price. It comes from a trusted manufacturer, ensuring reliable performance for complex AI algorithms and high-end gaming.

It's powered by the 11th Gen Intel Core i5-11400H processor, offering high speed and responsiveness. The laptop also features an Nvidia GeForce RTX 3050 graphics card, boosting its capacity to handle AI tasks. With 4GB GDDR6 memory and 1485 MHz boost clock speed, the laptop promises cutting-edge performance.

AI students will also benefit from Nvidia DLSS, a forward-thinking technology that uses AI to enhance graphical performance, providing sharper images, more precise details, and high frame rates. The laptop is equipped with 16GB RAM and a large 64GB memory, ensuring smooth operation without lag.

For storage, the 512GB SSD drive enhances performance by reducing loading times. The laptop's 15.6-inch thin bezel and FHD anti-glare display LSD offers immersive viewing. The X-rite Pantone Certification guarantees precise color reproduction, vital for graphics and visualization work.

Moreover, this laptop can run a variety of AI and machine learning tools such as TensorFlow, Keras, and PyTorch, which are integral for AI studies. Therefore, the Gigabyte G5 GD stands as a top pick for AI students looking for a blend of power, affordability, and compatibility.

Pros

- 16GB RAM
- 512GB SSD
- Windows 11
- 144Hz display
- 512GB SSD
- Intel Core i5 processor

Cons . Comparatively heavy

6. ASUS ZenBook 14

The Asus ZenBook 14 Ultra-slim is an exceptional laptop for AI and researchers. Featuring a 14-inch Full HD NanoEdge bezel display, it provides unparalleled visual clarity, ideal for complex data visualizations and analysis. Its powerful 11th Gen Intel Core i7-1165G7 processor, with a speed up to 4.7 GHz and 12MB cache, ensures high performance, essential for handling demanding AI applications. This laptop comes with a 512GB PCIe NVMe SSD, ensuring rapid loading times and ample storage for large datasets commonly used in AI and research tasks. Additionally, its IR camera offers facial recognition, providing enhanced security without the hassle of passwords.

The Asus ZenBook 14 Ultra-slim provides a perfect blend of powerful performance, security, comfort, and connectivity, making it a top pick for AI researchers.

Pros

- AI noise-cancellation
- Intel Core i7-1165G7 processor

Cons . Small trackpad

Ddouble screen ai powered laptop

Key Takeaways

Asus unveils the Zenbook Duo (2024), the world's first AI-powered dual-screen laptop with detachable keyboard and trackpad.

The laptop features a pair of 3K 120Hz ASUS Lumina OLED 16:10 displays with a 180-degree hinge, creating a 19.8-inch canvas.

Powered by an Intel Core Ultra 9 processor, the Zenbook Duo offers 32GB of RAM, up to 2TB of SSD storage, and a Dolby Atmos speaker system. .

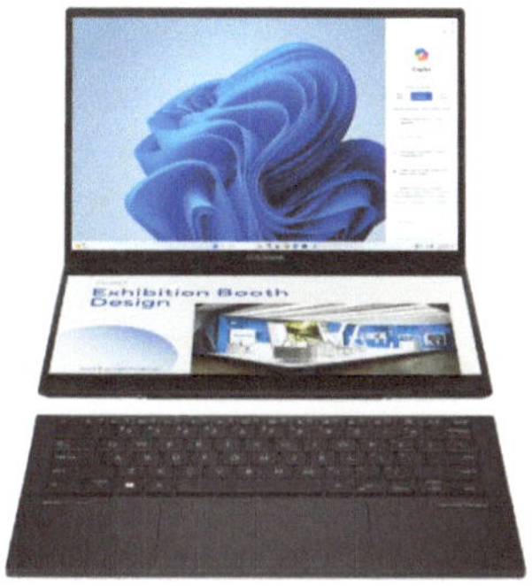

Fig 31..39 Asus unveils the Zenbook Duo (2024), the world's first AI-powered dual-screen laptop with detachable keyboard and trackpad.

Conclusion

In conclusion, the choice of the best laptop for AI tasks in 2023 primarily hinges on several core components that include a powerful processor, high-end graphics card, ample RAM, and substantial storage space. These are required to handle the intensive computational demands that come with running complex AI algorithms, processing large datasets, and executing machine learning tasks.

Among the laptops recommended are the Apple MacBook Pro, MSI P65 Creator-654, Lenovo Legion 5 15.6", Acer Predator Helios 300, GIGABYTE G5 GD – 15.6", and ASUS ZenBook 14. Each of these devices offers a balance of power, battery life, and value for money, catering to a range of users from students to professionals in the AI field.

In terms of hardware, the ideal specifications for handling AI tasks include a high-end CPU such as the Intel Core i9 or AMD Ryzen 9, a top-tier GPU like NVIDIA RTX 30 series or AMD Radeon RX 6000 series, at least 32GB of RAM, and 1TB or more of SSD storage. These specs are well-matched to the recommended laptops, which are equipped with high-performance CPUs, dedicated GPUs, and substantial RAM and storage.

Buying a top-rated AI laptop also involves consideration of software compatibility and the operating system, as many AI tools and libraries are built for specific platforms. Linux, for example, is commonly used in AI applications, but Windows and macOS are also viable options depending on the specific tools you plan to use.

Ultimately, the right laptop for AI will depend on your specific needs, preferences, and budget. High-performance laptops can provide the computational power required for many AI tasks, but they may come with trade-offs such as shorter battery life and less portability due to their powerful components. For some users, especially those who need to perform extremely resource-intensive tasks, desktop PCs or cloud-based AI services might be more appropriate options.

AI-powered robot dog looks like something from The Terminator

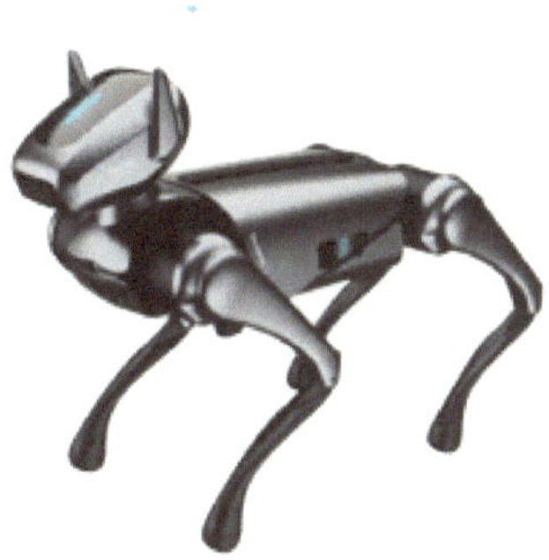

Fig 31..40 Tecno Mobile© Provided by Digital Trends

Tecno Mobile has taken to Mobile World Congress 2024 to announce the Tecno Dynamic 1, a robotic and AI-enhanced dog, reigniting the futuristic sci-fi dream for millions of nerds.

The Dynamic 1 has been painstakingly created to emulate a real dog as closely as possible, with its design based on the German Shepherd breed. A cooling system within the Dynamic 1's knees allows the robot to copy dog movements, letting it climb stairs, bow, and offer a paw for handshakes. Four microphones work with an AI algorithm within the dog's head to recognize audio prompts, so you can treat it just like a normal dog – but without any poop to pick up. Unlike normal dogs, though, the Dynamic 1 comes with a spec sheet. An 8-core ARM CPU powers the AI HyperSense Fusion System, which is tasked with making sure the robot can constantly correct itself while walking. Data from an Intel RealSense S430 depth camera, along with dual optical and infrared sensors, helps identify obstacles and guide the dog around them — and make sure it can get itself up when it does fall. Also included is 64GB of internal storage, Wi-Fi 6 and Bluetooth 5.2 support, and smartphone app controls. Fido certainly doesn't have that.

Envision Announces New Features for AI-Powered Smart Glasses

Envision announced several advanced features for its AI-powered Smart Glasses for the blind and visually impaired.

Envision's newly launched functionalities include greater Optical Character Recognition (OCR),

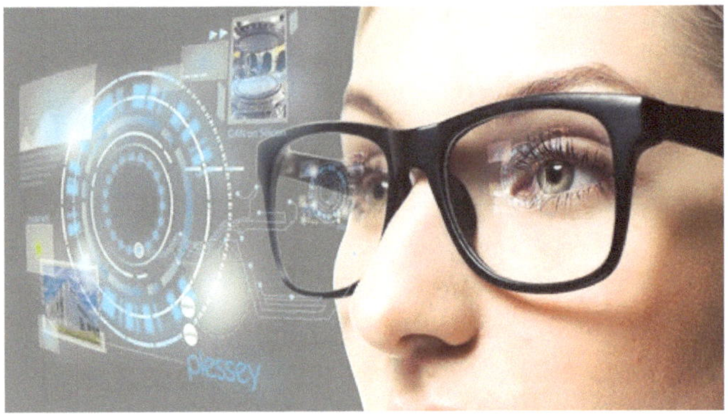

Fig 31..41 In 2017 google launched their first smart glass, it is also the first smart glass in the world of technology. Its framework is like any other normal glasses the only difference lies in its right-hand side strand, where the main technology is implemented due to which the glasses look asymmetrical. The right-hand strand projects out a prism which is indeed the actual glass of the spectacle and so it is also called optical head-mounted display. It does not hinder your normal vision as the prism is located in the right upper corner of the frame, you just need to look up a bit to have a vision over the glass.
According to google looking through the glass is like watching a 25inches screen from 8 feet away. To make the glass work it is needed to be connected to a MyGlass app in your smartphone through Bluetooth threading or WiFi. Very Google glass have some basic functions and those are 1. Taking Pictures, 2. Recording videos, 3. Navigation through google map, 4. Calling and messaging, 5. Google. All these functions could be controlled by voice action, we have to say "OK GLASS" and the tell the action we need to perform. For example to take a picture you need to say "OK GLASS TAKE THE PICTURE", or to call someone from google contacts we need to say "OK GLASS CALL JOHN". The same thing could be done for navigation and to search something in google. In google map navigation it would guild your direction with a real-time arrow in the map. You could also slide between windows or screens by using the touchpad of the glass.

improved text reading with contextual intelligence, the addition of new languages, and the creation of a third-party app ecosystem allowing the "easy integration of specialist services, such as indoor and outdoor navigation," to the Envision platform.
Developed on the Enterprise Edition of Google Glass, Envision made its debut at the 2020 CSUN Conference. It uses artificial intelligence (AI) to extract different kinds of information from images and then speaks the images out loud, enabling blind and low-vision users to read documents at work, recognize their friends, find personal belongings at home, use public transportation, and generally enjoy greater freedom, independence, and understanding of the world around them, according to the company's announcement."Our mission is to improve the lives of the world's two billion people who are blind or visually impaired by providing them with life-changing assistive technologies, products, and services," said Karthik Kannan, co-founder of Envision. "By analyzing real-time user data and direct feedback from across our communities, we are able to constantly enrich the Envision experience and innovate our products, most recently with the addition of our new capture and context features. Everyone is entitled to live in a world without boundaries and are thrilled to make Envision Glasses to as many people as possible."
Envision is available as an iOS and Android App and a Google Glass integration. According to Envision, it can read and translate any type of text (digital and handwritten) from any surface (eg, food packaging, posters, timetables, computer display screens, barcodes, etc..) into over 60 different languages. It can recognize faces, objects, and colors, and even describe scenes and connect users to contacts through its Ally function – a private video call solution built directly into the glasses. You can see it in action here.
Envision's new features include:

- Document Guidance for Accurate Capture – Removes the frustrations of taking multiple images to fully capture a document's complete text. Enhanced document guidance helps "provide verbal instructions to guide users to position documents to the optimal scanning position allowing capture in a single motion."
- Layout Detection – Helping to provide "a more realistic reading environment," Envision smart glasses will now help put a document into context for the reader. Whether a column-based document such as a newspaper, a shop window poster, road sign, or restaurant menu, Envision will "decipher the document layout and provide clear verbal guidance to the user." It recognizes headers, photo captions, and more, giving verbal layout context to the user, enabling a more natural flow to the audio read back of the document, the company says.
- Enhanced Offline Language Capabilities– Envision now adds four additional Asian languages, including Hindi, Japanese, Chinese, and Korean, which can be accurately captured and read offline. This addition brings the total of languages supported when offline to 26, with the number of languages supported when connected to more than 60.
- Third-Party App Development Support – Envision now adds a third-party ecosystem to its platform by allowing developers to build added value services to its users. Launching with the initial partner Cash Reader app, Envision can now recognize banknotes in over 100 currencies.
- Building Ally – One of the Envision Glasses' "most powerful and popular features" is the Ally function that enables a user to ask for assistance or share experiences with trusted contacts (Allys) via private video calls directly from the glasses. The new, improved version is optimized for both mobile network and WiFi hotspots, according to Envision.
- Optimizing Optical Character Recognition (OCR) – Leveraging tens of millions of data points processed by the Envision Glasses and apps has "significantly improved image capture and interpretation accuracy."

Envision Glasses are available at a recommended retail price of $3,500 directly from Envision and via its global distributor network.

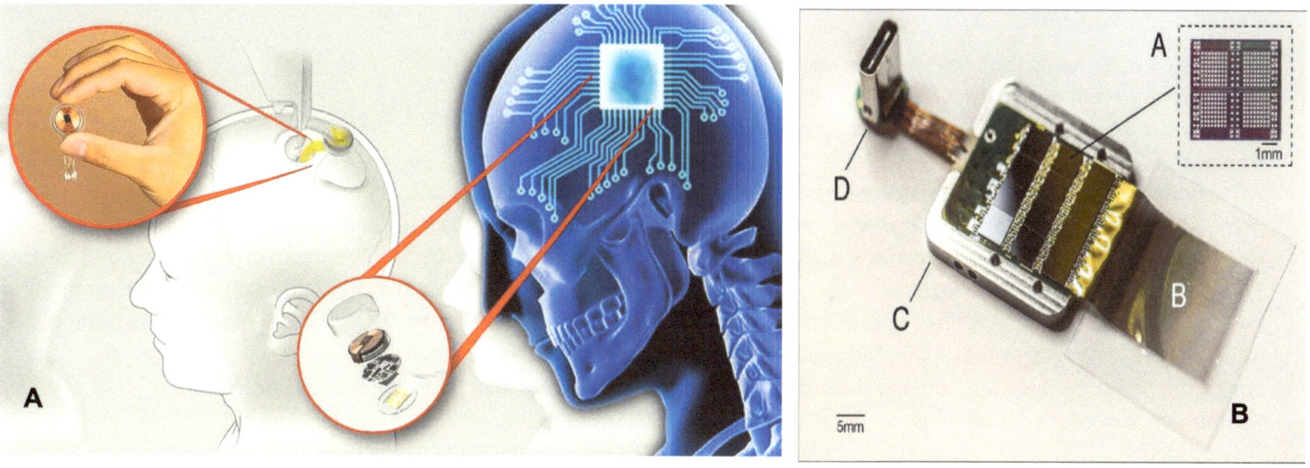

Fig. (A) Neuralink features a 4mm-square chip called N1 which will be implanted to users' skulls Neuralink has created a machine that is able to insert threads which are thinner than a strand of human hair directly into the human brain and these threads are able to detect brain activity. These threads are then connected into a device behind the ear which can then be connected to a PC or other smart device. **(B) Neuralink chip**

What Is Neuralink?

Neuralink is a technology company building a device "designed to connect human brains directly to computers," said Ramses Alcaide, CEO of Neurable, a neurotech company developing non-invasive, brain-computer interfaces in the form of headphones. "[Neuralink's technology] is capable of recording and decoding neural signals and then transmitting information back to the brain using electrical stimulation."

The implant itself is called "the Link." This coin-sized brain chip is surgically embedded under the skull, where it receives information from neural threads that fan out into different sections of a subject's brain in control of motor skills. Each wire contains sensors capable of recording and emitting electrical currents that are "so fine and flexible that they can't be inserted by the human hand," according to Neuralink's website. That's why Neuralink has built a neurosurgical robot that's designed to become fully automated.

The company is also developing an app that would allow a person to manipulate a keyboard and mouse using only their mind."Neuralink is really at the vanguard of creating the commercialized, scalable versions of what has been pioneered in academia," said Sumner Norman, a scientist at nonprofit startup Convergent Research and former chief brain-computer interface scientist at software firm AE Studio."There's been decades of academic research to push this [field] as far as it can go," he said, "but ultimately, it becomes a very expensive space to develop."

How Does Neuralink Work?

Neuralink's underlying technology works in the same way as electrophysiology, Norman explained.

The electrical chemical signals in our nervous system spark as neurons communicate with one another across gaps between nerve cells known as synapses. This brain activity is captured by electrodes, or sensors that detect voltages, measuring the change in "spikes" of when these voltages fire (or potentially fire).In other words, our brain activity data is captured not only when we take action, but also if we think about taking action.

That's not to say the brain-computer interfacing that Neuralink does is on the same level as mind reading.

"It simply measures the brain activity and interprets it as an action," said Sonal Baberwal, a Dublin City University-based researcher developing machine learning algorithms built into brain computer interface wearables.

Baberwal likened this procedure to how blood pressure interprets a patient's level of stress or relaxation.

"Similarly with your brain signals — eyes closed or opened, a relaxed or deep-sleep state, an action or focus state — all of these aspects can be detected," she added.

As these devices record complex data sets, machine learning algorithms and other artificial intelligence agents are then employed to make sense of the information.

What Will Neuralink Do?

According to Neuralink's website, the company's initial goal is to help those immobilized by paralysis regain lost skills of communication. Down the line, it intends to pursue restoring motor, sensory and visual functions as well as treatment of neurological disorders. "A Neuralink-like device has the potential to enhance human memory, processing speed and cognitive abilities by creating a direct interface between the human brain and digital devices," Alcaide said.

RESTORE MOBILITY

Brain-computer interfaces can be used to control prosthetics or exoskeletons. This use case would enable people with paralysis or amputations to regain a certain level of mobility and independence, according to Alcaide.

IMPROVE COMMUNICATION FOR NON-VERBAL INDIVIDUALS

Neuralink's main focus is to help people who are unable to speak or write communicate with others by allowing them to control a virtual mouse, keyboard or send messages by thought.
For example, someone with paraplegia would be able to manipulate a computer or mobile device using speech or text synthesis to surf the web and create digital art.

TREAT NEUROLOGICAL CONDITIONS

By monitoring brain activity, brain-computer interfaces can also detect changes that may indicate neurological conditions such as epilepsy, bipolar disorder, obsessive-compulsive disorder, Alzheimer's or Parkinson's disease, Alcaide said.
They can also be used to monitor mental health symptoms. Electrical stimulation could be delivered to targeted areas in the brain as a treatment for burnout, fatigue, anxiety and depression, which, unlike motor skills that are localized to one area, are spread throughout the brain, Norman noted.
"Treating or curing paralysis, neurological disorders and injuries could make the world a substantially nicer place, where very few people have untreatable forms of depression or anxiety," said Norman, who has spent a decade developing brain-computer interfaces and neuroprosthetics for people with neurological injury or disease. "Giving agency back to those who've lost it — that's an undeniable benefit."

ENHANCE COGNITIVE ABILITIES

This tech can also help people improve their focus, memory and attention by allowing them to train their brain using real-time biofeedback and other techniques. In Musk's words, the Link is a sort of "Fitbit in your skull" with "all the sensors you'd expect to see in a smartwatch."
"If suddenly you could get every neuron in the human brain and sense them all at once, what would you actually do with that data?" We don't know," Norman said. "There's 80 billion neurons in the brain with about 1,000 synapses in between them — how do you interpret that kind of data?"
Neuralink's technology is currently detecting up to 10,000 of these connections — a big step up from the hundreds being studied in academic trials, Norman said.

Is Neuralink FDA Approved?

Yes. Neuralink announced on May 25, 2023 that it has received U.S. Food and Drug Administration clearance for an in-human clinical trial. The company has not yet opened recruitment for the trial, but shared in a tweet that the company would "announce more information on this soon."

Is Neuralink Being Used on Humans?

A human patient received the first Neuralink implant on January 28, 2024. And according to the company's website, the first clinical trial is "open for recruitment." Previously, the neural implant has been tested on rats, mice, monkeys, sheep and pigs.

Frequently Asked Questions

What does Neuralink actually do?

Neuralink is an implant that can monitor and stimulate brain activity using electrical currents.
Neuralink aims to help people with paralysis communicate by allowing them to remotely control devices using brain activity.
In the future, Neuralink may help enhance user memory and cognitive abilities, restore a user's motor, sensory and visual functions as well as treat neurological disorders.

What are the risks of Neuralink?

The potential risks of Neuralink include:

- Brain injury or infection
- Physical side effects like bleeding, headaches, nausea or seizures
- Psychological side effects like mood changes
- Allergic reaction to implanted materials
- Movement of implanted threads and wires to other parts of the brain
- Cybersecurity, hacking and privacy vulnerabilities
- Unknown long-term effects of use

Who is eligible for Neuralink?

Those eligible for participating in future Neuralink clinical trials must:

- Be a U.S. citizen or permanent resident in the United States.
- Be at least 18 years old and the age of majority in their state.
- Have quadriplegia, paraplegia, visual impairment or blindness, hearing impairment or deafness and/or aphasia or the inability to speak.
- Be able to consent to participation.

How much will Neuralink cost?

Let's talk about the main question of this article: how much will Neuralink cost?
The Neuralink V0.09 chipset is one of the most high-tech products out there. It connects the human brain to its own computer processor. The advantages of the link are many and this comes at a cost. Exactly how much the Neuralink cost can be estimated at this moment. Given its high cost of development and installation, it costs $1000s of dollars.
This cost includes everything that is required to install the chip in the human skull. From the automated operation to implanting the aesthetically invisible chip.

Reference

Brooke Becher

APPENDIX

Other Conributors To This Manuscript

A. M. Turing (1950) Computing Machinery and Intelligence. Mind 49: 433-460.
Artificial Intelligence in Cardiology: Present and Future DOI:https://doi.org/10.1016/j.mayocp.2020.01.038

Bhakti Patel and Amgad N. Makaryus Daniele Giansanti, Academic Editor and Norbert Hosten, Academic Editor :Artificial Intelligence Advances in the World of Cardiovascular ImagingHealthcare (Basel). 2022 Jan; 10(1): 154. Published online 2022 Jan 14. doi: 10.3390/healthcare10010154 PMCID: PMC8776229 PMID: 35052317DOI: https://doi.org/10.7861/clinmed.2023-0078 Clin Med May 2023

Dranove, D. (1993). The Five W's of Utilization Review. In R. B. Helms (Ed.), American Health Policy: Critical Issues for Reform American Enterprise Institute Eijkenaar, Frank, Martin Emmert, Manfred Scheppach, and Oliver Schöffski. "Effects of pay for performance in health care: a systematic review of systematic reviews." Health policy 110, no. 2-3 (2013): 115-130.

Farah Yasmin Syed Muhammad Ismail Shah, Aisha Naeem, Syed Muhammad Shujauddin, Adina Jabeen, Sana Kazmi, Sarush Ahmed Siddiqui, Pankaj Kumar Shiza Salman, Syed Adeel Hassan, Chandrashekhar Dasari, Ali Sanaullah Choudhry , Ahmad Mustafa, Sanchit Chawla, Hassan Mehmood Lak, Artificial intelligence in the diagnosis and detection of heart failure: the past, present, and future Rev. Cardiovasc. Med. 2021, 22(4), 1095–1113; https://doi.org/10.31083/j.rcm2204121

Gurpreet S. Sandhu, MD, PhDConor Senecal, MDPaul A. Friedman, MDShow all authors
Hassan Mumtaz a, Muhammad Saqib b, Farrukh Ansar c, Durafshan Zargar d, Madiha Hameed d, Mohammad Hasan e, Pakiza Muskan f The future of Cardiothoracic surgery in Artificial intelligence. Annals of Medicine and Surgery Volume 80, August 2022, 104251

Karthik Seetharam Daniel Brito Peter D. Farjo Partho P. Sengupta* The Role of Artificial Intelligence in Cardiovascular Imaging: State of the Art Review Department of Cardiology, West Virginia University Medicine Heart & Vascular Institute, Morgantown, WV, United States

Konstantinos C. Siontis, Peter A. Noseworthy, Zachi I. Attia & Paul A. Friedman : Artificial intelligence-enhanced electrocardiography in cardiovascular disease management Nature Reviews Cardiology volume 18, pages465–478 (2021)

M. Al-Ani, Chen Bai, M. Mardini Artificial intelligence guidance of advanced heart failure therapies: A systematic scoping review Published in Frontiers in Cardiovascular... 24 February 2023

Maxime Sermesant, Hervé Delingette, Hubert Cochet, Pierre Jaïs & Nicholas Ayache: Applications of artificial intelligence in cardiovascular imagingNature Reviews Cardiology volume 18, pages600–609 (2021) Published: 12 March 2021 Medicine, Computer Science DOI:10.3389/fcvm.2023.1127716 Corpus ID: 257194146 Medicine, Computer Science. DOI:10.3389/fcvm.2022.949454 Corpus ID: 255968657

Nitesh Gautam , Prachi Saluja , Abdallah Malkawi , Mark G Rabbat , Mouaz H Al-Mallah , Gianluca Pontone , Yiye Zhang , Benjamin C Lee , Subhi J Al'Aref Current and Future Applications of Artificial Intelligence in Coronary Artery Disease Healthcare (Basel)2022 Jan 26;10(2):232. doi: 10.3390/healthcare10020232.

P. Kampaktsis, Maria Emfietzoglou, A. Karlas : Artificial intelligence in atherosclerotic disease: Applications and trends Published in Frontiers in Cardiovascular... 19 January 2023

Pedro Covas, Eison De Guzman, Ian Barrows , Andrew J Bradley , Brian G Choi , Joseph M Krepp , Jannet F Lewis , Richard Katz , Cynthia M Tracy , Robert K Zeman , James P Earls , Andrew D Choi : Artificial Intelligence Advancements in the Cardiovascular Imaging of Coronary Atherosclerosis Front Cardiovasc Med 2022 Mar 21:9:839400. doi: 10.3389/fcvm.2022.839400. eCollection 2022.

Rajesh Kabra MD,FHRS , Sharat Israni PhD , Bharat Vijay MS , Chaitanya Baru PhD , Raghuveer Mendu BTech, Mark Fellman BS , Arun Sridhar MD, FHRS #, Pamela Mason MD, FHRS , Jim W. Cheung MD, FHRS , Luigi Di Biase MD, PhD, FHRS , Srijoy Mahapatra MD, FHRS §§, Jerome Kalifa MD, PhD Steven A. Lubitz MD , PeterA. Noseworthy MD,FHRS , Rachita Navara MDDavidD. McManus MD,FHRS, Mitchell Cohen MDMinaK. Chung MD,FHRS , Natalia Trayanova PhD,FHRSRakesh Gopinathannair MD,FHRS Dhanunjaya Lakkireddy MD,FHRS : Emerging role of artificial intelligence in cardiac electrophysiology Cardiovascular Digital Health Journal Volume 3, Issue 6, December 2022, Pages 263-275

Sallam, M.; Salim, N.A.; Barakat, M.; Al-Tammemi, A.B.: ChatGPT applications in medical, dental, pharmacy, and public health education: A descriptive study. Narra J. 2023, 3, e103. [Google Scholar] [CrossRef] Sam Sedaghat DOI: https://doi.org/10.7861/clinmed.2023-0078 Clin Med May 2023

Sam Sedaghat: Early applications of ChatGPT in medical practice, education and research
Syed Naveed Mohsin, Abubakar Gapizov, Chukwuyem Ekhator, Noor U Ain, Saeed Ahmad, Mavra Khan, Chad Barker, Muqaddas Hussain, Jahnavi Malineni, Afif Ramadhan, and Raghu Halappa Nagaraj :The Role of Artificial Intelligence in Prediction, Risk Stratification, and Personalized Treatment Planning for Congenital Heart Diseases Cureus. 2023 Aug; 15(8): e44374.

Yashendra Sethi, Neil Patel, Nirja Kaka, Ami Desai, Oroshay Kaiwan, Mili Sheth, Rupal Sharma, Helen Huang, Hitesh Chopra, Mayeen Uddin Khandaker, Maha M. A. Lashin, Zuhal Y. Hamd, and Talha Bin Emran: Artificial Intelligence in Pediatric Cardiology: A Scoping Review J Clin Med. 2022 Dec; 11(23): 7072.Published online 2022 Nov 29. doi: 10.3390/jcm11237072PMCID: PMC9738645

Ikram U Haq Karanjot Chhatwal Krishna Sanaka & Bo Xu;- Artificial Intelligence in Cardiovascular Medicine: Current Insights and Future Prospects Pages 517-528 | Published online: 19 Nov 2022

R. Cau, Francesco Pisu, Jasjit S. Suri, Roberta Montisci, Marco Gatti, L. Mannelli, Xiangyang Gong, L. Saba: Artificial Intelligence in the Differential Diagnosis of Cardiomyopathy Phenotypes.
Published in Diagnostics 10 January 2024 Medicine, Computer Science

Shuroug A. Alowais Sahar S. AlghamdiNada Alsuhebany, Tariq Alqahtani, Abdulrahman I. Alshaya Sumaya N. Almohareb Atheer Aldairem, Mohammed Alrashed, Khalid Bin Saleh, Hisham A. Badreldin, Majed S. Al Yami, Shmeylan Al Harbi and Abdulkareem M. Albekairy: The Role Of Artificial Intelligence(AI) In Clinical Practice BMC Med Educ. 2023; 23: 689. Published online 2023 Sep 22. doi: 10.1186/s12909-023-04698-z

Nitesh Gautam Sai Nikhila Ghanta Joshua Mueller Munthir MansourZhongning Chen Clara Puente Yu Mi HaTushar Tarun Gaurav Dhar Kalai Sivakumar Yiye Zhang hmed Abu Halimeh Ukash Nakarmi Sadeer Al-Kindi Deeptankar DeMazumder and Subhi J. Al'Aref : Artificial Intelligence, Wearables and Remote Monitoring for Heart Failure: Current and Future Applications. Diagnostics 2022, 12(12), 2964; https://doi.org/10.3390/diagnostics12122964 . 26 November 2022

Paulo H. Leocadio: Cardiac Pacemakers: The Route to Implantable Artificial Intelligence Published 09 November 2023

Federico Greco, , Rodrigo Salgado, Wim Van Hecke, Romualdo Del Buono, Paul M. Parizel, 5 and Carlo Augusto Mallio: Epicardial and pericardial fat analysis on CT images and artificial intelligence: a literature review Quant Imaging Med Surg. 2022 Mar; 12(3): 2075–2089. doi: 10.21037/qims-21-945

Zeynettin Akkus, Yousof H. Aly, Itzhak Z. Attia, Francisco Lopez-Jimenez, Adelaide M. Arruda-Olson, Patricia A. Pellikka, Sorin V. Pislaru, Garvan C. Kane, Paul A. Friedman, and Jae K. Oh: Artificial Intelligence (AI)-Empowered Echocardiography Interpretation: A State-of-the-Art Review. Published online 2021 Mar 30. doi: 10.3390/ jcm10071391. PMID: 33808513

INDEX

A

B

C

D

E

F

G

H

I

K

L

M

N

O

P

R

S

T

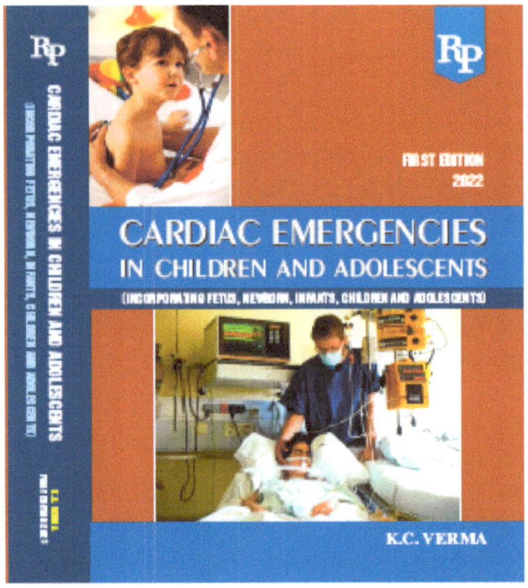
CARDIAC EMERGENCIES IN CHILDREN AND ADOLESCENTS
FIRST EDITION
2022
CARDIAC EMERGENCIES
IN CHILDREN AND ADOLESCENTS
(INCORPORATING FETUS, NEWBORN, INFANTS, CHILDREN AND ADOLESCENTS)
K.C. VERMA

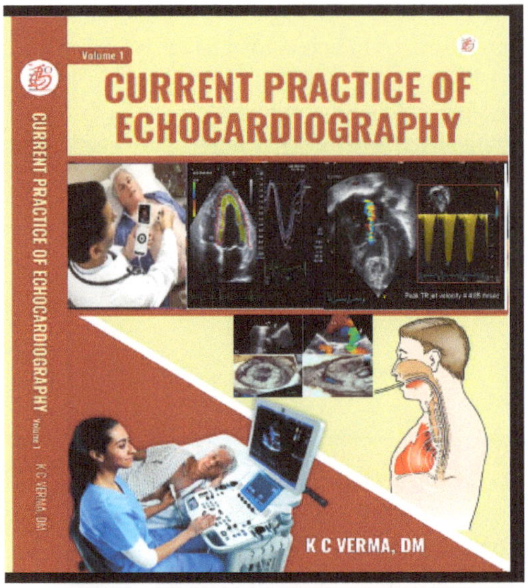
CURRENT PRACTICE OF ECHOCARDIOGRAPHY Volume 1 K C VERMA, DM
Volume 1
CURRENT PRACTICE OF
ECHOCARDIOGRAPHY
K C VERMA, DM

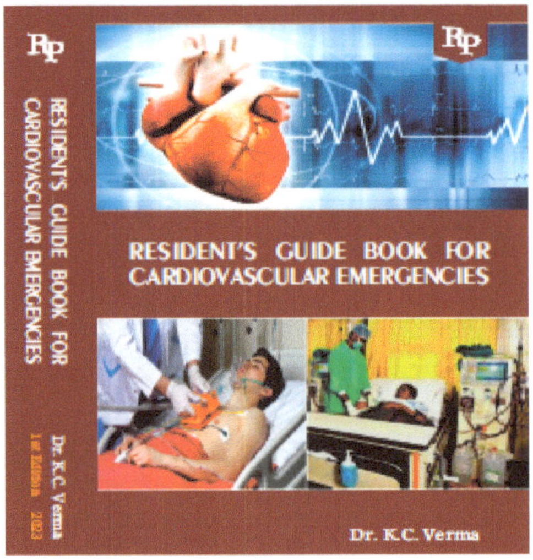
RESIDENT'S GUIDE BOOK FOR CARDIOVASCULAR EMERGENCIES
Dr. K.C. Verma
1st Edition 2023
RESIDENT'S GUIDE BOOK FOR
CARDIOVASCULAR EMERGENCIES
Dr. K.C. Verma

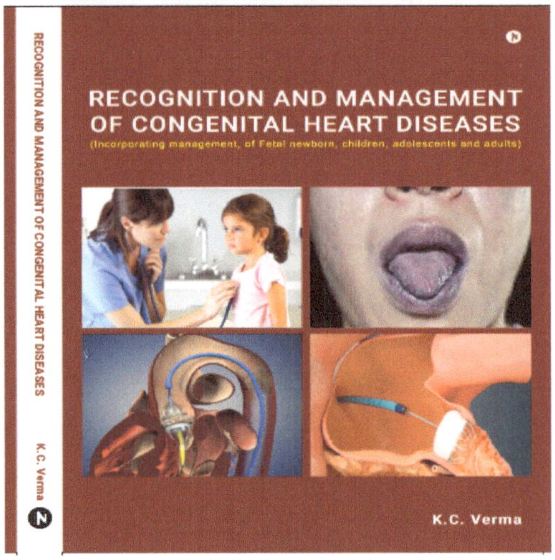
RECOGNITION AND MANAGEMENT OF CONGENITAL HEART DISEASES
K.C. Verma
RECOGNITION AND MANAGEMENT
OF CONGENITAL HEART DISEASES
(Incorporating management, of Fetal newborn, children, adolescents and adults)
K.C. Verma

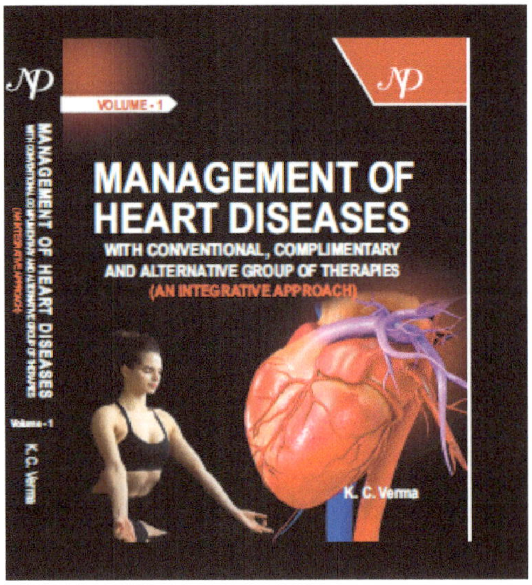
MANAGEMENT OF HEART DISEASES
Volume - 1
K.C. Verma
VOLUME - 1
MANAGEMENT OF
HEART DISEASES
WITH CONVENTIONAL, COMPLIMENTARY
AND ALTERNATIVE GROUP OF THERAPIES
(AN INTEGRATIVE APPROACH)
K. C. Verma

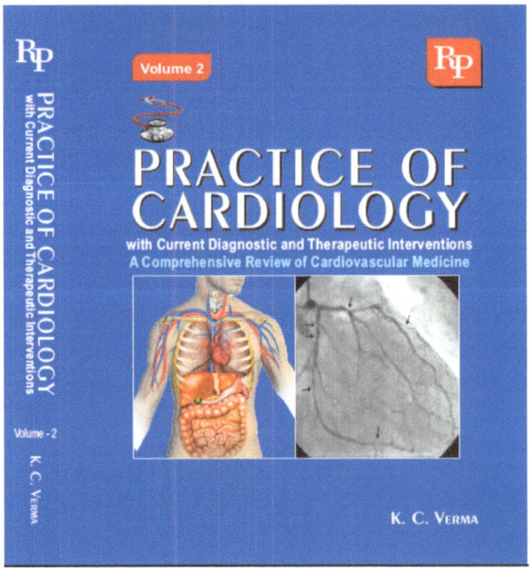
PRACTICE OF CARDIOLOGY
with Current Diagnostic and Therapeutic Interventions
Volume - 2
K. C. Verma
Volume 2
PRACTICE OF
CARDIOLOGY
with Current Diagnostic and Therapeutic Interventions
A Comprehensive Review of Cardiovascular Medicine
K. C. Verma

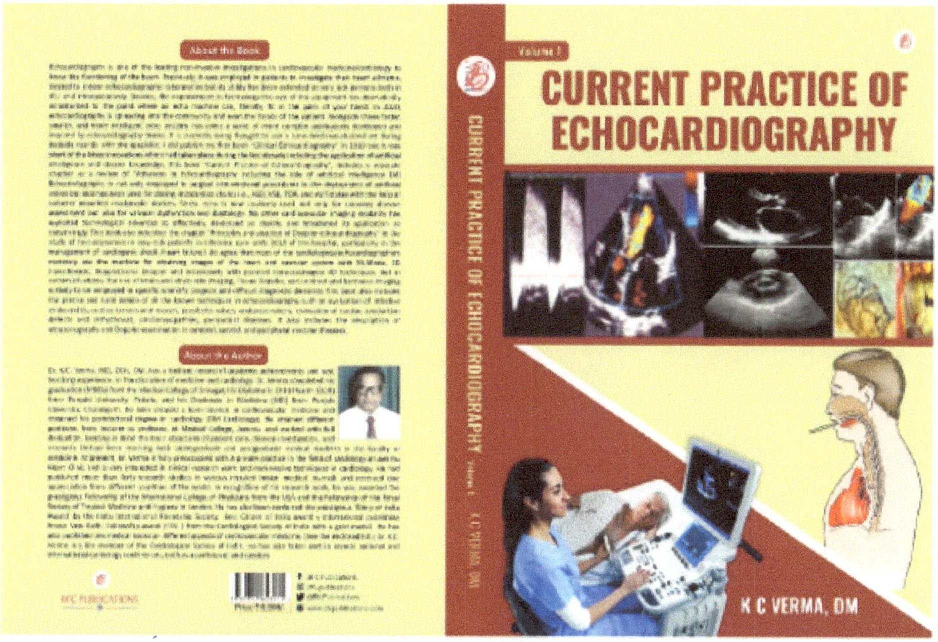
About the Book
About the Author
CURRENT PRACTICE OF ECHOCARDIOGRAPHY
Volume I
CURRENT PRACTICE OF ECHOCARDIOGRAPHY
K C VERMA, DM

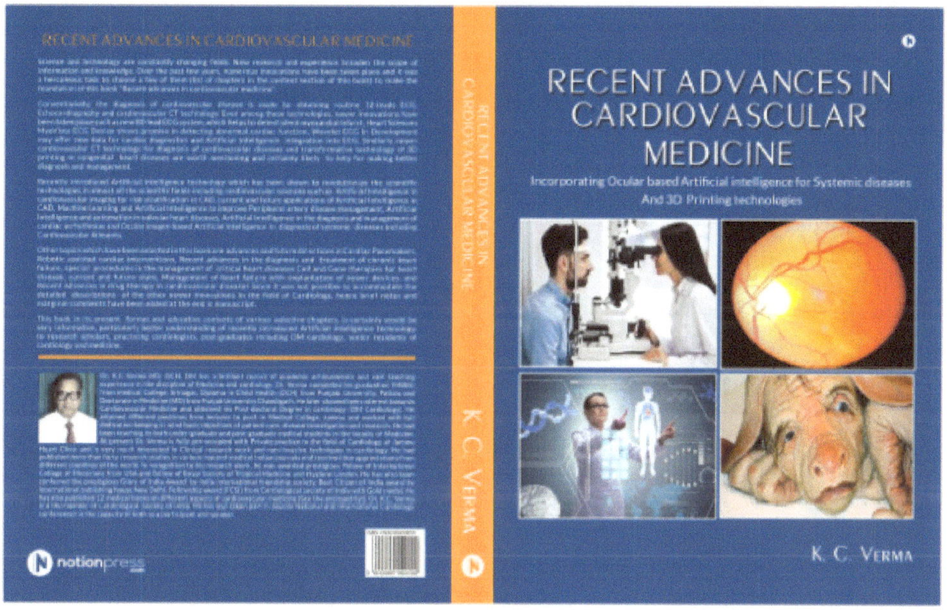
RECENT ADVANCES IN CARDIOVASCULAR MEDICINE
RECENT ADVANCES IN CARDIOVASCULAR MEDICINE
K. C. VERMA
RECENT ADVANCES IN CARDIOVASCULAR MEDICINE
Incorporating Ocular based Artificial intelligence for Systemic diseases And 3D Printing technologies
K. C. VERMA
notionpress

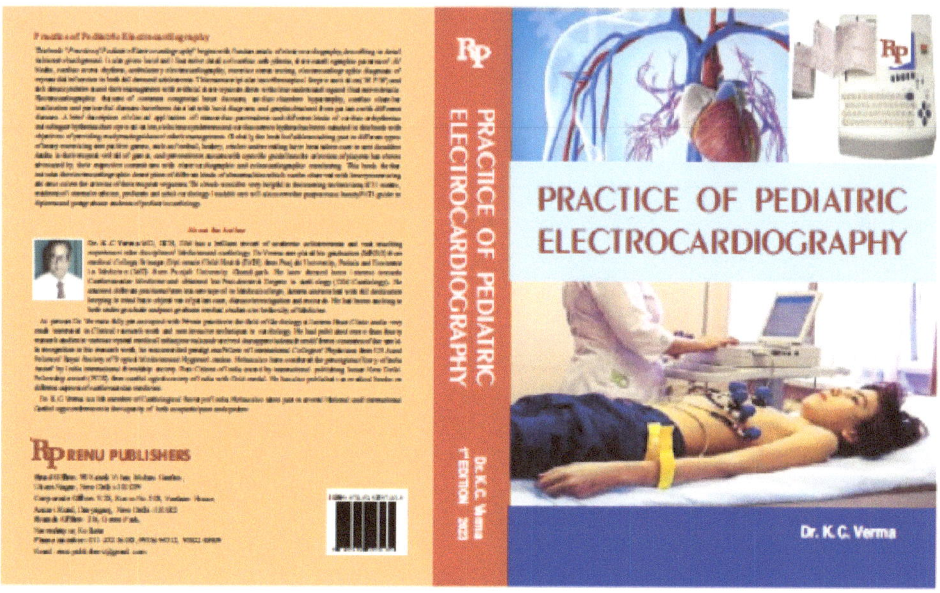
PRACTICE OF PEDIATRIC ELECTROCARDIOGRAPHY
Dr. K.C. Verma
PRACTICE OF PEDIATRIC ELECTROCARDIOGRAPHY
Dr. K.C. Verma
RENU PUBLISHERS

www.ingramcontent.com/pod-product-compliance
Ingram Content Group UK Ltd.
Pitfield, Milton Keynes, MK11 3LW, UK
UKHW060039010826
14090UKWH00041B/252
9798893228373